Whole Grains and Health

Whole Grains and Health

Second Edition

Edited by

Rikard Landberg
Head of Division Food and Nutrition Science
Department of Biology and Biological Engineering
Chalmers University of Technology
Gothenburg, Sweden

Nathalie Scheers
Food and Nutrition Science
Department of Biology and Biological Engineering
Chalmers University of Technology
Gothenburg, Sweden

WILEY Blackwell

This second edition first published 2021

Edition History: Blackwell Publishing (1e, 2007)

Registered Offices
John Wiley & Sons, Inc., 111 River Street, Hoboken, NJ 07030, USA
John Wiley & Sons Ltd, The Atrium, Southern Gate, Chichester, West Sussex, PO19 8SQ, UK

Editorial Office
The Atrium, Southern Gate, Chichester, West Sussex, PO19 8SQ, UK

For details of our global editorial offices, customer services, and more information about Wiley products visit us at www.wiley.com.

Wiley also publishes its books in a variety of electronic formats and by print-on-demand. Some content that appears in standard print versions of this book may not be available in other formats.

Library of Congress Cataloging-in-Publication Data

Names: Landberg, Rikard, editor. | Scheers, Nathalie, editor.
Title: Whole grains and health / Rikard Landberg, Nathalie Scheers.
Description: Second edition. | Hoboken : Wiley, 2021. | Includes bibliographical references and index.
Identifiers: LCCN 2020024775 (print) | LCCN 2020024776 (ebook) | ISBN 9781118939437 (cloth) | ISBN 9781118939413 (adobe pdf) | ISBN 9781118939406 (epub)
Subjects: LCSH: Health. | Grain–Therapeutic use. | Grain in human nutrition.
Classification: LCC RA776 .W4556 2020 (print) | LCC RA776 (ebook) | DDC 613–dc23
LC record available at https://lccn.loc.gov/2020024775
LC ebook record available at https://lccn.loc.gov/2020024776

Cover Design: Wiley
Cover Image: © Comaniciu Dan/Shutterstock

Set in 10/12pt Times by SPi Global, Pondicherry, India

10 9 8 7 6 5 4 3 2 1

Contents

Preface

Cereal foods constitute a backbone of the diet worldwide and are the major source of energy and nutrients in many populations. The most common way cereal foods are consumed have detrimental effects on human health. The largest proportion of the intake consists of refined-cereal products, generally associated with high glycemic index, reduced nutritional density and central in a dietary pattern associated with increased risk for non-communicable diseases (NCDs). However, shifting the intake towards whole grains is associated with a consistently reduced risk of developing NCDs, specifically cardiovascular disease, type 2 diabetes and certain cancers. In fact, a high whole grain intake is listed as one of the most important modifiable risk factors of NCDs (Global Burden of Disease). Whole grain cereals are rich sources of fibre, many minerals, vitamins and phytochemicals. Public health authorities in the European Union, United States and around the world encourage the increased intake of whole grain cereals based on the health benefits, but recently also for improved sustainability. Most of the evidence for their beneficial effects stem from observational studies, while dietary interventions have shown acute effects on glucose, hormonal and inflammatory responses, and long-term effects on insulin sensitivity, blood pressure and dyslipidaemia. Such effects have been linked to specific bioactive compounds, fibre components, gut microbiota, processing-induced changes and the structural features of whole grains and cereal-grain fractions. The dietary fibre complex, that is, dietary fibre and associated compounds, is believed to have a central role for the health effects of whole grain foods, but the mechanisms are to be elucidated in detail. The development of whole grain cereal foods has a potentially huge positive impact on the health of the global population, but there are important barriers to be torn down to succeed increasing the intake.

Since the first edition of the current book, the number of studies on whole grains and health have increased dramatically. In total, 2093 new publications on the search words *whole grain* AND *health* appeared in a Scopus search for the period 1 January 2007 to 26 March 2020. There has been a tremendous development of the field during the past decade, including definition and communication of whole grains to consumers, application of techniques to produce whole grain foods and studies of whole grain health effects. Such advancements are covered and discussed in detail in the different chapters of this book. For example, a large number of epidemiological studies have been carried out in different populations on the associations between whole grain consumption and risk of developing chronic diseases such as CVD, type 2 diabetes, some cancers, but also more rare diseases have been studied. Compared to older studies, more recent observational studies have investigated different grains separately and have also managed to estimate the intakes in g/d. Several large controlled human intervention studies have been conducted to investigate different aspects of whole grains on human health, including effects on cardiovascular and diabetes risk factors such as blood pressure, blood lipids, insulin sensitivity, body weight, body fat and inflammation. During the past decade, new biomarkers of whole grain wheat and rye intake has been developed and validated (alkylresorcinols and their metabolites).

These biomarkers have been adopted and shown useful to assess compliance in whole grain intervention studies and they have successfully been used as an independent measure of whole grain intake in observational studies in humans. Metabolomics has emerged as a new approach to address health effects and to find new biomarkers of both dietary exposures and health effects related to whole grain intake. Several metabolomics studies have been published recently to achieve better understanding of health effects underlying whole grain consumption. Such studies have recently shown a modest effect on microbial composition after whole grain/high-fibre cereal intake, which suggested several new mechanisms on why whole grain rye may have particular effects on insulin metabolism. Genomics have been applied in several large-scale intervention studies and have provided new knowledge on how gene expression profiles cause changes in response to whole grain intake. This will be of importance for the overall understanding of the physiological responses in relation to whole grain intake. Moreover, new bioactive compounds in whole grains and whole grain fractions have been identified and are currently studied. One example of such is the group of benzoxazinoids, which have recently been identified in whole wheat and rye grains and in bakery products of these cereals. These compounds, isolated from other sources or synthesized, have been studied for a number of bioactivities. Their uptake and elimination in animals and humans as well as their effects are currently extensively studied. Untargeted metabolomics approaches have facilitated the process of discovering new compounds. The role of gut microbiota for human health and disease has boomed the last 10 years, and important insights on the role of whole grains and dietary fibre and their interaction with gut microbiota for differential responses in human health outcomes have increased dramatically, although there is still much to improve concerning our understanding in this area. EU-regulations on health claims have been adopted with consequences for whole grain consumption. No health claim is allowed for whole grains but several specific claims, including grain components (reflecting beneficial physiological effects and disease risk reduction claims related to certain fibres) are allowed. No current worldwide definition of *whole grain intake* exists, but new definitions of both *whole grains* and *whole grain products* have been suggested.

The structure, outline and style of this book is designed to provide a comprehensive treatise on the subject covering the topic from the grains themselves, their components and distribution in different botanical fractions and products to the effect of whole grains on health and the molecular mechanisms/effects on risk factors underlying their health effects. The book also highlights the interest from the food industry and governmental and non-governmental authorities to develop new food products rich in whole grains as well as to educate consumers about the health benefits of consuming whole grain foods (the whole grain stamp is an example of this communication to the consumer and the whole grain campaigns launched in Denmark and The Netherlands are other examples). The chapters are comprehensive in their coverage with the aim to provide founded knowledge and information for researchers, research students, authority and industry personnel that gives them a multidisciplinary understanding of this important topic.

Recent advances will to a great extent be covered by the update of book chapters of the first edition. As in the previous edition, we divide the book into sections with a slight modification of the suggested sections. More emphasis will be put on the section "whole grains, cereal fibre and chronic disease" and "grain technology and health-related outcomes," whereas consumer aspects are given somewhat less attention compared with the first edition. We also provide comprehensive material on the whole grain morphology constituents,

Table 1 Brief description of the content of the sections.

Section	Content
1. Whole grain basics	Chemical composition and morphological structure of cereal grains and cereal fractions, such as bran, aleurone, germ and the endosperm, are described in detail as this is crucial for the understanding of physiological effects related to health. Differences and similarities among cereals are emphasized here. Important whole grain products are described with emphasis on traits and features that may be of importance for human health. This section also contains a chapter on the different definitions of *whole grain* and *whole grain products*. A chapter on consumption and description of lifestyle factors associated with whole grain intake as well as on tools for objective whole grain intake estimation through dietary biomarkers bridge this section to section two.
2. Evidences for disease prevention	The current literature on evidence for disease prevention derived from epidemiological – as well as intervention studies in humans and model – and animal studies have been reviewed and the evidence are evaluated in a systematic way focusing on the outcome of largest importance. Hard endpoints such as type 2 diabetes, CVD, cancer and mortality are at main focus in this section.
3. Whole grains mechanisms and effects on risk factors for chronic disease	This section bridges the section on whole grain basics and the section on chronic disease by discussing mechanisms and risk factors. This section contains chapters on whole grains and appetite, glycaemia, gut function as well as a chapter on bioactive compounds and effects that may be of relevance to human health. We have also included a chapter on potential negative aspects of whole grain consumption in which risk related to heavy metals, mycotoxins, acrylamide, gluten intolerance and wheat sensitivity are described and discussed.
4. Searching for new molecular mechanisms underlying health benefits of whole grains	In this section, the possibilities to use – OMICs to generate new hypotheses and to get better insights into new molecular mechanisms of the health effects of whole grains is presented. Metabolomics for discovery of new compounds and to monitor process changes in food products has been covered as well as its implementation in human studies to gain insights into molecular mechanisms and dissect biochemical pathways involved in processes with implication for health. Studies where changes in gene expression in response to interventions with whole grains in humans are also reviewed in a chapter.
5. Whole grains and the consumer	Barriers for whole grain consumption are at focus here. The industry's commitment to whole grains has also been discussed by representatives from major enterprises in Europe and the United States. The current regulation and labeling have been covered as well as a chapter describing the current situation on health claims in Europe and the United States, and strategies for consumer communication.

fractions and technology as well as products for readers coming from the medical or public-health sectors. The book comprises 5 sections and concluding remarks and future perspectives. In total, 23 chapters are included (Table 1).

We hope that the current edition of *Whole Grains and Health* will be of use and great pleasure for researchers, research students, industry personnel, governmental authorities (nutritionists, technologists, product developers, epidemiologists, health professionals) and others with wider interest in foods and health!

Rikard Landberg and Nathalie Scheers
Gothenburg, Sweden, March 2020.

Editors' Biographies

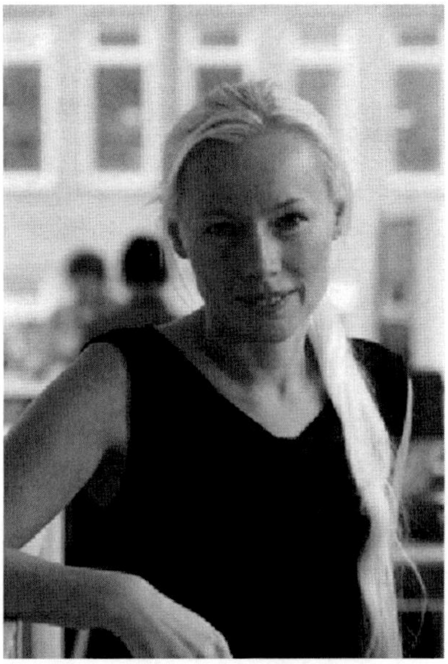

Nathalie Scheers
Associate Professor
Food and Nutrition Science
Department of Biology and Biological Engineering
Chalmers University of Technology
Gothenburg, Sweden

Associate Professor Nathalie Scheers and her research team conduct studies in the area of molecular nutrition with particular focus on metals, specific proteins, bioactive molecules and their physiological effects, on cellular or systemic level.

A core competence of Dr. Scheers includes human cell models. She investigates regulation of intestinal transport proteins, stress response and apoptosis, expression of cancer and inflammation markers, and bioavailability of nutrients. One of her main research topics is within iron nutrition, with a special focus on dietary iron supplements and fortificants. Together with collaborators, she is currently working on the mechanisms of cancer-promoting and pro-inflammatory effects of certain types of compounds used to fortify foods with iron. In addition, she is working on detoxification of gluten to celiacs. A few years back, she and her collaborators identified a food additive that can interfere with intestinal transglutaminase processing of gluten in vitro, which has the potential to render gluten non-immunogenic to celiacs. At present, Dr. Scheers is leading a human intervention trial in healthy volunteers to verify the previous findings in vivo, with the ultimate goal to provide celiac safe gluten products. Dr. Scheers is also active in research about the fish-protein parvalbumin beta and its association with physiological effects important for neurological diseases, toxicity of insects as human foods, and anti/pro-inflammatory effects of marine collagen and shellfish processing waste.

Associate Professor Scheers has authored 39 scientific publications including original research, book chapters, proceedings etc. Her main publication area is within molecular iron nutrition and she has an H-index of 10 according to Google Scholar.

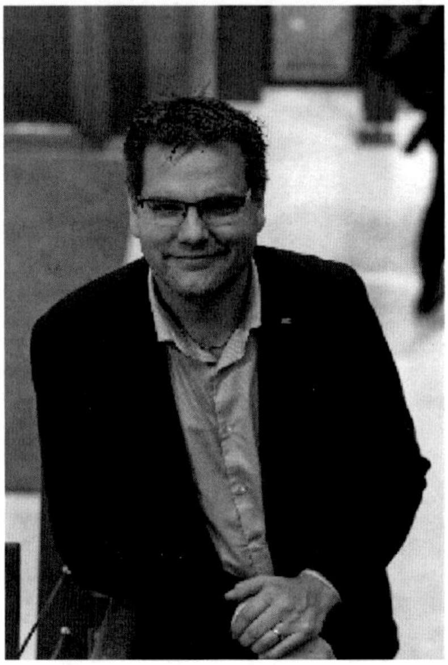

Rikard Landberg
Professor
Head of Division Food and Nutrition Science
Department of Biology and Biological Engineering
Chalmers University of Technology
Gothenburg, Sweden
Member of the Young Academy of Sweden

Affiliated Researcher

Department of Public Health and Clinical Medicine, Umeå University, Umeå, Sweden

Guest Researcher

Diet, Genes and Environment Group at Danish Cancer Society Research Center, Copenhagen, Denmark

Professor Rikard Landberg is the head of Division of Food and Nutrition Science at Chalmers University of Technology, Sweden. His group studies the preventive role of plant-based foods using observational and intervention studies as well as various model systems. Professor Landberg is the PI of several RCTs and molecular epidemiological studies on the role of whole grains and dietary fibre in appetite, body weight management, glycaemia, prostate cancer and on cardiometabolic risk. He is particularly interested in the health effects of rye and established the Nordic Rye Forum together with colleagues (https://www.nordicryeforum.info). Professor Landberg also leads studies to test novel OMICs-based personalized concepts for improved CVD prevention. Metabolomics is a key technique in Professor Landberg's research program, and it is developed and applied for discovery and validation of exposure and prediction biomarkers, and for molecular phenotyping as the basis for tailored dietary strategies for personalized nutrition. Novel biomarkers, from his lab, such as alkylresorcinolas, are extensively used by researchers all over the world. Professor Landberg has authored more than140 papers and over10 book chapters, and delivered more than 25 invited/keynote lectures. He has an H-index of 32 according to ISI web of science. Professor Landberg is an elected member of the Young Academy of Sweden and of the National Committee for Nutrition and Food Science at the Swedish Royal Academy of Sciences.

Acknowledgments

We would like to thank all the authors of the chapters in this book for their great contributions. The authors have generously provided their expertise and time to summarize the current knowledge within their respective field(s). We also would like to thank the following external experts for their help to review and provide input to some of the chapters in this book:

Dr. Carl Brunius, Dr. Susanna Larsson, Dr. Matti Marklund, Dr. Rob M. van Dam, and PhD-student Kia Nöhr-Iversen.

Rikard Landberg and Nathalie Scheers

Contributing Authors

Chapter 1

Maud Langton, Swedish University of Agricultural Sciences, Sweden
José Luis Vázquez Gutiérrex, Swedish University of Agricultural Sciences, Sweden and Centro Technológico ITENE, Spain

Chapter 2

Wenche Frølich, University of Stavanger, Norway
Per Åman, Swedish University of Agricultural Sciences, Sweden

Chapter 3

Cécile Barron, UMR IATE, CIRAD, INRAE, Université de Montpellier, France
Valérie Micard, UMR IATE, CIRAD, INRAE, Université de Montpellier, France
Valérie Lullien-Pellerin, UMR IATE, CIRAD, INRAE, Université de Montpellier, France

Chapter 4

Genyi Zhang, Jiangnan University, China
Bruce R. Hamaker, Purdue University, USA

Chapter 5

Alastair B. Ross, Chalmers University of Technology, Sweden and AgResearch Ltd, New Zealand
Cynthia Harriman, Oldways Whole Grains Council, USA
Roberto King, Nestlé Research Center, Switzerland

Chapter 6

Cecilie Kyrø, Danish Cancer Society Research Center, Denmark
Anja Olsen, Danish Cancer Society Research Center, Denmark

Chapter 7

Matti Marklund, Tufts University, USA
Izabela Biskup, Chalmers University of Technology, Sweden
Afaf Kamal-Eldin, United Arab Emirates University, UAE
Rikard Landberg, Chalmers University of Technology, Sweden

Chapter 8

Nicola McKeown, Tufts University, USA
Mette Bredal Kristensen, University of Copenhagen, Denmark

Chapter 9

Shilpa N. Bhupathiraju, Harvard T. Chan School of Public Health, USA
Frank B. Hu, Harvard T. Chan School of Public Health, USA

Chapter 10

Chris J. Seal, Newcastle University, UK
Iain A. Brownlee, Northumbria University, UK

Chapter 11

Anja Olsen, Danish Cancer Society Research Center, Denmark
Cecilie Kyrø, Danish Cancer Society Research Center, Denmark

Chapter 12

Guri Skeie, The Arctic University of Norway, Norway
David R. Jacobs Jr., University of Minnesota, USA

Chapter 13

Sabine Ibrügger, University of Copenhagen, Denmark
Kia Nøhr Iversen, Chalmers University of Technology, Sweden
Mette Kristensen, University of Copenhagen, Denmark
Rikard Landberg, Chalmers University of Technology, Sweden

Chapter 14

Marion G. Priebe, University Medical Center Groningen, The Netherlands
Coby Eelderink, University Medical Center Groningen, The Netherlands
Roel J. Vonk, University Medical Center Groningen, The Netherlands

Chapter 15

Johan Dicksved, Swedish University of Agricultural Sciences, Sweden
Emma Ivarsson, Swedish University of Agricultural Sciences, Sweden

Chapter 16

Anne-Maria Pajari, University of Helsinki, Finland
Riitta Freese, University of Helsinki, Finland
Susanna Kariluoto, University of Helsinki, Finland

Anna-Maija Lampi, University of Helsinki, Finland
Vieno Piironen, University of Helsinki, Finland

Chapter 17

Afaf Kamal-Eldin, United Arab Emirates University, UAE
Agneta Åkesson, Karolinska Institutet, Sweden
Maria Kippler, Karolinska Institutet, Sweden
Karl-Erik Hellenäs, National Food Agency, Sweden
Nathalie Scheers, Chalmers University of Technology, Sweden
Ann-Sofie Sandberg, Chalmers University of Technology, Sweden

Chapter 18

Amanda J. Lloyd, Aberystwyth University, UK
Kathleen Tailliart, Aberystwyth University, UK
Manfred Beckmann, Aberystwyth University, UK
John Draper, Aberystwyth University, UK

Chapter 19

Kati Hanhineva, University of Turku, Finland, University of Eastern Finland, Finland and Chalmers University of Technology, Sweden

Chapter 20

Marjukka Kolehmainen, University of Eastern Finland, Finland

Chapter 21

Frank Thielecke, Thielecke Consulting, Switzerland
Wolfgang Bindzus, Cereal Partners Worldwide S.A., Switzerland

Chapter 22

Heddie Mejborn, Technical University of Denmark, Denmark
Caroline Sluyter, Oldways Whole Grains Council, USA

Supplementary Material

Additional materials, including multiple choice questions and supplementary chapters, can be found under the "Downloads" section online at https://www.wiley.com/en-gb/Whole+Grains+and+Health-p-9781118939437

1 The Structure of Cereal Grains and Their Products

Maud Langton[1] and José Luis Vázquez Gutiérrex[1,2]

[1]Department of Molecular Sciences, Swedish University of Agricultural Sciences, Uppsala, Sweden
[2]Department of Molecular Sciences, Swedish University of Agricultural Sciences, Uppsala, Sweden Present address: Centro Technológico ITENE, Valencia, Spain

1.1 Introduction

Through the senses, consumers can subjectively detect properties in food. However, other qualities such as long-term health benefits of food that cannot be easily detected. A deep knowledge of cereal grain structure and how it is modified by processing is necessary to understand the physical and health properties of the different cereal products. This chapter focuses on the microstructure, at different levels, of cereal grains and their products. The structure of the grain is briefly overviewed and followed by the effect of processing on the structure of different food products. Based on the microstructure of the final product, three groups are distinguished: rolled cereals and porridge, protein network-based products and starch network-based products. This different organization is important for food production and technological aspects. The impact on the health-related aspects of the product is currently investigated.

1.2 Grain structure

Cereals are the most important crops in the world and are destined to become both human food and animal feed. Cereals, which belong to the grass family (*Gramineae*), produce dry, one-seeded fruits. These fruits are, botanically speaking, caryopses, but they are commonly referred as "grains" or "kernels." The cereal grains such as wheat, rice, maize, barley, oats, rye, sorghum and millet provide 50% of the food energy and 50% of the protein consumed on earth. Wheat, rice and corn constitute around 75% of world's grain production (Ramaswamy and Riahi 2003). In this chapter, wheat is used as reference to explain the structure of cereal grain. Its kernels contain three main parts: embryo, endosperm and their covering layers. The last are, in milling, often separated as the bran fraction (Figure 1.1A). If all the parts of the kernel are retained in processing, one can speak of whole grain. If either the bran or germ is separated from the kernel during milling, then it is a "refined grain."

Whole Grains and Health, Second Edition. Edited by Rikard Landberg and Nathalie Scheers.

Additional materials available for download online at https://www.wiley.com/en-gb/Whole+Grains+and+Health-p-9781118939437

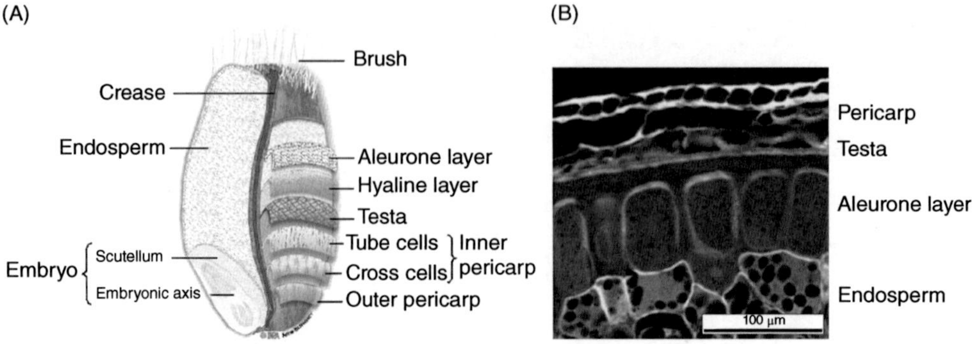

Figure 1.1 A: General structure of a cereal grain); B: Epifluorescence micrograph of parts of rye grain. The sections were stained with Acid Fuchsin and Calcofluor: protein appears red, cell walls rich in β-glucan appear light blue and lignified cell walls of the pericarp appear yellowish-orange. Structure of cereal foods (Source: Hemery et al. 2007). (*See color representation of this figure in the color plate section*).

1.3 Embryo

The embryonic axis (rudimentary root and shoot of the next generation) and the scutellum (storage organ) together constitute the embryo, which makes up 2.5% to 3.5% of the weight of the entire kernel in wheat. It is often referred to as germ, although, strictly speaking, the germ is the embryo-rich fraction of the kernel produced during milling. Wheat germ contains protein (25%), sugar (18%), oil (16% of the embryonic axis and 32% of the scutellum), and it is also rich in vitamins B and E (Delcour and Hoseney 2010a). In the case of rye, the embryo constitutes about 3.8% of the weight of the grain and contains 37.2% of protein, 13.4% of lipids and 43.6% of carbohydrates (Lasztity 1999; Ellis 2007).

1.4 Endosperm

The endosperm is the largest tissue of the grain. It is the primary starch and protein storage site and the source for white flour. It contains protein, carbohydrates, iron and B-vitamins, such as riboflavin, niacin and thiamine. However, it is nutritionally inferior to the whole grain. The endosperm comprises two different parts: the starchy endosperm and the aleurone layer. The aleurone is botanically part of the endosperm. However, in practice, it is most often part of the bran since it is removed together with the pericarp and testa during the milling process. The main part of the grain constitutes the starchy endosperm, which consists of cells packed with nutrients, mainly starch, to support the growth of the embryonic axis after germination. It is also rich in protein. In all cereals, there is an inverse gradient involving these two components. The protein content increases towards the periphery, while starch is more predominant towards the center of the kernel. Cell size also decreases towards the outside and this is accompanied by increasing cell wall thickness. The endosperm cell walls of wheat are mainly composed of arabinoxylans, while in barley and oats (1-3)- and (1-4)-β-D glucans predominate. The contribution of cellulose to the cereal endosperm cell wall is low except in the case of rice.

1.5 Bran

The bran consists of the hard outer layers of the kernel and, depending on the milling process, constitutes around 14% of the grain. Generally, wheat bran comprises approximately 12% water, 13–18% protein, 3.5% fat and 56% carbohydrates. Wheat bran can be chemically differentiated by the occurrence of complex structures of either C6-sugars like cellulose or C5-sugars like xylans. Phenolic compounds and their polymer lignin are found in different concentrations within the bran. It also contains a large quantity of B-vitamins as well as insoluble dietary fibre (Prückler et al. 2014). From the histological point of view, wheat bran is composed of the pericarp, testa and aleurone layer.

1.5.1 Pericarp

The pericarp consists of several complete and incomplete layers of dry, largely empty cells. During development, it serves to protect and support the growing endosperm and embryo. The outer layers of wheat bran, pericarp and testa are formed by thick cell walls containing cellulose, lignin and complex xylans with high arabinose to xylose ratios and substitution by ferulic acid dehydromers as cross-linkers between polymer chains (Hemery et al. 2007).

1.5.2 Testa

The testa is a hydrophobic, semipermeable layer under the pericarp, which contains a cuticle rich in lipidic compounds. The testa is the outermost tissue of the seed and may consist of one or two cellular layers. Almost all of the alkylresorcinols in the grain are localized in the testa of wheat, rye, triticale and, at much lower levels, in barley (Ross et al. 2003b; Landberg et al. 2008). Alkylresorcinols are antioxidant compounds whose main function is to protect the membrane against lipid peroxidation. They are commonly used as biomarkers for whole grain intake since they are absorbed and at least partially metabolized in the human intestine (Ross et al. 2003a; Linko et al. 2005).

1.5.3 Aleurone layer

The aleurone layer surrounds the starchy endosperm and part of the embryo, and makes up 5–8% of the kernel. It is usually constituted by a single cell layer except in the case of barley, which contains two to three layers. Aleurone cells do not contain starch but they have high protein content and they are rich in lipids. They release active enzymes that help the cereal grain grow into a plant. The main component of wheat and rye aleurone cell walls is arabinoxylan (Karin 2006). The aleurone cell walls in wheat are relatively thick (3–4 μm) and have been reported to possess high cellulose content and relatively linear arabinoxylans with low arabinose-xylose ratio (Saulnier et al. 2007). Whole grain wheat contains less than 1% β-glucan and the majority is located in the aleurone and subaleurone layers, while in whole grain rye (Figure 1.1B), β-glucan accounts for 1.5% of dry matter and seems to be more evenly distributed throughout the grain (Dornez et al. 2011; Frølich et al. 2013). The content of β-glucan is higher in other cereals such as oat and barley, which contain 5% and 4.6%, respectively (Frølich et al. 2013). β-Glucan in oat is more concentrated in the sub-aleurone layers, while in barley it is evenly distributed across the starchy endosperm (Cui and Wang 2009). The aleurone layer also contains an important amount of minerals like magnesium and phosphorus, vitamins, and phenolic compounds, such as ferulic acid, and p-coumaric acid. For instance, the aleurone layer contains almost all of the niacin and almost one-third of the lysine found in wheat (Delcour and Hoseney 2010a).

Cereal grains possess a well-organized microstructure. The endosperm is rich in starch and storage proteins located in protein bodies, and the cells are compartmentalized by cell wall polysaccharides (Figure 1.2A). Indeed, especially refined cereal foods may be considered at the structural scale as a composite of starch and proteins blended with other ingredients such as fat, sugar and fibre. Processes such as milling, dough mixing, baking, rolling and extrusion cause large changes in the structure of proteins, starch and cell wall components and therefore affect the structure and quality of the end product (Autio and Salmenkallio-Marttila 2001; Della Valle et al. 2014). The organization of the grain components at different structural levels contributes to the different characteristics among cereal products, as shown in Figure 1.2, and Figure 1.2B shows the microstructure of a rye porridge, where fragments are easily detected. The effect of

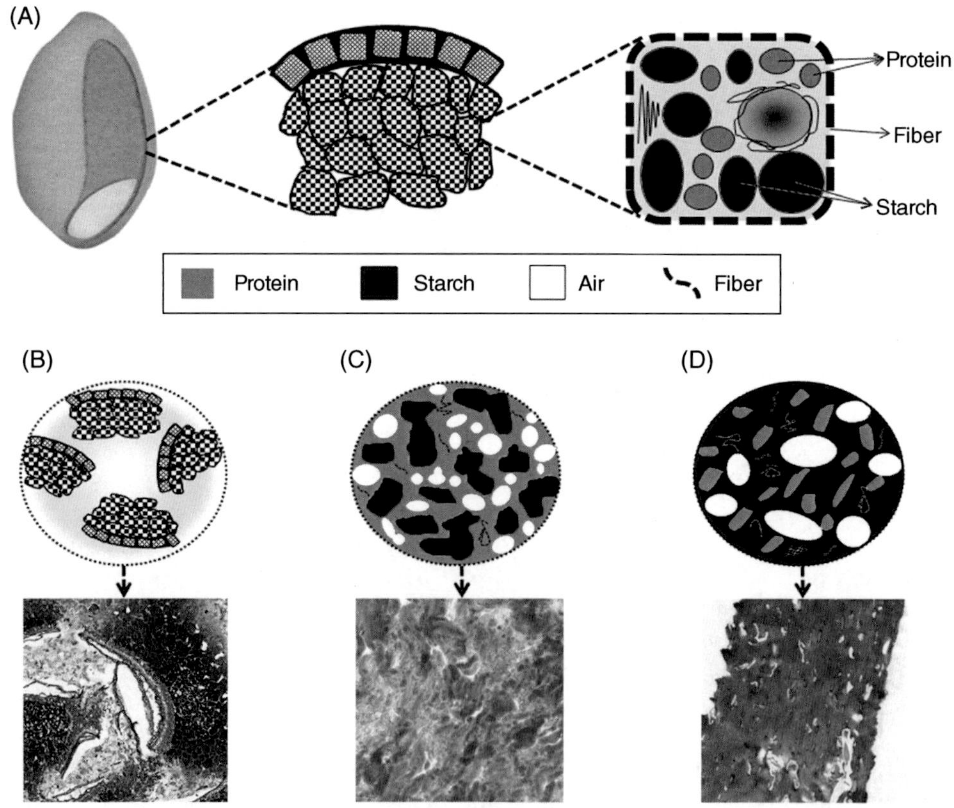

Figure 1.2 Schematic representation of a typical endosperm cell (A) and microstructure of different cereal products such as rye porridge (B), wheat bread (C) and extruded rye breakfast cereal (D). Starch and protein can be observed in blue/purple and green, respectively. (*See color representation of this figure in the color plate section*).

baking and extrusion on the microstructure is shown in Figures 1.2C and 1.2D, where dough mixing and baking provides a continuous protein network while extrusion provides a continuous starch phase. In both cases, the generation of an aerated structure and the presence of pores are essential for the desired properties of this kind of products. The mechanical properties, which are highly associated with texture and to a great extent consumer acceptance, depend on the morphology of the product. For instance, the structure of porridge is composed of grain fragments in a continuous phase of released amylose from the starch granules and storage proteins (Figure 1.2B). Wheat bread and cakes obtain their solid foam structure due to the continuous gluten network being able to retain air in open or closed cellular network (Figure 1.2C), while many crispbread products and most ready-to-eat cereals, which include extruded products, obtain their crunchiness from the multiple air cell layers retained in a continuous starch phase (Figure 1.2D).

Structure is also essential for nutritional properties since it influences the bolus structure before swallowing as well as further gastrointestinal digestion. Most studies have been focused on defining or creating food structures, but knowledge on food structure breakdown during consumption is also needed. In this way, gelatinized starch is more rapidly digested than in its native crystalline form and compact products such as pasta or porridge are more slowly digested than porous ones. At the molecular level, the amylose component of starch is more slowly digested than amylopectin, and the use of high-amylose raw materials helps lowering the glycaemic response (Alminger and Eklund-Jonsson 2008; Poutanen et al. 2014). This could be partly due to the lower swelling capacity of high amylose starch granules compared to waxy starch granules (Lii et al. 1996). The presence of sucrose or emulsifiers has also been shown to delay the swelling of starch granules (Richardson et al. 2003). The length of the amylose chains and interactions between starch and other components in the product such as proteins, dietary fibre or lipids can also influence the digestibility of starch (Sajilata et al. 2006).

Structural characteristics of cells and tissues influence grain quality and performance in food processes. These microstructural changes can be studied using a variety of microscopy techniques such as light microscopy, confocal laser scanning microscopy (CLSM) and electron microscopy. Light microscopy provides lower magnification than, for instance electron microscopy but it allows specific staining of different chemical components. This is particularly useful in cereal products, which are complicated multicomponent multiphase materials. For instance, amylose and amylopectin can be identified under the light microscopy by staining with iodine (Langton and Hermansson 1989; Autio and Salmenkallio-Marttila 2001). Iodine staining also allows subsequent image analyses and obtaining quantitative results (Srikaeo et al. 2006). Some staining systems can also be used in CSLM, which requires a lower degree of sample preparation compared to other microscopy techniques (Autio and Salmenkallio-Marttila 2001). Moreover, the use of fluorescently labelled antibodies has high potential due to the combination of immunological specificity with the sensitivity of fluorescence (Vázquez-Gutiérrez and Langton 2015). Scanning electron microscopy (SEM) permits three-dimensional observation of a wide spectrum of food structures. Since this technique does not require sectioning, it is appropriate for visualization of porous structures and sample preparation is easier compared to light microscopy (Sanchez-Pardo et al. 2008). SEM has been used to observe cooking-induced changes in starch granules and protein matrix (Srikaeo et al. 2006; Sanchez et al. 2008).

1.6 Rolled cereals and porridge

The structure of cereal products such as muesli and porridge, just before their consumption, is composed of rolled whole grains or grain fragments in a continuous aqueous phase. The confinement of a great part of the starch inside the cellular structure of the grain fragments (which are semi-intact inside the cells) is an efficient way of slowing down starch digestion, compared to other products with higher proportion of gelatinized starch such as bread (Poutanen et al. 2014). However, it has also been suggested that porridge, due to its semi-solid nature, could be emptied faster from the gastric compartment. In cases where porridge is made from flour rather than flakes, this could result in faster intestinal hydrolysis of starch and release of glucose (Johansson et al. 2018).

Rolled cereal, such as oat, rye or wheat, is one of the main components of muesli. The elaboration of rolled cereal involves steaming, pressing between rollers and drying of the grains. Light microscopy images of rolled rye show that cell walls are partially disrupted after the rolling process, gluten bodies are deformed developing a more network-like structure within the particulate fragments, and starch is partially gelatinized after the drying (Figure 1.3). In this way, the resulting rolled grains absorb water more quickly and, in the case of those consumed as porridge, the cooking time decreases as the thickness of the rolled grains decreases. There is also a relationship between the rolled grain size and its subsidiary effects on digestion and colonic microbiota fermentation. The thickness would determine the availability and types of dietary fibre that are able to avoid digestion, and this would in turn have a consequence in the fermentation profile (Connolly et al. 2010).

Porridge is a dish made by boiling rolled or crushed cereal, usually oats, in water, milk or both, usually served hot in a bowl or dish. From the structural point of view, porridge is a compact cereal product where insoluble fragments of grain are dispersed in viscous grain extract. The boiling process favors the partial release of amylose from the starch granules and their swelling which, together with the amounts of β-glucan solubilized from the cell walls, directly affect the viscosity and the texture of the product (Source: Yiu et al. 1987; Vázquez-Gutiérrez et al. 2015) (Figure 1.2B).

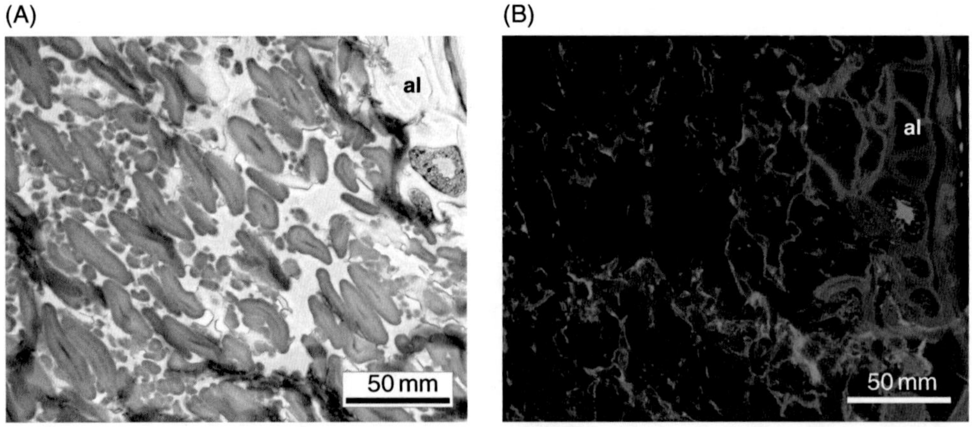

Figure 1.3 Microstructure of rolled rye grain. A: bright field micrograph with iodine and light green staining for observation of starch (purple) and protein (green), respectively; B: epifluorescence micrograph with Calcofluor and Acid Fuchsin staining for observation of cell walls (blue) and protein (red), respectively. (*See color representation of this figure in the color plate section*).

1.7 Protein network-based products

The formation of gluten is essential for the structure and texture of bread, cakes and pasta.

1.7.1 Bread

With the addition of water to wheat flour and subsequent mixing, the storage proteins of the wheat endosperm (glutenin and gliadin) hydrate and interact to develop the gluten matrix, which provides viscoelastic properties to the dough and allows the incorporation of air (Autio and Salmenkallio-Marttila 2003; Boitte et al. 2013). The gluten forms the continuous phase in which starch granules, lipid, added yeast cells, and cell wall fragments are dispersed (Figure 1.2C). The aggregation of gliadins and glutenins are greatly determined by noncovalent bonds and define the structural and physical properties of the dough. The quantity and quality of gluten proteins largely determine dough mixing requirements and the rheological properties, which influences the gas retention properties and the volume and crumb structure of the resulting bread (Chavan and Chavan 2011). Apart from gluten, the other components affecting the distribution of water in the dough, such as starch and cell walls, have a direct influence on the final texture of bread, too (Flander 2012).

During yeast fermentation, carbon dioxide is generated and the dough expands. At the beginning of the fermentation process, the gas cells are embedded in the starch-protein matrix. At a later stage of expansion, the matrix fails to enclose the gas cells and areas containing only liquid film are formed between adjacent gas cells. The end of dough expansion is marked by the rupture of the film, and not that of the starch–protein matrix (Gan et al. 1995). The major structural changes at the microscopic level during baking are starch gelatinization, denaturation of protein, melting of fat crystals and their incorporation into the surface of air cells and, sometimes, fragmentation of the cell walls (Autio and Salmenkallio-Marttila 2001). Therefore, the final crumb structure is dependent not only on the shape, number and size of gas bubbles, but also on the structural properties of gluten-starch matrix and probably on liquid film composed of surface-active material (Autio and Salmenkallio-Marttila 2003). The addition of shortenings stabilizes the gas cells. The fat crystals from the shortenings migrate towards the gas-liquid interface and they melt during baking, allowing the bubbles to grow without rupture (Brooker 1996). Light microscopy is the most commonly used technique to determine bread structure (Jakubczyk et al. 2008). Scanning and transmission electron microscopy have also been used to study the effect of baking on starch granule structure (Bechtel 1985).

Water evaporation occurs at the surface layers of the dough once it is placed in the oven. The lower water content in the surface compared to the core, together with the enhanced release of gasses due to the proximity to the interface with the oven air, generating smaller-sized cells are structural characteristics of the crust that contribute to its mechanical properties (Vanin et al. 2009). The distribution of protein and partially gelatinized starch in the bread crust affects its fracturability (Primo-Martín et al. 2006; Primo-Martín et al. 2007). Migration of water, which acts as plasticizer, from the crumb to the crust during storage of bread can be influenced by the morphology of the product (porosity, gas cell size). The firmness of the bread increases during storage, which is called staling. It is mainly caused by the retrogradation of starch, specifically of the short amylopectin side chains (Gray and Bemiller 2003).

One of the main challenges in breadmaking is to increase the content of whole grain and dietary fibre to improve the nutritional value of the product. However, the presence of the outer bran layers of the grain alters not only the continuity and rheological properties of the starch–protein matrix, but also the water availability for lamellar film formation. This has an effect on gas cell stabilization and gas retention in wholemeal dough (Poutanen et al. 2014). Rye flour, which is typically used for baking in Northern and Eastern Europe, is suitable for making bread but it has marked differences in rheological properties and gas retention capacity compared to wheat bread. The elasticity of rye gluten is lower than that of wheat gluten and it holds less moisture. In this way, the increase of volume in rye dough during fermentation and baking is lower and resulting bread is more compact than wheat bread. Furthermore, rye starch gelatinizes at lower temperatures and is more susceptible of enzymatic degradation during baking than wheat starch (Weipert 1997). Oat can only be used in limited quantities for bread production because of its inferior baking quality, too. This is due to the lack of gluten proteins and the high content of β-glucan and other dietary fibres (Flander 2012). Brown rice provides better nutritional properties than white rice since it contains considerably higher amounts of proteins and minerals (Lamberts et al. 2007), and is naturally gluten-free and hypoallergenic. However, rice proteins lack the visco-elastic properties necessary for the production of yeast-leavened products. For this reason, the addition of hydrocolloids and gums (Sivaramakrishnan et al. 2004; Sciarini et al. 2010), and more recently, enzymatic processing of rice flour (Gujral and Rosell 2004; Renzetti and Arendt 2009) have been investigated in order to improve the breadmaking performance of rice and brown rice flour. Enzymatic processing promotes protein cross-linking, and thus increases the elastic and viscous behavior of batters. As shown by Renzetti and Arendt (2009), treatment with protease affected the crumb microstructure, where smaller protein aggregates were more widely dispersed in the dominating starch phase, in comparison to the large aggregates of the control bread (Figure 1.4). The enrichment of gluten-free breads with soluble fibres improves not only nutritional quality but also physicochemical characteristics, such as specific volume, crumb cohesiveness and cell density (Martínez et al. 2014).

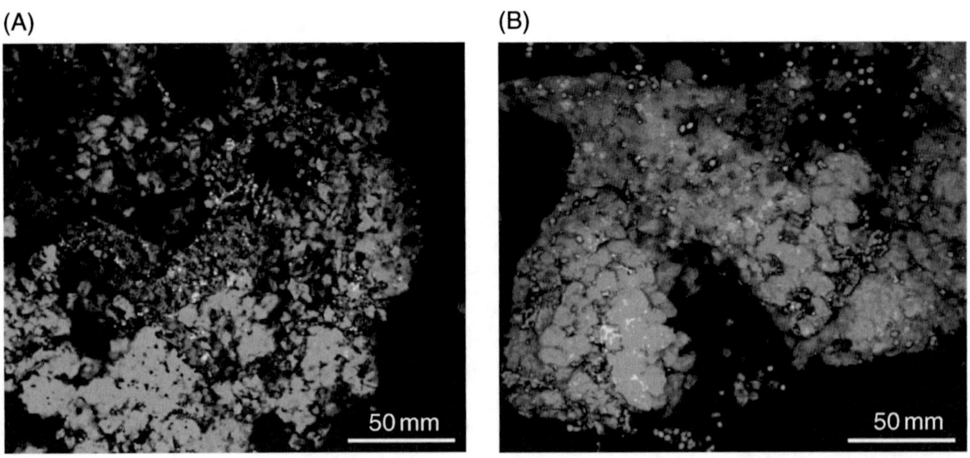

Figure 1.4 CLSM images of untreated (A) and 0.01% protease-treated (B) brown rice bread crumbs (40x magnification) showing starch (green) and proteins (red-yellow). Adapted from Renzetti and Arendt 2009. (*See color representation of this figure in the color plate section*).

1.7.2 Sourdough bread

Sourdough fermentation provides improved flavour and structure to rye and wheat bread. In the case of rye, the swelling of flour constituents is favoured and the enzyme activity is limited under acid conditions, which prevents early staling (Narvhus and Sørhaug 2012). The interest in the significant potential of sourdough fermentation to improve the nutritional properties of rye, oat and wheat products is increasing nowadays (Komlenić et al. 2012). The whole grain or fractions of cereal grain can be modified by sourdough fermentation to improve nutritional value or promote healthfulness of cereal foods (Chavan and Chavan 2011). Sourdough fermentation has been associated to positive effects in whole grain bread such as improved of palatability, mineral bioavailability and levels of bioactive compounds, and reduction of starch digestibility (Poutanen et al. 2009). The ability of sourdough processing to reduce starch digestibility is assumed to be mainly due to formation of organic acids, especially lactic acid, during fermentation (Liljeberg et al. 1995).

Specific modifications in baked product texture can be achieved by development of new sourdough cultures, and by optimizing acidity and interactions with grain components. As reported by Katina et al. (2005), the changes in dough structure over time can not only be detected by small deformation viscoelastic measurements, but also by confocal laser-scanning microscopy. The protein fraction of the gluten-free sourdough is degraded over time, although this process is more obvious in wheat sourdough (Clarke et al. 2004). However, the addition of sourdough to gluten-free batters does lead to an improvement of the gluten-free-bread (Katina et al. 2005).

1.7.3 Cakes

Cakes are characterized by high levels of sugar and fat in the formula. Since they also contain relatively high levels of water, the molar sugar concentration is not high enough to prevent starch gelatinization during baking. Because of that, cakes set when baked, giving a light product. The presence of α-crystalline emulsifiers increases the incorporation of air and the batter volume (Richardson et al. 2002). During conventional baking, cake batter undergoes structural transformations, including starch gelatinization, protein denaturation, volume increase, liberation of carbon dioxide from leavening agents, water evaporation, crust formation and non-enzymatic browning. Sucrose regulates starch gelatinization and protein denaturation during baking, causing a shift towards higher temperature values (Kim and Walker 1992). Partial or total substitution of sucrose has been studied using sorbitol, wheat starch and inulin (Baeva et al. 2003; Rodríguez-García et al. 2014). However, the replacement of sucrose in sponge cake batters with other water-retaining agents may affect the physical and chemical transformations in the sponge cake system (Rodríguez-García et al. 2014).

Rice flour, which does not contain gluten, is one of the alternatives to wheat flour in order to obtain gluten-free cereal products. However, due to its low gas retention capacity, rice products have some quality problems such as low volume, poor texture, color and crumb structure. Gums such as xanthan, guar, κ-carrageenan can be added to gluten-free cake formulation in order to emulate the viscoelastic properties of glutenin. Different effects on the porosity are obtained depending on the gum type (Turabi et al. 2010).

1.7.4 Pasta

Two important transformations in the main components of durum wheat pasta take place during cooking: gluten polymerization and starch gelatinization. The competition of both components for water determines the final texture properties of the product (Fuad and Prabhasankar 2010). Microscopy techniques such as scanning electron microscopy and light microscopy of stained sections have helped to increase knowledge regarding the induced structural changes of pasta during cooking (Heneen and Brismar 2003). There is a moisture distribution gradient from the surface to the center due to the penetration of water and the progress of starch gelatinization. This moisture gradient is essential for the texture properties of pasta. In this way, the ideal texture of pasta, known as "al dente" is characterized by a soft outer region and a very thin hard core (Sekiyama et al. 2012). Pasta is usually made from durum wheat semolina and is a good source of low glycaemic index carbohydrate (Brennan 2008). Bran and germ particles in semolina produce a less homogeneous mixture and the particles can physically interfere with gluten development (Manthey and Schorno 2002). For this reason, bran and germ, commonly referred to as pollard, are largely removed during milling of durum wheat. However, nutritionally-enriched pasta is also available commercially, prepared using wholemeal, semolina/flour or ground whole-wheat. Although negative effects in the cooking and sensory properties of whole-wheat or bran enriched pasta have been frequently reported, spaghetti dried at high temperature can be prepared with pollard, with 10% substitution of semolina, causing minimal impact on sensory and technological properties (Aravind et al. 2012). High molecular weight inulin can also be incorporated with minimal effect on the technological and sensory properties below 20% incorporation (Aravind et al. 2012b).

Nuclear magnetic resonance imaging (MRI) is a non-invasive and nondestructive method to visualize the water distribution and to study its influence in the properties of pasta (Bonomi et al. 2012). It has proved particularly useful in combination with microscopy techniques such as light microscopy or epifluorescence. This way, the water distribution has been related to differently cooked zones in pasta (Sekiyama et al. 2012) and the influence of raw materials in the microstructure of cooked pasta (Steglich et al. 2014). In pasta, the gluten network is continuous throughout the whole tissue encapsulating starch granules and fibre particles. However, according to the study carried out on spaghetti by Steglich et al. (2014), microstructure is not homogeneous throughout the product after cooking since starch granules are affected by heat differently depending on their distance to the surface. Starch granules in the core region did not gelatinize, while granule distortion and amylose leakage increased towards the surface (Figure 1.5A). The MRI and microscopy results of this study proved that the local water content and microstructure differed due to locally varying raw materials. The whole grain pasta showed lower (darker) T_2^* values, which was attributed to faster exchange of water protons with exchangeable fibre protons or to less swelled starch granules in the areas close to the fibre particles or both (Figure 1.5 B–D). Rice, being low in protein, has relatively poor technological properties for interacting and developing a cohesive network for gluten-free pasta products. Severe parboiling, extrusion cooking and/or addition of pre-gelatinized flour are required in order to obtain the desired texture and avoid excessive leaching of solids during cooking (Marti et al. 2013).

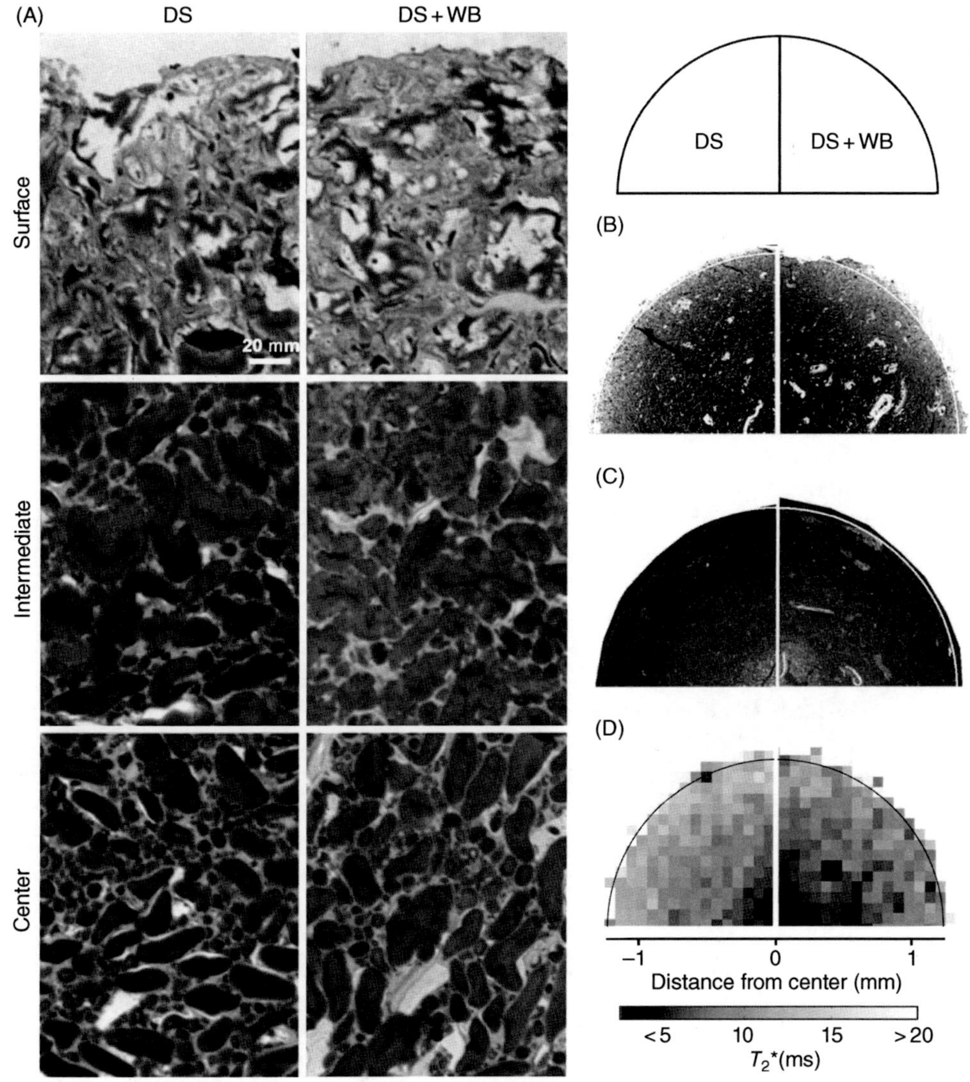

Figure 1.5 Representative cross-sections of 10-min cooked spaghetti made of 100% fine durum wheat semolina (DS) and durum whole grain flour (DS+WG). A: Bright field light micrographs at high magnification from three regions; B–D: Bright field light micrographs (B), polarized light micrographs (C), and T_2^* maps (D) of cross-sections at lower magnification. Sections in A and B were stained with Light Green and Lugol's iodine solution for observation of protein (green) and starch (blue/violet), respectively, while fibre particles were not stained (Source: (B) and (D): Modified from Steglich et al. 2014). (*See color representation of this figure in the color plate section*).

1.8 Starch network-based products

Most ready-to-eat cereals (RTEC) possess a starch network-based structure. These products are processed cereals suitable for human consumption with or without further cooking at home and are usually eaten at breakfast or as snacks. RTEC constitutes an important contribution to daily nutrient intake and breakfast quality according to recent analyses on previous studies and evidence (Kosti et al. 2010; Williams 2014). RTEC are typically grouped by cereal form rather than the type of grain used. Apart from rolled cereals, the main types are whole grain flakes, puffed grain cereals and extruded cereals. Unlike rolled cereals, the later types of RTEC go through a step that cooks the grain in combination with flavor materials, sweeteners and/or nutritional fortifying agents. Gelatinization of the starch grain fractions is the main purpose of the cooking stage and is essential for the development of the desired textural and organoleptic properties of these products.

Crispbread, which traditionally has been elaborated with rye flour, have a continuous starch network which encapsulates the protein, due to the inability of the later to form a gluten network. This network consists of highly swollen starch granules with some leaked amylose (Johansson et al. 2015 and Johansson et al 2018).

1.8.1 Whole grain flakes

Flaked cereals are made directly from whole grain kernels or parts of kernels. Corn flakes are made with maize endosperm. The maize grits are pressure cooked with a solution containing sugar, malt (nonenzymatic), and salt. The cooked grits are partially dried to remove stickiness and then tempered for 24 hours to allow the moisture to equilibrate. The grits are subsequently submitted to flaking and toasting, where the moisture decreases to less than 3%, and the product is browned and blistered. After cooling, the flakes are sprayed with a solution of vitamins and minerals. To make wheat or rye flakes, the whole kernel is used and each kernel makes one flake. A heating step is applied before the flaking to plasticize the kernel. Instead of cooked grains, flakes may also be made from extruded pellets in a similar way.

Collapse of structure and formation of rubbery and crystalline states affects strongly physical properties of cereal products (Boitte et al. 2013). The mechanical and sensory properties of grain flakes are affected by water content. Crunchiness is lost upon water adsorption and it is attributed to the plasticizing effect of water. However, water adsorption has either plasticizing or antiplasticizing effect depending on the water activity (Gondek and Lewicki 2006).

The type of grain affects the internal structure of the product. For instance, corn flakes present a porous structure with thick, continuous and homogenous air bubbles, whereas wheat bran flakes have a heterogeneous structure with many discontinuities, cracks and ruptures. These structural differences influence the behavior of the products against compression. Fragile breaking of the matrix occurs in corn flakes, while dislocations of one piece of wheat bran against the others manifest in the wheat bran flakes (Gondek and Lewicki 2006).

1.8.2 Puffed-grain cereals

Puffed-grain cereals are commonly used as ready-to-eat breakfast foods or as ingredients in snack formulations. They have characteristic lightness and crispness, qualities related to their cellular structure (Peleg 1997) and degree of expansion (Owusu-Ansah et al. 1984). Moreover, the effect of the puffing treatment is strongly influenced by the morphology and composition of the kernel (Mariotti et al. 2006). Two technological processes are generally used in order to decrease the bulk density of puffed cereals. Oven puffing involves the sudden application of heat at atmospheric pressure to a prewetted cereal. The product expands due to the vaporization of water inside the kernel. Gun puffing is based on the sudden transfer of a piece containing superheated water to a lower pressure, thus allowing the water to suddenly vaporize (Delcour and Hoseney 2010b). The degree of expansion with gun-puffing is 15–20 times, much greater than with oven puffing (2–5 times). Oven-puffed cereals are made almost exclusively using whole grain rice or maize, while rice and wheat are the only types of grain used in gun-puffed whole grain production (Fast 2000). Puffed products must keep less than 3% moisture to maintain crispness, but due to their high porosity, they absorb moisture rapidly. The greater the expansion, the more difficult is to maintain the moisture. In this way, gun-puffed cereals require special packaging.

The ultrastructure of the grains is severely affected by puffing and is reflected in some physical properties such as bulk density and water uptake. Puffed rye and rice presents a very porous matrix made up of numerous cavities of increasing size from the center of the kernel outwards, whereas wheat and barley show a more compact and non-homogeneous structure (Mariotti et al. 2006). The changes in the structure after compression of puffed cereals have also been studied (Roopa et al. 2009).

1.8.3 Extruded breakfast cereals and snacks

Extrusion cooking handles cereal flours at relatively low moisture contents (12–20%) and limited amounts of fibre and fat. It is a continuous process that uses both temperature and pressure to expand the product (Delcour and Hoseney 2010b). The dough is forced through an extruder to give it a specific shape and dried. This process causes starch gelatinization and mechanical damage in cell walls (Salmenkallio-Marttila et al. 2004). The presence and gelatinization of starch is essential for optimal sensory properties of extruded products. Porosity is a key characteristic that determines quality properties such as crispness in this kind of products. Crispness is indeed the result of breaking behavior of complex structures at different length scales (Chanvrier et al. 2014). Extruded flours of maize or oat are usually puffed by extrusion at high temperature. In extruded whole grain rye, all starch granules are completely destroyed during processing, resulting in a continuous homogenous starch phase consisting of a mixture of amylose and amylopectin (Figure 1.2D). This also results in a very low content of resistant starch, according to Johansson et al. (2018). This recent study on rye has established a relationship between microstructure and product composition and in vitro glucose release. A later glucose peak was detected in extruded whole grain rye compared to wheat bread and fermented crisp rye bread. This was partially attributed to less degraded fibres, such as β-glucans and arabinoxylans, in the extruded rye contributing to higher viscosity of the food digesta which would favor a slower diffusion of enzymes. Additionally, it was suggested that the extruded rye was more resistant to disintegration in the gastric compartment.

Although extrusion cooking can be used for the production of fibre-rich products, bran particles act as inert fillers within the extrudate matrix, and thus affect the mechanical and physical properties (Robin et al. 2012). The addition of dietary fibre can affect the density and textural properties of the product since it can limit the extent of starch gelatinization and the proper formation of air cells (Stojceska 2013). Fibres such as pericarp cell wall remnants are not easily plasticized and, therefore, are not readily expandable under normal commercial extrusion conditions. Fibre particles disrupt the amorphous regions of plasticized starch and protein, decreasing the gas-holding capacity and generating denser and less expanded products (Lue et al. 1991; Jin et al. 1995; Robin et al. 2012). Therefore, the cereal fibre content either isolated or in the form of whole grains, is a key factor in extruded products. Structural differences are obtained in extruded cereals depending on the type and level of fibre as well as on the base recipe (Chanvrier et al. 2013). As revealed by X-ray tomography and 3D image analysis, higher porosity is obtained in whole wheat products compared to corn products (Chanvrier et al. 2014). Moreover, it could also be observed in the same study that porosity decreases with the amount of added fibres (Figure 1.6). The structural differences of the walls depending on the amount of added fibres induced also different breaking behaviors and noise creation. In this way, according to Chanvrier et al. (2014), the organization of the wall would have a greater impact on the breaking properties than the wall thickness. For instance, the presence of soy protein may induce different molecular interactions between fibres and the corn/soy matrix. As a result, the viscoelasticity of the extrudate changes and the interactions between all the components may be modified (Chanvrier et al. 2014).

1.8.4 Crispbread

Crispbread is a dry cereal-based baked and extruded product very popular in the Nordic countries. It is a light, flat and dry type of cracker with relatively long shelf life. Crispbread traditionally consists of wholemeal rye flour, salt, and water. However, different crispbread products containing wheat, other grains and spices can be found nowadays. The air cells can be introduced using leavening, mechanically or submitting the dough under pressure in an extruder. The traditional method involved rolling, sheeting and baking the dough. However, the introduction of the extrusion process has complemented and often replaced the traditional methods. Extrusion process conditions have a great influence in the porosity and texture of crispbread (Gondek et al. 2013). Furthermore, differences in insulin response between leavened and non-leavened (whipped) whole grain rye crispbread have been recently reported (Johansson et al. 2015). Crispbread contains only about 5–8% water. However, this product is hygroscopic, depending on the process, due to its chemical composition, porosity and presence of starch in the amorphous state (Colonna et al. 1984). If the moisture of these crispy products increases due to water sorption during storage, loss of crispness may occur, leading to consumer rejection. Adsorbed water is supposed to behave as a lubricant at high water activities and reduce the friction between surfaces, which results in low strength. This can be explained by differences in the microstructure of the products (Jakubczyk et al. 2008). Therefore, mechanical properties and fracture behavior of crispbread are strongly affected by its structure.

One of the most commonly used technique to determine bread structure is based on light microscopy (Jakubczyk et al. 2008). However, the observation of crispbread by light microscopy is complicated due to the dry and brittle structure of the product. X-ray microcomputed tomography (micro-CT) is a non-invasive technique that enables the visualization of the internal microstructure of food products and has been applied for the characterization of extruded crispbread microstructure (Gondek et al. 2013). Extruded crispbread has a highly porous structure (porosity is higher than 90%), with numerous thin cell walls surrounding a multitude of irregular air inclusions in various shapes, sizes and orientations (Figures 1.7A and 1.7B). Scanning electron micrographs of extruded crispbread show that the structure of the surface layer is different than that of the interior due to the extrusion process (Marzec et al. 2007). The surface structure consists of numerous

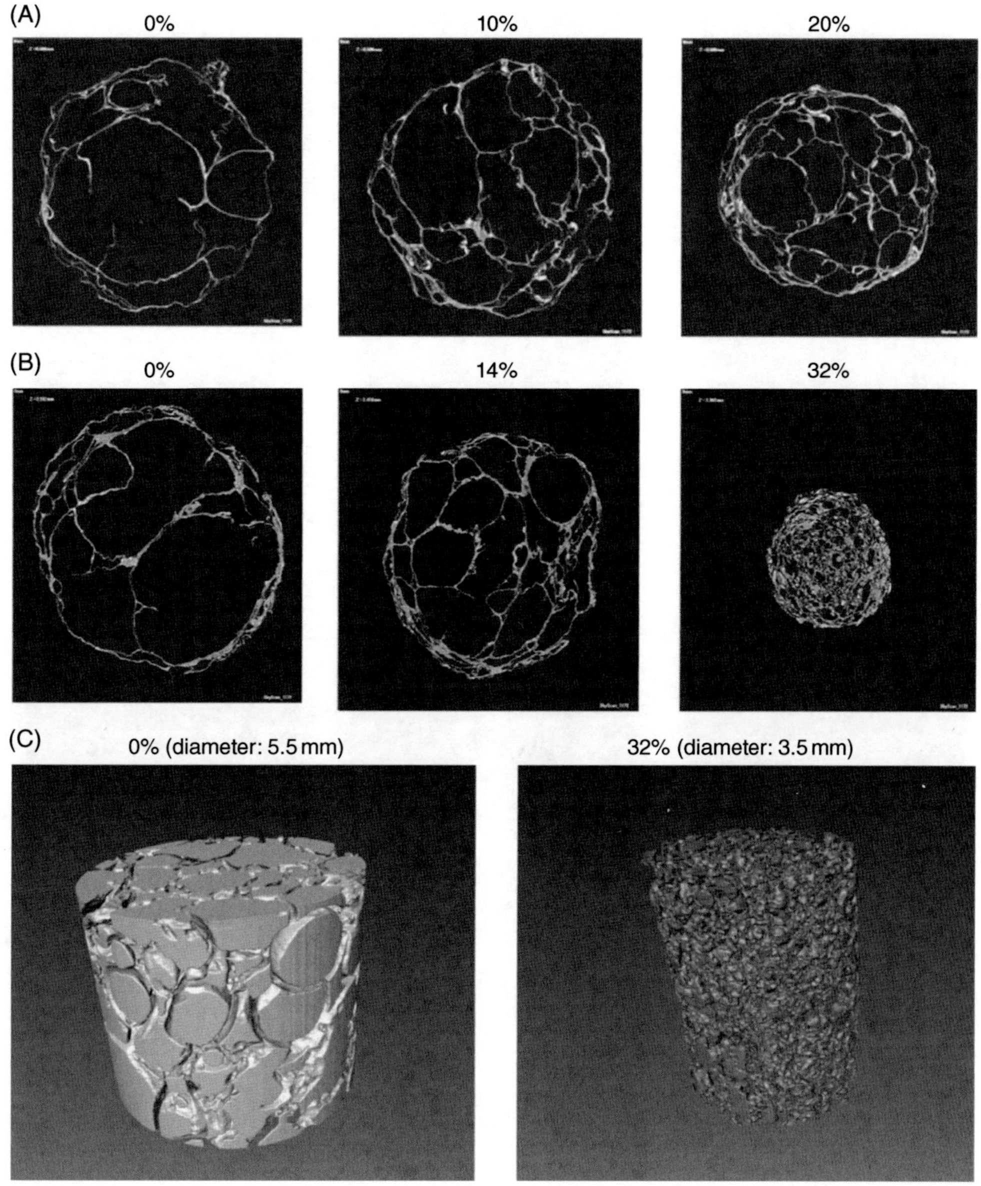

Figure 1.6 Cross-sectional X-ray tomography images (10 mm × 10 mm) of extruded cereals with added fibres (wheat bran. A: wheat recipe with 40% whole wheat; B: corn recipe; C: corn recipe in 3D rendering (carrot cut in the extruded ball). Adapted from (Chanvrier et al. 2014).

small air cells with rather thick cell walls, while the interior is highly porous with large air cells and thin cell walls (Figure 1.7C). Scanning electron microscopy has also been used to study the improvement of consistency and refinement of crispbread by addition of sodium stearoyl lactylate to the dough (Li et al. 2013) and the effect of different water activities on the mechanical properties of the product (Jakubczyk et al. 2008).

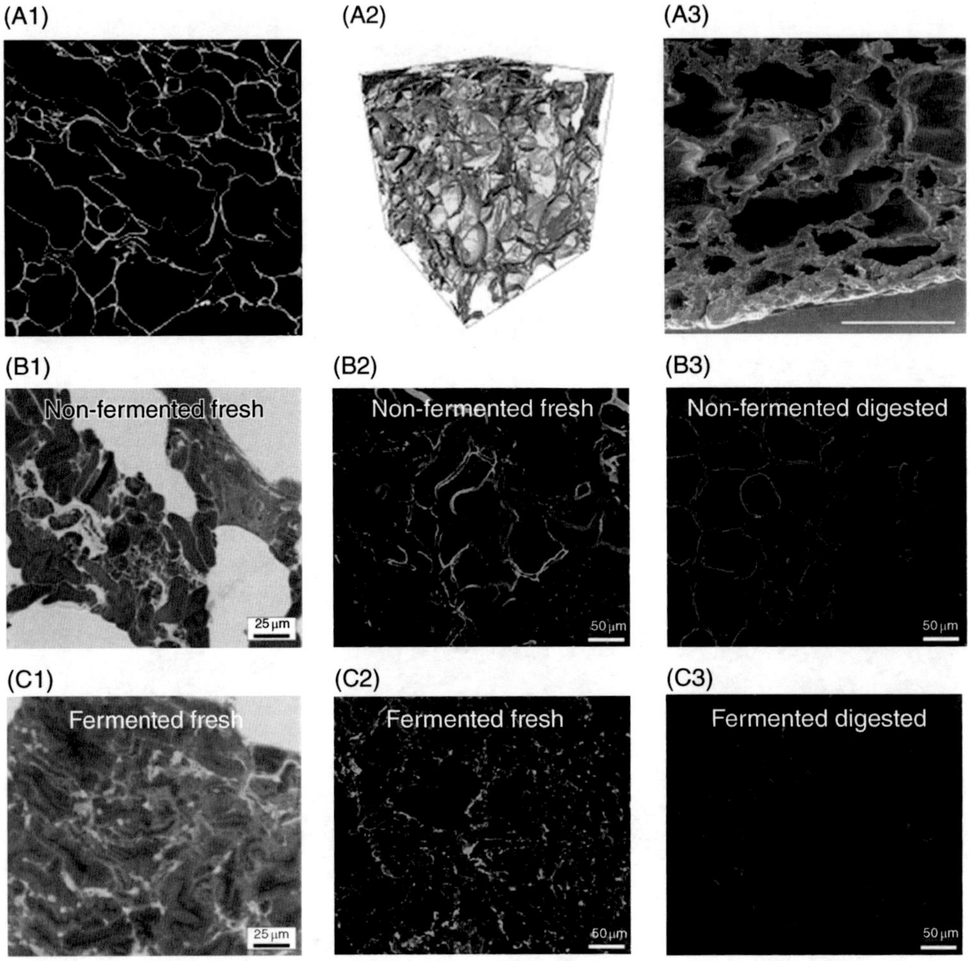

Figure 1.7 Microstructure of rye crisp bread. A1 and A2: Reconstructed X-ray micro-CT cross-sections and 3-D structure of extruded rye crispbread (Gondek et al. 2013). A3: Scanning electron micrograph of extruded rye crispbread (Marzec et al. 2007). B1–C3: bright field (B1 and C1) and confocal (B2, B3, C2, C3) micrographs of non-fermented and fermented (yeast leavened) rye crisp bread before and after in vitro digestion. Amylose in blue, amylopectin in purple, protein in yellow, β-glucan in green fluorescence. Images from B1 to C3 kindly provided by Daniel Johansson (Source: Department of Molecular Sciences, SLU, Uppsala). (*See color representation of this figure in the color plate section*).

As suggested by Johansson et al. (2018), factors related to the microstructure of cereal products can influence the digestive process and the release and absorption of nutrients, with possible later implications for the postprandial responses in vivo. Some microstructural differences between whipped (non-fermented) and leavened (fermented) rye crispbread can be observed under confocal microscopy (Figure 1.7). Due to the inability of rye proteins to properly develop gluten, both types of crispbread present a continuous starch network consisting of highly swollen starch granules with some leaked amylose that encapsulates the protein (Figures 1.7 B1 and 1.7 C1). Visualization of the β-glucans by using immunolabeling and confocal microscopy show that β-glucans (green fluorescence) appear to be more degraded or solubilized in fermented rye crispbread (Figure 1.7 C2) compared to non-fermented rye crispbread (Figure 1.7 B2). This has also been confirmed by analysis of the calcofluor average molecular weight of β-glucans in these products (Johansson et al. 2018). Yeast fermentation has been shown to decrease the molecular weight of β-glucans (Andersson et al. 2004; Tiwari and Cummins 2009; Rakha et al. 2010). In the same way, digested samples of non-fermented rye crispbread show less degraded β-glucans than the leavened one (Figures 1.7 B3 and 1.7 C3). Lower degradation of fibres could contribute to higher viscosity of the digesta and slower diffusion rates of enzymes, which has been related to later glucose peaks registered in in vitro experiments and lower insulin responses in human trials for non-fermented rye crispbread compared to leavened rye crispbread (Johansson et al. 2015, 2018).

1.9 Conclusions

Cereal products constitute complex systems and lack of understanding of the mechanisms involved in the generation of cereal product structures may result in detrimental changes in texture and functionality. Microstructural characteristics of cereal products help define and predict their physical and health properties. The wide range of microscopy techniques available in combination with other analytical tools make it possible to increase the knowledge on structure-functionality relationship of cereal products.

1.10 References

Alminger, M., and Eklund-Jonsson, C. (2008). Whole-grain cereal products based on a high-fibre barley or oat genotype lower post-prandial glucose and insulin responses in healthy humans. *European Journal of Nutrition*, 47, 294–300.

Andersson, A.A.M., Armö, E., Grangeon, E., Fredriksson, H., Andersson, R. and Åman, P. (2004). Molecular weight and structure units of (1→3, 1→4)-β-glucans in dough and bread made from hull-less barley milling fractions. *Journal of Cereal Science*, 40, 195–204.

Aravind, N., Sissons, M., Egan, N., and Fellows, C. (2012). Effect of insoluble dietary fibre addition on technological, sensory, and structural properties of durum wheat spaghetti. *Food Chemistry*, 130, 299–309.

Autio, K., and Salmenkallio-Marttila, M. (2001) Light microscopic investigations of cereal grains, doughs and breads. *LWT – Food Science and Technology*, 34, 18–22.

Autio, K., and Salmenkallio-Marttila, M. (2003). Understanding microstructural changes in biopolymers using light and electron microscopy. In Characterization of Cereals and Flours: Properties, Analysis And Applications (eds. G. Kaletunc and K.J. Breslauer), pp. 387–408. CRC Press.

Baeva, M.R., Terzieva, V.V., and Panchev, I.N. (2003). Structural development of sucrose-sweetened and sucrose-free sponge cakes during baking. *Food/Nahrung*, 47, 154–160.

Bechtel, D.B. (1985). The microstructure of wheat: Its development and conversion into bread. *Food Microstructure*, 4, 125–133.

Boitte, J.B., Hayert, M., and Michon, C. (2013). Observation of wheat flour doughs under mechanical treatment using confocal microscopy and classification of their microstructures. *Journal of Cereal Science*, 58, 365–371.

Bonomi, F., D'Egidio, M.G., Iametti, S., Marengo, M., Marti, A., Pagani, M.A., and Ragg, E.M. (2012). Structure–quality relationship in commercial pasta: A molecular glimpse. *Food Chemistry*, 135, 348–355.

Brennan, C.S. (2008). High-fibre pasta products. In Technology of Functional Cereal Products (ed. B.R. Hamaker), pp. 428–445. Woodhead Publishing.

Brooker, B.E. (1996). The role of fat in the stabilisation of gas cells in bread dough. *Journal of Cereal Science*, 24, 187–198.

Chanvrier, H., Desbois, F., Perotti, F., Salzmann, C., Chassagne, S., Gumy, J.-C., and Blank, I. (2013). Starch-based extruded cereals enriched in fibers: A behavior of composite solid foams. *Carbohydrate Polymers*, 98, 842–853.

Chanvrier, H., Jakubczyk, E., Gondek, E., and Gumy, J.-C. (2014). Insights into the texture of extruded cereals: Structure and acoustic properties. *Innovative Food Science & Emerging Technologies*, 24, 61–68.

Chavan, R.S., and Chavan, S.R. (2011). Sourdough technology—A traditional way for wholesome foods: A review. *Comprehensive Reviews in Food Science and Food Safety*, 10, 169–182.

Clarke, C.I., Schober, T.J., Dockery, P., O'Sullivan, K., and Arendt, E.K. (2004). Wheat sourdough fermentation: Effects of time and acidification on fundamental rheological properties. *Cereal Chemistry Journal*, 81, 409–417.

Colonna, P., Doublier, J.P., Melcion, F., and De Monredon and Mercier, C. (1984). Extrusion cooking drum drying of wheat starch. I. Physical and macromolecular modifications. *Cereal Chemistry*, 61, 538–541.

Connolly, M.L., Lovegrove, J.A., and Tuohy, K.M. (2010). In vitro evaluation of the microbiota modulation abilities of different sized whole oat grain flakes. *Anaerobe*, 16, 483–488.

Cui, S.W., and Wang, Q. (2009). Cell wall polysaccharides in cereals: chemical structures and functional properties. *Structural Chemistry*, 20, 291–297.

Delcour, J.A., and Hoseney, R.C. (2010a). Structure of Cereals. In Principles of Cereal Science and Technology (eds. J.A. Delcour and R.C. Hoseney), pp. 1–22. AACC International, Inc.

Delcour, J.A., and Hoseney, R.C. (2010b). Breakfast Cereals. In: Principles of Cereal Science and Technology. (eds. J.A. Delcour and R.C. Hoseney), pp. 241–248. AACC International, Inc.

Della Valle, G., Chiron, H., Cicerelli, L., Kansou, K., Katina, K., Ndiaye, A., Whitworth, M., and Poutanen, K. (2014). Basic knowledge models for the design of bread texture. *Trends in Food Science & Technology*, 36, 5–14.

Dornez, E., Holopainen, U., Cuyvers, S., Poutanen, K., Delcour, J.A., Courtin, C.M., and Nordlund, E. (2011). Study of grain cell wall structures by microscopic analysis with four different staining techniques. *Journal of Cereal Science*, 54, 363–373.

Ellis, R.H. (2007). The encyclopaedia of seeds: Science, technology and uses. *Annals of Botany*, 100, 1379–1379.

Fast, R.B. (2000). Manufacturing technology of ready-to-eat cereals. In Breakfast Cereals and How They Are Made (eds. R.B. Fast and E.F. Caldwell), pp. 17–54. AACC International, Inc.

Flander, L. (2012). "Bioprocessing to improve oat bread quality," University of Helsinki.

Frølich, W., Åman, P., and Tetens, I. (2013). Whole grain foods and health – A Scandinavian perspective. *Food & Nutrition Research*, 57, 10.3402/fnr.v3457i3400.18503.

Fuad, T., and Prabhasankar, P. (2010). Role of ingredients in pasta product quality: A review on recent developments. *Critical Reviews in Food Science and Nutrition*, 50, 787–798.

Gan, Z., Ellis, P.R,. and Schofield, J.D. (1995). Gas cell stabilisation and gas retention in wheat bread dough. *Journal of Cereal Science*, 21, 215–230.

Gondek, E., and Lewicki, P.P. (2006). Antiplasticization of cereal-based products by water. Part II: breakfast cereals. *Journal of Food Engineering*, 77, 644–652.

Gondek, E., Jakubczyk, E., Herremans, E., Verlinden, B., Hertog, M., Vandendriessche, T., Verboven, P., Antoniuk, A., Bongaers, E., Estrade, P., and Nicolaï, B.M. (2013). Acoustic, mechanical and microstructural properties of extruded crisp bread. *Journal of Cereal Science*, 58, 132–139.

Gray, J.A., and Bemiller, J.N. (2003). Bread staling: Molecular basis and control. *Comprehensive Reviews in Food Science and Food Safety*, 2, 1–21.

Gujral, H.S., and Rosell, C.M. (2004). Improvement of the breadmaking quality of rice flour by glucose oxidase. *Food Research International*, 37, 75–81.

Hemery, Y., Rouau, X., Lullien-Pellerin, V., Barron, C., and Abecassis, J. (2007). Dry processes to develop wheat fractions and products with enhanced nutritional quality. *Journal of Cereal Science*, 46, 327–347.

Heneen, W.K., and Brismar, K. (2003). Structure of cooked spaghetti of durum and bread wheats. *Starch - Stärke*, 55, 546–557.

Jakubczyk, E., Marzec, A., and Lewicki, P.P. (2008). Relationship between water activity of crisp bread and its mechanical properties and structure. *Polish Journal of Food and Nutrition Sciences*, 58, 45–51.

Jin, Z., Hsieh, F., and Huff, H.E. (1995). Effects of soy fiber, salt, sugar and screw speed on physical properties and microstructure of corn meal extrudate. *Journal of Cereal Science*, 22, 185–194.

Johansson, D.P., Lee, I., Risérus, U., Langton, M., and Landberg, R. (2015). Effects of unfermented and fermented whole grain rye crisp breads served as part of a standardized breakfast, on appetite and postprandial glucose and insulin responses: A randomized cross-over trial. *PLoS ONE*, 10, e0122241.

Johansson, D.P., Vázquez-Gutiérrez, J.L., Landberg, R., Alminger, M., and Langton, M. (2015b). Impact of food processing on rye products properties and their in vitro digestion. (2018) *Eur J Nutr* 57:1651–1666

Karin, A. (2006). Functional aspects of cereal cell-wall polysaccharides. In Carbohydrates in Food, Second Edition, pp. 167–207. CRC Press.

Katina, K., Arendt, E., Liukkonen, K.H., Autio, K., Flander, L., and Poutanen, K. (2005). Potential of sourdough for healthier cereal products. *Trends in Food Science & Technology*, 16, 104–112.

Kim, C.S., and Walker, C.E. (1992). Interactions between starches, sugars, and emulsifiers in high ratio cake model systems. *Cereal Chemistry*, 69, 206–212.

Komlenić, D.K., Slačanac, V., and Jukić, M. (2012). Influence of acidification on dough rheological properties In Rheology (ed. J. de Vicente), pp. 265–292. InTech.

Kosti, R.I., Panagiotakos, D.B., and Zampelas, A. (2010). Ready-to-eat cereals and the burden of obesity in the context of their nutritional contribution: Are all ready-to-eat cereals equally healthy? A systematic review. *Nutr. Res. Rev.*, 23, 314–322.

Lamberts, L., De Bie, E., Vandeputte, G.E., Veraverbeke, W.S., Derycke, V., De Man, W., and Delcour, J.A. (2007). Effect of milling on colour and nutritional properties of rice. *Food Chemistry*, 100, 1496–1503.

Landberg, R., Kamal-Eldin, A., Salmenkallio-Marttila, M., Rouau, X., and Åman, P. (2008). Localization of alkylresorcinols in wheat, rye and barley kernels. *Journal of Cereal Science*, 48, 401–406.

Langton, M., and Hermansson, A.M. (1989). Microstructural changes in wheat starch dispersions during heating and cooling. *Food Microstructure*, 8, 29–39.

Lasztity, R. (ed.) (1999). Cereal Chemistry. Akademiai Kiado.

Li, W., Li, G., Su, B., Tian, X., and Xu, S. (2013). Effect of sodium stearoyl lactylate on refinement of crisp bread and the microstructure of dough. *Advance Journal of Food Science and Technology*, 5, 682–687.

Lii, C.-Y., Tsai, M.-L., and Tseng, K.-H. (1996). Effect of amylose content on the rheological property of rice starch. *Cereal Chemistry*, 73, 415–420.

Liljeberg, H.G.M., Lönner, C.H., and Björck, I.M.E. (1995). Sourdough fermentation or addition of organic acids or corresponding salts to bread improves nutritional properties of starch in healthy humans. *The Journal of Nutrition*, 125, 1503–1511.

Linko, A.-M., Juntunen, K.S., Mykkänen, H.M., and Adlercreutz, H. (2005). Whole-grain rye bread consumption by women correlates with plasma alkylresorcinols and increases their concentration compared with low-fiber wheat bread. *The Journal of Nutrition*, 135, 580–583.

Lue, S., Hsieh, F., and Huff, H.E. (1991). Extrusion cooking of corn meal and sugar beet fiber: Effects on expansion properties, starch gelatinization, and dietary fiber content. *Cereal Chemistry*, 68, 227–234.

Manthey, F.A., and Schorno, A.L. (2002). Physical and cooking quality of spaghetti made from whole wheat durum. *Cereal Chemistry Journal*, 79, 504–510.

Mariotti, M., Alamprese, C., Pagani, M.A., and Lucisano, M. (2006). Effect of puffing on ultrastructure and physical characteristics of cereal grains and flours. *Journal of Cereal Science*, 43, 47–56.

Marti, A., Caramanico, R., Bottega, G., and Pagani, M.A. (2013). Cooking behavior of rice pasta: Effect of thermal treatments and extrusion conditions. *LWT – Food Science and Technology*, 54, 229–235.

Martínez, M.M., Díaz, Á., and Gómez, M. (2014). Effect of different microstructural features of soluble and insoluble fibres on gluten-free dough rheology and bread-making. *Journal of Food Engineering*, 142, 49–56.

Marzec, A., Lewicki, P.P., and Ranachowski, Z. (2007). Influence of water activity on acoustic emission of flat extruded bread. *Journal of Food Engineering*, 79, 410–422.

Narvhus, J.A., and Sørhaug, T. (2012). Bakery and Cereal Products. In Food Biochemisty and Food Processing. Second Edition (ed. B.K. Simpson), pp. 594–612. Wiley-Blackwell.

Owusu-Ansah, J., van de Voort, F.R., and Stanley, D.W. (1984). Textural and microstructural changes in corn starch as a function of extrusion variables. *Canadian Institute of Food Science and Technology Journal*, 17, 65–70.

Peleg, M. (1997). Review: Mechanical properties of dry cellular solid foods. *Food Science and Technology International*, 4, 227–240.

Poutanen, K., Flander, L., and Katina, K. (2009). Sourdough and cereal fermentation in a nutritional perspective. *Food Microbiology*, 26, 693–699.

Poutanen, K., Sozer, N., and Della Valle, G. (2014). How can technology help to deliver more of grain in cereal foods for a healthy diet? *Journal of Cereal Science*, 59, 327–336.

Primo-Martín, C., van de Pijpekamp, A., van Vliet, T., de Jongh, H.H.J., Plijter, J.J., and Hamer, R.J. (2006). The role of the gluten network in the crispness of bread crust. *Journal of Cereal Science*, 43, 342–352.

Primo-Martín, C., van Nieuwenhuijzen, N.H., Hamer, R.J., and van Vliet, T. (2007). Crystallinity changes in wheat starch during the bread-making process: Starch crystallinity in the bread crust. *Journal of Cereal Science*, 45, 219–226.

Prückler, M., Siebenhandl-Ehn, S., Apprich, S., Höltinger, S., Haas, C., Schmid, E., and Kneifel, W. (2014). Wheat bran-based biorefinery 1: Composition of wheat bran and strategies of functionalization. *LWT – Food Science and Technology*, 56, 211–221.

Rakha, A., Åman, P., and Andersson, R. (2010). Characterisation of dietary fibre components in rye products. *Food Chemistry*, 119, 859–867.

Ramaswamy, H.S., and Riahi, E. (2003). Structure and composition of cereal grains and legumes. In Handbook of Postharvest Technology. Cereals, Fruits, Vegetables, Tea, and Spices (eds. H.S. Ramaswamy, G.S.V. Raghavan, A. Chakraverty and A.S. Mujumdar), pp. 1–16. CRC Press.

Renzetti, S., and Arendt, E.K. (2009). Effect of protease treatment on the baking quality of brown rice bread: From textural and rheological properties to biochemistry and microstructure. *Journal of Cereal Science*, 50, 22–28.

Richardson, G., Langton, M., Fäldt, P., and Hermansson, A.M. (2002). Microstructure of α-crystalline emulsifiers and their influence on air incorporation in cake batter. *Cereal Chemistry Journal*, 79, 546–552.

Richardson, G., Langton, M., Bark, A., and Hermansson, A.-M. (2003). Wheat starch gelatinization — The effects of sucrose, emulsifier and the physical state of the emulsifier. *Starch – Stärke*, 55, 150–161.

Robin, F., Schuchmann, H.P., and Palzer, S. (2012). Dietary fiber in extruded cereals: Limitations and opportunities. *Trends in Food Science and Technology*, 28, 23–32.

Rodríguez-García, J., Salvador, A., and Hernando, I. (2014). Replacing fat and sugar with inulin in cakes: Bubble size distribution, physical and sensory properties. *Food and Bioprocess Technology*, 7, 964–974.

Roopa, B.S., Mazumder, P., and Bhattacharya, S. (2009). Fracture behavior and mechanism of puffed cereal during compression. *Journal of Texture Studies*, 40, 157–171.

Ross, A.B., Kamal-Eldin, A., Lundin, E.A., Zhang, J.-X., Hallmans, G., and Åman, P. (2003a). Cereal alkylresorcinols are absorbed by humans. *The Journal of Nutrition*, 133, 2222–2224.

Ross, A.B., Shepherd, M.J., Schüpphaus, M., Sinclair, V., Alfaro, B., Kamal-Eldin, A., and Åman, P. (2003b). Alkylresorcinols in cereals and cereal products. *Journal of Agricultural and Food Chemistry*, 51, 4111–4118.

Sajilata, M.G., Singhal, R.S., and Kulkarni, P.R. (2006). Resistant starch – A review. *Comprehensive Reviews in Food Science and Food Safety*, 5, 1–17.

Salmenkallio-Marttila, M., Heiniö, R.-L., Myllymäki, O., Lille, M., Autio, K., and Poutanen, K. (2004). Relating microstructure, sensory and instrumental texture of processed oat. *Agricultural and Food Science*, 13, 14.

Saulnier, L., Sado, P.-E., Branlard, G., Charmet, G., and Guillon, F. (2007). Wheat arabinoxylans: Exploiting variation in amount and composition to develop enhanced varieties. *Journal of Cereal Science*, 46, 261–281.

Sciarini, L.S., Ribotta, P.D., León, A.E., and Pérez, G.T. (2010). Effect of hydrocolloids on gluten-free batter properties and bread quality. *International Journal of Food Science and Technology*, 45, 2306–2312.

Sekiyama, Y., Horigane, A.K., Ono, H., Irie, K., Maeda, T., and Yoshida, M. (2012). T2 distribution of boiled dry spaghetti measured by MRI and its internal structure observed by fluorescence microscopy. *Food Research International*, 48, 374–379.

Sivaramakrishnan, H.P., Senge, B., and Chattopadhyay, P.K. (2004). Rheological properties of rice dough for making rice bread. *Journal of Food Engineering*, 62, 37–45.

Srikaeo, K., Furst, J.E., Ashton, J.F., and Hosken, R.W. (2006). Microstructural changes of starch in cooked wheat grains as affected by cooking temperatures and times. *LWT – Food Science and Technology*, 39, 528–533.

Steglich, T., Bernin, D., Röding, M., Nydén, M., Moldin, A., Topgaard, D., and Langton, M. (2014). Microstructure and water distribution of commercial pasta studied by microscopy and 3D magnetic resonance imaging. *Food Research International*, 62, 644–652.

Stojceska, V. (2013). Fibre-enriched snack foods. In Fibre-Rich and Wholegrain Foods (eds. K. Poutanen and J.A. Delcour), pp. 389–406. Woodhead Publishing.

Tiwari, U., and Cummins, E. (2009). Factors influencing β-glucan levels and molecular weight in cereal-based products. *Cereal Chemistry Journal*, 86, 290–301.

Turabi, E., Sumnu, G., and Sahin, S. (2010). Quantitative analysis of macro and micro-structure of gluten-free rice cakes containing different types of gums baked in different ovens. *Food Hydrocolloids*, 24, 755–762.

Vanin, F.M., Lucas, T., and Trystram, G. (2009). Crust formation and its role during bread baking. *Trends in Food Science & Technology*, 20, 333–343.

Vázquez-Gutiérrez, J.L., Johansson, D.P., and Langton, M. (2015). Effects of added inulin and gluten on rheology and structure of rye porridge. *LWT – Food Science and Technology*.

Vázquez-Gutiérrez, J.L., and Langton, M. (2015). Current potential and limitations of immunolabeling in cereal grain research. *Trends in Food Science & Technology*, 41, 105–117.

Weipert, D. (1997). Processing performance of rye as compared to wheat. *Cereal Foods World*, 42, 706–712.

Williams, P.G. (2014). The benefits of breakfast cereal consumption: A systematic review of the evidence base. *Advances in Nutrition: An International Review Journal*, 5, 636S–673S.

Yiu, S.H., Wood, P.J., and Weisz, J. (1987). Effects of cooking on starch and beta-glucan of rolled oats. *Cereal Chemistry*, 64, 373–379.

2 Definition of *Whole Grain* and Determination of Content in Cereal Products

Wenche Frølich[1] and Per Åman[2]

[1]Norwegian School of Hotel Management, University of Stavanger, Lindebergveien 39, N-1358 Jar, Norway
[2]Department of Molecular Sciences, Swedish University of Agricultural Sciences, Uppsala, Sweden

2.1 Introduction

Worldwide, dietary recommendations are given for increasing the intake of whole grain to improve health and well-being. There has been a strong international trend to develop and market whole grain foods; however, it has been difficult to obtain reliable and required information for selecting the most desirable products from a nutritional point of view. Even if an increasing number of consumers are well aware that whole grain foods are healthy, they are less informed about the nutritional differences in composition between cereals as well as pseudocereals. In Western populations, whole grain intake comes mainly from wheat, oats, rye, barley and corn. The estimated health risk reductions observed for whole grain in existing studies are therefore most likely due to intake of these particular cereals. It is well known that large regional differences exist in types of grains eaten both within and between countries although reliable and exact information on this intake is scarce (Kyrø et al. 2014). In order to provide consumers with appropriate dietary advices and to give the industry the opportunity to develop and market innovative and healthy foods, well-defined definitions not only of whole grain but also of whole grain foods are needed. This will help authorities to encourage the producers (industries) to label foods with correct and understandable amounts of whole grain. A common definition of whole grain foods is also important as international research and trade with foods are increasing.

Whole grain cereals are major sources of dietary carbohydrate and protein as well as containing high amounts of a variety of dietary fibres, minerals, vitamins and other bioactive components (Fardet 2010; Andersson et al. 2014). The latter components are mainly present in the outer parts of the grain or in the germ and are therefore removed to a large extent during extraction of sifted flours. As a result, health authorities in many countries are recommending exchanging the sifted flours with whole grain flours. However, evidence-based recommendations on the exact amounts and types of whole grains to be consumed are still lacking.

Questions that ought to be raised in this context are therefore: Do consumers know what is meant by *whole grain*? Do they know which grains are included in this group? Are all whole grains or whole grain foods the same when it comes to nutritional content and health effects?

Whole Grains and Health, Second Edition. Edited by Rikard Landberg and Nathalie Scheers.

Additional materials available for download online at https://www.wiley.com/en-gb/Whole+Grains+and+Health-p-9781118939437

2.2 Definition of *whole grain* in different countries

With the growing interest in whole grain, not only among researchers and health authorities but also among the consumers and the food industries, an exact and strict definition of *whole grain* is urgently needed (Frølich and Åman 2010).

The scientific community has for many years been involved in the discussions regarding an international common definition, including issues such as the types and parts of grains that should be included in such a definition. Important aspects in finding an applicable definition is different for target groups: the consumers to facilitate their choice of healthy food alternatives; the scientific community to establish uniform food frequency questioners and standardized dietary factors to study in relation to health; the authorities to be able to make recommendations; and the food industries to produce a variety of new whole grain products. A common international definition of *whole grain* would certainly benefit all these interests. However, for a definition to be useful in a long-term perspective for all these groups, it must be grounded on evidence-based nutritional aspects rather than simply classification of food items. In addition to short definitions launched some decades ago, more recent compressive definitions have been developed in several countries. In these definitions, lists of cereals and pseudocereals are included as well as specifications of the processes allowed to be used (van der Kamp and Lupton 2013).

Cereals are members of the grass family (*Poaceae* or previously *Gramineae*) and produce dry one-seeded fruits (caryopsis) that are commonly called a kernel or grain (Delcour and Hoseney 2010). All cereals consist of a fruit coat (pericarp) surrounding the seed. The seed contains an embryo (germ) and an endosperm surrounded by a nucellar epidermis and a seed coat (testa). In general, all cereals have broadly similar proportions of these botanical structures. However, it is not possible to specify a standard ratio for the different botanical structures since these vary within and between cereals. In addition, some cereals such as rice, oats and barley retain their husk during threshing and this must be removed to produce acceptable foods for humans. Bran is a technical fraction from the milling industry. It generally comprises the fruit wall, seed wall, aleurone layer, germ and smaller amounts of the starchy endosperm. The composition of a bran fraction is highly dependent on the milling technology and type of grain used (Kamal-Eldin et al. 2009).

Pseudocereals such as amaranth, quinoa and buckwheat are not members of the grass family, but because of the high starch content in their seeds and their use in cereal-like products, it has been suggested that they should be classified as whole grain together with the cereals in the grass family (Frølich and Åman 2010). These seeds contain no gluten and are therefore suitable alternatives for people with celiac disease. Certain pulses or grain legumes are other seeds with a high content of starch that can be used in different types of cereal-like products. Because of the characteristics of these, it could be argued if they should also be included in the definition of *whole grain*; however, they are generally not regarded as such.

2.2.1 AACC International and American Whole Grain *Council definitions of* whole grain

Whole grain was defined by AACC International (1999): "Whole grain shall consist of the intact, ground, cracked or flaked caryopsis whose principal anatomical components – the starchy endosperm, germ and bran – are present in the same relative proportion as they exist in the intact caryopsis." From this, it is clear that inclusion or non-inclusion of grains in this definition is not based on the dietary fibre contents. Pseudocereals (buckwheat, amaranth and quinoa), on the other hand, are included since they are considered to have similar macronutrient composition as whole grain cereals and they are also eaten in similar ways.

The AACC International definition of *whole grain* was adopted by the US Food and Drug Administration in the document "Whole Grain Label Statements" in 2006, to provide guidance for the industry (Anon. 2006). The American Whole Grain Council (2004) defines *whole grain* in a similar way to AACC International, using the following wording: "Whole grains or foods made from them contain all the essential parts and naturally-occurring nutrients of the entire grain seed in their original proportions. If the grain has been processed (e.g., cracked, crushed, rolled, extruded and/or cooked), the food product should deliver approximately the same rich balance of nutrients that are found in the original grain seed."

This definition includes the following cereals and pseudocereals (and forms of these): Amaranth; barley; buckwheat; corn, including whole cornmeal and popcorn; millet; oats, including oatmeal; quinoa; rice, both brown rice and colored rice; rye; sorghum (also called milo); teff; triticale; wheat, including varieties such as spelt, emmer, farro, einkorn, Kamut®, durum and forms such as bulgur, cracked wheat and wheat berries and wild rice. It also includes more unusual cereals belonging to the grass family such as canary seed, Job's tears, montana, and fonio when consumed with all of their bran, germ and endosperm.

2.2.2 Whole grain *definition in Denmark and the Scandinavian Keyhole*

A Danish Task Force from 2008 defined *whole grain* as intact, ground, cracked or flaked kernels after removal of the husks (Mejborn et al. 2008). In this definition, the nine main cereals within the grass family (barley, oats, wheat, rye, rice, millet, maize, sorghum and triticale) are included, but not the pseudocereals. It is permissible to combine different milling fractions, but the relative proportions of bran, starchy endosperm and germ must be the same as in the intact kernels. Only dry flour of whole maize is included, but not fresh maize and popcorn. The three Scandinavian countries Denmark, Sweden and Norway have agreed on common rules for declaration of healthy foods in a system entitled "The Scandinavian Keyhole" (Anon. 2009). These rules, accepted by the health authorities in the three countries, include the following definition of *whole grain.* "Whole grain is defined as intact and processed (dehulled, ground, cracked, flaked or the like) products where endosperm, germ, and bran are present in the same proportions as in the intact grain. If these fractions are separated under processing, they should be added back so that the final product has approximately the same relative proportions of the three parts as in the intact grain. The whole grain definition includes the following whole grain cereals: wheat, rye, oats, barley, maize (dry seeds), rice, millet, and sorghum. Wild rice, quinoa, amaranth, and buckwheat are not included."

2.2.3 The HealthGrain definition of whole grain

In Europe, a definition of *whole grain* was recently launched by a group of researchers from the HealthGrain EU project (2005–2010) (van der Kamp et al. 2014). This definition is based on the following scopes

1. More comprehensive than existing definitions
2. Pan – European
3. Reflecting current industrial flour manufacturing practices
4. Useful mainly for nutritional guidelines and labeling purposes

The main part of this definition states: "Whole grain shall consist of the intact ground, cracked, or flaked kernel after the removal of inedible parts such as the hull and husk. The principal anatomical components (the starchy endosperm, germ, and bran) are present in the same relative proportion as they exist in the intact kernel. Small losses of components (that is less than 2% of the grain/10 % of the bran) that occur through processing methods consistent with safety and quality are allowed."

The following cereals are included: wheat, (including spelt and emmer, faro, einkorn, khorahan wheat, durum), rice (including brown, black and other colored rice varieties), barley (including hull-less or naked barley but not pearled), maize (corn), rye, oats (including hull-less or naked oats), millet, sorghum, teff (tef), triticale, canary seed, Job's tears and fonio (black fonio, Asian millet) as well as the pseudocereals amaranth, buckwheat tartar buckwheat, quinoa and wild rice.

In Europe, the European Food Safety Authority states that the term whole grain is not sufficiently defined to be used for health claims and therefore the explanatory text of the HEALTHGRAIN definition claims: "This whole grain definition is expected to be useful in the context of nutritional recommendations and guidelines, and nutrition claims. Health claims on the other hand must be based on documentation of specific effects of grains or grain components of the diet."

This summary of some existing definitions of *whole grain* indicates main similarities between different countries. One clear difference however is that the Nordic countries do not include pseudocereals. Which grains are to be included are sometimes determined by the grains that dominate on the market in a region. Another determining factor is what the definition should be used for: scientific studies (where consumption should be related to health effects), consumer information or product development.

2.3 Definition of *whole grain food*

As no generally accepted definition of whole grain foods is available, several working groups in different countries have dealt with this issue. A review by Ferruzzi et al. (2014) stated that qualification standards for whole grain foods vary among countries, governments and regulatory authorities, resulting in lack of standardization when it comes to labeling. This review also stated that the terms *whole grain* and *dietary fibre* are often used interchangeably in labeling, resulting in confusion for many consumers when buying whole grain foods. Establishing a whole grain food definition is therefore critical for moving the field forward not only to improve dietary guidelines, but also to provide standards to the food industries when producing tasty foods with high content of whole grain. A common definition would also aid the standardization of studies on health effects of whole grain foods.

Recently, HealthGrain Forum, a non-for-profit consortium of academics and industry working with cereal foods, established a working group to gather input from academics and industry to develop guidance on labeling the whole grain content of foods (Ross et al. 2017). The aim was to come up with a simple whole grain food definition that aligns with whole grain intake recommendations and can be applied for all product categories.

The HealthGrain Forum recommends that a food may be labeled as "whole grain" if it contains 30% whole grain ingredients in the overall product and if it contains more whole grain than refined grains (both on dry weight basis). It also provided recommendations on labeling whole grain content in mixed-cereal foods such as pizza and ready meals, and highlighted a need to meet health nutrition criteria. The definition allow comparison across product categories since it is based on dry weight and is a move away from generic whole grain labels and instead encourages reporting the actual percentage of whole grain in a product.

2.4 Recommendations for intake of whole grain foods

As previously discussed, definitions exist for *whole grain*, however, a consistent official and international definition for which components should be included in whole grain foods has not been agreed on, although recent suggestions have been made (Ross et al. 2017). Studies have consistently shown that dietary fibre is one important contributor to the health benefits in whole grain, but it does not explain all of the effects of whole grain (Fardet 2010; Reynolds et al. 2019). The vast amounts of bioactive components are, as mentioned before, found in much greater concentrations in whole grains compared to the refined counterparts, but vary however highly between grains and botanical fractions (Spaggiari et al. 2020; Zhu and Sang 2017). The multitude of different bioactive components in whole grains is present in different proportions of germ, starchy endosperm and bran. Sometimes fractionated germ and bran are added to the refined flour. Both of these fractions contain different bioactive components with putative health effects, but these ingredients alone do not qualify as whole grain food and should not be described as such (Ferruzzi et al. 2014).

2.5 Dietary recommendations for whole grain intake

Many countries have recommendations for the intake of whole grain. In these recommendations, the specific quantities of whole grains to be consumed per day varies considerably (Frølich and Åman 2010; Ferruzzi et al. 2014). Also, recommendations of whole grain products are given in many guidelines internationally, either quantitatively (g) or qualitatively (eat more) (van der Kamp and Lupton 2013). The quantitative recommendation varies between a minimum of 48 g (US) and 75 g (Denmark) of whole grain per day.

Inconsistency in labeling and large variation in the amount of whole grain in products labeled as whole grain foods makes it difficult for the consumers to choose whole grain products. The consumers often believe that a high dietary fibre content is equivalent to high amounts of whole grain, which is not always the case since the content of dietary fibre in different whole grains vary considerably (from about 3% in rice to about 20% in rye). Isolated and synthesized dietary fibre from different sources could also be added to the products and wrongly indicating high whole grain content on the label.

What qualifies as whole grain products varies greatly in different populations and makes it challenging to determine the true intake of whole grain as g per day. Various classifications have been used in different studies such as:

1. whole grains listed as first ingredient on the label
2. dietary fibre rich products
3. products with more than 25% or 50% of whole grain
4. dark bread

The content of whole grain may be based either on dry weight or on fresh weight of the product. Foods with a high content of water will show much lower figure of whole grain than if this figure was based on dry weight. In some countries, declared/labeled content of whole grain is based on the total flour base, not including other food ingredients present in the product. It will therefore be misleading if the content of flour accounts for only a minor part compared to other ingredients in the product.

Today, little information is available on the intake of different whole grain types, which is important since different grain contains different nutrients and bioactive components. This will be a challenge in the future when health effects of individual whole grains will be studied in nutrition and population studies (Biskup et al. 2016). A study on subgroups in Scandinavia showed distinct national differences in the source of whole grain intake (Kyrø et al. 2012) and subsequent epidemiological studies have tried to analyze the role of whole grains from different grains separately in relation to disease outcomes (Wu et al. 2019; Kyrø et al. 2018; Johnsen et al. 2015).

2.6 Markers for whole grain wheat and rye content in food

Currently, the content of total dietary fibre has been suggested as a benchmark for determining whether a product is whole grain or not. However, as previously discussed, the total content of dietary fibre varies highly between different cereals, and this marker is therefore very uncertain for foods with mixed cereals and fractions. Alkylresorcinols have been suggested as a marker for whole grain wheat and rye content in cereal products (Chen et al. 2004). A range of Swedish cereal raw materials have been analyzed for total and individual alkylresorcinols. Results have shown that bran and whole grain of wheat and rye are the only main ingredients containing significant amounts of alkylresorcinols (Menzel et.al 2012). It was also shown that by using the alkylresorcinol homologue composition it was possible to determine if the whole grain in a food was from wheat or rye or a mixture of the two. By plotting analyzed alkylresorcinol content against calculated alkylresorcinol content from mean values of ingredients, a good correlation (R^2 =0.91) can be obtained despite a wide variation within the individual ingredients (Chen et al. 2004). A good correlation between and high compliance between calculated and analyzed alkylresorcinol levels in Norwegian soft wheat and rye breads has also been found (Andersson et al. 2010) as well as findings suggesting that whole grain content and the proportion of rye and wheat may be predicted from alkylresorcinol content and the ratio of specific alkylresorcinol homologues, respectively (Menzel 2012). Alkylresorcinols therefore appear to be good markers of whole grain wheat and rye, and their analysis may be an objective way to identify foods rich in whole grain wheat and/or rye or brans thereof.

2.7 Effects of processing on whole grain

The structure of cereal foods has for a long time been recognized as a parameter of importance for health benefits of whole grain foods that was pointed out among others by Frølich and Åman (2013). Studying flours comprising whole grains, cracked grains, course and fine whole grain wheat flour, it was found that the smaller the particle size of the food, the lower the satiety rating (Holt and Miller (1994). Also, glycemic responses are highly dependent on particle size (Tosh and Shu 2015).

Whole grain wheat bread, but not whole grain wheat pasta, has been shown to reduce appetite measures compared to refined wheat bread (Kristensen et al. 2010). This study indicates that the complexity and the interaction between the cereal source and the processing need to be raveled. Later studies have shown that preserving the natural initial fibrous network more or less intact, especially in wheat, rye, oats and barley kernels seems to be of importance for the physiological responses like satiety. Also formed compact structures, like in pasta and dumplings, can give positive responses on the same parameter (Riccardi et al. 2003).

Amount, molecular weight distribution, structure and conformation of fermentable dietary fibre are of importance for the physiological effects in the intestine (Poutanen et al. 2017). The solubility of the dietary fibre varies greatly between whole grain cereals and is as high as 37 % for rye but lower for the other cereals (Andersson et al. 2009). During wet processing, such as baking, endogenous β-glucan degrading enzymes may reduce the molecular weight of the polymer. This will lead to changed properties such as reduced viscosity and modified gelling properties. Similar modifications may take place with extractable arabinoxylans, but this polymer is more resistant to degradation/fermentation than β-glucan maybe due to a more complex structure requiring several enzymatic activities. It has been shown in a human study that a lower average molecular weight of the β-glucan is less effective in reducing the cholesterol concentrations compared to more inert β-glucan present in oats (Wolever et al. 2010). A scientific opinion by the European Food Safety Authority (EFSA) also states that oat β-glucan may be degraded during purification and manufacturing of foods, affecting considerably its physiochemical properties (EFSA 2010). Consequently, the cholesterol-lowering effect of oat β-glucan in food may be weakened or may even disappear during processing.

Resistant starch is naturally present in some foods with intact botanical structures, like in intact barley and rye kernels, but can also be formed during heat treatment. During hydrothermal processing, resistant starch can be formed due to crystallization of amylose, resulting in a higher dietary fibre content in the cereal foods. It has, for example, been shown that preparation of whole grain rye flour porridge will increase the content of resistant starch compared to the raw ingredients (Rakha et al. 2011). Whole grain cereals, especially rye, are a rich source of fructan, but the content of fructan may be decreased during breadmaking. Also, sourdough baking reduces the fructan content, up to 62% (Andersson et al. 2009). Processes such as germination and fermentation will have a large impact on phytochemicals in grains, which may have consequences for the health effects of the grains (Koistinen and Hanhineva 2017; Singh and Sharma 2017; Fardet 2015). Whole grain foods are valuable sources of minerals. A high content of phytate in these products has been considered a factor for limited bioavailability of these important nutrients (Hunt 2003). Degradation of phytate may, however, result in an increased bioavailability of the minerals (Schlemmer et al. 2009). This could be done during food processing like soaking, germination, malting and fermentation. The acidity of the dough during breadmaking is of great importance for phytate degradation, both during scalding and sourdough fermentation.

To summarize, processing will highly influence that content and properties of certain bioactive components in whole grain foods. However, these changes will generally only have a smaller effect on total whole grain mass and therefore only have a minimal effect on *whole grain* definitions and contents.

2.8 References

American Association of Cereal Chemists International. (1999). Whole grain definition. *Cereals Foods World*, 45, 79.

Andersson, A.A.M., Åman, P., Wandel, M., and Frølich, W. (2010). Alkylresorcinols in wheat and rye flour and bread. *J. Food Comp. Anal.*, 23, 794–801.

Andersson, A.A.M., Dimberg, L., Åman, P., and Landberg, R. (2014). Recent findings on certain bioactive components in whole grain wheat and rye. *J. Cereal Sci.*, 59, 294–311.

Andersson, R., Fransson, G., Tietjen, M., and Åman, P. (2009). Content and molecular weight distribution of dietary fiber components in whole grain rye flour and bread. *J. Agric. Food Chem.*, 57, 2004–2008.

Anon. (2006). Health claims meeting significant scientific agreement (SSA) http://www.fda.gov/Food/LabelingNutrition/Label Claims (cited September 2014).

Anon. (2009). Guidelines for the Scandinavian keyhole. http://www.norden.org/en/nordic-council-of-ministers/council-of-ministrs/council-of-ministrs -for-fisheries-and-aquaculture-agriculture-food-and-forestry-mr-fjls/keyhole-nutrition-label (cited Sept. 2014).

Biskup, I., Kyrø, C., Marklund, M., Olsen, A., van Dam, R.M., Tjønneland, A., Overvad, K., Lindahl, B., Johansson, I., and Landberg, R. (2016). Plasma alkylresorcinols, biomarkers of whole-grain wheat and rye intake, and risk of type 2 diabetes in Scandinavian men and women. *Am. J. Clin. Nutr., July*, 104(1), 88–96. doi:10.3945/ajcn.116.133496

Chen, Y., Ross, A., Åman, P., and Kamal-Eldin, A. (2004). Alkylresorcinols as markers of whole grain wheat and rye in cereal products. *J. Cereal Food Chem.*, 52, 8242–8256.

Delcour, J.A., and Hoseney, R.C. (2010). *Principles of food science and technology*, 3rd ed. pp.1–2. St. Paul, MN: AACC International.

EFSA. (2010). Scientific opinion on the substantiation of a health claim related to oat beta-glucan and lowering blood cholesterol and reduced risk of (coronary) hearth disease pursuant to article 24 of regulation (EC) No 1924/206. *EFSA J.*, 12, 3381–3393.

Fardet, A. (2010). New hypothesis for the health-protective mechanisms of whole grain cereals: What is beyond fiber? *Nutr. Res. Rev.*, 320, 65–134.

Fardet A. (2015). A shift toward a new holistic paradigm will help to preserve and better process grain products' food structure for improving their health effects. *Food Funct.*, Feb., 6(2), 363–382. doi:10.1039/c4fo00477a

Ferruzzi, M., Jonnalagadda, S.S., Liu, S., et al. (2014). Developing a standard definition of whole –grain foods for dietary recommendations: Summary reports of a multidisciplinary expert round table discussion. *Am. Soc. Nutr. Adv. Nutr.*, 5, 164–176.

Frølich, W., and Åman, P. (2013). Whole grain for whom and why? *Food Nutr. Res.*, 54, 5056.

Frølich, W., Åman, P., and Tetens, I. (2013). Whole grain foods and health – A Scandinavian perspective. *Food Nutr. Res.*, 57, 18503.

Holt, S.H., and Miller J.B. (1994). Particle size, satiety and the glycemic response. *Eur. J. Clin. Nutr.*, 48, 496–502.

Hunt, J.R. (2003). Bioavailability of iron, zinc, and other trace minerals from vegetarian diets. *Am. J. Clin. Nutr.* 78(Suppl.), 633S–9S.

Johnsen, N.F., Frederiksen, K., Christensen, J., Skeie, G., Lund, E., Landberg, R., Johansson, I., Nilsson, L.M., Halkjær, J., Olsen, A., Overvad, K., and Tjønneland, A. (2015). Whole-grain products and whole-grain types are associated with lower all-cause and cause-specific mortality in the Scandinavian HELGA cohort. *Br. J. Nutr., Aug. 28*, 114(4), 608–23. doi:10.1017/S0007114515001701

Kamal-Eldin, A., Nygaard Laerke, H., Knudsen, K.E.B., et al. (2009). Physical, microscopic and chemical characterization of industrial rye and wheat brans from the Nordic countries. *Food Nutr. Res.*, 53, 1912.

Koistinen, V.M., and Hanhineva, K. (2017). Microbial and endogenous metabolic conversions of rye phytochemicals. *Mol. Nutr Food Res.*, Juy, 61(7). doi:10.1002/mnfr.201600627

Kristensen, M., Jensen, M.G., Riboldi, G., et al. (2010). Wholegrain vs refined wheat bread and pasta. Effect on post prandial glycemia, appetite, and subsequent ad libitum energy intake in young healthy adults. *Appetite*, 54, 63–69.

Kyrø, C., Tjønneland, A., Overvad, K., Olsen, A., and Landberg, R. (2018). Higher whole-grain intake is associated with lower risk of type 2 diabetes among middle-aged men and women: The Danish Diet, Cancer, and Health Cohort. *J. Nutr.*, Sept. 1, 148(9), 1434–1444. doi:10.1093/jn/nxy112

Kyrø, C., Olsen, A., Bueno-de-Mesquita, B., et al. (2014). Plasma alkylresorcinol concentrations, biomarkers of whole-grain wheat and rye intake, in the European prospective investigation into cancer (EPIC) cohort. *Br. J. Nutr.*, 111, 1881–1890.

Kyrø, C., Skeie, G., Dragsted, L.O., et al. (2012). Intake of whole grain in Scandinavia: intake, sources and compliance with new national recommendations. *Scand. J. Publ. Health.*, 40, 76–84.

Mejborn, H., Biltoft-Jensen, A., Trolle, E., and Tetens, I. (2008). Fuldkorn. Definition og vidensgrundlag for anbefaling af fuldkornsindtag i Danmark (Whole grain. Definition and scientific background for a recommendation for whole grain intake in Denmark). Available at: http://www.fuldkorn.dk/files/Rapporter/Fuldkorn%20definition%20og%20vidensgrundlag.pdf (accessed Feb. 2012).

Menzel, C., Kamal-Eldin, A., Marklund, M., Andersson, A., Åman, P. snf Landberg, R. (2012). Alkylresorcinols in Swedish cereal foods products. *J. Food Comp. Anal.*, 28, 119–125.

Poutanen, K.S., Dussort, P., Erkner, A., Fiszman, S., Karnik, K., Kristensen, M., Marsaux, C.F., Miquel-Kergoat, S., Pentikäinen, S.P., Putz, P., Slavin, J.L., Steinert, R.E., and Mela, D.J. (2017). A review of the characteristics of dietary fibers relevant to appetite and energy intake outcomes in human intervention trials. *Am. J. Clin. Nutr., Sept.* 106(3), 747–754. doi:10.3945/ajcn.117.157172

Rakha, A., Åman, P., and Andersson, R. (2011). How does the preparation of rye porridge affect molecular weight distribution of extractable dietary fibers. *Int. J. Mol. Sci.*, 12, 3381–3393.

Riccardi, G., Clemente, G., and Giacco, R. (2003). Glycemic index of local foods and diets: The Mediterranean experience. *Nutr. Rev.*, 61, 56–60.

Ross, A.B., Van der Camp J.W., King, R., Le, K.A., Mejborn, H., Seal, C.J, Thielecke, F. (2017). Perspective: A Definition for Whole-Grain Food Products – Recommendations from the Healthgrain Forum. *American Society for Nutrition. Adv. Nutr.*, 8, 525–531; doi:https://doi.org/10.3945/an.116.014001

Reynolds, A., Mann, J., Cummings, J., Winter, N., Mete, E., Te Morenga, L. (2019). Carbohydrate quality and human health: A series of systematic reviews and meta-analyses. *Lancet*, Feb. 2, 393(10170), 434–445. doi:10.1016/S0140-6736(18)31809-9

Schlemmer, U., Frølich, W., Preto, R., and Grases, F. (2009). Phytate in foods – Bioavailability and significance for humans. *Mol. Nutr. Food Res.*, 53, S330–S375.

Singh, A., and Sharma, S. (2017). Bioactive components and functional properties of biologically activated cereal grains: A bibliographic review. *Crit. Rev. Food Sci. Nutr., Sept. 22*, 57(14), 3051–3071. doi:10.1080/10408398.2015.1085828

Spaggiari, M., Calani, L., Folloni S., Ranieri, R., Dall'Asta, C., and Galaverna, G. (2020). The impact of processing on the phenolic acids, free betaine and choline in Triticum spp. L. whole grains and milling by-products. *Food Chem., May* 1, 311, 125940. doi:10.1016/j.foodchem.2019.125940

Tosh, S.M., and Chu, Y. (2015). Systematic review of the effect of processing of whole-grain oat cereals on glycaemic response. *Br. J. Nutr.*, Oct. 28, 114(8), 1256–1262. doi:10.1017/S0007114515002895

The American Whole Grain Council (2004). http://wholegrainscouncil.org/whole-grain s -101/definition-of-whole-grains (cited Oct 2020).

Van der Kamp, J.W., and Lupton, J. (2013). Definitions, regulations and health claims associated with dietary fiber and wholegrain foods. In Fiber Rich and Wholegrain Foods (eds. J. Delcour and K. Poutanen). pp. 3–24. Woodhead.

Van der Kamp, J.W., Poutanen, K., Seal, C.J., and Richardson, D.P. (2014). The HEALTHGRAIN definition of "whole grain". *Food & Nutr. Res.*, 58, 22100.

Wolever, T.M.S., Tosh, S.M., Gibbs, A.L., et al. (2010). Physiochemical properties of oat β-glucan influence its ability to reduce serum LDL cholesterol in humans: A randomized clinical trial. *Am. J. Clin. Nutr.*, 92, 723–732.

Wu, H., Kyrø, C., Tjønneland, A., Boll, K., Olsen, A., Overvad, K., and Landberg, R. (2019). Long-term whole grain wheat and rye intake reflected by adipose tissue alkylresorcinols and breast cancer: A case-cohort study. *Nutrients*, Feb. 22, 11(2), E465. doi:10.3390/nu11020465

Zhu, Y., and Sang, S. (2017). Phytochemicals in whole grain wheat and their health-promoting effects. *Mo.l Nutr. Food Res., July*, 61(7). doi:10.1002/mnfr.201600852

3 Whole grain Fractions and Their Utilization in Foods

Cécile Barron, Valérie Micard, and Valérie Lullien-Pellerin

UMR IATE, INRAE, CIRAD, Institut Agro, University of Montpellier, Montpellier, France

3.1 Introduction

Due to their richness in starch and proteins, as well as in fibres and micronutrients, cereal grains are considered as an interesting nutritional source to promote better health (Poutanen 2012). Grains are made of numerous tissues with distinct composition, structure and physiological role for the future plant. The major part of the grain (60–85% of the dry grain mass) corresponds to the starchy endosperm (Evers and Millar 2002) and contains the storage compounds, as starch and proteins, for the plant growth. Depending on the cereal, it is covered with one or several aleurone layers (2–10% of the grain mass) containing the major part of the grain vitamins, minerals and molecules with antioxidant activities. Aleurone also plays a critical role in germination with the production of hydrolytic enzymes for the degradation of the storage compounds. It is surrounded by several tissues, called envelopes, with the nucellus, testa and pericarp acting as barriers to water and pathogens for the grain protection as well as being rich in insoluble fibres and phenolic compounds. The last part of the grain (3–7% depending on the cereal) corresponds to the germ and includes the scutellum, the plumule, the radicle and the embryonic axis that leads to the new plant.

Cereal grains are rarely consumed without prior transformation. Envelopes, especially the more external ones, and the germ have to be removed from the endosperm to maintain safety, high shelf-life and good technological and taste properties of the cereal products. The most external grain tissues may indeed be contaminated by microorganisms (Laca et al. 2006) and undesirable compounds, such as pesticides, heavy metals and mycotoxins (Balinova et al. 2006; Rios et al. 2009; Cheli et al. 2010). Moreover, the germ, which is rich in lipids, can suffer from oxidation.

Grain processing methods are mainly focused on the isolation of the starchy endosperm to produce flour or semolina, the remaining products being recovered in the technological bran and short fractions. Technologies can differ depending on the country, cereal type, food product and industry considered. They range from small batch milling units to continuous milling of large amount of grains. They also differ according to the grain anatomy (presence or absence of a crease) and are dependent on differences between tissue mechanical properties. Semolina and flour fractions therefore mainly derive from the

Whole Grains and Health, Second Edition. Edited by Rikard Landberg and Nathalie Scheers.

Additional materials available for download online at https://www.wiley.com/en-gb/Whole+Grains+and+Health-p-9781118939437

endosperm, whereas bran and shorts mainly come from the envelopes, aleurone layer and germ. However, each fraction also respectively contains part of the other grain tissues in proportions depending on the processing methodology and steps as well as on the sample variability inherent to genetic background and environmental conditions. This means that a comparison between fractions with the same denomination remains difficult without proper characterization of the tissue composition. Traditional methods monitoring ash content or color properties of semolina or flour are found to be limited to monitor the presence of the outer layers (Greffeuille et al. 2005). Moreover, new analytical methods have shown that bran obtained from grain debranning or milling displays a distinct proportion of grain tissues (Hemery et al. 2009).

Recently, efforts have been made to increase our understanding of the grain tissue behavior throughout the fractionation process and to answer the consumer and social demands with the aim to produce cereal fractions with desired properties but without losses of nutritionally interesting compounds. These efforts have led to the development of new tools and strategies to isolate tissues or molecules in order to better exploit the grain resource and increase the nutritional value of corresponding food products. This chapter points out and summarizes this progress, mainly focusing on dry fractionation.

3.2 Cereal technologies to obtain fractions from whole grains

Fractionation diagrams are adapted according to cereal species, cereal grain structure and targeted end-products. Harvested cereal grains can be naked or surrounded by a husk formed by the palea and lemma and mainly composed of cell wall material (cellulose, hemicelluloses and a high amount of lignin [10–15%]) associated with minerals such as hydrated silica as shown in rice (Hoije et al. 2005; Miller and Fulcher 2011; Friedman 2013). Therefore, when present, a dehulling step is needed to remove the husks, prior to the fractionation diagram. This is encountered for rice but also for barley and oat processing. In rice, the hull is not tightly stuck onto the grain and can therefore be easily removed using rubber roll huskers and an aspirator. This first step produces brown rice from paddy rice. In oat milling, dehulling is based on both impact and abrasion forces using rotors with fins or blades in the dehuller (Girardet and Webster 2011). The objective of this step in the cereal processing chain is to maximize the dehulling efficiency but to minimize the kernel breakage. The hull fraction, which accounts for about 15–25% of the initial grain weight, can be used as a high-fibre animal feed or for biofuels or furfural production, or incinerated (Girardet and Webster 2011; Friedman 2013). When processing dehulled or naked grains, two main types of fractionation diagrams can be described in relation to the kernel shape, and more specifically with the presence of a crease, where the outer layers are invaginated (see Figure 3.1).

For cereal grains without a crease (e.g., rice), the starchy endosperm is surrounded by the peripheral layers easily removed from the outside. In that case, brown rice, issued from the dehulling step, is used in the whitening step of the process leading to the separation of the envelopes and germ tissues from the harder starchy endosperm to recover entire polished grains. Several mechanisms are used, alone or in combination, to obtain the removal of the outer layers. For example, grains can come into contact with an abrasive roll (abrasion-type system) or rub against each other (friction-type system). This friction processing leads to white grains with a more polished and smoother surface, but induces a higher proportion of broken grains that may have implication for later product quality. Pearling machines are

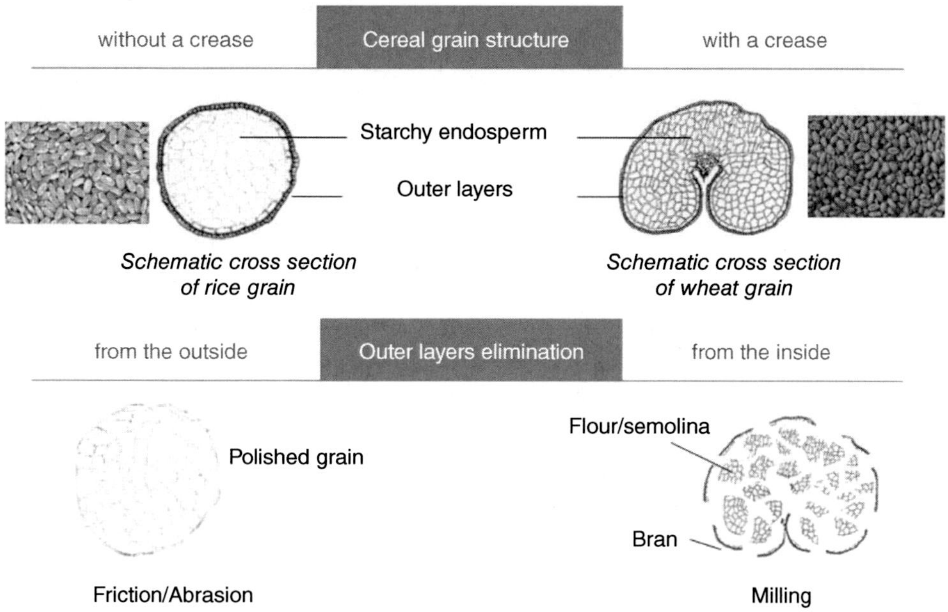

Figure 3.1 Main fractionation diagrams according to the cereal-grain structure. Source: Rikard Landberg.

equipped with a rotating abrasive stone and a surrounding screen. The degree of pearling is determined by different parameters such as the feeding rate, the distance between the stone and the screen, the retention time as well as the stone abrasiveness (Bottega et al. 2009). After rice processing, fractions consisting of about 20% of hull, 8–12% of bran and 68–72% of white rice (whole and broken) are obtained, depending on the degree of polishing. Hull, bran, germ and fine broken kernels are considered as by-products. In such a diagram, the starchy endosperm hardness is considered as an important factor that can affect the white rice yield (Lu and Siebenmorgen 1995). Indeed, the percentage of grain breakage is commonly related to the endosperm mechanical resistance. The endosperm hardness appears dependent on genetic and environmental factors, but also on the water content of the grain.

For cereal grains displaying a crease (i.e., barley, wheat, oat and rye) in which up to 25% of the outer layers can be invaginated, another diagram is needed. These grains are split by grinding and the starchy endosperm is recovered from the inside to the outside. The milling process, which is the most effective in the wheat industry, is made of successive controlled grinding and separation steps. At each grinding step, particles are sorted out based on their size and/or density, and further sent to an additional grinding step, leading to a complex flow scheme. In such a fractionation diagram, differences in mechanical properties between the starchy endosperm, the envelopes and germ are key factors in the grain fractionation behavior. In particular, a grain conditioning step is generally carried out to increase the moisture level and plasticize the envelopes leading to bigger bran particles that are easier to sieve. The number of grinding/sieving steps can differ according to the type of cereal and the goals in terms of endosperm extraction yield (the diagram length being directly related to the efficiency of this gradual separation). As an example, in oat milling, only two steps of size reduction are often encountered, whereas a typical wheat milling process combines at least 14 to 17 breaking/reduction grinders (with different configurations) (Wang et al. 2007). A typical rye milling consists of 5–7 breaks and 4–7 reduction steps (Lorenz 2000). The mill flow-scheme is also different according to the targeted end-product. For example, contrary to common wheat milling, no reduction steps using smooth roller mills are used in durum wheat milling where flour is considered as a by-product and semolina the targeted product.

In addition to the processing step selection, depending on the crease presence, dry fractionation strategies also depend on the relative proportion of the different parts of the grain. For example, in corn grain, emphasis can be given to the germ extraction as it accounts for about 10–12% of the grain weight (Watson 1987), whereas it only represents 2–3% in wheat. Corn grain water content is thus first adjusted to about 20% and then processed in a de-germinator where the bran and the germ are stripped away from the endosperm through abrasion. Parts of the outer layers can still remain attached to the endosperm and are further purified through the milling process, including a subsequent step of grinding and a separation step using gravity tables (Alexander 1987).

If the processing steps mainly allow the extraction of the starchy endosperm from the envelopes and germ, none of the mill streams can be considered as a pure tissue. Therefore, the degree of purity of flour and semolina, coupled to the milling yield, is evaluated to express the global milling efficiency. In the French wheat milling industry, ash content in flour or semolina is used as a conventional marker of the presence of the envelopes or germ as these tissues contain a higher concentration of minerals. However, if minerals are effectively concentrated in these tissues, they are also still present in the endosperm and their amount and distribution varies according to environmental conditions (Lempereur et al. 1997). Therefore, compounds with more specific localization have been identified to better monitor the behavior of each grain tissue during the fractionation process (Pussayanawin et al. 1988; Peyron et al. 2002; Hemery et al. 2009). These tools have been developed for wheat but generalization to other cereals is not straightforward (Barron et al. 2011).

3.3 The starchy endosperm fraction – a good source of energy

Starchy endosperm accounts for about 60–85% of the harvested cereal grain by weight (Hettiarachchy et al. 2000; Evers and Millar 2002; Barron et al. 2007; Miller and Fulcher 2011) and can be recovered with milling, as described briefly for wheat in the previous paragraph. The milling fractions can be used as raw material for cereal food making or directly consumed as whole grains after debranning (e.g., white rice or pearled barley). The size of the endosperm particles generated by milling clearly depends on the grain mechanical resistance and on the number of reduction steps. Flours are therefore the main expected product obtained from common wheat, whereas semolina or hominies are produced from durum wheat or corn, respectively.

The starchy endosperm fractions are mainly composed of starch (75–85%) and protein (10–15%), which make cereal food products a major source of energy. These macronutrients also display techno-functional properties that can be exploited when making food products. In the case of wheat, and rye to a lesser extent, but not with other cereal grains, the storage proteins are able to form a network, known as gluten, when flour is mixed with water. This gluten network displays unique viscoelastic properties, which are particularly important for entrapping carbon dioxide in bread leavening (Shewry 2009). The protein content and protein nature of the starchy endosperm vary within and between cereals. Endosperm fractions are low in vitamins, minerals and total fibre (less than 3–5%) but concentrate the most part of grain soluble fibre fraction (Hemery et al. 2007). Barley and oat endosperm cell walls are rich in β-glucans, while wheat or rye endosperm cell walls mainly contain arabinoxylans (Evers and Millar 2002). Rice is unique among the cereals in the sense of having significant amount of cellulose in its endosperm. In general, starchy endosperm fractions are also low in lipids (about 0.5–2%), except for oat where the endosperm lipid range 8–18% of the grain weight and corresponds up to 90% of the grain lipids (Barthole et al. 2012). These lipids are not encountered in individual entities (oil bodies), as observed in the aleurone layer or the embryo, but tend to fuse together into a continuous oil matrix located between starch and protein (Heneen et al. 2008).

Different quality criteria are taken into consideration to characterize the flour or semolina fractions to meet the requirements of the end-use. Protein and ash content, the percentage of damaged starch, the particle size distribution and the product color are typical parameters considered. The flour or semolina quality does not only depend on the grain genetic background and environmental growth conditions, but also on the production parameters, process type and extraction rate. Differences in the flour particle size and starch damage are noticed depending on the mechanical solicitations (impact vs. roll mill, e.g.) during process (Posner 2000). Particle size distribution is also found to be related to the grain mechanical resistance. This character is both dependent on genetic locus Ha (Hardness) that differentiates soft and hard common wheats and the environmental conditions that affects the endosperm porosity, known as vitreousness (Greffeuille et al. 2006; Greffeuille et al. 2007). A higher degree of starch damage is observed in flours from hard common wheat in comparison with soft wheat (Brites et al. 2008). Wheat hardness also affects the flour composition due to differences in milling behavior. Thus, a greater amount of phytic acid, a cellular compound from the aleurone layer, is measured in flour from hard common wheat grains in comparison with the soft wheat (Greffeuille et al. 2005). Moreover, differences in protein content are observed according to the grain structure between the floury and vitreous part of maize or durum wheat (Alexander 1987; Samson et al. 2005).

Flours, with specific characteristics and properties, can be extracted at different stages of the milling process. All of the produced flours are generally blended to obtain the straight run grade flour, but each flour stream can also be mixed in specific proportions to obtain more dedicated flour. Their specific composition has been related to the compositional heterogeneity of the starchy endosperm. Typically, a reverse gradient of protein and starch is observed in starchy endosperm cells with higher protein concentration in the most external part (Pomeranz and Shellenberger 1961). Therefore, as the milling process progresses from the inside to the outside, starch content decreases but protein and ash content increases regardless of the cereal (Gomez et al. 2009; Gomez et al. 2011). This gradient can be accompanied by a change in the protein nature with, for example more β- and ϒ-zeins in the outermost part of the starchy maize endosperm or more low-molecular-weight subunits of glutenin (LMW-GS), alfa- and omega-gliadins in the similar location of the wheat endosperm (Shewry and Halford 2002; Tosi et al. 2011; He et al. 2013).

Different physical post-treatments (e.g., hydro-thermal, micronization, air classification) of flours can be carried out in order to either stabilize or modify their functional properties. These treatments can affect both the rheological properties and the biochemical composition of the product. For example, Protonotariou et al. (2014) have demonstrated that the reduction of flour particle size by further regrinding led to an increase the starch damage level and also modify the flour rheology. Superfine powders can be obtained by jet-milling or more classical grinding technologies, and further air classification allows enriching flour in protein content whatever the cereal species (Mattern et al. 1970; Stringfellow et al. 1976; Dick et al. 1977; Vose and Youngs 1978).

3.4 The germ fraction – the most unstable of cereal fractions

The percentage of dry grain mass corresponding to the germ, taking into account both the embryonic axis and the scutellum, differs depending on the cereal. Maize or sorghum have the highest germ mass values, in the range 12–15% (Evers et al. 1999), essentially due to the scutellum weight. The embryonic axis only represents 1–2%. However, as it is easily detached from the grain by mechanical impact (Posner and Li 1991), embryonic axis is generally called the germ in the milling industry. Germ fractions are known to be rich in proteins, lipids, sugars and minerals as well as tocopherols with vitamin E activity, B-vitamins (mainly thiamin and riboflavin) and other bioactive compounds with antioxidant properties (Hemery et al. 2007; Brandolini and Hidalgo 2012).

Wheat germ lipids constitute around 10–15% of the germ dry mass and are rich in free fatty acids (5–25%), but are mainly composed of triglycerides with the unsaturated linoleic acid (18:2) being the most abundant fatty acid. Differences in the relative composition and amount of fatty acids are dependent on wheat cultivars, growth and storage conditions as well as methods of extraction. Germ fractions also contain compounds whose nutritional values are always under debate, like phytic acid or lectin-type proteins (as the wheat germ agglutinin, WGA). Indeed, phytic acid is known to infer the availability of minerals, but also to display antioxidant and anticancer properties and possibly other health effects (Kumar et al. 2010). WGA is generally considered to have adverse health effects principally due to its binding and damaging of the gut epithelial cell layer. However, a recent review on lectins points out the possible difference in effects according to the WGA amount and the lack of toxic evidence when consumed in transformed products after cooking, baking or extrusion (van Buul and Brouns 2014). Enzymes with adverse hydrolytic and oxidative activities, mainly lipases and lipoxygenases, are also unwanted activities responsible for storage damaging of germ and derived products (Sjovall et al. 2000). As other fractions, germ also contains undesirable compounds from grain contaminated with fungi. Recent studies analyzing the distribution of mycotoxins (Gimenez et al. 2013) reveal that wheat germ and derived oil contain deoxynivalenol (DON), but do not represent a significant source considering the tolerable daily intake. Analyses of mycotoxins in maize give low level of fumonisins and DON in refined oil and margarine even if present in the germ fraction. A significant amount of ZEA is detected, on the contrary, probably due to its lipophilic nature (Escobar et al. 2013). However, these authors estimate the dietary exposure to be less than 0.2% tolerable daily intake.

Differences in the distribution of some chemical compounds are observed between different cereal grains. For example, phytic acid is mainly found in the embryo in maize (87% of the total), whereas it is mainly located in the aleurone layer in wheat (Evers et al. 1999). Therefore, precise allocation of a specific compound in a cereal germ sample, as well as its quantification, must pay attention to the isolation method and the considered tissue as the embryonic axis and scutellum do not have identical composition (Pomeranz 1988) due to a distinct difference in physiological role in grain. Hand dissection of tissues and identification of biochemical markers specific for each tissue (Hemery et al. 2009) allow improvement in the characterization of cereal fraction.

Degerming prior to milling is more common and easier in maize than for other grains due to the larger size of the grain and germ and the importance of the germ oil extraction for further use. It is realized either using dry or wet processes. In the dry processing, the embryonic axis can be dislodged from the endosperm without grinding by mechanically shearing or impacting the grain. Mehra and Eckhoff (1997) have used a degerminator (Beall, Decatur, Illinois, U.S) to recover maize embryo, but other methods are also described to isolate a germ fraction (Gerschwiler et al. 2006; Hemery et al. 2007). A wheat germ by-product, mainly corresponding to germ axis, is possibly recovered from a germ separator or traditional roller mills but with a low efficiency (15–20% of the total germ [Hemery et al. 2007]). Posner and Li (1991) have developed a two-step tempering and processing procedure that allows the recovering of both the embryonic axis and the scutellum reaching 50–100% of the total germ. Isolation of a germ enriched fraction is also effective from hull-less barley using a Fitzpatrick comminuting mill followed by sieving (Moreau and Hicks 2013).

In the wet-milling process, a germ fraction is separated from a protein, starch or fibre-enriched fraction. This method classically uses denaturing solutions for proteins as it generally proceeds in presence of sulphur dioxide and lactic acid at a low pH (Vignaux et al. 2006). However, Singh and Eckhoff (1996) have combined a dry and wet procedure to quicker recover the germ with an equivalent yield but avoiding the use of sulphur dioxide. Singh et al. (2001) compare different processing methods and have described significant differences in the corn germ oil yield and biochemical composition.

The efficiency of germ isolation is generally not evaluated due to difficulties to give a precise quantification of each tissue in recovered milling fractions. Different approaches have therefore been developed in order to monitor germ isolation during fractionation. Using transgenic maize lines expressing the green fluorescent protein (GFP) either in the endosperm or germ, Shepherd et al. (2008) compared the efficiency of different processing strategies through the analysis of this fluorescence marker. Specific biochemical markers such as tocopherols and a wheat germ agglutinin (WGA) also allow the monitoring of the germ composing oil (Morrison et al. 1982) or the embryonic axis (Hemery et al. 2009). Barnes and Jorgensen (1987) and Barnes and Tester (1987) developed spectral methods to quantify wheat germ in milling products based on the detection of the fluorescence emission of glycoflavones, which are the phenolic compounds known to be present at higher concentration in germ than in other tissues. Hsi-Mei (1999) has compared the relative germ content in different millstream flour samples using this method.

Germ isolation aims first to reduce the lipid content of flour and thus avoid possible oxidation during storage. It is also used for oil recovery that is achieved by mechanical pressing (Al-Obaidi et al. 2013) or solvent extraction (Piras et al. 2009) removing, respectively, 50% or 90% of the total grain lipids. Alternative approaches have been developed where supercritical carbon dioxide is used for extraction instead of toxic solvents (Zacchi et al. 2006; Piras et al. 2009; Ko et al. 2012; Ozcan et al. 2013). This method is found very efficient to extracts lipids as well as fat-soluble compounds like tocopherols. Gelmez et al. (2009) defined the optimal pressure, temperature and time of CO_2 extraction based not only on yield, but also on the efficiency of phenolic compounds and tocopherols as well as antioxidant activities retained throughout the extraction. More recently, Fang and Moreau

(2014) have developed an aqueous enzymatic method to extract oil from wheat germ with high yield prior (72%) and after demulsification (around 60%).

Since germ lipids are mainly unsaturated, they are prone to oxidation and degradation under the conditions used for oil extraction and storage. Autoxidation of unsaturated lipids in germ or derived oil occurs rapidly, which leads to possible off-flavors and formation of even toxic products. The most common classical method to prevent germ spoilage is dry heating or steaming (Srivastava et al. 2007), but other efficient methods have also been developed such as continuous microwave (Sjovall et al. 2000; Xu et al. 2013) or gamma irradiation (Jha et al. 2013). Krings et al. (2000) demonstrated the potential of roasting germ to delay the increase of peroxide value and conjugated diene hydro-peroxide concentration as well as decomposition of tocopherol. Germ oil oxidation is potentially reduced by vacuum packaging, packing under an inert gas and refrigeration/freezing (Naz et al. 2005). Other methods like addition of antioxidant molecules from other plants, as those found in rosemary methanolic extracts, also prevent oxidation (Yesil-Celiktas et al. 2009).

Extraction of oil releases a germ fraction enriched in protein (>30%) with well-balanced amino acid content, notably including lysine. This remaining fraction is also rich in flavonoids, minerals (potassium, magnesium and calcium mainly) and phenolic acids (Zhu et al. 2006; Zhu et al. 2011). Therefore, defatted wheat germ can be used as an interesting nutritional food additive or as a raw matter for extraction of molecules with health functionalities.

As germ can be easily isolated, it has even been used as a bioreactor for recombinant protein production allowing an easy recovery of the produced heterogeneous protein (Zhang et al. 2009; Paraman et al. 2010). The only disadvantage is that the target recombinant protein is isolated with a number of proteins from germ and a high level of lipids especially in corn. Choice of the dry or wet fractionation process in this case has to pay attention to the recombinant protein sensitivity towards the generally harsh conditions used in the latter. Recently, it has also been shown possible to increase the germ size and therefore seed oil content by introducing wheat puroindolines into corn (Zhang et al. 2010).

3.5 Bran fractions – a source of micronutrients to exploit?

Bran fractions are considered by millers as by-products and are therefore not standardized. They correspond to classical fractions obtained by debranning or milling from grains concomitantly with flours and semolina or hominies. They are mainly constituted of outer layers of grains ranging from the aleurone layer to the outer pericarp, without the eventual hulls, with a minor proportion of remaining starchy endosperm. Bran fractions differ greatly in tissue composition and thus biochemical composition and functional properties, depending on grains (oat vs. wheat), process (debranning vs. milling) and extraction rate used. Oat bran, but no other bran, is defined by AACC (http://www.aaccnet.org) based on its chemical composition and extraction rate, but not from the anatomical point of view. According to this definition "the oat bran fraction is no more than 50% of the original starting grain, and displays a total β-glucan content of at least 5.5% (dry weight basis) and a total dietary fibre content of at least 16.0% (dry weight basis) such as at least one-third of the total dietary fibre corresponds to soluble fibre.

A typical wheat bran contains about 60–70% carbohydrates, 13–18% proteins, 12% water, 3–4% lipids (Apprich et al. 2014). However, composition is variable according to the extraction rate (varying between 18–40%), the grain cultivar, but also environmental conditions (Lempereur et al. 1997; Shewry et al. 2010). Present carbohydrates are mainly arabinoxylans (around 25–35%), (Delcour et al. 1998; Wang et al. 2006), cellulose, and β-glucans (Hemery et al. 2007). Brans are thus relatively rich in dietary fibre (50–60%, (Hell et al. 2014), but also contain variable proportions of starch from the remaining starchy endosperm, depending on the extraction rate. The amount of protein in bran can reach higher contents than those found in starchy endosperm or in whole grain (Sullivan et al. 2010), but the protein nature is different as shown by its amino acid composition. The starchy endosperm contains mainly the storage proteins richer in cysteine and amido-acids whereas the aleurone layer contains more soluble functional proteins richer in lysine (Rhodes and Stone 2002; Buri et al. 2004). Moreover, bran fractions are also rich in phytic acid and minerals (Tabekhia and Luh 1979; Anson et al. 2012), vitamins B and E (niacin, folates, tocopherols and tocotrienols) (Watson 1987; Pomeranz 1988; Wang et al. 1993; Edelmann et al. 2012) as well as phenolic compounds such as phenolic acids, lignans, and alkylresorcinols (Tabekhia and Luh 1979; Anson et al. 2012; Landberg et al. 2014; Wang et al. 2014), betaine and choline (Bruce et al. 2010), and sterols (Nystrom et al. 2007b; Nurmi et al. 2012). Pigmented grains, rice, for example, are rich in phenolic acids and other bioactive compounds such as anthocyanins and proanthocyanins (Min et al. 2012; Shao et al. 2014) mainly recovered in bran (Paiva et al. 2014).

Bran fractions are commonly recovered as a by-product of the milling industry. Extraction rate first influences the amount of starchy endosperm adherent to the whole outer layers and therefore the amount of starch in bran. Fractions recovered after processes such as pearling or peeling as well as those recovered after milling of peeled/pearled grains are also called bran fractions even if they do not have the same histological composition (Hemery et al. 2009; Chandra Lohani et al. 2012). Debranning technologies have first been developed from rice technology and have then further adapted to other cereal grains such as wheat (Fellers et al. 1976; Dexter and Wood 1996), barley (Izydorczyk et al. 2003), rye (Lampi et al. 2004), oat (Doehlert and Moore 1997; Peterson et al. 2001), millet (Chandra Lohani et al. 2012), sorghum (Viraktamath et al. 1971) and triticale (Lorenz and Al-Husaini 1980) to remove hulls but also bran. Debranning is based on a sequential removal of the most peripheral layers through successive steps in modified rice polishing equipment allowing the control of the target debranning yield. However, taking into account the grain form (ovoid vs. elongate) and possible presence of a crease, the efficiency of the debranning process to successively recover the different outer layers surrounding the starchy endosperm varies. The histological composition is different between bran fractions obtained with distinct processing steps such as debranning, milling or milling after debranning (Hemery et al. 2009), as illustrated in Figure 3.2 for the last two processes. In consequence, the bran biochemical composition is also different. Low degree of debranning (< 2%) is used in the wheat milling industry to decontaminate grains by removing about 90% of heavy metal such as Pb or Hg, but also microbial load (Eugster 2005; Laca et al. 2006). The resulting brans are discarded taking into account their content in undesirable compounds.

A bran stabilization step is often carried out in order to avoid any rancidity problem caused mainly by lipase, in particular, in rice. Different technologies are used such as thermal treatment (dry heat treatment, microwave, ohming heating, toasting), gamma-irradiation or infrared radiation, or treatment coupling thermal and mechanical processes such as extrusion. Grinding post-treatments, such as micronization, can also be carried out. Regrinding bran modifies its functional properties when incorporating in

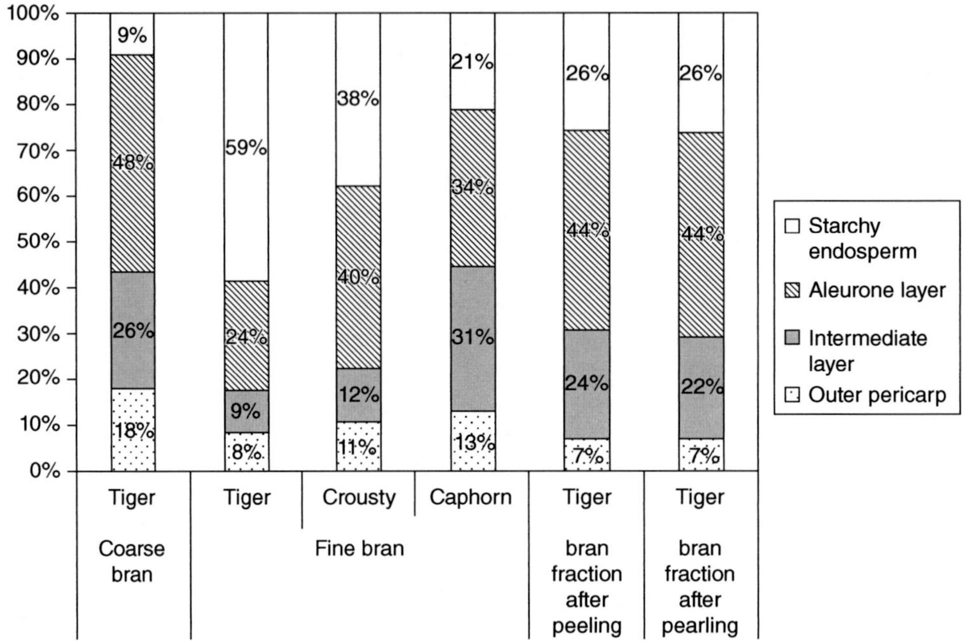

Figure 3.2 Tissue composition of different bran issues obtained from different processes (conventional milling technologies with or without previous peeling or pearling pre-treatment), and for similar process but with different grain cultivars (Tiger, Crousty and Caphorn).

food products (Noort et al. 2010; Kim et al. 2013), but can also modify its nutritional properties. Indeed, an ultrafine grinding increases the bioaccessibility of phenolic acids (mainly sinapic and ferulic acids) from wheat bran (Hemery et al. 2010). The specific surface area of wheat bran powder also appears to be positively correlated to its antioxidant capacity (Rosa et al. 2013a). Mechanical and biological bran pre-treatments are the most efficient to increase the phenolic acid accessibility (Wang et al. 2014). Treatment with enzymes hydrolyzing the cell walls also appears to increase sterols accessibility (Nystrom et al. 2007a).

Until recently, bran has mostly been used in the animal feed industry. However, considering its richness in compounds of high nutritional value mainly located in the aleurone layer, the food industry has begun to use it as a food ingredient, especially in cereal products. Bran fraction is commonly added in a fixed proportion to white flours to obtain whole-meal flour from wheat, barley, rye, oat and maize (van der Kamp et al. 2014). The addition of bran generally impacts technological properties (e.g., bread volume, color), but also the shelf-life and sensory attributes (texture, bitter taste) of the food product. Various available processes can overcome such problems but also impact nutritional properties (Katina et al. 2007). Bran consumption has also increased for non-food uses such as bioethanol production (Friedman 2013; Apprich et al. 2014; Pruckler et al. 2014). It has also been used as a raw material to produce ingredients by wet extraction, for example, proteins (Youngs 1974), oil (Friedman 2013) or dietary fibres such as β-glucans from oat or barley (Knuckles et al. 1992).

3.6 Innovative fractions

Due to the aleurone's richness in compounds with large nutritional potential, different strategies to increase the amount of this tissue in fractions have been developed during the last years. This has been possible due to the improvement of fractionation methods and tissue monitoring with the measurement of specific molecules. These methods have also opened the way to molecular fractionation in order to particularly isolate molecules with specific end-uses in dry conditions, that is, starch, storage proteins, dietary fibres such as β-glucans.

3.6.1 The aleurone fraction – richest in micronutrients and phytochemicals

Aleurone develops from surface endosperm cells and is therefore located in the outer part of the cereal grain starchy endosperm. A unicellular layer made from block-shaped cells in wheat (37–65 x 25–75 micrometre; Evers and Bechtel 1988), the aleurone layer is multilayered in other cereals such as barley (2–3 parallel cell layers), rice and oat (Stone 1985). Aleurone represents 7–9% (w/w) of the wheat kernel (Buri et al. 2004). In wheat, the cell-wall of its constitutive cells are larger and thicker than in other cereals (Xiong et al. 2013).

The biochemical composition of the wheat aleurone fraction has been recently reviewed in Rosa-Sibakov et al. (2015) and Brouns et al. (2012). Even if this fine composition depends on the wheat sample and the fractionation processes used, the aleurone fraction is always particularly rich in fibres (44–50% dm, Amrein et al. (2003)), mainly arabinoxylans (65%) and β-glucans (30%) coming from the non-lignified cell-walls (Bacic and Stone 1981; Saulnier et al. 2007). The main part of these arabinoxylans (95%) are water unextractable (Saulnier et al. 2007; Rosa et al. 2013b) and esterified with ferulic acid that is the main phenolic acid compound found in the aleurone layer (constitutes 95%). Ferulic acid is mainly bound to arabinoxylans and only minor amounts of ferulic acid are under free or even conjugated forms (Rosa et al. 2013b). Beside ferulic acid, *p*-coumaric, sinapic, vanillic acid and caffeic acids are detected in small amounts (Rhodes et al. 2002; Parker et al. 2005; Barron et al. 2007; Li et al. 2008). The aleurone fraction generally also contains the intracellular compounds of the aleurone layer (60–70% of the aleurone layer dry mass) which are proteins (15% of the total protein and 30% of the total wheat grain lysine content), minerals (40–60% of the total wheat grain content) associated with phytic acid (around 80% of the total phytic acid content), B-vitamins (notably 80% of the total niacin) and phytosterols (Evers and Bechtel 1988; Pomeranz 1988; Buri et al. 2004; Brouns et al. 2012).

According to Chen et al. (2013a), the antioxidant capacity is higher in aleurone than in bran (412 vs. 205 micromol TE/gram; ORAC oxygen radical absorbance capacity test) and also presents higher oxidation inhibition (42% vs. 30%). Ferulic acid, tocol and other phenolic acids (vanillic, *p*-coumaric acid, benzoic and caffeic acids) contribute to the antioxidant properties of wheat aleurone fraction in given order (Chen et al. 2013a). Beside ferulic acid located in the aleurone cell walls, two main carotenoids, lutein and zeaxanthin, are present in the lipid fraction of the aleurone layer in wheat, oat and corn grains (Hentschel et al. 2002; Adom et al. 2003; Panfili et al. 2004; Konopka et al. 2006; Ndolo and Beta 2013). Their total content has been positively correlated to the antioxidant properties of the aleurone (Ndolo and Beta 2013). Due to its high nutritional composition, several processes have been developed to produce enriched or pure aleurone fractions using wheat bran, ranging from lab to industrial scale (Hemery et al. 2007; Brouns et al. 2012). The first developed protocols to isolate aleurone from wheat and barley used a prior step of bran maceration in solvents followed by milling, sieving, air classification and centrifugation steps (Bacic and Stone 1981; Pomeranz 1988). Mechanical treatments of grains (successive debranning or pearling steps) have also been used to obtain bran fractions enriched in aleurone (Dexter and Wood 1996; Harris et al. 2005; Liyana-Pathirana and Shahidi 2006). More recently, new large dry-fractionation processes have been attempted in order to obtain aleurone enriched fraction with a percentage of enrichment over 60% (Hemery et al. 2007; Brouns et al. 2012).

Dry processes, avoiding solvents, may better preserve aleurone structure integrity and composition, and thus, preserves the content of phytochemicals and functional properties. Dry processes are mainly based on the differences in mechanical properties between the aleurone layer and the other tissues composing bran. They include two main steps composed of one or several grinding steps followed by one or several separation steps according to the size and/or density of the generated particles. Milling is realized with roller, hammer or centrifugal impact devices (Stone and Minifie 1988; Bohm et al. 2003; Chen et al. 2013b). Separation methods based on electrostatic properties have been developed to sort out aleurone particles from bran (Hemery et al. 2007; Hemery et al. 2011b) based on the differences in charging properties between aleurone and pericarp tissues (Antoine et al. 2004a). These processes consist of two steps, tribo-charging then electrostatic separation in an electric field. Electrostatic separation allows to obtain an aleurone enriched fraction with high aleurone purity. This method has been first described in 1988 (Stone and Minifie 1988). It has allowed the recovery of an almost pure (95%) fraction, however with a yield hardly reaching 10%. In the last ten years, Bühler company has patented (Bohm et al. 2003; Bohm and Kratzer 2008) a dry fractionation process using an electric field separation step in order to recover a fraction containing from 60–90% aleurone tissue in particles made of 5 to 40 intact cells (Amrein et al. 2003; Hemery et al. 2009). Chen et al. (2014b) used a non-uniform electric field to isolate tribo-charged particles allowing the enrichment of aleurone cell-cluster with a final yield reaching 42%. The same authors (Chen et al. 2014a) have demonstrated the importance of process conditions such as air flow rate and nature of the tribo-charging device (Teflon vs. Nylon or stainless steel pipe) in the efficiency of electrostatic separation.

Due to high and diverse content of micronutrients and dietary fibres, the aleurone layer may contribute to health effects (Brouns et al. 2012) and could therefore be of interest for food enrichment. Price et al. (2012), for example have prepared ready-to-eat products and bread rolls enriched with aleurone (to deliver about 27 g/day of aleurone per person) to feed healthy, older, overweight adults. These authors have demonstrated a significant lowering of one of the inflammatory markers in plasma, the C-reactive protein of which a high level is associated with the risk of cardiovascular disease. Wheat aleurone or sub-aleurone enriched flours have also been produced in order to enrich pasta in protein and fibre (Bagdi et al. 2014). This addition has appeared more applicable in value-added pasta production than those of wheat bran fractions or whole grain flour.

Depending on the degree of integrity of the aleurone layer, modification of the bioaccessibility and bioavailability of compounds of interest has been observed (Figure 3.3). Indeed, reduction of the aleurone particle size has increased the iron bioaccessibility (Latunde-Dada et al. 2014) and ferulic acid bioaccessibility as shown with the in vitro gastrointestinal Caco-2 model (Hemery et al. 2010). An ultrafine grinding of an aleurone

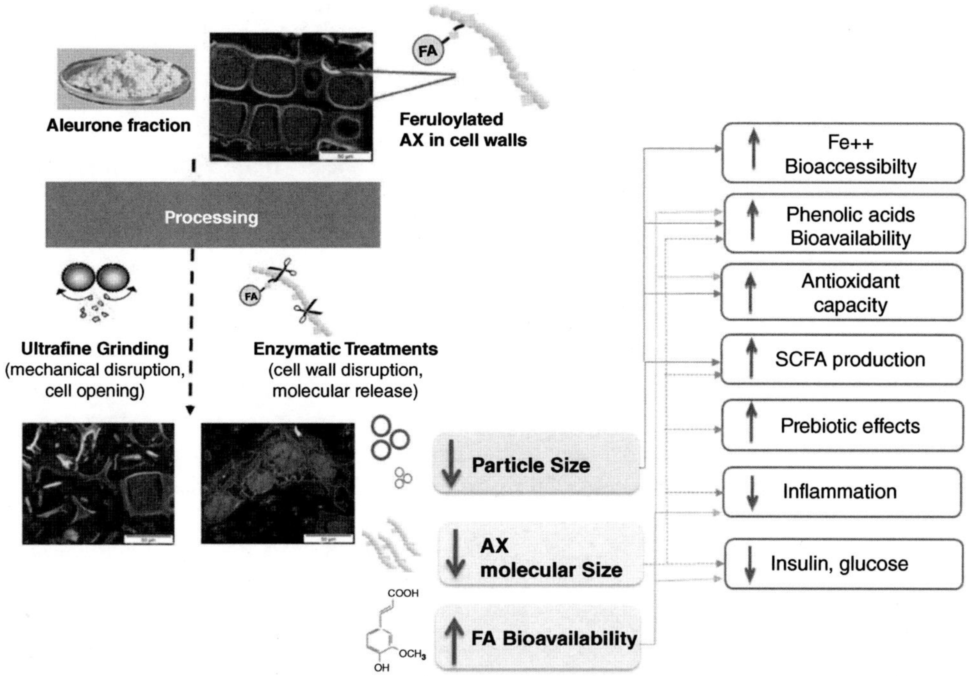

Figure 3.3 Processing of wheat fractions leads to changes in their structural parameters which can improve their health effects. Adapted from Rosa-Sibakov et al. 2015. © 2015 Elsevier.

fraction (particle size under 50 micrometre, Rosa et al. 2013b) increased its antioxidant capacity by a two-fold factor (44 mmol TEAC/kg). This change was linked to the opening of 50% of the aleurone cells, which increased the accessibility of ferulic acid, the major contributor to the antioxidant properties in cereals (Anson et al. 2008). Degrading the aleurone cell to a higher extent with enzymes such as xylanase, coupled or not with ferulate esterase, drastically increases (by a four-fold factor) the aleurone antioxidant capacity. This additional increase was due to the release of 85% of the ferulic acid in its bio-accessible form and possibly also to additional antioxidant compounds released from the aleurone cells with the enzymatic treatment (Rosa et al. 2013b).

The effect of aleurone disintegration, especially its ability to counteract metabolic disorders in diet-induced obesity and its effect on weight reduction, adiposity, inflammation and oxidative stress has been studied in mice (Rosa et al. 2014). The aleurone grinding does not positively affect these health parameters and has even been demonstrated to slightly increase mice body weight gain. On the contrary, the enzymatic aleurone disintegration with both xylanase and ferulate esterase has a tendency to lower the mice weight gain, reduce the accumulation of fat in internal organs and also the fasting plasma insulin and leptin levels (Rosa et al. 2014). These positive effects are probably related to the high content of soluble AX and bioavailable FA of enzymatically treated aleurone (Rosa et al. 2014). AX depolymerization is indeed often related with a better degradation in colon and in high SCFA production even if the relationship between AX structure and SCFA production remains unclear (Rosa et al. 2014). FA enzymatically released from AX by esterase appears available in the upper intestinal tract (Zhao and Moghadasian 2008; Anson et al. 2009;

Rosa-Sibakov et al. 2015) and rapidly transformed in metabolites by colonic microflora. Some of these metabolites have possible anti-inflammatory properties (Rosa et al. 2014). Recently, it has been demonstrated that enzymatically treated aleurone displaying a high amount of ferulic acid under free form allows to change the metabolite profile in urine of obese mice (Pekkinen et al. 2014). However, even if positive effects have been registered to counteract some of the metabolic disorders caused by obesity in mice, they remain limited probably because obesity was already settled before aleurone introduction in the mice diet. Native or enzymatically–treated aleurone should be more efficient when introduced into the diet as prevention, before obesity is established.

3.6.2 From a grain tissue separation to isolation of macromolecules

The improvement of dry fractionation methods in order to decrease the size of the obtained particles and the development of separation methods based on different physical properties allows sub-cellular constituent (e.g., cell wall material from bran tissue) or even macromolecule isolation besides histological fractionation. In order to achieve dissociation at this scale size, superfine grinding is essential to disrupt the cellular structure. This can be obtained by modifying the grinding mode as done with jet milling where size reduction is the result of inter-particle collision, or by changing the brittleness of the raw material with a strong decrease in temperature as occurred with cryogenic grinding (Hemery et al. 2007). Purity of the product can be lowered in comparison with the one obtained after wet fractionation but its structure and properties are expected to be better preserved. According to the purified macromolecule and its distribution in cereal grain, dry fractionation diagrams are carried out from different mill streams (e.g., flour for protein/starch extraction) or specific cereal species (e.g., oat or barley for β-glucan production).

Subcellular fractionation of the aleurone tissue has been targeted taking into account its richness in compounds with nutritional interest (dietary fibres in the cell walls and micro-nutrients and phyto- chemicals in the cell content). This approach allows the isolation of dietary fibres and their co-passengers such as hydroxycinnamic acid that is known to display antioxidant properties. Coupling different steps of pin-milling, sieving and air-classification on wheat bran separate a fraction rich in fibrous components (coming from the aleurone and the pericarp) and a fraction rich in aleurone cell content (Antoine et al. 2004b). Subcellular fractionation has been further improved by using ultra-fine grinding (either in cryogenic condition or at room temperature) coupled with tribo-charging electrostatic separation (Hemery et al. 2011a; Hemery et al. 2011b). Based on different charging properties between fibrous components (aleurone cell walls vs. pericarp tissue) and cellular components, tribo-charging electrostatic separation has successfully been carried out to recover around 65% of the initial aleurone cell walls in a unique fraction.

Macromolecular fractionation has been mainly focused on starch and protein extraction using air-classification from cereal endosperm fractions (flours, groats) to recover a fraction enriched in proteins (up to 54%) in the finest particle class (Wu and Stringfellow 1973; Wu and Stringfellow 1992). Letang et al. (2002) have carried out jet-milling for flour regrinding coupled with air classification in order to purify starch in the medium-coarse fractions of hard and soft wheat flours. Residual protein content in the starch rich fraction has been reduced to 2% for both types of common wheat, but the workflow sheet is longer for hard wheat and the level of starch damage higher.

Considering the LDL-cholesterol lowering effect of β-glucan, lot of works have been carried out to extract this macromolecule either from barley flour (Knuckles et al. 1992; Wu et al. 1994) or oat flakes or bran (Wu and Doehlert 2002) to produce value-added commercial products. Dry fractionation has the advantage to recover β-glucan with a molecular weight close to the native one (Sibakov et al. 2014) contrary to wet extraction, which induces a significant de-polymerization that impacts its nutritional properties negatively (Wolever et al. 2010). If conventional dry fractionation (including fine grinding, sieving and air classification) allows the enrichment of β-glucan up to 20–25% (Knuckles et al. 1992; Wu and Doehlert 2002), higher enrichment has been achieved including in the process of bran/flakes defatting with super critical carbon dioxide (Stevenson et al. 2008; Sibakov et al. 2011) or new separation technologies such as tribo-charging electrostatic separation (Sibakov et al. 2014). Fractions containing 34–54% of β-glucans have then been obtained.

3.7 Conclusion

Dry fractionation processes have been developed based on know-how mainly to isolate the starchy endosperm rich in macronutrients as starch and storage proteins but thus lead to a loss of most of the healthy micronutrients, phytochemicals and fibres present in cereal grains. In comparison with wet fractionation, it presents the advantage of reducing effluents, avoiding post-drying and additional energy cost. Depending on the processing steps, it is possible to control the tissue structure integrity and the enrichment of molecules with functional properties.

During the last years, a huge amount of data about the characterization and localization of compounds with nutritional interest have been obtained. Different strategies have been developed to limit the germ and aleurone removal or to reintroduce part of the bran and co-fractions or isolated compounds of interest into the endosperm fractions in order to increase the nutritional value of the product. These new fractionation diagrams are now possible due to the development of rapid methods for characterization and identification of biochemical markers to monitor the tissue behavior during processing. However, introduction of bran or germ fractions in flour or semolina cannot only alter the technological properties of the final products (i.e., texture, volume, color, shelf-life), but also their sensory properties and thus the general acceptability of the products. Depending on the tissue introduced it is also important to re-evaluate the products' safety. As an example, if the increase of heath beneficial component can be reach by substituting 10% of flour by debranning fractions enriched in the aleurone layer, this percentage could not be further increased without dramatically altering the technological properties of the bread, and accumulating the contaminating deoxynivalenol mycotoxin (Blandino et al. 2013).

If strategies exist to enrich cereal foods with compounds with nutritional interest, recent data have also noted that the limiting factor is not only the average amount of such compounds but also their accessibility. Therefore, recent studies have shown that physical (mechanical) or biological (enzymatical) pre-treatment of the fractions used for enrichment (bran or aleurone layer) are efficient to increase the micronutrient accessibility.

The enrichment of a target compound in the final product depends on (a) the considered cereal, as differences in amount and location exists between distinct cereal grains; (b) its accumulation in grains, which relies on the genetic background of the chosen cultivar and the environmental conditions along growth; (c) the choice of fractionation steps, which impact the compound distribution in the fractions. The health potential will depend on the molecule bioavailability depending both on its chemical form and its interactions with other components in the food matrix. Consumer acceptance of the product finally depends on a number of parameters (sensory properties, price, convenience, etc.), which are strongly affected by socio-economical and ethnical factors.

Therefore, future research has to select the most adapted cereal grains, cultivars and samples in relation with processing steps. However, to build both the best healthy cereal food and the most suitable for consumer acceptance, it has not only to optimize the first transformation but to consider the overall chain, from the field to the fork.

3.8 References

Adom, K.K., Sorrells, M.E., and Liu, R.H. (2003). Phytochemical profiles and antioxidant activity of wheat varieties. *Journal of Agricultural and Food Chemistry,* 51, 7825–7834.

Al-Obaidi, L., Dunford, N.T., and Goad, C. (2013). Mechanical extraction of wheat germ oil *Transactions of the Asabe,* 56, 1871–1876.

Alexander, R.J. (1987). Corn dry milling : processes, products, and applications. In *Corn: Chemistry and Technology* (eds. S.A. Watson and P.E. Ramstad), pp. 351–375. AACC.

Amrein, T.M., Gränicher, P., Arrigon, E., and Amadò, R. (2003). In vitro digestibility and colonic fermentability of aleurone isolated from wheat bran. *Lebensmittel-Wissenschaft un-d Technology,* 36, 451–460.

Anson, N.M., Hemery, Y.M., Bast, A., and Haenen, G.R.M.M. (2012). Optimizing the bioactive potential of wheat bran by processing. *Food & Function,* 3, 362–375.

Anson, N.M., Selinheimo, E., Havenaar, R., Aura, A.M., Mattila, I., Lehtinen, P., Bast, A., Poutanen, K., and Haenen, G. (2009). Bioprocessing of wheat bran improves in vitro bioaccessibility and colonic metabolism of phenolic compounds. *Journal of Agricultural and Food Chemistry,* 57, 6148–6155.

Anson, N.M., van den Berg, R., Havenaar, R., Bast, A., and Haenen, G. (2008). Ferulic acid from aleurone determines the antioxidant potency of wheat grain (Triticum aestivum L.). *Journal of Agricultural and Food Chemistry,* 56, 5589–5594.

Antoine, C., Castellon, J., Toureille, A., Rouau, X., and Dissado, L. (2004a). Comparison of constitutive wheat bran tissues by dielectric spectroscopy and effect of their moisture content. *Polymer International,* 53, 2169–2177.

Antoine, C., Peyron, S., Lullien-Pellerin, V., Abecassis, J., and Rouau, X. (2004b). Wheat bran tissue fractionation using biochemical markers. *Journal of Cereal Science,* 39, 387–393.

Apprich, S., Tirpanalan, Ö., Hell, J., Reisinger, M., Böhmdorfer, S., Siebenhandl-Ehn, S., Novalin, S., and Kneifel, W. (2014). Wheat bran-based biorefinery 2: Valorization of products. *LWT – Food Science and Technology,* 56, 222–231.

Bacic, A., and Stone, B.A. (1981). Chemistry and organisation of aleurone cell wall components from wheat and barley. *Australian Journal of Plant Physiology,* 8, 475–495.

Bagdi, A., Szabo, F., Gere, A., Kokai, Z., Sipos, L., and Tomoskozi, S. (2014). Effect of aleurone-rich flour on composition, cooking, textural, and sensory properties of pasta. *Lwt-Food Science and Technology,* 59, 996–1002.

Balinova, A., Mladenova, R., and Obretenchev, D. (2006). Effect of grain storage and processing on chlorpyrifos-methyl and pirimiphos-methyl residues in post-harvest-treated wheat with regard to baby food safety requirements. *Food Additives and Contaminants,* 23, 391–397.

Barnes, P.J., and Jorgensen, K.G. (1987). Fluorimetric measurement of wheat-germ in milling products. 2. Sodium tetraborate reagent. *Journal of Cereal Science,* 5, 149–154.

Barnes, P.J., and Tester, R.F. (1987). Fluorimetric measurement of wheat-germ in milling products. 1. Boron-trifluoride methanol reagent. *Journal of Cereal Science,* 5, 139–148.

Barron, C., Samson, M.F., Lullien-Pellerin, V., and Rouau, X. (2011). Wheat grain tissue proportions in milling fractions using biochemical marker measurements: Application to different wheat cultivars. *Journal of Cereal Science,* 53, 306–311.

Barron, C., Surget, A., and Rouau, X. (2007). Relative amounts of tissues in mature wheat (Triticum aestivum L.) grain and their carbohydrate and phenolic acid composition. *Journal of Cereal Science,* 45, 88–96.

Barthole, G., Lepiniec, L., Rogowsky, P.M., and Baud, S. (2012). Controlling lipid accumulation in cereal grains. *Plant Science,* 185–186, 33–39.

Blandino, M., Sovrani, V., Marinaccio, F., Reyneri, A., Rolle, L., Giacosa, S., Locatelli, M., Bordiga, M., Travaglia, F., Coisson, J.D., and Arlorio, M. (2013). Nutritional and technological quality of bread enriched with an intermediated pearled wheat fraction. *Food Chemistry,* 141, 2549–2557.

Bohm, A., Bogoni, C., Behrens, R., and Otto, T. (2003). Method for the extraction of aleurone from bran. A.G., B. *US Patent application publication US 2003/0175384.*

Bohm, A., and Kratzer, A. (2008). Method forisolating aleurone particles. A.G., B. *US Patent application publication US 2008/02577787 A1.*

Bottega, G., Caramanico, R., Lucisano, M., Mariotti, M., Franzetti, L., and Pagani, M.A. (2009). The debranning of common wheat (Triticum aestivum L.) with innovative abrasive rolls. *Journal of Food Engineering,* 94, 75–82.

Brandolini, A., and Hidalgo, A. (2012). Wheat germ: Not only a by-product. *International Journal of Food Sciences and Nutrition,* 63, 71–74.

Brites, C.M., dos Santos, C.A.L., Bagulho, A.S., and Beirao-Da-Costa, M.L. (2008). Effect of wheat puroindoline alleles on functional properties of starch. *European Food Research and Technology,* 226, 1205–1212.

Brouns, F., Hemery, Y., Price, R., and Mateo Anson, N. (2012). Wheat aleurone: Separation, composition, health aspects, and potential food use. *Critical Reviews in Food Science and Nutrition,* 52, 553–568.

Bruce, S.J., Guy, P.A., Rezzi, S., and Ross, A.B. (2010). Quantitative measurement of betaine and free choline in plasma, cereals and cereal products by isotope dilution LC-MS/MS. *Journal of Agricultural and Food Chemistry,* 58, 2055–2061.

Buri, R.C., von Reding, W., and Gavin, M.H. (2004). Description and characterization of wheat aleurone. *Cereal Foods World, 49,* 274+.

Chandra Lohani, U., Prakash Pandey, J., and Chandra Shahi, N. (2012). Effect of degree of polishing on milling characteristics and proximate compositions of barnyard millet (Echinochloa frumentacea). *Food and Bioprocess Technology,* 5, 1113–1119.

Cheli, F., Campagnoli, A., Ventura, V., Brera, C., Berdini, C., Palmaccio, E., and Dell'Orto, V. (2010). Effects of industrial processing on the distributions of deoxynivalenol, cadmium and lead in durum wheat milling fractions. *LWT – Food Science and Technology,* 43, 1050–1057.

Chen, Y.F., Dunford, N.T., and Goad, C. (2013a). Phytochemical composition of extracts from wheat grain fractions obtained by tangential abrasive dehulling. *Lwt-Food Science and Technology,* 54, 353–359.

Chen, Z.W., Liu, F.R., Wang, L., Li, Y.F., Wang, R., and Chen, Z.X. (2014a). Tribocharging properties of wheat bran fragments in air-solid pipe flow. *Food Research International,* 62, 262–271.

Chen, Z.W., Wang, L., Wang, R., Li, Y.F., and Chen, Z.X. (2014b). Triboelectric separation of aleurone cell-cluster from wheat bran fragments in nonuniform electric field. *Food Research International,* 62, 111–120.

Chen, Z.W., Zha, B.P., Wang, L., Wang, R., Chen, Z.X., and Tian, Y.N. (2013b). Dissociation of aleurone cell cluster from wheat bran by centrifugal impact milling. *Food Research International,* 54, 63–71.

Delcour, J.A., Van Win, H., and Grobet, P.J. (1998). Distribution and structural variation of arabinoxylans in common wheat mill streams. *Journal of Agricultural and Food Chemistry,* 47, 271–275.

Dexter, J.E., and Wood, P.J. (1996). Recent applications of debranning of wheat before milling. *Trends in Food Science & Technology,* 7, 35–41.

Dick, J.W., Shuey, W.C., and Banasik, O.J. (1977). Adjustment of rheological properties of flour by fine grinding and air classification *Cereal Chemistry,* 54, 246–255.

Doehlert, D.C., and Moore, W.R. (1997). Composition of oat bran and flour prepared by three different mechanisms of dry milling. *Cereal Chemistry,* 74, 403–406.

Edelmann, M., Kariluoto, S., Nyström, L., and Piironen, V. (2012). Folate in oats and its milling fractions. *Food Chemistry,* 135, 1938–1947.

Escobar, J., Loran, S., Gimenez, I., Ferruz, E., Herrera, M., Herrera, A., and Arino, A. (2013). Occurrence and exposure assessment of Fusarium mycotoxins in maize germ, refined corn oil and margarine. *Food and Chemical Toxicology,* 62, 514–520.

Eugster, W. (2005). Avantages commerciaux réalisés grâce au process de décorticage "Peeling." *Industrie des Céréales,* 143, 31–32.

Evers, A.D., and Bechtel, D.B. (1988). Microscopic structure of the wheat grain. In *Wheat : Chemistry and Technoloy* (ed. Y. Pomeranz), pp. 47–95 AACC.

Evers, A.D., Blakeney, A.B., and O'Brien, L. (1999). Cereal structure and composition. *Australian Journal of Agricultural Research,* 50, 629–650.

Evers, A.D., and Millar, S. (2002). Cereal grain structure and development: Some implications for quality. *Journal of Cereal Science,* 36, 261–284.

Fang, X.Z., and Moreau, R.A. (2014). Extraction and demulsification of oil from wheat germ, barley germ, and rice bran using an aqueous enzymatic method. *Journal of the American Oil Chemists Society,* 91, 1261–1268.

Fellers, D.A., Mossman, A.P., Johnston, P.H., and Wheeler, E.L. (1976). Mechanical debranning of whole-kernel wheat. III. Composition, cooking characteristics, and storage stability. *Cereal Chemistry,* 53, 308–317.

Friedman, M. (2013). Rice brans, rice bran oils, and rice hulls: Composition, food and industrial uses, and bioactivities in humans, animals, and cells. *Journal of Agricultural and Food Chemistry* 61, 10626–10641.,

Gelmez, N., Kincal, N.S., and Yener, M.E. (2009). Optimization of supercritical carbon dioxide extraction of antioxidants from roasted wheat germ based on yield, total phenolic and tocopherol contents, and antioxidant activities of the extracts. *Journal of Supercritical Fluids,* 48, 217–224.

Gerschwiler, O., Eugster, W., and Zwahlen, U. (2006). Method and device for husking and degerminating cereals. A.G., B. *US Patent application publication US 2006/0053764 A.*

Gimenez, I., Herrera, M., Escobar, J., Ferruz, E., Loran, S., Herrera, A., and Arino, A. (2013). Distribution of deoxynivalenol and zearalenone in milled germ during wheat milling and analysis of toxin levels in wheat germ and wheat germ oil. *Food Control,* 34, 268–273.

Girardet, N., and Webster, F.H. (2011). Oat milling : specification, storage, and processing. In *Oats: Chemistry and technology* (ed. F.H. Webster), pp. 301–319. AACC.

Gomez, M., Pardo, J., Oliete, B., and Caballero, P. (2009). Effect of the milling process on quality characteristics of rye flour. *Journal of the Science of Food and Agriculture,* 89, 470–476.

Gomez, M., Ruiz-Paris, E., and Oliete, B. (2011). Influence of wheat milling on low-hydration bread quality developed by sheeting rolls. *Food Science and Technology International,* 17, 256–265.

Greffeuille, V., Abecassis, J., Bar L'Helgouach, C., and Lullien-Pellerin, V. (2005). Differences in the aleurone layer fate between hard and soft common wheats at grain milling. *Cereal Chemistry,* 82, 138–143.

Greffeuille, V., Abecassis, J., Barouh, N., Villeneuve, P., Mabille, F., Bar L'Helgouac'h, C., and Lullien-Pellerin, V. (2007). Analysis of the milling reduction of bread wheat farina: physical and biochemical characterisation. *Journal of Cereal Science,* 45, 97–105.

Greffeuille, V., Abecassis, J., Rousset, M., Oury, F.X., Faye, A., Bar L'Helgouac'h, C., and Lullien-Pellerin, V. (2006). Grain characterization and milling behaviour of near-isogenic lines differing by hardness. *Theoretical and Applied Genetics,* 114, 1–12.

Harris, P.J., Chavan, R.R., and Ferguson, L.R. (2005). Production and characterisation of two wheat-bran fractions: an aleurone-rich and a pericarp-rich fraction. *Molecular Nutrition & Food Research,* 49, 536–545.

He, J.B., Penson, S., Powers, S.J., Hawes, C., Shewry, P.R., and Tosi, P. (2013). Spatial patterns of gluten protein and polymer distribution in wheat grain. *Journal of Agricultural and Food Chemistry,* 61, 6207–6215.

Hell, J., Kneifel, W., Rosenau, T., and Böhmdorfer, S. (2014). Analytical techniques for the elucidation of wheat bran constituents and their structural features with emphasis on dietary fiber – A review. *Trends in Food Science & Technology,* 35, 102–113.

Hemery, Y., Chaurand, M., Holopainen, U., Lampi, A.M., Lehtinen, P., Piironen, V., Sadoudi, A., and Rouau, X. (2011a). Potential of dry fractionation of wheat bran for the development of food ingredients, part I: Influence of ultra-fine grinding. *Journal of Cereal Science,* 53, 1–8.

Hemery, Y., Holopainen, U., Lampi, A.M., Lehtinen, P., Nurmi, T., Piironen, V., Edelmann, M., and Rouau, X. (2011b). Potential of dry fractionation of wheat bran for the development of food ingredients, part II: Electrostatic separation of particles. *Journal of Cereal Science,* 53, 9–18.

Hemery, Y., Lullien-Pellerin, V., Rouau, X., Abecassis, J., Samson, M.F., Aman, P., von Reding, W., Spoerndli, C., and Barron, C. (2009). Biochemical markers: Efficient tools for the assessment of wheat grain tissue proportions in milling fractions. *Journal of Cereal Science,* 49, 55–64.

Hemery, Y., Rouau, X., Lullien-Pellerin, V., Barron, C., and Abecassis, J. (2007). Dry processes to develop wheat fractions and products with enhanced nutritional quality. *Journal of Cereal Science,* 46, 327–347.

Hemery, Y.M., Anson, N.M., Havenaar, R., Haenen, G., Noort, M.W.J., and Rouau, X. (2010). Dry-fractionation of wheat bran increases the bioaccessibility of phenolic acids in breads made from processed bran fractions. *Food Research International,* 43, 1429–1438.

Heneen, W.K., Karlsson, G., Brismar, K., Gummeson, P.O., Marttila, S., Leonova, S., Carlsson, A.S., Bafor, M., Banas, A., Mattsson, B., Debski, H., and Stymne, S. (2008). Fusion of oil bodies in endosperm of oat grains. *Planta,* 228, 589–599.

Hentschel, V., Kranl, K., Hollmann, J., Lindhauer, M.G., Boehm, V., and Bitsch, R. (2002). Spectrophotometric determination of yellow pigment content and evaluation of carotenoids by high-performance liquid chromatography in durum wheat grain. *Journal of Agricultural and Food Chemistry,* 50, 6663–6668.

Hettiarachchy, N.S., Ju, Z.Y., Siebenmorgen, T., and Sharp, R.N. (2000). Rice : production, processing and utilization. In *Handbook of Cereal Science and Technology, Second Edition, Revised and Expanded* (eds. K. Kulp and J.G. Ponte), pp. 203–221. Dekker.

Hoije, A., Grondahl, M., Tommeraas, K., and Gatenholm, P. (2005). Isolation and characterization of physicochemical and material properties of arabinoxylans from barley husks. *Carbohydrate Polymers,* 61, 266–275.

Hsi-Mei, L. (1999). A simple procedure for the measurement of wheat germ in the milling products by fluorescence spectroscopy. *Food Science and Agricultural Chemistry,* 1, 47–54.

Izydorczyk, M.S., Jacobs, M.S., and Dexter, J.E. (2003). Distribution and structural variation of nonstarch polysaccharides in milling fractions of hull-less barley with variable amylose content. *Cereal Chemistry,* 80, 645–653.

Jha, P.K., Kudachikar, V.B., and Kumar, S. (2013). Lipase inactivation in wheat germ by gamma irradiation. *Radiation Physics and Chemistry,* 86, 136–139.

Katina K., Laitila A., Juvonen R., Liukkonen K.H., Kariluoto S., Piironen V., Landberg R., Åman P., and Poutanen K. (2007). Bran fermentation as a means to enhance technological properties and bioactivity of rye. *Food Microbiology,* 24(2), 175–186.

Kim, B.K., Cho, A.R., Chun, Y.G., and Park, D.J. (2013). Effect of microparticulated wheat bran on the physical properties of bread. *International Journal of Food Sciences and Nutrition,* 64, 122–129.

Knuckles, B.E., Chiu, M.M., and Betschart, A.A. (1992). Beta-glucan-enriched fractions from laboratory-scale dry milling and sieving of barley and oats. *Cereal Chemistry,* 69, 198–202.

Ko, S.N., Ha, T.Y., Hong, S.I., Yoon, S.W., Lee, J., Kim, Y., and Kim, I.H. (2012). Enrichment of tocols from rice germ oil using supercritical carbon dioxide. *International Journal of Food Science and Technology,* 47, 761–767.

Konopka, I., Czaplicki, S., and Rotkiewicz, D. (2006). Differences in content and composition of free lipids and carotenoids in flour of spring and winter wheat cultivated in Poland. *Food Chemistry,* 95, 290-300.

Krings, U., El-Saharty, Y.S., El-Zeany, B.A., Pabel, B., and Berger, R.G. (2000). Antioxidant activity of extracts from roasted wheat germ. *Food Chemistry,* 71, 91–95.

Kumar, V., Sinha, A.K., Makkar, H.P.S., and Becker, K. (2010). Dietary roles of phytate and phytase in human nutrition: A review. *Food Chemistry,* 120, 945–959.

Laca, A., Mousia, Z., Diaz, M., Webb, C., and Pandiella, S.S. (2006). Distribution of microbial contamination within cereal grains. *Journal of Food Engineering,* 72, 332–338.

Lampi, A.M., Moreau, R.A., Piironen, V., and Hicks, K.B. (2004). Pearling barley and rye to produce phytosterol-rich fractions. *Lipids,* 39, 783–787.

Landberg, R., Marklund, M., Kamal-Eldin, A., and Aman, P. (2014). An update on alkylresorcinols – Occurrence, bioavailability, bioactivity and utility as biomarkers. *Journal of Functional Foods,* 7, 77–89.

Latunde-Dada, G.O., Li, X., Parodi, A., Edwards, C.H., Ellis, P.R., and Sharp, P.A. (2014). Micromilling enhances iron bioaccessibility from wholegrain wheat. *Journal of Agricultural and Food Chemistry,* 62, 11222–11227.

Lempereur, I., Rouau, X., and Abecassis, J. (1997). Genetic and agronomic variation in arabinoxylan and ferulic acid content of durum wheat (*Triticum durum* L.) grains and its milling fractions. *Journal of Cereal Science,* 25, 103–110.

Letang, C., Samson, M.F., Lasserre, T.M., Chaurand, M., and Abecassis, J. (2002). Production of starch with very low protein content from soft and hard wheat flours by jet milling and air classification. *Cereal Chemistry,* 79, 535–543.

Li, L., Shewry, P.R., and Ward, J.L. (2008). Phenolic acids in wheat varieties in the HEALTHGRAIN diversity screen. *Journal of Agricultural and Food Chemistry,* 56, 9732–9739.

Liyana-Pathirana, C.M., and Shahidi, F. (2006). Importance of insoluble-bound phenolics to antioxidant properties of wheat. *Journal of Agricultural and Food Chemistry,* 54, 1256–1264.

Lorenz, K. (2000). Rye. In *Handbook of Cereal Science and Technology, Second Edition, Revised and Expanded.* (eds. K. Kulp and J.G. Ponte), pp. 223–256. Dekker.

Lorenz, K., and Al-Husaini, S.S. (1980). Mechanical debranning of whole kernel triticale. I. Proximate compositions and properties of fractions. *Lebensmittel-Wissenschaft und -Technologie* 13, 25–29.

Lu, R., and Siebenmorgen, T. (1995). Correlation of head rice yield to selected physical and mechanical properties of rice kernels. *Transactions of the ASAE,* 38, 889–894.

Mattern, P.J., Johnson, V.A., and Schmidt, J.W. (1970). Air-classification and baking characteristics of high-protein Atlas 66 * Comanche lines of hard red winter wheat. *Cereal Chemistry,* 47, 309–316.

Mehra, S.K., and Eckhoff, S.R. (1997). Single-stage short-duration tempering of corn for dry-milling. *Cereal Chemistry,* 74, 484–488.

Miller, S.S., and Fulcher, R.G. (2011). Microstructure and chemistry of the oat kernel. In *Oats. Chemistry and echnology. Second edition* (eds. F.H. Webster and P.J. Wood), pp. 77–94. AACC.

Min, B., Gu, L.W., McClung, A.M., Bergman, C.J., and Chen, M.H. (2012). Free and bound total phenolic concentrations, antioxidant capacities, and profiles of proanthocyanidins and anthocyanins in whole grain rice (Oryza sativa L.) of different bran colours. *Food Chemistry,* 133, 715–722.

Moreau, R.A., and Hicks, K.B. (2013). Removal and isolation of germ-rich fractions from hull-less barley using a Fitzpatrick comminuting mill and sieves. *Cereal Chemistry,* 90, 546–551.

Morrison, W.R., Coventry, A.M., and Barnes, P.J. (1982). The distribution of acyl lipids and tocopherols in flour millstreams. *Journal of the Science of Food and Agriculture,* 33, 925–933.

Naz, S., Siddiqi, R., Sheikh, H., and Sayeed, S.A. (2005). Deterioration of olive, corn and soybean oils due to air, light, heat and deep-frying. *Food Research International,* 38, 127–134.

Ndolo, V.U., and Beta, T. (2013). Distribution of carotenoids in endosperm, germ, and aleurone fractions of cereal grain kernels. *Food Chemistry,* 139, 663–671.

Noort, M.W.J., Haaster, D.V., Hemery, Y., Schols, H.A., and Hamer, R.J. (2010). The effect of particle size of wheat bran fractions on bread quality – evidence for fibre-protein interactions. *Journal of Cereal Science,* 52, 59–64.

Nurmi, T., Lampi, A.M., Nystrom, L., Hemery, Y., Rouau, X., and Piironen, V. (2012). Distribution and composition of phytosterols and steryl ferulates in wheat grain and bran fractions. *Journal of Cereal Science,* 56, 379–388.

Nystrom, L., Lampi, A.M., Rita, H., Aura, A.M., Oksman-Caldentey, K.M., and Piironen, V. (2007a). Effects of processing on availability of total plant sterols, steryl ferulates and steryl glycosides from wheat and rye bran. *Journal of Agricultural and Food Chemistry,* 55, 9059–9065.

Nystrom, L., Paasonen, A., Lampi, A.M., and Piironen, V. (2007b). Total plant sterols, steryl ferulates and steryl glycosides in milling fractions of wheat and rye. *Journal of Cereal Science,* 45, 106-115.

Ozcan, M.M., Rosa, A., Dessi, M.A., Marongiu, B., Piras, A., and Al-Juhaimi, F.Y.I. (2013). Quality of wheat germ oil obtained by cold pressing and supercritical carbon dioxide extraction. *Czech Journal of Food Sciences,* 31, 236–240.

Paiva, F.F., Vanier, N.L., Berrios, J.D.J., Pan, J., Villanova, F.D.A., Takeoka, G., and Elias, M.C. (2014). Physicochemical and nutritional properties of pigmented rice subjected to different degrees of milling. *Journal of Food Composition and Analysis,* 35, 10–17.

Panfili, G., Fratianni, A., and Irano, M. (2004). Improved normal-phase high-performance liquid chromatography procedure for the determination of carotenoids in cereals. *Journal of Agricultural and Food Chemistry,* 52, 6373–6377.

Paraman, I., Fox, S.R., Aspelund, M.T., Glatz, C.E., and Johnson, L.A. (2010). Recovering corn germ enriched in recombinant protein by wet-fractionation. *Bioresource Technology,* 101, 239–244.

Parker, M.L., Ng, A., and Waldron, K.W. (2005). The phenolic acid and polysaccharide composition of cell walls of bran layers of mature wheat (Triticum aestivum L. cv. Avalon) grains. *Journal of the Science of Food and Agriculture,* 85, 2539–2547.

Pekkinen, J., Rosa, N.N., Savolainen, O.I., Keski-Rahkonen, P., Mykkanen, H., Poutanen, K., Micard, V., and Hanhineva, K. (2014). Disintegration of wheat aleurone structure has an impact on the bioavailability of phenolic compounds and other phytochemicals as evidenced by altered urinary metabolite profile of diet-induced obese mice. *Nutrition & Metabolism,* 11.

Peterson, D.M., Emmons, C.L., and Hibbs, A.H. (2001). Phenolic antioxidants and antioxidant activity in pearling fractions of oat groats. *Journal of Cereal Science,* 33, 97–103.

Peyron, S., Surget, A., Mabille, F., Autran, J.C., Rouau, X., and Abecassis, J. (2002). Evaluation of tissue dissociation of durum wheat grain (Triticum durum desf.) generated by the milling process. *Journal of Cereal Science,* 36, 199–208.

Piras, A., Rosa, A., Falconieri, D., Porcedda, S., Dessi, M.A., and Marongiu, B. (2009). Extraction of oil from wheat germ by supercritical CO2. *Molecules,* 14, 2573–2581.

Pomeranz, Y. (1988). Chemical composition of kernel structures. In *Wheat: Chemistry and Technoloy* (ed. Y. Pomeranz), pp. 97–158. AACC.

Pomeranz, Y., and Shellenberger, J.A. (1961). Histochemical characterization of wheat and wheat products. II. Mapping of protein distribution in the wheat kernel. *Cereal Chemistry,* 38, 109–113.

Posner, E.S. (2000). Wheat. In *Handbook of Cereal Science and Technology, Second Edition, Revised and Expanded* (eds. K. Kulp and J.G. Ponte), pp. 1–30. Dekker.

Posner, E.S., and Li, Y.Z. (1991). A technique for separation of wheat germ by impacting and subsequent grinding. *Journal of Cereal Science,* 13, 49–70.

Poutanen, K. (2012). Past and future of cereal grains as food for health. *Trends in Food Science & Technology,* 25, 58–62.

Price, R.K., Wallace, J.M.W., Hamill, L.L., Keaveney, E.M., Strain, J.J., Parker, M.J., and Welch, R.W. (2012). Evaluation of the effect of wheat aleurone-rich foods on markers of antioxidant status, inflammation and endothelial function in apparently healthy men and women. *British Journal of Nutrition,* 108, 1644–1651.

Protonotariou, S., Drakos, A., Evageliou, V., Ritzoulis, C., and Mandala, I. (2014). Sieving fractionation and jet mill micronization affect the functional properties of wheat flour. *Journal of Food Engineering,* 134, 24–29.

Pruckler, M., Siebenhandl-Ehn, S., Apprich, S., Holtinger, S., Haas, C., Schmid, E., and Kneifel, W. (2014). Wheat bran-based biorefinery 1: Composition of wheat bran and strategies of functionalization. *LWT – Food Science and Technology,* 56, 211–221.

Pussayanawin, V., Wetzel, D.L., and Fulcher, R.G. (1988). Fluorescence detection and measurement of ferulic acid in wheat milling fractions by microscopy and HPLC. *Journal of Agricultural and Food Chemistry,* 36, 515–520.

Rhodes, D.I., Sadek, M., and Stone, B.A. (2002). Hydroxycinnamic acids in walls of wheat aleurone cells. *Journal of Cereal Science,* 36, 67–81.

Rhodes, D.I., and Stone, B.A. (2002). Proteins in walls of wheat aleurone cells. *Journal of Cereal Science,* 36, 83–101.

Rios, G., Pinson-Gadais, L., Abecassis, J., Zakhia-Rozis, N., and Lullien-Pellerin, V. (2009). Assessment of dehulling efficiency to reduce deoxynivalenol and Fusarium level in durum wheat grains. *Journal of Cereal Science,* 49, 387–392.

Rosa-Sibakov, N., Poutanen, K., and Micard, V. (2015). How does wheat grain, bran and aleurone structure impact their nutritional and technological properties? *Trends in Food Science & Technology,* 41, 118–134.

Rosa, N.N., Barron, C., Gaiani, C., Dufour, C., and Micard, V. (2013a). Ultra-fine grinding increases the antioxidant capacity of wheat bran. *Journal of Cereal Science,* 57.

Rosa, N.N., Dufour, C., Lullien-Pellerin, V., and Micard, V. (2013b). Exposure or release of ferulic acid from wheat aleurone: Impact on its antioxidant capacity. *Food Chemistry,* 141, 2355–2362.

Rosa, N.N., Pekkinen, J., Zavala, K., Fouret, G., Korkmaz, A., Feillet-Coudray, C., Atalay, M., Hanhineva, K., Mykkanen, H., Poutanen, K., and Micard, V. (2014). Impact of wheat aleurone structure on metabolic disorders caused by a high-fat diet in mice. *Journal of Agricultural and Food Chemistry,* 62, 10101–10109.

Samson, M.F., Mabille, F., Cheret, R., Abecassis, J., and Morel, M.H. (2005). Mechanical and physicochemical characterization of vitreous and mealy durum wheat endosperm. *Cereal Chemistry,* 82, 81–87.

Saulnier, L., Sado, P.-E., Branlard, G., Charmet, G., and Guillon, F. (2007). Wheat arabinoxylans: Exploiting variation in amount and composition to develop enhanced varieties. *Journal of Cereal Science,* 46, 261–281.

Shao, Y., Xu, F., Sun, X., Bao, J., and Beta, T. (2014). Identification and quantification of phenolic acids and anthocyanins as antioxidants in bran, embryo and endosperm of white, red and black rice kernels (Oryza sativa L.). *Journal of Cereal Science,* 59, 211–218.

Shepherd, C.T., Vignaux, N., Peterson, J.M., Scott, M.P., and Johnson, L.A. (2008). Dry-milling and fractionation of transgenic maize seed tissues with green fluorescent protein as a tissue marker. *Cereal Chemistry,* 85, 196–201.

Shewry, P.R. (2009). *Wheat. Journal of Experimental Botany*, 60, 1537–1553.

Shewry, P.R., and Halford, N.G. (2002). Cereal seed storage proteins: Structures, properties and role in grain utilization. *Journal of Experimental Botany,* 53, 947–958.

Shewry, P.R., Piironen, V., Lampi, A.M., Edelmann, M., Kariluoto, S., Nurmi, T., Fernandez-Orozco, R., Ravel, C., Charmet, G., Andersson, A.A.M., Aman, P., Boros, D., Gebruers, K., Dornez, E., Courtin, C.M., Delcour, J.A., Rakszegi, M., Bedo, Z., and Ward, J.L. (2010). The HEALTHGRAIN wheat diversity screen: effects of genotype and environment on phytochemicals and dietary fiber components. *Journal of Agricultural and Food Chemistry,* 58, 9291–9298.

Sibakov, J., Abecassis, J., Barron, C., and Poutanen, K. (2014). Electrostatic separation combined with ultra-fine grinding to produce β-glucan enriched ingredients from oat bran. *Innovative Food Science and Emerging Technologies.*

Sibakov, J., Myllymäki, O., Holopainen, U., Kaukovirta-Norja, A., Hietaniemi, V., Pihlava, J.M., Poutanen, K., and Lehtinen, P. (2011). Lipid removal enhances separation of oat grain cell wall material from starch and protein. *Journal of Cereal Science,* 54, 104–109.

Singh, V., and Eckhoff, S.R. (1996). Effect of soak time, soak temperature, and lactic acid ore germ recovery parameters. *Cereal Chemistry,* 73, 716–720.

Singh, V., Moreau, R.A., Hicks, K.B., and Eckhoff, S.R. (2001). Effect of alternative milling techniques on the yield and composition of corn germ oil and corn fiber oil. *Cereal Chemistry,* 78, 46–49.

Sjovall, O., Virtalaine, T., Lapvetelainen, A., and Kallio, H. (2000). Development of rancidity in wheat germ analyzed by headspace gas chromatography and sensory analysis. *Journal of Agricultural and Food Chemistry,* 48, 3522–3527.

Srivastava, A.K., Sudha, M.L., Baskaran, V., and Leelavathi, K. (2007). Studies on heat stabilized wheat germ and its influence on rheological characteristics of dough. *European Food Research and Technology,* 224, 365–372.

Stevenson, D.G., Eller, F.J., Jane, J.L., and Inglett, G.E. (2008). Structure and physicochemical properties of defatted and pin-milled oat bran concentrate fractions separated by air-classification. *International Journal of Food Science and Technology,* 43, 995–1003.

Stone, B.A. (1985). Aleurone cell walls – Structure and nutritional significances. In *New approaches to research on cereal carbohydrates* (eds. R.D. Hill and L. Munck), pp. 349–354. Elsevier Science Publishers.

Stone, B.A., and Minifie, J. (1988). Recovery of aleurone cells from wheat bran. University, L. T. *US patent 4,746,073* US patent 4,746,073.

Stringfellow, A.C., Wall, J.S., Donaldson, G.L., and Anderson, R.A. (1976). Protein and amino-acid compositions of dry-milled and air-classified fractions of triticale grain. *Cereal Chemistry,* 53, 51–60.

Sullivan, P., O'Flaherty, J., Brunton, N., Gee, V.L., Arendt, E., and Gallagher, E. (2010). Chemical composition and microstructure of milled barley fractions. *European Food Research and Technology,* 230, 579–595.

Tabekhia, M.M., and Luh, B.S. (1979). Effect of milling on macro and micro minerals and phytate of rice. *Deutsche Lebensmittel-Rundschau,* 75, 57–62.

Tosi, P., Gritsch, C.S., He, J.B., and Shewry, P.R. (2011). Distribution of gluten proteins in bread wheat (Triticum aestivum) grain. *Annals of Botany,* 108, 23–35.

van Buul, V.J., and Brouns, F. (2014). Health effects of wheat lectins: A review. *Journal of Cereal Science,* 59, 112–117.

van der Kamp, J.W., Poutanen, K., Seal, C.J., and Richardson, D.P. (2014). The HEALTHGRAIN definition of 'whole grain'.

Vignaux, N., Fox, S.R., and Johnson, L.A. (2006). A 10-g laboratory wet-milling procedure for maize and comparison with larger scale laboratory procedures. *Cereal Chemistry,* 83, 482–490.

Viraktamath, C.S., Raghavendra, G., and Desikachar, H.S.R. (1971). Use of rice milling machinery for commercial pearling of grain sorghum (jowar) and culinary uses for pearled sorghum products. *Journal of Food Science and Technology (Mysore),* 8, 11–13.

Vose, J.R., and Youngs, C.G. (1978). Fractionation of barley and malted barley flours by air classification. *Cereal Chemistry,* 55, 280–286.

Wang, L., Xue, Q., Newman, R.K., and Newman, C.W. (1993). Enrichment of tocopherols, tocotrienols, and oil in barley fractions by milling and pearling. *Cereal Chemistry,* 70, 499–501.

Wang, M.W., Sapirstein, H.D., Machet, A.S., and Dexter, J.E. (2006). Composition and distribution of pentosans in millstreams of different hard spring wheats. *Cereal Chemistry,* 83, 161–168.

Wang, R., Koutinas, A.A., and Campbell, G.M. (2007). Effect of pearling on dry processing of oats. *Journal of Food Engineering,* 82, 369–376.

Wang, T., He, F.L., and Chen, G.B. (2014). Improving bioaccessibility and bioavailability of phenolic compounds in cereal grains through processing technologies: A concise review. *Journal of Functional Foods,* 7, 101–111.

Watson, S.A. (1987). Structure and composition. In: Corn : Chemistry and Technology (eds. S.A. Watson and P.E. Ramstad), pp. 53–82. AACC.

Wolever, T.M., Tosh, S.M., Gibbs, A.L., Brand-Miller, J., Duncan, A.M., Hart, V., Lamarche, B., Thomson, B.A., Duss, R., and Wood, P.J. (2010). Physicochemical properties of oat β-glucan influence its ability to reduce serum LDL cholesterol in humans: A randomized clinical trial. *The American Journal of Clinical Nutrition,* 92, 723–732.

Wu, Y.V., and Doehlert, D.C. (2002). Enrichment of β -glucan in Oat Bran by Fine Grinding and Air Classification. *LWT - Food Science and Technology,* 35, 30–33.

Wu, Y.V., and Stringfellow, A.C. (1973). Protein concentrates from oat flours by air classification of normal and high-protein varieties. *Cereal Chemistry,* 50, 489–496.

Wu, Y.V., and Stringfellow, A.C. (1992). Air classification of flours from wheats with varying hardness-proteins shifts. *Cereal Chemistry,* 69, 188–191.

Wu, Y.V., Stringfellow, A.C., and Inglett, G.E. (1994). Protein- and beta-glucan enriched fractions from high-protein, high beta-glucan barleys by sieving and air classification. *Cereal Chemistry,* 71, 220–223.

Xiong, F., Yu, X.R., Zhou, L., Wang, Z., Wang, F., and Xiong, A.S. (2013). Structural development of aleurone and its function in common wheat. *Molecular Biology Reports,* 40, 6785–6792.

Xu, B., Zhou, S.L., Miao, W.J., Gao, C., Cai, M.J. and Dong, Y. (2013). Study on the stabilization effect of continuous microwave on wheat germ. *Journal of Food Engineering,* 117, 1–7.

Yesil-Celiktas, O., Isleten, M., Karagul-Yuceer, Y., Bedir, E., and Vardar-Sukan, F. (2009). Influence of supercritical carbon dioxide and methanolic extracts of rosemary on oxidation and sensory properties of wheat germ oil. *Journal of Food Quality,* 32, 709–724.

Youngs, V.L. (1974). Extraction of a high-protein layer from oat groat bran and flour. *Journal of Food Science,* 39, 1045–1046.

Zacchi, P., Daghero, J., Jaeger, P., and Eggers, R. (2006). Extraction/fractionation and deacidification of wheat germ oil using supercritical carbon dioxide. *Brazilian Journal of Chemical Engineering,* 23, 105–110.

Zhang, C., Glatz, C.E., Fox, S.R., and Johnson, L.A. (2009). Fractionation of transgenic corn seed by dry and wet milling to recover recombinant collagen-related proteins. *Biotechnology Progress,* 25, 1396–1401.

Zhang, J.R., Martin, J.M., Beecher, B., Lu, C.F., Hannah, L.C., Wall, M.L., Altosaar, I., and Giroux, M.J. (2010). The ectopic expression of the wheat Puroindoline genes increase germ size and seed oil content in transgenic corn. *Plant Molecular Biology,* 74, 353–365.

Zhao, Z.H., and Moghadasian, M.H. (2008). Chemistry, natural sources, dietary intake and pharmacokinetic properties of ferulic acid: A review. *Food Chemistry,* 109, 69–702.

Zhu, K.X., Lian, C.X., Guo, X.N., Peng, W., and Zhou, H.M. (2011). Antioxidant activities and total phenolic contents of various extracts from defatted wheat germ. *Food Chemistry,* 126, 1122–1126.

Zhu, K.X., Zhou, H.M., and Qian, H.F. (2006). Comparative study of chemical composition and physicochemical properties of defatted wheat germ flour and its protein isolate. *Journal of Food Biochemistry,* 30, 329–341.

4 Whole grain Carbohydrates

Genyi Zhang[1] and Bruce R. Hamaker[2]

[1]State Key Laboratory of Food Science and Technology, School of Food Science and Technology, Jiangnan University, Wuxi, China
[2]Whistler Center for Carbohydrate Research, Department of Food Science, Purdue University, West Lafayette, Indiana, USA

4.1 Introduction

Whole grains or whole grain foods, based on the Whole Grains Council (2004), contain "all the essential parts and naturally-occurring nutrients of the entire grain seed in their original proportions" and its carbohydrates include endosperm starch and non-starch polysaccharides (dietary fibre), and minor amounts of inulin (Van Loo et al. 1995, in wheat, rye, barley) and simple sugars. Whole grains comprise cereals and pseudocereals, but not legumes or oilseeds. Starch, as a semi-crystalline entity, is presented in a granular form in the endosperm of different shapes and sizes. In cereals, there are pores leading to channels within the starch granules that facilitate more rapid enzyme digestion of raw starch than is the case in granules without channels such as in tubers. Molecularly, starch is composed of essentially linear amylose and highly branched amylopectin that are both homopolymers providing energy to the body in the form of glucose. The nutritional character of starch is represented by the rate and extent of its digestion in the small intestine and, based on an in vivo-supported in vitro digestion method (Englyst et al. 1992), it is described by its content of rapidly digestible starch (RDS), slowly digestible starch (SDS) and resistant starch (RS). The latter is considered as a type of dietary fibre with a prebiotic property (Bird et al. 2010). Whole grain dietary fibre is composed of a heterogeneous class of mostly polysaccharides with high complexity in their sugar unit and linkage compositions, molecular structures, and 3-dimensional conformations, which lead to different physiochemical properties as well as human body functions, including modulation of starch digestion and glucose absorption, and, through changes of the gut microbiota, impacting of the immune system and intestinal epithelial barrier function (Anderson et al. 2009). The physiological quality of available or glycemic carbohydrates is captured in a number of ways with the most common being glycemic index (GI) (Jenkins et al. 1981), which is based on postprandial glycemic response. Many low GI foods have a high amount of dietary fiber (Björck and Elmstathl 2003), suggesting that dietary fibres may lower glycemic response. The combination of glycemic and non-glycemic carbohydrates, as indispensable parts of whole grains, is related to the concept of whole grain foods having good "carbohydrate quality."

Whole Grains and Health, Second Edition. Edited by Rikard Landberg and Nathalie Scheers.

Additional materials available for download online at https://www.wiley.com/en-gb/Whole+Grains+and+Health-p-9781118939437

A good understanding of the mechanism and role carbohydrates play in the health benefits associated with whole grain foods is a necessary basis to develop strategies to optimize their impact in unprocessed and processed foods. This is of particular importance for the starch component, as whole grains that are further processed to commercial products often significantly increase glycemic response. Many whole grain foods, as approved in regulatory systems, are also composed of recombined flour streams. The outcome of these processes on the health-related property of final whole grain food products is not well understood and conceivably could be neutral, negative or positive in regards to glycemic response, as well as on the action of the dietary fiber component in the gastrointestinal tract, including its effect on the gut microbiota. The study of Mozaffarian et al. (Mozaffarian et al. 2013) on whole grain products showed that a ratio of total carbohydrate (i.e., mainly glycemic carbohydrate) to dietary fibre of ≤ 10:1 was characteristic of healthy whole grain food products. In addition to the composition of dietary carbohydrates, the spatial arrangement of starch and dietary fibre in the food matrix is also important to the digestion property of starch and probably to the health benefit of whole grain foods (Heaton et al. 1988; Björck et al. 1994).

4.2 General composition of whole grain carbohydrates

There are different ways to classify whole grain carbohydrates (Table 4.1) focusing on different aspects, including chemical structure and complexity as well as nutritional bioavailability (rate, extent and location of digestion/fermentation). While simple monosaccharides can be directly absorbed, they are in very low amount in whole grain foods. The main carbohydrates are starch and non-starch polysaccharides with highly complex structures (Table 4.2). Their contribution to carbohydrate quality in whole grain foods is the focus of this chapter.

4.3 Dietary fibre

Historically, *dietary fibre* was a term first used by Hipsley (1953) to describe nondigestible food constituents referring to plant cell wall materials, including cellulose, hemicelluloses and lignin. With the advancement of scientific investigation, as well as new methodologies for dietary fibre measurement, dietary fibre is essentially now considered another food

Table 4.1 Classification of whole grain carbohydrates.

Carbohydrate	2nd Level Classification		Examples	Digestibility
Simple Carbohydrate	Monosaccharide		Glucose, fructose, galactose	Direct Absorption
	Disaccharide		Sucrose	Rapid
Complex Carbohydrate	Starch (glycemic carbohydrate)	RDS	Cooked waxy starch	Rapid
		SDS	Raw corn starch	Slow
		RS	Retrograded amylose	Fermented
	Non-starch polysaccharides (dietary fibre)	Soluble	β-glucan, arabinoxylan, pectin	Partially fermented
		Insoluble	Cellulose, hemicelluloses	
Oligosaccharide			Fructans	Fermented

Table 4.2 The composition of whole grain carbohydrates (% dry weight) (Choct 1997; Collins et al. 2010).

Cereal	Starch	Arabinoxylan	β-Glucan	Cellulose	Glucomannan	Galactan	
Wheat	68	8.1	0.8	2.0	–*	0.3	Barley
60	7.9	4.3	3.9	0.2	0.2	Rye	69
8.9	2.0	1.5	0.3	0.3	Triticale	53	10.8
1.7	2.5	0.6	0.5	Sorghum	77	2.1	0.2
2.2	0.1	0.15	Corn	78	5.2	–	2.0
0.2	0.6	Oats	50	3.1	4.3	2.3	–
–	Brown rice	66	2.6	0.13	2.6	–	–
Pearl millet	63	2.5	–	1.5	–	–	

macronutrient. Organizations and regulatory agencies have their own definitions, such as the American Association of Cereal Chemists (AACC 2001), CODEX Alimentarius Commission (CODEX 2009), European Food Safety Authority (EFSA 2010), US Food and Drug Administration (FDA 2016) and the Institute of Medicine (IOM 2001). Among these definitions, CODEX Alimentarius is broadly accepted and represents a relatively comprehensive and flexible definition reflecting the current knowledge of dietary fibre. *Dietary fibre* as defined by CODEX Alimentarius is as follows:

"Dietary fibre means carbohydrate polymers with ten or more monomeric units,* which are not hydrolysed by the endogenous enzymes in the small intestine of humans and belong to the following categories:

1. Edible carbohydrate polymers naturally occurring in the food as consumed,
2. Carbohydrate polymers, which have been obtained from food raw material by physical, enzymatic or chemical means and which have been shown to have a physiological effect of benefit to health as demonstrated by generally accepted scientific evidence to competent authorities,
3. Synthetic carbohydrate polymers which have been shown to have a physiological effect of benefit to health as demonstrated by generally accepted scientific evidence to competent authorities.

*Decision on whether to include carbohydrates from three to nine monomeric units should be left to national authorities.

By this definition, dietary fibres that have been isolated or synthesized and used as ingredients must also be shown to have a physiological benefit, but importantly whole grain fibres do not have this requirement. This fibre requirement of physiological benefit is also incorporated into the new FDA *dietary fibre* definition of 2016 (US FDA 2016). Cellulose, hemicellulose, lignin, gums, modified celluloses, mucilages, oligosaccharides, pectins and associated minor substances such as waxes, cutin, and suberin all fall within the scope of dietary fibre. By the late 1990s, the methodologies for dietary fibre analysis had been refined by AOAC and AACC (DeVries et al. 1999). However, novel digestion-resistant materials developed by the food industry were not always within their scope, and a new method, (AOAC Official Method 2009.01, 2009), was developed to capture analytically all fibre materials meeting the definitions. Based on Footnote 2 found in the AOAC method, resistant oligosaccharides, resistant starch and resistant maltodextrin all satisfy the definition of *dietary fibre* (Jones 2014).

Dietary fibre is, in a general way, often separated into water-soluble and water-insoluble types. Some water-soluble dietary fibres, such a β-glucans and pectins, have a high viscosity property that can slow the transit of food in the gastrointestinal tract, reduce the postprandial glucose spike, and aid in the excretion of bile acids and cholesterol. They are also readily fermented in the colon and produce short chain fatty acids (acetate, propionate and butyrate) that have certain health benefits and modulate the microbiota. Some water-insoluble dietary fibres have water retention capacity to promote bowel movement and generally have a lesser degree of fermentation. In whole grain foods, β-glucans and some arabinoxylans are the main water-soluble dietary fibres in cereals (Carpita and Gibeaut 1993) and xyloglucans and pectins in pseudocereals like amaranth and quinoa (Lamothe et al. 2015), while the major water-insoluble dietary fibres are cellulose, the insoluble cross-linked arabinoxylans, and lignin (Table 4.2). Depending on the botanical source of the dietary fibre as well as individual genotypes and growth conditions, there may be variability in degree of heterogeneity in structure within the same type of fibre polysaccharide type. Such a wide range of fibre structures in whole grains could differentially influence the gut microbiome and resulting metabolic and physiological responses (Hamaker and Tuncil 2014). Additionally, as illustrated from the molecular architecture of the plant cell wall (Figure 4.1), dietary fibre polysaccharides in whole grain usually exist in a cell wall form consisting of a fibrillar phase of cellulose microfibrils in a matrix composed of non-cellulosic polysaccharides with a variety of different structures along with structural proteins, glycoproteins

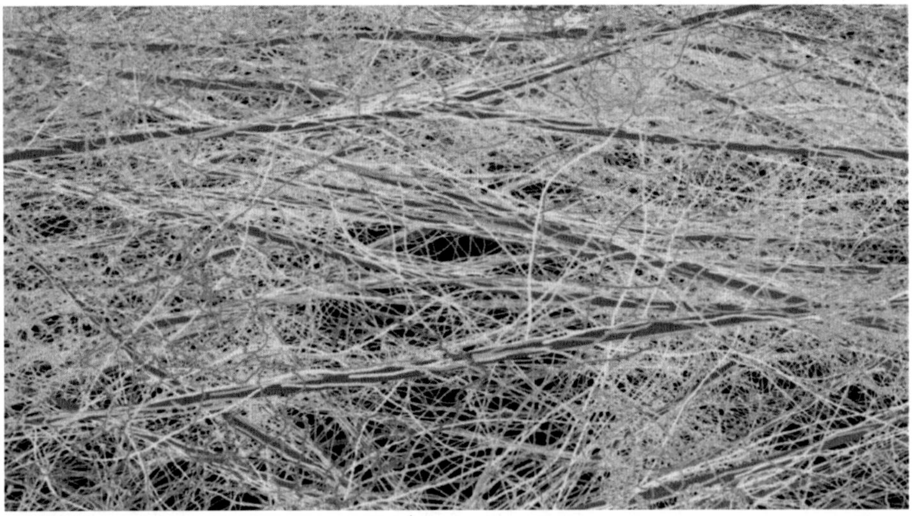

Figure 4.1 Depiction of plant cell wall structure consisting of cellulose microfibrils (blue), non-cellulosic polysaccharides, termed hemicelluloses (green), and pectins (yellow/brown). Source: Johnson et al. 2018. (*See color representation of this figure in the color plate section*).

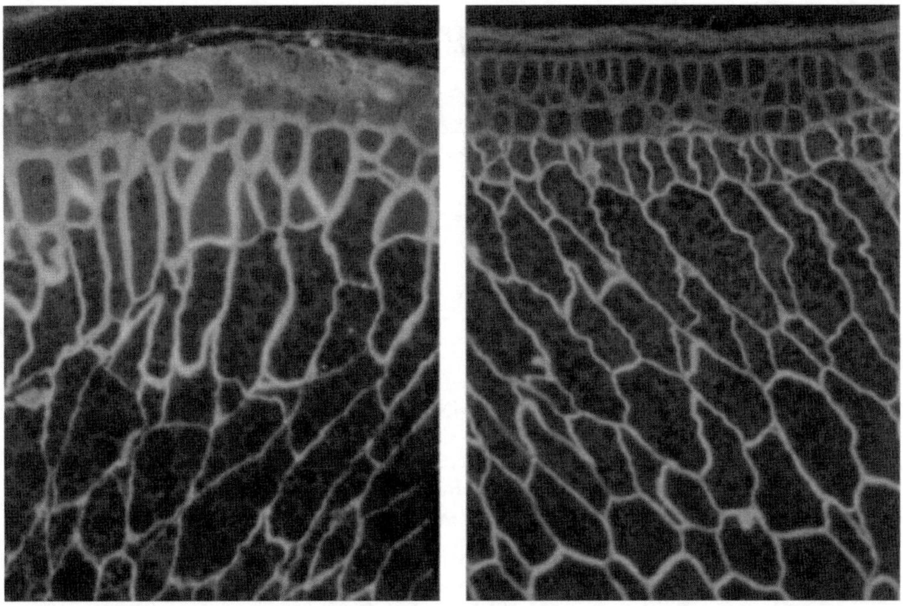

Figure 4.2 The endosperm cell wall in oats and barley as it contains starch (dark spheres) and other constituents. Source: Tosh 2013.

and phenolic components. At a more macro-level, whole grain cell wall structures may contain starch (Figure 4.2), and make it more difficult to access, and thus slowing its digestion or making it resistant. The principal whole grain non-starch polysaccharides and their molecular structures (shown in Figure 4.3) are briefly discussed in the following, along with their potential association with starch in the context of the whole grain food matrix as related to carbohydrate quality in whole grain foods.

4.3.1 Arabinoxylan

Arabinoxylans belong to the hemicellulose component of the cell wall of cereals, and are also termed pentosans as they are composed of the 5-carbon monosaccharides of arabinose and xylose. In cereal grains, they are in highest concentration in the bran layer, though are also found in the endosperm cell walls. Structurally, the simplest arabinoxylan consists of a backbone of D-xylanopyranosyl units linked through β-(1→4) bonds with branches to single L-arabinofuranose by α-(1→2) and/or α-(1→3) linkages (Izydorczyk and Biliaderis 1995; Ebringerová and Heinze 2000) (Figure 4.4). Thus, the structural property of arabinoxylan is often expressed by the ratio of arabinose and xylose (Ara/Xyl). Although most of side branches are single arabinose, there are side chains consisting of arabinose residues and other sugar units such as xylose and galactose and glucuronic acid. Depending on the botanical source of the arabinoxylan, the branch pattern may be of low or high complexity depending on the substituent position and density and composition of the side chains (Rumpagaporn et al. 2015). Additional to the sugar units, there are also phenolic compounds, mainly ferulic acid linked to arabinoxylans. In whole grain foods, arabinoxylans, in most cases, are

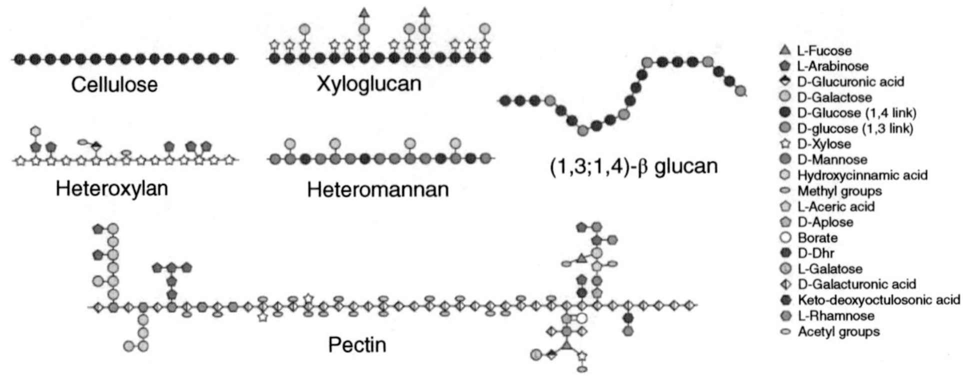

Figure 4.3 The molecular structure of the major non-starch polysaccharides found in plant cell walls. Heteroxylan (arabinoxylan), (1,3/1,4)-β-glucan and cellulose are the major non-starch polysaccharides in whole grain cereals; and pectin, xyloglucan, and cellulose are the major non-starch polysaccharides in whole grain pseudocereals (amaranth, quinoa). Source: Burton et al. 2010. © 2010 Springer Nature. (*See color representation of this figure in the color plate section*).

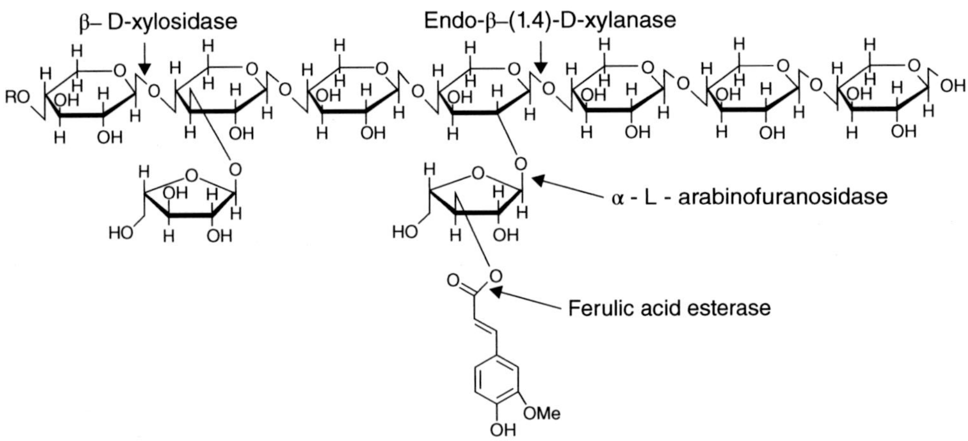

Figure 4.4 The general structure of arabinoxylan composed of side chains of L-arabinose, glucuronic acid, galactose and xylose, and a backbone of xylose. Sources: Based on Ebringerová and Heinze 2000; Mendis and Simsek 2014.

cross-linked with themselves and other polysaccharides in a cell wall form, which further increases its complexity lowering gut microbiota fermentability (Rose et al. 2010).

4.3.2 β-glucans

The β-glucans are composed of D-glucopyranose units with β-1→4 and 1→3 linkages types. The number of adjacent glucose units with the same linkage determines the complexity of β-glucans with its various molecular weights, solubilities, viscosities and three-dimensional configurations. For the water-soluble β-glucans such as the (1,3/1,4) β-glucan that is rich in oats and barley, the (1,4)-β-linkages are present mainly in groups of two or

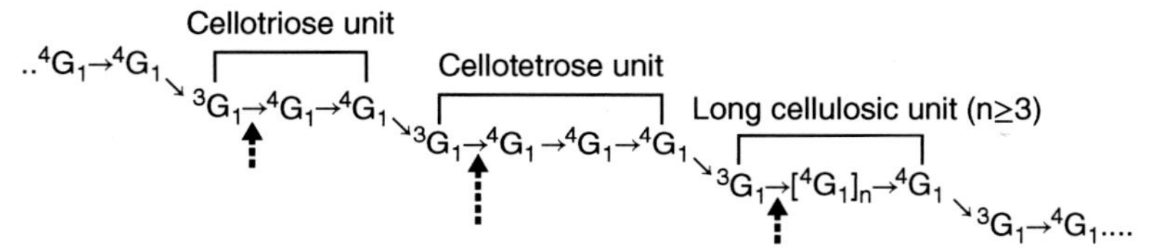

Figure 4.5 The general structure of cereal mixed linkage (1→3) (1→4)-β-D-glucan (Source: Lazaridou and Biliaderis 2007)

three adjacent linkages (Figure 4.5). The ratio of randomly arranged cellotriosyl (DP3) and cellotetraosyl residues (DP4) is used to represent the structural property of (1,3/1,4) β-glucan, and β-glucans with a ratio of 1.5-2.5 tends to form a gel-like matrix, while lower and higher ratios tend to form aggregates (Burton et al. 2010). The ratio of DP3/DP4 from oats is in the range of 1.5–2.3, while a ratio of 1.8–3.5 was found for barley-sourced β-glucan, while the ratio is even higher in wheat (3.0–4.5) (Lazaridou and Biliaderis 2007). There are also long cellulosic oligomers (DP>4), such as in barley. The structural diversity of β-glucans determines differences in physiochemical properties and related health benefits.

4.3.3 Other Cereal Dietary Fibres

While arabinoxylan and β-glucan are the major non-starch polysaccharides in whole cereal grains, pectin and xyloglucan are mainly present in whole grain pseudocereals (amaranth, quinoa) (Lamothe et al. 2015). A low amount of xyloglucan was found in rice (Choct 1997). Also, glucomannans comprised of β-(1→4)-linked glucose and mannose is in cereal grains and galactomannan in low amounts is found in amaranth and quinoa (Gartaula et al. 2018; Lamothe et al. 2015). Arabinogalactan, a polymer of β-(1→4) galactan (comprised of (1→4)-β-D-galactose) substituted with arabinose side chains was found in wheat flour. Although RS does not belong to the non-starch polysaccharides, it is regarded as dietary fibre (Phillips and Cui 2011). Depending on the origin of RS, different types are recognized. RS1is physically inaccessible starch; RS2 refers to raw starch granule types that are resistant to digestion such as potato and banana; RS3 is retrograded starch, namely, of amylose after cooking to gelatinization; and RS4 is a chemically-modified resistant starch. Although they are all termed resistant starch, processing can affect their resistance to digestion as RS1, RS2 and RS3 can disappear during some types of thermal and shear-induced processing, while RS4 is generally not sensitive to such treatments.

Cellulose is a linear polymer of β-(1→4)-linked D-glucopyranosyl residues with a dimer of anhydrocellobiose as the repeating unit (Brown et al. 1996). The strongly associated cellulose molecules into crystalline structures are one component of water-insoluble dietary fibre in whole grains. The cellulose content of cereal grain cell walls varies among cereal species and location in the grain. In endosperm cell walls of wheat and barley, cellulose accounts for only a few percent of the total cell wall material, while in the outer, lignified layers it may comprise up to 20% of the cell wall weight (Fincher and Stone 1986). Lignin is a polymer of phenyl-propanoides deposited in secondary thickened cells walls (Vanholme et al. 2010). As it is an intrinsic component of cell wall, it is considered as another component of dietary fibre.

4.3.4 Starch

Granular starch is the most abundant material in whole grains with variation of size shape, and surface properties depending on its source and processing treatment (Krok et al. 2000). Starch granules have different levels of structural features and the granule is a semi-crystalline material. Whole grain cereal and pseudocereal (quinoa and amaranth) starches are of the A-type showing peaks at 2θ of 9.9, 11.2, 15, 17, 18.1 and 23.3°, which differentiates them from B-type tuber starches showing peaks at 5.6, 15, 17, 22 and 24°. A- and B-type starches reflect the difference in the geometry of their unit cells, the packing density of double helices and the amount of bound water within the crystal structure (Buléon et al. 1998; Qian and Kuhn 1999). When starch is gelatinized and dispersed, the linear amylose (essentially α-(1→4) linked) and highly branched amylopectin [containing both α-(1→4) and α-(1→6) linkages] can be separated by their structural difference and size. The percentage of α-(1→6) linkage is one aspect of the fine structure of amylopectin, for example, 4.6% for normal maize starch and 5.7% for waxy maize starch (Shin et al. 2008).

4.4 Carbohydrate quality of whole grain foods

The term *carbohydrate quality* refers to the health-associated aspects of carbohydrates in foods and generally is more specifically related to the quality of glycemic carbohydrates in foods. It is not usually used in reference to the dietary fibre component. For whole grain foods, the glucose-generating starch is the glycemic carbohydrate. While the entire whole grain package is generally considered important to the beneficial health outcome of whole grains (Fardet et al. 2008), the nutritional property of its starch is an essential though understudied component.

4.5 Slow digestion property of starch

Much about the notion of carbohydrate quality of whole grains is centered on the idea that whole grain foods have a low GI compared to refined grain foods. In this case, low GI is equated with a slow digestion property of starch that moderates and extends glycemic response. Low GI foods (GI<55) are considered to be beneficial to health by preventing or therapeutically addressing obesity and associated metabolic diseases (Ludwig 2002; Livesey 2005; Fabricatore et al. 2011). High GI foods (GI >75), which have been associated with consumption of refined grain products (Ludwig et al. 1999). Thus, whole grain foods with starch of the same chemical structure can generate different nutritional outcomes based on their digestion profile or carbohydrate quality property. A positive correlation between GI and RDS-derived glucose (Englyst et al. 1999) and a negative correlation between RDS and SDS (Zhang et al. 2008) indicate that SDS is the structural basis for cereal-based low GI foods. It should be noted that whether there remains a controversy regarding the relationship between GI and health, though a recent international consensus report supports that low GI or glycemic load foods in diets reduce certain chronic metabolic diseases such as diabetes and heart disease (Augustin et al. 2015).

Although *SDS* is defined by an in vitro starch digestion method (Englyst et al. 1992), studies on raw corn starch, which is a naturally pure source of SDS, showed it to produce a prolonged and sustained low postprandial glycemic and insulinemic responses similar to those of low GI foods (Seal et al. 2003; Wachters-Hagedoorn et al. 2006). Indeed, the health benefits of SDS are also assumed to be similar to low GI foods (Lehmann and Robin 2007). Literature reports have shown metabolic and physiological effects of SDS consumption. SDS epigenetically caused a shift of the gene expression peak of SGLT1 from the upper jejunum to ileum (Shimada et al. 2009), leading to an increased glucose transporters in the ileum (Woodward et al. 2012), and consumption of SDS in the form of raw normal corn starch resulted in sustained release of incretin hormone of GLP-1 (Wachters-Hagedoorn et al. 2006), which is important for body weight regulation and insulin sensitivity (Larsen 2008). Our recent animal study (Hasek et al. 2018) using a slowly digestible starch-entrapped microsphere that digests starch into the ileum showed reduced food intake behavior and decreased expression of hypothalamic orexigenic neuropeptides NPY and AgRP, which are appetite stimulators. Thus, SDS not only generates a modulated postprandial glycemic response, but also influences a variety of processes that may be important to human health.

The making of efficacious healthy SDS materials requires an understanding of the in vivo process of starch digestion related glycemic response, and also to physiological response. Our group has pursued a path of research relating location of digestion and glucose release in the ileal region of the small intestine to activation of the gut-brain axis and ileal brake (Hasek et al. 2018; Lee et al. 2013; Romijn et al. 2008). Yet, not all SDS materials necessarily digest into the ileum, and this is also true with digestion of starch in whole grain foods. For instance, using a pig model, normal corn starch, which is a standard SDS material, was nearly all digested in the duodenum and upper jejunum with little measurable amount of starch getting to the ileum (Hasjim et al. 2010). More research needs to be done on the factors that moderate starch digestion in whole grain foods and, in particular, the role of whole grain matrices in digestion.

4.6 Physical form of whole grain foods

Food structure is a key factor affecting starch digestion, and any disruption of the physical or botanical structure of cereal grains can increase the rate of digestion and postprandial glycemic response (Björck et al. 1994). Coarse particles of whole grains were found to reduce the rate of starch digestion more than fine whole grain flour (Liljeberg et al. 1992). Particle size of grains from wheat, corn and oat were likewise found to influence in vitro starch digestion rate, with larger particles being slower digesting (Heaton et al. 1988). Thus, the physical structure in whole grain foods is an important factor contributing to the starch digestion property and is likely related physiological effect. The botanical structure of grain kernels provides a nature-produced physical barrier to protect the nutritive contents from environment influences. Starch, as the energy provider for seed germination, is mainly located in the endosperm cellular compartment that is embedded in a matrix formed by proteins and cell wall material (Kamal-Eldin et al. 2009). Depending on the type of endosperm, a dense packing of starch granules in the protein matrix of the vitreous endosperm significantly decreases the rate of starch digestion (Lopes et al. 2009). The influence of the protein matrix, even after cooking, still affects starch digestibility with the report of SDS content of 20% in a cooked flour compared to 0–2% in cooked isolated starch (Zhang et al. 2008). Soluble fibre in the endosperm cell wall of oats was shown to affect starch digestion, where different degrees of β-glucan solubilization using cooking methods caused that different degrees of starch digestion (Yiu et al. 1987). Whole grain kernels also have fibre-rich multiple-layered bran that may decrease the accessibility of hydrolytic enzyme to some starch granules. Accordingly, the ordered botanical structure of whole grain kernels is a natural way to produce slowly digestible or perhaps even some degree of resistant starches.

Although the whole grain botanical structure provides some degree of physical barrier to starch hydrolytic enzymes, most whole grain foods are further processed before consumption. An understudied area is how to effectively process whole grain foods to retain or minimize the loss of physical barrier function important to slow starch digestion properties and moderated postprandial glycaemia. Food processing with high temperatures and shear conditions may completely disrupt grain structure and disperse gelatinize starch, leading to a high content of RDS, which from the starch perspective differs little from processed refined grain products. On the other hand, moderate processing such as with rolled oats can lead to reduced rate of starch digestion due to a minimal disruption of the physical structure of the grain (Mishra and Monro 2009). Similarly, food processing to produce a dense packing of food form may create a physical barrier property to starch digestion, such as in pasta that can contain a significant SDS.

4.7 Digestibility of dietary fibre

Dietary fibres such as arabinoxylan, pectin, cellulose, β-glucan and resistant starch are often mentioned regarding the health benefit of whole grain foods (Lattimer and Haub 2010; Cho et al. 2013). Related to starch digestion and glucose absorption, viscous-forming fibres (e.g., β-glucans, water-soluble arabinoxylans) in some whole grain foods have been shown to moderate diffusion kinetics of α-amylase and its digested products to the small intestine epithelial cells for glucose production by the mucosal α-glucosidases (Blackburn and Johnson 1981; Johnson and Gee 1981; 2013). High viscosity of β-glucans lowered in vitro starch digestion (Kim and White 2013), and the zero-shear viscosity of jejunal digest containing β-glucans was found to negatively correlate with glucose absorption in a pig study (Ellis et al. 1995). Other whole grain sources do not have appreciable amounts of viscous-forming fibres, though cellulose as an insoluble fibre has been shown to inhibit α-amylase activity to reduce starch digestion (Dhital et al. 2015).

Short chain fatty acids generated through fibre fermentation by the colon microbiota induce the release of the gut hormone peptide YY (PYY) (Wen et al. 1998) and GLP-1 (Tollhurst et al. 2012) to slow gastric emptying, promote insulin secretion and moderate glycemic response. This creates a "second-meal effect" first described by Jenkins et al. (1982; Brighenti et al. 2006). Thus, dietary fibres can slow the absorption of glucose or other nutrients from both its physiochemical property such as high viscosity (Zijlstra et al. 2012) and the ileo-colonic brake systems, which enhance carbohydrate quality of whole grain foods.

4.8 Phytochemicals

Phytochemicals mostly reside at the outer layers of cereal grains, particularly in the pericarp seed coat and aleurone layers, and can affect carbohydrate digestion and absorption in the gastrointestinal tract. Polyphenols such as phenolic acids found in whole grains have affinity to proteins like enzymes (Bandyopadhyay et al. 2012), and their inhibiting function on the activity of the α-amylases and α-glucosidases (maltase-glucoamylase and sucrase-isomaltase) have been documented (Shihabudeen et al. 2011; Forester et al.

2012; Mkandawire et al. 2013; Tu et al. 2013; et al. 2013; Simsek et al. 2015). In addition to their inhibition effect on hydrolytic enzymes, they also have been shown to interrupt the uptake of glucose by binding to the sodium-glucose linked transporter, SGLT1 (Kobayashi et al. 2000) and glucose transporter 2, GLUT2 (Kwon et al. 2007; Stelmanska 2009; Manzano and Williamson 2010), or by reducing the expression of glucose transporters (Alzaid et al. 2013). Thus, both starch digestion and glucose absorption may be interfered by whole grain polyphenols, which could result in a reduction of postprandial glycemic response.

4.9 Future perspectives

Whole grain carbohydrates consist principally of dietary fibres and starch. They are considered to be the main contributors of the health benefits ascribed to whole grain foods. While starch is quantitatively the major component of whole grains, relatively less is known relating starch quality to the health attributes of whole grains. Whole grain foods are broadly considered low GI foods, though their processing can change this attribute. Thus, the quality of starch is an important factor requiring further investigation, particularly in the area of glucose release kinetics and location of digestion in the gut related to potential gut-brain axis and ileal brake responses. The role of whole grain dietary fibres on the gut microbiome is large and a growing area of research, and likely an expanded research effort is needed for a more precise and fundamental understanding of the action of different fibres and their physical forms on the microbiota and their consequent effect on health. Last, the complex interactions in whole grain foods among starch, dietary fibre and other food components require more studies to develop novel food processing technologies for processed foods to maximize the health benefits.

4.10 References

AACC. (2001). The definition of dietary fiber. *Cereal Foods World*, 46, 112–126.

Alzaid, F., Cheung, H.M., Preedy, V.R., and Sharp, P.A. (2013). Regulation of glucose transporter expression in human intestinal Caco-2 cells following exposure to an anthocyanin-rich berry extract. *PLoS ONE*, 8(11), e78932. doi:10.1371/journal.pone.0078932

Anderson, J.W., Baird, P., Davis, R.H., Ferreri, S., Knudtson, M., Koraym, A., Waters, V., and Williams, C.L. (2009). Health benefits of dietary fiber. *Nutrition Reviews*, 67, 188–205.

AOAC Official Method 2009.01. (2009). Total dietary fiber in foods, enzymatic–gravimetric–chromatographic method, first action. AOAC Official Methods of Analysis *(18th ed.)*. AOAC International, Gaithersburg, USA.

Augustin, L.S.A., Kendall, C.W.C., Jenkins, D.J.A., Willett, W.C., Astrup, A., Barclay, A.W., Björck, I., Brand-Miller, J.C., Brighenti, F., Buyken, A.E., Ceriello, A. La Vecchia, Livesey, G. Liu, S., Riccardi, G., Rizkalla, S.W., Sievenpiper, J.L., Trichopoulou, A., Wolever, T.M.S., Baer-Sinnott, S., and Poli, A. (2015). Glycemic index, glycemic load and glycemic response: An International Scientific Consensus Summit from the International Carbohydrate Quality Consortium (ICQC). *Nutrition, Metabolism and Cardiovascular Diseases*, 25, 795e815.

Bandyopadhyay, P., Ghosh, A.K., and Ghosh, C. (2012). Recent developments on polyphenol-protein interactions: effects on tea and coffee taste, antioxidant properties and the digestive system. *Food & Function*, 3, 592–605.

Bird, A.R., Conlon, M.A., Christophersen, C.T., and Topping, D.L. (2010). Resistant starch, large bowel fermentation and a broader perspective of prebiotics and probiotics. *Beneficial Microbes*, 1, 423–431.

Björck, I., and Elmstahl, H.L. (2003). The glycaemic index: Importance of dietary fibre and other food properties. *Proceedings of the Nutrition Society*, 62, 201–206.

Björck, I., Granfeldt, Y., Liljeberg, H., Tovar, J., and Asp, N.G. (1994). Food properties affecting the digestion and absorption of carbohydrates. *American Journal of Clinical Nutrition*, 59, 699S–705S.

Blackburn, N.A., and Johnson, I.T. (1981). The effect of guar gum on the viscosity of the gastrointestinal contents and on glucose uptake from the perfused jejunum in the rat. *British Journal of Nutrition*, 46, 239–246.

Brighenti, F., Benini, L., Del Rio, D., Casiraghi, C., Pellegrini, N., Scazzina, F., Jenkins, D.J.A., and Vantini, I. (2006). Colonic fermentation of indigestible carbohydrates contributes to the second-meal effect. *American Journal of Clinical Nutrition*, 83, 817–822.

Brown, M.R., Saxena, I.M., and Kudlicka, K. (1996). Cellulose biosynthesis in higher plants. *Trends in Plant Science*, 1, 149–156.

Buléon, A., Colonna, P., Planchot, V., and Ball, S. (1998). Starch granules: Structure and biosynthesis. *International Journal of Biological Macromolecules*, 23, 85–112.

Burton, R.A., Gidley, M.J., and Fincher, G.B. (2010). Heterogeneity in the chemistry, structure and function of plant cell walls. *Nature Chemical Biology*, 6, 724–732.

Carpita, N.C., and Gibeaut, D.M. (1993). Structural models of primary cell walls in flowering plants: Consistency of molecular structure with the physical properties of the walls during growth. *Plant Journal*, 3, 1–30.

Cho, S.S., Qi, L., Fahey, G.C., and Klurfeld, D.M. (2013). Consumption of cereal fiber, mixtures of whole grains and bran, and whole grains and risk reduction in type 2 diabetes, obesity, and cardiovascular disease. *American Journal of Clinical Nutrition*, doi:10.3945/ajcn.113.067629

Choct, M. (1997). Non-starch polysaccharides: chemical structures and nutritional significance. *Feed Milling International*, June, 13–26.

Codex. (2009). Alinorm 09/32/26, Report of the 30th Session of the Codex Committee on nutrition and foods for special dietary uses. *Joint FAO/WHO Food Standards Programme Codex Alimentarius Commission* 47.

Collins, H.M., Burton, R.A., Topping, D.L., Liao, M-L., Bacic, A., and Fincher, G.B. (2010). Variability in fine structures of noncellulosic cell wall polysaccharides from cereal grains: Potential importance in human health and nutrition. *Cereal Chemistry*, 87, 272–282.

DeVries, J.W., Prosky, L., Li, B., and Cho, S. (1999). A historical perspective on defining dietary fiber. *Cereal Foods World*, 44, 367–369.

Dhital, S., Gidley, M.J., and Warren, F.J. (2015). Inhibition of alpha-amylase activity by cellulose: Kinetic analysis and nutritional implications. *Carbohydrate Polymers*, 123, 305–312.

Ebringerová, A., and Heinze, T. (2000). Xylan and xylan derivatives – biopolymers with valuable properties, 1. Naturally occurring xylans structures, isolation procedures and properties. *Macromolecular Rapid Communications*, 21, 542–556.

EFSA. (2010). European Food Safety Authority: outcome of the public consultation on the draft opinion of the Scientific Panel on Dietetic Products, Nutrition, and Allergies (NDA) on dietary reference values for carbohydrates and dietary fibre. *EFSA Journal* 8, 1508–1569.

Ellis, P.R., Roberts, F.G., Low, A.G., and Morgan, L.M. (1995). The effect of high-molecular-weight guar gum on net apparent glucose absorption and net apparent insulin and gastric inhibitory polypeptide production in the growing pig: relationship to rheological changes in jejunal digesta. *British Journal of Nutrition*, 74, 539–556.

Englyst, H.N., Kingman, S.M., and Cummings, J.H. (1992). Classification and measurement of nutritionally important starch fractions. *European Journal of Clinical Nutrition*, 46, S33–50.

Englyst, K.N., Englyst, H.N., Hudson, G.J., Cole, T.J., and Cummings, J.H. (1999). Rapidly available glucose in foods: An in vitro measurement that reflects the glycemic response. *American Journal of Clinical Nutrition*, 69, 448–454.

Fabricatore, A.N., Wadden, T.A., Ebbeling, C.B., Thomas, J.G., Stallings, V.A., Schwartz, S., and Ludwig, D.S. (2011). Targeting dietary fat or glycemic load in the treatment of obesity and type 2 diabetes: A randomized controlled trial. *Diabetes Research and Clinical Practice*, 92, 37–45.

Fardet, A., Llorach, R., Orsoni, A., Martin, J.F., Pujos-Guillot, E., Lapierre, C., and Scalbert, A. (2008). Metabolomics provide new insight on the metabolism of dietary phytochemicals in rats. *The Journal of Nutrition*, 138, 1282–1287.

Fincher, G.B., and Stone, B.A. (1986). Cell walls and their components in cereal grain technology. In Advances in Cereal Science and Technology (ed. Y. Pomeranz), pp. 207–295. AACC International.

Forester, S.C., Gu, Y., and Lambert, J.D. (2012). Inhibition of starch digestion by the green tea polyphenol, (-)-epigallocatechin-3-gallate. *Molecular Nutrition and Food Research*, 56, 1647–1654.

Gartaula, G., Dhital, S., Netzel, G., Flanagan, B.M., Yakubov, G.E., Beahan, C.T., Collins, H.M., Burton, R.A., Bacic, A., and Gidley, M.J. (2018). Quantitative structural organisation model for wheat endosperm cell walls: Cellulose as an important constituent. *Carbohydrate Polymers*, 196, 199–208.

Gidley, M.J. (2013). Hydrocolloids in the digestive tract and related health implications. *Current Opinion in Colloid & Interface Science*, 18, 371–378.

Hamaker, B.R., and Tuncil, Y.E. (2014). A perspective on the complexity of dietary fiber structures and their potential effect on the gut microbiota. *Journal of Molecular Biology*, 426, 3838–3850.

Hasek, L.Y., Phillips, R.J., Zhang, G., Kinzig, K.P., Kim, C.Y., Powley, T.L., and Hamaker, B.R. (2018). Dietary slowly digestible starch triggers the gut–brain axis in obese rats with accompanied reduced food intake. *Molecular Nutrition and Food Research*, 62, 1700117.

Hasjim, J., Lavau, G.C., Gidley, M.J., and Gilbert, R.G. (2010). In vivo and in vitro starch digestion: Are current in vitro techniques adequate? *Biomacromolecules*, 11, 3600–3608.

Heaton, K.W., Marcus, S.N., Emmett, P.M., and Bolton, C.H. (1988). Particle size of wheat, maize, and oat test meals: effects on plasma glucose and insulin responses and on the rate of starch digestion in vitro. *American Journal of Clinical Nutrition*, 47, 675–682.

Hipsley, E.H. (1953). Dietary "fibre" and pregnancy toxaemia. *British Medical Journal*, 2, 420–422.

IOM. (2001). Institute of Medicine (IOM). U.S. National Academy of Sciences: Dietary Reference Intakes: Proposed Definition of Dietary Fiber. Washington, D.C: National Academy Press.

Izydorczyk, M.S., and Biliaderis, C.G. (1995). Cereal arabinoxylans: Advances in structure and physicochemical properties, *Carbohydrate Polymers*, 28, 33–48.

Jenkins, D.J., Wolever, T.M., Taylor, R.H., Barker, H., Fielden, H., Baldwin, J.M., Bowling, A.C., Newman, H.C., Jenkins, A.L., and Goff, D.V. (1981). Glycemic index of foods: A physiological basis for carbohydrate exchange. *American Journal of Clinical Nutrition*, 34, 362–366.

Jenkins, D.J., Wolever, T.M., Taylor, R.H., Griffiths, C., Krzeminska, K., Lawrie, J.A., Bennett, C.M., Goff, D.V., Sarson, D.L., and Bloom S.R. (1982). Slow release dietary carbohydrate improves second meal tolerance. *American Journal of Clinical Nutrition*, 35, 1339–1346.

Johnson, I.T., and Gee, J.M. (1981). Effect of gel-forming gums on the intestinal unstirred layer and sugar transport in vitro. *Gut*, 22, 398–403.

Johnson, J.L., Gidley, M.J., Bacic, A., and Doblin, M.S. (2018). Cell wall biomechanics: A tractable challenge in manipulating plant cell walls "fit for purpose"! *Current Opinion in Biotechnology*, 49, 163–171.

Jones, J.M. (2014). CODEX-aligned dietary fiber definitions help to bridge the "fiber gap." *Nutrition Journal*, 13, 1475–2891.

Kamal-Eldin, A., Laerke, H.N., Knudsen, K.E., Lampi, A.M., Piironen, V., Adlercreutz, H., Katina, K., Poutanen, K., and Man, P. (2009). Physical, microscopic and chemical characterisation of industrial rye and wheat brans from the Nordic countries. *Food Nutrition Research*, 53, doi:10.3402/fnr.v53i0.1912

Kim, H.J., and White, P.J. (2013). Impact of the molecular weight, viscosity, and solubility of beta-glucan on in vitro oat starch digestibility. *Journal of Agricultural and Food Chemistry*, 61, 3270–3277.

Kobayashi, Y., Suzuki, M., Satsu, H., Arai, S., Hara, Y., Suzuki, K., Miyamoto Y., and Shimizu, M. (2000). Green tea polyphenols inhibit the sodium-dependent glucose transporter of intestinal epithelial cells by a competitive mechanism. *Journal of Agricultural and Food Chemistry*, 48, 5618–23.

Krok, F., Szymońska, J., Tomasik, P., and Szymoński, M. (2000). Non-contact AFM investigation of influence of freezing process on the surface structure of potato starch granule. *Applied Surface Science*, 157, 382–386.

Kwon, O., Eck, P., Chen, S., Corpe, C. P., Lee, J.-H., Kruhlak M., and Levine, M. (2007). Inhibition of the intestinal glucose transporter GLUT2 by flavonoids. *FASEB Journal*, 21, 366–377.

Lamothe, L.M., Srichuwong, S., Reuhs, B.L., and Hamaker, B.R. (2015). Quinoa (Chenopodium quinoa W.) and amaranth (Amaranthus caudatus L.) provide dietary fibres high in pectic substances and xyloglucans. *Food Chemistry*, 167, 490–496.

Larsen, P.J. (2008). Mechanisms behind GLP-1 induced weight loss. *British Journal of Diabetes, & Vascular Disease*, 8, S34–S41.

Lattimer, J.M., and Haub, M.D. (2010). Effects of dietary fiber and its components on metabolic health. *Nutrients*, 2, 1266–1289.

Lazaridou, A., and Biliaderis, C.G. (2007). Molecular aspects of cereal β-glucan functionality: Physical properties, technological applications and physiological effects. *Journal of Cereal Science*, 46**,** 101–118.

Lee, B.-H., Bello-Perez, L.A., Lin, A. H.-M., Kim, C.Y., and Hamaker, B.R. (2013). Importance of location of digestion and colonic fermentation of starch related to its quality. *Cereal Chemistry*, 90, 335–343.

Lehmann, U., and Robin, F. (2007). Slowly digestible starch-its structure and health implications: A review. *Trends in Food Science & Technology*, 18, 346–355.

Liljeberg, H., Granfeldt, Y., and Björck, I. (1992). Metabolic responses to starch in bread containing intact kernels versus milled flour. *European Journal of Clinical Nutrition*, 46, 561–575.

Livesey, G. (2005). Low-glycaemic diets and health: Implications for obesity. *Proceedings of the Nutrition Society*, 64, 105–113.

Lopes, J.C., Shaver, R.D., Hoffman, P.C., Akins, M.S., Bertics, S.J., Gencoglu, H., and Coors, J.G. (2009). Type of corn endosperm influences nutrient digestibility in lactating dairy cows. *Journal of Dairy Science*, 92, 4541–4548.

Ludwig, D.S. (2002). The glycemic index: Physiological mechanisms relating to obesity, diabetes, and cardiovascular disease. *Journal of the American Medical Association*, 287, 2414–2423.

Ludwig, D.S., Majzoub, J.A., Al-Zahrani, A., Dallal, G.E., Blanco, I., and Roberts, S.B. (1999). High glycemic index foods, overeating, and obesity. *Pediatrics*, 103, E26.

Manzano, S., and Williamson, G. (2010). Polyphenols and phenolic acids from strawberry and apple decrease glucose uptake and transport by human intestinal Caco-2 cells. *Molecular Nutrition & Food Research*, 54, 1773–1780.

Mendis, M., and Simsek, S. (2014). Arabinoxylans and human health. *Food Hydrocolloids*, 42, 239-243.

Mishra, S., and Monro, J.A. (2009). Digestibility of starch fractions in wholegrain rolled oats. *Journal of Cereal Science*, 50, 61–66.

Mkandawire, N.L., Kaufman, R.C., Bean, S.R., Weller, C.L., Jackson, D.S., and Rose, D.J. (2013). Effects of Sorghum (Sorghum bicolor (L.) Moench) Tannins on α-Amylase Activity and in Vitro Digestibility of Starch in Raw and Processed Flours. *Journal of Agricultural and Food Chemistry*, 61, 4448–4454.

Mozaffarian, R.S., Lee, R.M., Kennedy, M.A., Ludwig, D.S., Mozaffarian, D., and Gortmaker, S.L. (2013). Identifying whole grain foods: A comparison of different approaches for selecting more healthful whole grain products. *Public Health Nutrition*, 16, 2255–2264.

Phillips, G.O., and Cui, S.W. (2011). An introduction: Evolution and finalisation of the regulatory definition of dietary fibre. *Food Hydrocolloids*, 25, 139–143.

Qian, J., and Kuhn, M. (1999). Characterization of Amaranthus cruentus and Chenopodium quinoa starch. *Starch – Stärke*, 51, 116–120.

Romijn, J.A., Corssmit, E.P., Havekes, L.M., and Pijl, H. (2008). Gut-brain axis. *Current Opinion in Clinical Nutrition & Metabolic Care*, 11, 518–521.

Rose, D.J., Patterson, J.A., and Hamaker, B.R. (2010). Structural differences among alkali-soluble arabinoxylans from maize (Zea mays), rice (Oryza sativa), and wheat (Triticum aestivum) brans influence human fecal fermentation profiles. *Journal of Agricultural and Food Chemistry*, 58, 493–499.

Rumpagaporn, P., Reuh, B.L., Kaur, A., Patterson, J.A., Keshavarzian, A., and Hamaker, B.R. (2015). Structural features of soluble cereal arabinoxylan fibers associated with a slow rate of in vitro fermentation by human fecal microbiota. *Carbohydrate Polymers*, 130, 191–197.

Seal, C.J., Daly, M.E., Thomas, L.C., Bal, W., Birkett, A.M., Jeffcoat, R., and Mathers, J.C. (2003). Postprandial carbohydrate metabolism in healthy subjects and those with type 2 diabetes fed starches with slow and rapid hydrolysis rates determined in vitro. *British Journal of Nutrition*, 90, 853–864.

Shihabudeen, H.M.S., Priscilla, D.H., and Thirumurugan, K. (2011). Cinnamon extract inhibits alpha-glucosidase activity and dampens postprandial glucose excursion in diabetic rats. *Nutrition & Metabolism*, 8, 1–11.

Shimada, M., Mochizuki, K., and Goda, T. (2009). Feeding rats dietary resistant starch shifts the peak of SGLT1 gene expression and histone H3 acetylation on the gene from the upper jejunum toward the ileum. *Journal of Agricultural and Food Chemistry*, 57, 8049–8055.

Shin, J.E., Simsek, S., Reuhs, B.L., and Yao, Y. (2008). Glucose release of water-soluble starch-related alpha-glucans by pancreatin and amyloglucosidase is affected by the abundance of alpha-1,6-glucosidic linkages. *Journal of Agricultural and Food Chemistry*, 56, 10879–10886.

Simsek, M., Quezada-Calvillo, R., Ferruzzi, M.G., Nichols, B.L., and Hamaker, B.R. (2015). Dietary phenolic compounds selectively inhibit the individual subunits of maltase-glucoamylase and sucrase-isomaltase with the potential of modulating glucose release. *Journal of Agricultural and Food Chemistry*, 63, 3873–3879.

Stelmanska, E. (2009). The important role of GLUT2 in intestinal sugar transport and absorption. *Postepy Biochem*, 55, 385–387.

Tolhurst, G., Heffron, H., Lam, Y.S., Parker, H.E., Habib, A.M., Diakogiannaki, E., Cameron, J., Grosse, J., Reimann, F., and Gribble, F.M. (2012). Short-chain fatty acids stimulate glucagon-like peptide-1 secretion via the G-protein-coupled receptor FFAR2. *Diabetes*, 61, 364–371.

Toth S. (2013). The research legacy of Peter J. Wood. *Bioactive Carbohydrates and Dietary Fibre*, 2 (2), 170–180.

Tu, J., Chen, J., Zhu, S., Zhang, C., Chen, H., and Liu, Y. (2013). Inhibition of wheat bran and it's active components on α-glucosidase in vitro. *Pharmacognosy Magazine*, 9, 309–314.

United States Food and Drug Administration (USFDA). (2016). Nutrition and Supplement Facts label final rule. Federal Register, May 27.

Van Loo, J., Coussement, P., De Leenheer, L., Hoebregs, H., and Smits, G. (1995). On the presence of insulin and oligofructose as natural ingredients in the Western diet. *Critical Reviews in Food Science & Nutrition*, 35, 525–552.

Vanholme, R., Demedts, B., Morreel, K., Ralph, J., and Boerjan, W. (2010). Lignin biosynthesis and structure. *Plant Physiology*, 153, 895–905.

Wachters-Hagedoorn, R.E., Priebe, M.G., Heimweg, J.A.J., Heiner, A.M., Englyst, K.N., Holst, J.J., Stellaard F., and Vonk, R.J. (2006). The rate of intestinal glucose absorption is correlated with plasma glucose-dependent insulinotropic polypeptide concentrations in healthy men. *Journal of Nutrition*, 136, 1511–1516.

Wang, Y., Xiang, L., Wang, C., Tang, C., and He, X. (2013). Antidiabetic and antioxidant effects and phytochemicals of mulberry fruit (*Morus alba L.*) polyphenol enhanced extract. *PLoS ONE*, 8, e71144.

Wen, J., Luque-de Leon, E., Kost, L.J., Sarr, M.G., and Phillips, S.F. (1998). Duodenal motility in fasting dogs: Humoral and neural pathways mediating the colonic brake. *American Journal of Physiology*, 274, G192–G195.

Whole Grain Council. (2004). Whole grain definition from Whole Grain Council. http://wholegrainscouncil.org/whole-grains-101/definition-of-whole-grain

Woodward, A.D., Regmi, P.R., Ganzle, M.G., van Kempen, T.A., and Zijlstra, R.T. (2012). Slowly digestible starch influences mRNA abundance of glucose and short-chain fatty acid transporters in the porcine distal intestinal tract. *Journal of Animal Science*, 90(Suppl. 4), 80–82.

Yiu, S.H., Wood, P.J., and Weisz, W.J. (1987). Effects of cooking on starch and β-glucan of rolled oats. *Cereal Chemistry*, 64, 373–379.

Zhang, G., Ao, Z., and Hamaker, B.R. (2008) .Nutritional property of endosperm starches from maize mutants: A parabolic relationship between slowly digestible starch and amylopectin fine structure. *Journal of Agricultural and Food Chemistry*, 56, 4686–4694.

Zhang, G., Sofyan, M., and Hamaker, B.R. (2008). Slowly digestible state of starch: Mechanism of slow digestion property of gelatinized maize starch. *Journal of Agricultural and Food Chemistry*, 56, 4695–4702.

Zijlstra, R.T., Jha, R., Woodward, A.D., Fouhse, J., and van Kempen, T.A. (2012). Starch and fiber properties affect their kinetics of digestion and thereby digestive physiology in pigs. *Journal of Animal of Science*, 90(Suppl.4), 49–58.

5 Whole grain Content of Cereal Products

Alastair B. Ross[1,2], Cynthia Harriman[3], and Roberto King[4]

[1]Food and Nutritional Science, Department of Biology and Biological Engineering, Chalmers University of Technology, Gothenburg, Sweden
[2]Food and Biobased Products, AgResearch Ltd, Lincoln, New Zealand
[3]Oldways Whole Grains Council, Boston, Massachusetts, USA
[4]Nestlé Research Center, Vers chez les Blanc, 1000, Lausanne, 26, Switzerland

5.1 Introduction

After the approval of a health claim for whole grains and the prevention of cardiovascular disease and some cancers by the US Food and Drug Administration in 1999, and the inclusion of specific recommendations to "make at least half your grains whole" in the US Dietary Guidelines of 2005, there has been a rapid increase in the number of products available that contain whole grains, and that make whole grain related claims. Yet, in parallel with this increase, there has been a concern over how to estimate the amount of whole grains in foods, and how to accurately report this, both for labeling purposes and for scientific research. This chapter covers the issues around reporting and measuring whole grains in food products, and why this is an important challenge to meet.

5.2 Why is it important to know the whole grain content of food?

Accurate quantification of whole grains in food is of fundamental importance for research on whole grains and for regulatory and labeling policies, including for checking compliance with regulations around labeling and health claims based on whole grain content. Estimation of whole grain intake requires information about the whole grain content of available foods, yet many products contributing whole grains to the diet do not state the amount or proportion of whole grains present. Since whole grain content in foods can vary from very little to 100%, a large amount of guesswork may go into estimating whole grain content, potentially reducing the accuracy of associations between whole grains and health. Quantifying whole grains in foods is also important for clearly and honestly marketing whole grains to consumers, to ensure consumer confidence that a product labeled as containing whole grains does actually contain what is stated.

In some food cultures, only those foods that contain close to or 100% whole grain ingredients can be called "whole grain,"(1) while in other food cultures, products labeled as "whole grain" may contain <20% of whole grains.(2) Scientifically, it is the overall intake of whole grain ingredients that is important for understanding the relationship between

Whole Grains and Health, Second Edition. Edited by Rikard Landberg and Nathalie Scheers.

Additional materials available for download online at https://www.wiley.com/en-gb/Whole+Grains+and+Health-p-9781118939437

whole grains and health, rather than the overall amount of products classified as containing whole grains. Yet, while it is feasible to weigh a slice of bread, it is impossible to know the amount of whole grain ingredients in that slice of bread unless you have access to the recipe or it is stated on the packaging. Ideal methods of quantification would provide accurate estimation of whole grain amount for a wide variety of foods containing whole grains, as even foods with more refined grain flour than whole grain flour may make an important contribution of whole grains to some diets.(2) Recognition of whether a product is "whole grain" or contains whole grains is often done based on product appearance. A bread or pasta may be brown, there may be visible bran in the product, or there may be intact grains or seeds visible in the food. These visual cues do not, in fact, tell anything about whether a product is whole grain or not, nor about the proportion of whole grains in a product. Bread can be made to look dark by the addition of caramel coloring; the addition of a small amount of bran can give a product a "grainy" look; and common seeds are not whole grains. The ingredients list may give important clues, as ingredients must be labeled in descending order of amount. This means that a cereal-based product listing whole grain flour first is quite likely to have >50% of its grain as whole grains. However, this still leaves a large margin of error, especially in foods with multiple refined- and whole grain ingredients. In the European Union, ingredients lists follow Quantitative Ingredients Declaration (QUID) law, where, for example, a product labeled as whole grain would need to state the percentage of any whole grain(s) in the ingredients list. This gives the proportion of whole grains in a product, though there is still some leeway for inaccuracy based on the amount of water in a product (see the following).

5.2.1 How whole grain content of cereal products has been reported

Whole grains are a diverse group of cereals and pseudocereals that are on one level well defined as ingredients, but at the level of food products, poorly defined due to no universally accepted definition of what constitutes a whole grain food product. This is further clouded by a wide range of definitions used by scientists, regulatory authorities, private labeling initiatives and what is reported "on pack" for food products containing cereals.

In the scientific literature, the use of "whole grains" to identify foods of potential interest for reducing disease risk, first used a cut-off point of 25% whole grains (as a percent of total weight as consumed) in a product.(3,4,5) Deciding on a threshold for whether a product would count as being "whole grain" or not was necessary to establish whether there was a relationship between foods containing whole grains and health. However, this also means that a food included as whole grain for the purposes of estimating intake could contain anywhere between 25% and 100% of its total weight as whole grains. A product that contained 26% whole grains would be considered to contribute the same amount of whole grains to overall whole grain intake as a food with 100% whole grain ingredients. Further, using this threshold does not account for products that contain <25% whole grains, so it would not be possible to determine whether such foods make an important contribution to whole grain intake. So while a 25% threshold was a good starting point, as research on whole grains has progressed since the early studies associating whole grain intake with reduced disease risk, it has been necessary to further develop how whole grain intake is estimated and how whole grain content in foods is measured and used to estimate intake.

In 1999, the United States Food and Drug Administration (FDA) allowed a health claim to be made for whole grain foods and cardiovascular disease and some types of cancer. With this health claim came the first set of criteria to define what a whole grain food product was: a food with ≥51% whole grains (by total weight as consumed), low in fat, sugar and salt. Determination of whether a product was whole grain or not was based on the dietary fibre content of wheat – a laudable attempt, but problematic as many commonly consumed cereals have a lower dietary fibre content than wheat – notably rice and corn/maize. The water content of whole grain foods was not addressed, allowing dry foods like RTE breakfast cereal, crackers and pasta to qualify for the FDA health claim much more easily than moist foods like bread. In contrast, a definition developed by the Swedish Nutrition Foundation to support a Swedish health claim for whole grain foods specified that foods needed to have at least 50% whole grain ingredients on a dry weight basis, but that foods could claim "whole grain" on their packaging if they had at least 25% on a dry weight basis, and stated the proportion of whole grains.[6]

5.2.2 Quantifying whole grain content

Much of what is known about whole grain content of food is based on what is reported on food packaging or in recipe books. Few countries have clear guidelines for labeling whole grain content, which limits the value of a product labeled as "whole grain" for estimating intake or for consumer communication. There are three main approaches to quantifying whole grain content in food:

- The percentage of the grain ingredients that are whole grain (i.e., whole grain vs. refined grain)
- The percentage of the product dry weight that is whole grain (i.e., without the influence of water added during food processing or cooking)
- The percentage of the product as consumed that is whole grain (i.e., accounting for non-grain-based ingredients)

The United States Dietary Guidelines for Americans, in their practical advice for helping consumers select whole grain products, advise that selecting products with "whole grains as the first ingredient" is a good consumer shortcut for choosing foods that will provide a substantial proportion of whole grains. However, it still falls short as a quantitative tool, and from a regulatory and consumer perspective, requires knowledge about ingredient lists and close-up investigation of the back of the packaging to make this crude measurement of whole grain content.

Most cereal foods have water added, and depending on what is quantified, this may make a big difference to a whole grain label that is based on percentage of a product's weight as consumed. For example, dried pasta contains essentially no water, and if made from only whole grain durum wheat, could be labeled as "100% whole grain pasta." The same pasta cooked and frozen for a ready meal would be only 33% whole grain if reported on a fresh weight basis, although the amount of dry pasta in a serving would be the same. This highlights the need to account for water content when reporting whole grain content in foods.

A further issue is that of the effect of processing – at what point do whole grains become so highly processed that they are no longer whole grain? There are few guidelines and this topic is somewhat out of scope here, though it is worth mentioning that the United States

Department of Agriculture (USDA), in 2008, stated that when a shoot from a sprouted cereal seed is longer than the seed itself, then it is no longer considered a grain, but has become a vegetable. Others have also suggested that once more than 10% of the dietary fibre has been removed or disintegrated then the resulting ingredient or product can no longer be considered to be whole grain.[1] However, this is complicated, as total dietary fibre may not reflect the effect of processing that can have a major impact on biological function[7] even if total fibre does not change. For example, some water soluble compounds may be leached out during boiling of cereal products.

Currently, two "user friendly" and accurate ways to report whole grain content are available in different parts of the world, helping researchers, consumers and policy-makers alike. The first is the QUID labeling used in Europe (see earlier), which clearly documents any whole grains as a percentage of the product as consumed.[1] The second is the Whole Grain Stamp, a labeling certification programme offered through the non-profit Oldways Whole Grains Council, which displays the grams of whole grain ingredients per serving of more than 13,000 products in 63 countries.

An important additional aspect of quantifying whole grain content is to report the proportion of different grains. As interest in understanding the differential effects of different grains increases, breaking down daily whole grain intake into different types of grain is necessary[8,9]: whole grain oats or rye, for instance, may be associated with different health benefits than whole grain wheat or barley. This is usually done with QUID labeling, and is recommended as part of guidelines for whole grain food labeling.[1]

5.2.3 Whole grain contents in different cereal foods

Cereal-based foods are highly diverse and in most categories of cereal products it is possible to have products that are (or are close to) 100% whole grain. Until the past 150 or so years, most flour produced was whole grain, due to the difficulty of cleanly separating bran and germ from the endosperm. As white flour has become readily available and cheap, it has dominated cereal products for more than a century, and food manufacturers have grown accustomed to the ease of making uniform products, and consumers have adapted to the flavor and texture of refined grains. These habits present challenges for reintroducing a wide range of whole grain foods. In this section, we summarize the range of whole grain content in different cereal food categories, and in Table 5.1, average amounts of whole grains in different food products are presented.

a. Bread

Bread is one of the most common cereal foods, and intake is nearly ubiquitous among all people. Bread as a product is highly diverse, both in terms of ingredients (e.g., wheat, rye, corn/maize, barley, gluten-free dough mixes) and processing (yeast leavened, sourdough, crispbread and unleavened flatbreads; short or long fermentation; use of enzymes and additives to improve shelf-life and loaf properties). The whole grain content of bread varies between 0% and 100% of the flour component, with the increasing amount of whole grain in bread usually leading to denser loaf volume. However, the addition of baking improvers such as vital gluten or enzymes can give acceptable volume to breads with 100% or close to 100% whole grain. Some baking enzymes are known to have side activities that break down dietary fibre, which may be a concern as dietary fibre is sometimes used as a reference for whole grains in a product.

Table 5.1 Flour content and potential contribution to whole grain intake of common grain-based products, based on Marquart et al 2006. Alkylresorcinol content is included to give an idea of how one proposed marker for whole grain reflects the proportion of whole grains in a product. Note that as alkylresorcinols are only present in wheat, rye, barley and quinoa, they do not universally reflect the whole grain content of foods.

Product	Flour/grain %	Type of grains	Serving size (fresh weight)	Maximum contribution to whole grain intake per serving (g)	Total alkylresorcinol content (µg/g dry weight)
Bread					
White-wheat bread	51	Wheat	28	0	20[a]
Whole-wheat bread	51	Wheat	28	14	438[a]
Rye bread	42	Rye and wheat	30	12	412[a]
Breakfast cereal					
Corn flakes		Corn	30	0	0
Whole wheat/rice flakes	80	Wheat and rice	30	24	251
Whole-wheat biscuits	100	Wheat	40	40	478[a]
Bran-based cereal	85	Wheat bran	40	0	1700
Rolled oats/oatmeal (not cooked)	100	Oats	30	30	0
Main meals					
Pizza	23	Wheat	140	32	100
Refined pasta	40	Wheat	140	0	49[a]
Whole grain pasta	40	Wheat	140	56	290[a]
Refined couscous	40	Wheat	140	0	69
Whole grain couscous	40	Wheat	140	56	402
White rice (cooked)	40	Rice	140	0	0
Brown rice (cooked)	40	Rice	140	56	0
Quinoa	40	Quinoa	140	56	58[b]
Snacks					
Biscuit/cookie	22	Wheat	15	3.3	5.6[a]
Digestive	70 (16% WG)	Wheat	15	2.4	57
Muesli/granola bar	40	Wheat and oats	30	12	49[a]
Popcorn	100	Corn	30	30	0
Refined wheat cracker	85	Wheat	14	0	16
Whole grain wheat cracker	85	Wheat	14	12	340[a]

[a]Average based on products with the same designation but different amounts of cereal ingredients.
[b]Alkylresorcinols only, not including methyl and branched chain alkylresorcinols.
Sources: Ross AB, Svelander C, Karlsson G et al. (2017) Identification and quantification of even and odd chained 5-n alkylresorcinols, branched chain-alkylresorcinols and methylalkylresorcinols in Quinoa (Chenopodium quinoa). *Food Chem* 220, 344–351; Chen Y, Ross AB, Åman P et al. (2004) Alkylresorcinols as markers of whole grain wheat and rye in cereal products. *JAgricFood Chem* 52, 8242–8246; Ross AB (2012) Analysis of alkylresorcinols in cereal grains and products using ultrahigh-pressure liquid chromatography with fluorescence, ultraviolet, and coulArray electrochemical detection. *J Agric Food Chem* 60, 8954–8962; Ross AB, Kochhar S (2009) Rapid and sensitive analysis of alkylresorcinols from cereal grains and products using HPLC-Coularray-based electrochemical detection. *J Agric Food Chem* 57, 5187–5193; Andersson AAM, Åman P, Wandel M et al. (2010) Alkylresorcinols in wheat and rye flour and bread. *J Food Compost Anal* 23, 794–80.

In some countries, it is common practice to add syrup or caramel coloring to give bread a darker appearance, or to add bran, intact grains or seeds in bread dough made from largely white flour to get a bread with good loaf volume and soft texture, but with the appearance of "wholesomeness" (Figure 5.1). This makes it very difficult to judge the whole grain content of bread based on appearances alone. Information on-pack, or from manufacturers, is necessary to get an accurate measure of the whole grain content of individual breads. In some countries, such as the Netherlands and Germany, there are clear guidelines for labeling bread as whole grain, requiring 90–100% of flour to be whole grain flour,(1) though in other countries, it may be difficult or impossible to determine whole grain content for "dark bread."

Due to the highly variable nature of bread, and the fact that the use of whole grain flour may be highly specific for different countries or regions, it is necessary to carry out on-the-ground surveys of both pre-packaged bread and bread bought directly from local bakeries to get an idea of whole grain content.

b. Breakfast cereals

Breakfast cereals represent a diverse range of products and in some countries, notably in North America, the United Kingdom and Ireland,(10,11,12,13,14,15) are one of the main sources of whole grains in people's diet. Breakfast cereals encompass "ready to eat" (RTE) breakfast cereals that are often based on flour (frequently with added sugar) that is mixed with water, then heated and extruded, as well as cooked porridges and mueslis. As with bread, breakfast cereals range from 0–100% whole grain with no reasonable "average" for whole grain content of a whole grain–containing breakfast cereal.

Recent years have seen efforts to promote the whole grain content of packaged cereals so that, in many countries, this is either prominently displayed on the packaging or clearly indicated in the ingredients list. Importantly, breakfast cereals often include grains that are otherwise not so commonly consumed. Due to the dominance of wheat in bread and pasta-type products, the frequent use of oats for breakfast cereals, porridges and mueslis provides some diversity in the types of cereals eaten. Specialty cereals often contain less common grains, and while on a population basis median intake may be negligible, intake by those who *do* consume these cereals may be important for health outcomes. As with all cereal foods, it is important that information on the type of cereal in the diet is recorded, not just the total amount.

Several well-known RTE breakfast cereals are 90–100% whole grain, and with serving sizes ranging from 30–60 g dry cereal, these can represent an important part of daily whole grain intake. Although breakfast cereals are more likely than other cereal-food categories to be high in whole grain content, making assumptions about whole grain content based solely on color or texture is fraught. A further complication in some breakfast cereals is the inclusion of cereal bran, an ingredient that is sometimes mistakenly thought to be a whole grain. Although the focus of this chapter is not to discuss the relative merits of whole grains versus bran, it should be noted that in the most widely accepted whole grain definitions,(16,17) bran is not considered to be a whole grain, and nor is there any equivalency assumed. Bran-based cereals are an important source of dietary fibre, and efforts should be made to separate intake of cereal bran as an ingredient (as opposed to estimating cereal bran coming from both whole grains and as a separate ingredient, which has been done previously,(18,19) but suffers from the high degree of collinearity between whole grain intake and bran intake estimated in this manner).

Porridge is a common food in many countries, consisting of cereal (intact, rolled and heat treated, or flour) and water or milk, boiled until a thick consistency is reached. In many cases, the grains used are whole grains, such as oat porridge, but others may be refined, such as wheat semolina and degerminated cornmeal. Estimating intake of whole grains from porridge is greatly affected by whether the product is reported on a dry- or wet-weight basis, as cooked porridge is generally 80–90% water.

c. Cooked cereal foods

While bread and breakfast cereals make up the bulk of whole grain intake worldwide, a potentially substantial portion can come from meals that include whole grain pasta, noodles, pizza, tortillas or couscous, or "intact" grains such as brown rice, quinoa or wheatberries.

A standard dry weight serving of these foods is between 45–70 g, which is around the minimum (48 g) recommended intake of whole grains in the United States, and close to the 75 g/2000 kcal recommended in Denmark and Sweden. Since all cereals – from wheat, rye, barley and rice to pseudocereals such as buckwheat, amaranth and quinoa – can be easily incorporated "intact" into main dishes and salads, this category can contribute to greater diversity of whole grain consumption and enjoyment.

Unlike bread and breakfast cereals, whose whole grain content is hard to ascertain, "main meal" carbohydrates such as brown rice or quinoa are easily identifiable as 100% whole grain. Pasta is generally made from either 0%, 50% or 100% whole grain flour, while noodles can also be made from 100% whole grain flour, though sometimes "whole grain noodles" are made with less than 50% whole grain in order to maintain a similar texture to noodles made with 100% refined grain flour.

Fresh corn/maize is usually included as a vegetable in dietary surveys, although corn/maize is a cereal (and dried corn in the form of popcorn is included as a whole grain cereal). The contribution of fresh corn/maize to whole grain intake is not well established to date, and should be estimated (on a dry-weight basis) as part of efforts to understand the intake and potential health impact of different cereal species. As for other whole grain foods, reporting on dry or wet weight can make a big difference to estimates of whole grain intake, especially for products such as fresh pasta or noodles, or frozen ready meals.

d. Sweet baked goods, snacks and other products

Although sweet foods are often not considered to be suitable for whole grain claims, many sweet foods such as buns and muesli/granola bars include whole grain ingredients, and determining intake from these sources is important for understanding how much they contribute to overall whole grain intake, and how this may impact on health. Generally, few pastries and cakes contain whole grain flour due to the difficulties in making pastry or batter with the desired properties.

Sweet products such as some types of biscuits/cookies or muesli/granola bars may contain a significant amount of whole grain per serving. In general, though, high levels of fat, sugar and inclusions like nuts and dried fruit mean that foods in this category contain relatively low amounts of whole grain as a percentage of weight as consumed (Table 5.1).

One of the most commonly consumed whole grains among "non-whole grain" consumers is corn/maize in the form of popcorn. While not always recognized as a whole grain food, popcorn is a dried intact kernel of corn, and while the starch in the kernel expands and pops with heat, all the components of the grain are still generally attached. Some studies have found that popcorn intake is associated with reduced disease risk,[20,21] suggesting that popcorn deserves more attention as a healthy whole grain food. Other savory snack foods may also contain a relatively high amount of whole grains. This includes crisp-type products (called snack chips in the United States) made from cereal flours and crackers. However, recommended serving sizes for whole grain snack foods are often limited, so as a category, should be considered fairly limited as a sole source of whole grains in a diet. However, it is positive that there are a wide range of whole grain snacks available as an alternative to those based on refined carbohydrate sources.

5.2.4 Measuring the whole grain content of foods

To date, there are no validated instrumental methods to independently determine the whole grain content of food. Thus, labeling claims for whole grains are difficult to police, and are ultimately dependent on the honesty of the food manufacturer – who may be tempted to "healthwash" a product, to make it seem healthy while still maintaining organoleptic properties similar to a non-whole grain product. For both research and regulatory purposes, it would be useful to have a method for measuring whole grain intake by determining the amount of whole grain content in unknown samples.

There are no officially accepted methods for monitoring compliance to reported whole grain content or levels. The FDA in its whole grain health claim guidance directs that fibre content of at least 11% be used for this purpose, though this approach does not account for the wide range of dietary fibre contents in different cereal grains (e.g., wheat, used as a reference by the FDA as it is one of the most commonly consumed grains in the United States, has a dietary fibre content of around 10–11%, while brown rice has just 3–3.5% dietary fibre). A ratio of 10:1 carbohydrate to fibre has also been proposed as an index to help consumers choose foods with the highest whole grain content in foods[22] though this is essentially the same as the FDA proposal, and is not effective for foods with whole grain rice or corn/maize or foods with added fibre.

One simple method for regulators to monitor whether the whole grain content of foods matches that which is reported on packaging is to check the paper trail in relation to the making of that product – that is, following good manufacturing practice standards. In food manufacturing, there should be clear documentation detailing what ingredients have gone into making a batch of a product, including the weight. Thus, an audit of this documentation should reveal if the reported whole grain content accurately reflects what is in the product. This should work well where such record keeping is normal, but still requires a method that could highlight such products. Nor will it help in detecting the whole grain content in foods where the proportion of whole grains is not publicly available.

Independent methods are needed that can be used for both regulatory purposes and screening, including for food composition databases and work on whole grain intake. The major problem is finding a method that is able to differentiate between the addition of bran and whole grain flour. Measures such as that proposed by the USFDA that are based on dietary fibre are limited because of the inability of simple methods of measuring dietary fibre that distinguish between fibre from bran or other sources. Other more complex methods have been proposed for measuring the whole grain content of foods. These include the analysis of components that are derived from bran, germ and endosperm, and checking the relative ratios.[23] This has proven to be effective, but requires many different types of analyses so is expensive and too slow for screening or monitoring. Other more simple measures include the use of biomarker compounds such as the alkylresorcinols. These phenolic lipids are present as several homologues that differ between common wheat, durum wheat, rye, barley and quinoa, and represent a fingerprint that distinguishes between these cereals.[24,25] However, alkylresorcinols are not present in other cereals, and they are mainly present in the bran fraction, so they cannot distinguish between whole grain flour or flour with added bran. In Table 5.1, it is possible to see the potential problems of using alkylresorcinols as markers of whole grain content, as several whole grain foods contain no alkylresorcinols, while wheat bran-based breakfast cereal has the highest amount by some margin, even though for wheat- and rye-based products they are strongly correlated to whole grain content.[26]

The question of whether it is possible to develop a method that can distinguish between whole grain flour and flour with bran and germ added from another batch of flour, and is both rapid and cheap, remains open. That there are some methods available that are able to give some indication does at least help to reinforce measures such as auditing of good manufacturing practice documentation.

5.2.5 Reporting whole grain content in foods in clinical trials

The plethora of different ways of reporting whole grains in clinical trials has led to great difficulty in directly comparing different studies. This, in turn, hampers meta-analyses pooling data from different studies to increase the statistical power for finding differences due to dietary interventions that include whole grains. Reports of whole grain intake may be as basic as people who report "eating more brown bread" through to a detailed breakdown of the gram amounts of different cereal types in the diet.

As scientists working in the field struggle to reconcile the consistent and strong evidence that whole grains reduce disease risk with the mixed intervention-study evidence, it is clear that few studies offer both a clear idea of exactly which specific grains people were eating and in what amount, and whether the subjects were actually eating what they reported. One study using dietary biomarkers found major discrepancies between what people reported eating in an intervention study and what they plausibly ate based on an unbiased biomarker measurement of intake,[27] which raises questions about other studies where compliance was not rigorously cross-checked. Another large study found that although average biomarker concentrations increased, individual variation suggested that a large proportion of subjects were likely not compliant, in spite of major efforts to ensure compliance using suitably packaged food and questionnaires.[28] In essence, the entire field has a cloud of uncertainty over it due to the fact that there are several different ways that intake of whole grains is reported, and we cannot confirm whether study volunteers are actually eating the products they are supposed to. Of some comfort is the observation that generally those studies where overall compliance has been judged to have been good based on biomarker measurements, have also been those where effects on risk markers have been observed.[29,30, 31,32]

These issues led to recommendations for reporting whole grain intake in both intervention and population-based studies.[33] The proposed guidelines for reporting whole grains in foods and whole grain intake are as follows:

- Report whole grain intake as grams of whole grain ingredients rather than absolute amounts of a particular food or poorly defined measures such as servings.
- Note which definition is being used to define whole grain ingredients – for example, the AACCI or HealthGrain definition.

- State the proportion of different cereal grains that have been provided or are consumed so that it is possible to separate effects of, for example, whole grain wheat or oats.
- For intervention studies, describe the type of processing the intervention foods have undergone, including the structure of the flour (e.g., fine or coarse flour).
- If bran or germ are of interest, clearly state what is added bran or germ versus bran and germ coming from whole grain flour.
- Use an appropriate control group in intervention studies, such as an equivalent amount of similar foods based on refined flour. Avoid situations that may lead to the "addition" of intervention foods, rather than replacement of normal foods with intervention foods.
- If possible, use a biomarker of whole grain intake to improve estimates of compliance or intake.

These recommendations aim to standardize reporting of whole grain intake and also allow greater nuances to be applied to our understanding of the effects of whole grains on health – in particular, around the different types of cereals and cereal processing. The requirement to report on food processing also increases the requirement for scientists running such trials to have some knowledge about food processing, or to include food scientists when designing and preparing for such studies.

5.3 How can we better measure whole grain content and intake in the future?

For there to be comparability, consistency and credibility among whole grain research and regulation, there need to be agreed standard measures for estimating the whole grain content of foods. New technologies may enable rapid measurement of whole grain content, and the development of such techniques should go hand in hand with efforts to define regulations around labeling whole grain foods. There also needs to be greater information availability and transparency around whole grain content in foods. For example, the reporting of whole grain content in national food composition databases would greatly enhance the ability to make better estimates of the whole grain content of different food categories. The Swedish Food Composition Database includes "whole grain" as one of the composition variables, reported on a percentage of dry-weight basis, while the USDA has also recently included coding to capture foods that contain more than 50% whole grains (reported as "ounce equivalents"). The Oldways Whole Grains Council, with a large database of whole grain content of thousands of foods, can also provide publicly available data to researchers. Although these different approaches highlight the issues around standardization of reporting, it is positive that there are moves to make information about the whole grain content of foods readily available.

As part of efforts to improve reporting standards, scientific journals must clearly state that measurements of whole grain intake must meet recommended criteria. The recommended criteria, of course, need to be defined and agreed upon, and this only underlines the urgency of doing so.

Accurate estimation of whole grain intake is at the core of strong, science-based recommendations for whole grains, and for there to be accurate estimation, there needs to be clear and reliable information about the whole grain content of foods that is consistently applied by scientists when doing research on whole grains. Further, clear information about whole grain foods will lead to standardized reporting of whole grain content on food packaging,[1] making it easier for consumers to compare products based on whole grain content.

5.4 References

1 Ross, A.B., van der Kamp, J.W., King, R., and et al. (2017). Perspective: A definition for whole-grain food products – Recommendations from the Healthgrain Forum. *Adv. Nutr.*, 8, 525–531.

2 Jones, A.R., Mann, K.D., Kuznes of SA, et al. (2017). The whole grain content of foods consumed in the UK. *Food Chem.*, 214, 453–459.

3 Jacobs, D.R., Jr., Meyer, H.E., and Solvoll, K. (2001). Reduced mortality among whole grain bread eaters in men and women in the Norwegian County Study. *Eur. J. Clin. Nutr.*, 55, 137–143.

4 Jacobs, D.R., Jr., Meyer, K.A., Kushi, L.H., et al. (1998). Whole-grain intake may reduce the risk of ischemic heart disease death in postmenopausal women: The Iowa Women's Health Study. *Am. J. Clin. Nutr.*, 68, 248–257.

5 Jacobs, J., Marquart, L., Slavin, J., et al. (1998). Whole-grain intake and cancer: An expanded review and meta-analysis. *Nutr. Cancer*, 30, 85–96.

6 Asp, N.-G., and Bryngelsson, S. (2007). Health claims in the labelling and marketing of food products: The Swedish food sector's Code of Practice in a European perspective. *Scandinavian Journal of Food & Nutrition*, 51, 107–126.

7 Frank, J., Sundberg, B., Kamal-Eldin, A., et al. (2004). Yeast-leavened oat breads with high or low molecular weight beta-glucan do not differ in their effects on blood concentrations of lipids, insulin, or glucose in humans. *J. Nutr.*, 134, 1384–1388.

8 Ross, A.B., Pineau, N., Kochhar, S., et al. (2009). Validation of a FFQ for estimating whole-grain cereal food intake. *Br. J. Nutr.*, 102, 1547–1551.

9 Hollaender, P.L., Ross, A.B., and Kristensen, M. (2015). Whole-grain and blood lipid changes in apparently healthy adults: A systematic review and meta-analysis of randomized controlled studies. *Am. J. Clin. Nutr.*, 102, 556–572.

10 Thane, C.W., Jones, A.R., Stephen, A.M., et al. (2007). Comparative whole-grain intake of British adults in 1986–7 and 2000–1. *Br. J. Nutr.*, 97, 987–992.

11 Bazzano, L.A., Song, Y., Bubes, V., et al. (2005). Dietary intake of whole and refined grain breakfast cereals and weight gain in men. *Obes. Res.*, 13, 1952–1960.

12 Thane, C.W., Jones, A.R., Stephen, A.M., et al. (2005). Whole-grain intake of British young people aged 4–18 years. *Br. J. Nutr.*, 94, 825–831.

13 Lang, R., Thane, C.W., Bolton-Smith, C., et al. (2003). Consumption of whole-grain foods by British adults: Findings from further analysis of two national dietary surveys. *Public Health Nutr.*, 6, 479–484.

14 O'Donovan, C.B., Devlin, N.F., Buffini, M., et al. (2019). Whole grain intakes in Irish adults: Findings from the National Adults Nutrition Survey (NANS). *Eur. J. Nutr.*, 58, 541–550.

15 Devlin, N.F.C., McNulty, B.A., Gibney, M.J., et al. (2013). Whole grain intakes in the diets of Irish children and teenagers. *Br. J. Nutr.*, 110, 354–362.

16 van der Kamp, J.W., Poutanen, K., Seal, C.J., et al. (2014). The HEALTHGRAIN definition of "whole grain." *Food Nutr. Res.*, 58, 22100.

17 AACCI. (2013). AACI's Whole Grains Working Group Unveils New Whole Grain Products Characterization. http://www.aaccnet.org/about/newsreleases/Pages/WholeGrainProductCharacterization.aspx (accessed April 29, 2016).

18 Jensen, M.K., Koh-Banerjee, P., Hu, F.B., et al. (2004). Intakes of whole grains, bran, and germ and the risk of coronary heart disease in men. *Am. J. Clin. Nutr.*, 80, 1492–1499.

19 Franz, M., and Sampson, L. (2006). Challenges in developing a whole grain database: Definitions, methods and quantification. *J. Food Compost Anal.*, 19, S38–S44.

20 Burgess-Champoux, T.L., Larson, N.I., Neumark-Sztainer, D.R., et al. (2010). Longitudinal and secular trends in adolescent whole-grain consumption, 1999–2004. *Am. J. Clin. Nutr.*, 91, 154–159.

21 Grandjean, A.C., Fulgoni, V.L., III, Reimers, K.J., et al. (2008). Popcorn consumption and dietary and physiological parameters of US children and adults: Analysis of the National Health and Nutrition Examination Survey (NHANES) 1999–2002 dietary survey data. *J. Am. Diet. Assoc.*, 108, 853–856.

22 Mozaffarian, R.S., Lee, R.M., Kennedy, M.A., et al. (2013). Identifying whole grain foods: A comparison of different approaches for selecting more healthful whole grain products. *Public Health Nutr.*, 16, 2255–2264.

23 Hemery, Y., Lullien-Pellerin, V., Rouau, X. et al. (2009). Biochemical markers: Efficient tools for the assessment of wheat grain tissue proportions in milling fractions. *Journal of Cereal Science.* 49, 55–64.

24 Ross, A.B. (2012). Present status and perspectives on the use of alkylresorcinols as biomarkers of wholegrain wheat and rye intake. *J. Nutr. Metab.*, 2012, 1–12.

25 Ross, A.B., Svelander, C., Karlsson, G., et al. (2017). Identification and quantification of even and odd chained 5-n alkylresorcinols, branched chain-alkylresorcinols and methylalkylresorcinols in Quinoa (Chenopodium quinoa). *Food Chem.*, 220, 344–351.

26 Chen, Y., Ross, A.B., Åman, P., et al. (2004). Alkylresorcinols as markers of whole grain wheat and rye in cereal products. *J. Agric. Food Chem.*, 52, 8242–8246.
27 Kristensen, M., Pelletier, X., Ross, A.B., et al. (2017). A high rate of non-compliance confounds the study of whole grains and weight maintenance in a randomised intervention trial – The case for greater use of dietary biomarkers in nutrition intervention studies. *Nutrients*, 9.
28 Ross, A.B., Bourgeois, A., Macharia, H.N., et al. (2012). Plasma alkylresorcinols as a biomarker of whole grain food consumption in a large population – Results from the WHOLEheart intervention study. *Am. J. Clin. Nutr.*, 95, 204–211.
29 Harris Jackson, K., West, S.G., Vanden Heuvel, J.P., et al. (2014). Effects of whole and refined grains in a weight-loss diet on markers of metabolic syndrome in individuals with increased waist circumference: A randomized controlled-feeding trial. *The American Journal of Clinical Nutrition*, 100, 577–586
30 Kirwan, J.P., Malin, S.K., Scelsi, A.R., et al. (2016). A Whole-grain diet reduces cardiovascular risk factors in overweight and obese adults: A randomized controlled trial. *The Journal of Nutrition*, 146, 2244–2251.
31 Kristensen, M., Toubro, S., Jensen, M.G., et al. (2012). Whole grain compared with refined wheat decreases the percentage of body fat following a 12-week, energy-restricted dietary intervention in postmenopausal women. *J. Nutr.*, 142, 710–716.
32 Ross. A.B., Bruce, S.J., Blondel-Lubrano, A., et al. (2011). A whole-grain cereal-rich diet increases plasma betaine, and tends to decrease total and LDL-cholesterol compared with a refined-grain diet in healthy subjects. *Br. J. Nutr.*, 105, 1492–1502.
33 Ross, A.B., Kristensen, M., Seal, C.J., et al. (2015). Recommendations for reporting whole-grain intake in observational and intervention studies. *Am. J. Clin. Nutr.*, 101, 903–907.
34 Ross, A.B. (2012). Analysis of alkylresorcinols in cereal grains and products using ultrahigh-pressure liquid chromatography with fluorescence, ultraviolet, and coulArray electrochemical detection. *J. Agric. Food Chem.*, 60, 8954–8962.
35 Ross, A.B., and Kochhar, S. (2009). Rapid and sensitive analysis of alkylresorcinols from cereal grains and products using HPLC-Coularray-based electrochemical detection. *J. Agric. Food Chem.*, 57, 5187–5193.
36 Andersson, A.A.M., Åman, P., Wandel, M., et al. (2010). Alkylresorcinols in wheat and rye flour and bread. *J. Food Compost Anal.*, 23, 794–801.

6 Whole grain consumption and associated lifestyle and sociodemographic factors

Cecilie Kyrø and Anja Olsen

Danish Cancer Society Research Center, Copenhagen, Denmark

6.1 Introduction

The extent of whole grain consumption differs substantially worldwide. The health benefits of dietary fibre have been in focus for a while, but it was not until recently that the focus has been turned to health benefits of whole grains as such. Today, many national authorities are advising the general population to increase the consumption of whole grains in relation to refined grains. The cereals wheat, barley, rye and oats originate from the Middle East; corn/maize, from Central America; millet and sorghum (Durra), from West Africa, while rice originates from Asia (Bjørnstad 2010). These staples are now cultivated throughout the world, the location depending on climate and other cultivation conditions. Due to globalization, cereals are commodities that are traded internationally, and the type consumed in different countries depends on availability, preference and traditional food habits. Besides differences in whole grain intake between countries, whole grain intake also varies within countries. Like other healthy foods, intake is associated with other health-related factors such as fruit and vegetable consumption, socioeconomic status, societal trends, and so on. The outcomes of observational studies of whole grain intake are therefore sensitive to these confounding factors and may lead to an over- or underestimation of the true association (Rothman and Greenland 1998).

The main problem gathering information on global whole grain intake is that it is usually collected by the national authorities, and if made publicly available, it is often made available only in the native language. Thus, few countries report information on whole grain intake in peer-reviewed journals. We have found one publication that has systematically collected information on whole grain intake from national health authorities (Micha et al. 2015). We present the main results from this paper as well as data obtained from peer-reviewed papers in English.

6.2 Global whole grain intake

A paper was published in 2015 in which data were used from 35 surveys in 25 countries, representing 41% of the world's adult population. The data was supplemented with FAO food balance sheets (Micha et al. 2015), thus the results are rather crude and should be interpreted with caution. In the next section, we present the main results from Micha et al. (2015). We have also identified peer-reviewed single studies reporting whole grain intake.

Whole Grains and Health, Second Edition. Edited by Rikard Landberg and Nathalie Scheers.

Additional materials available for download online at https://www.wiley.com/en-gb/Whole+Grains+and+Health-p-9781118939437

For these studies, the generalizability of the findings is questionable because cohort studies often suffer from over-representation of participants with higher socioeconomic positions or participants in certain age groups. Furthermore, different *whole grain* definitions are used in the studies in relation to which cereal types that are included as well as (in some cases) how much whole grains a product must contain in order to be classified as a whole grain product (i.e., whole grain quantifier). Finally, the studies are based on different ways to assess whole grain intake. In some studies, whole grain intake is assessed as *whole grain servings* or as *whole grain products*. Lately, several studies have used the calculated whole grain content (i.e., *whole grain intake in g/day*) to describe whole grain intake. Generally, one serving is equivalent to 16 g of whole grain intake or 28 g of whole grain product intake.

6.3 Whole grain intake according to Mica et al. (2015)

In the study of the global whole grain intake (Micha et al. 2015), the whole grain intake was given as *whole grain products*. The global mean intake (95% uncertainty interval) was 38 g (36–42) *whole grain products/day*. Very large variation was observed, with a fifteen-fold difference across regions. The highest intakes were observed in Southeast Asia, and in East and West Sub-Saharan Africa, and the lowest intake was observed in high-income Asia Pacific, East Asia and Tropical Latin America (Figure 6.1). Details on the country-specific intake can be found in the original paper (Micha et al. 2015).

6.4 Single studies of whole grain intake

In Table 6.1, an overview of single studies on whole grain intake is shown. Note that the studies differ in regard to year of dietary assessment, age ranges, generalizability, whole grain classification method, and so on. In some cases, the whole grain intake is given in servings per day. In these cases, the intake is recalculated to whole grain intake in g/day, based on general accepted conversions, assuming that a serving was equal to 16 g. If data on whole grain intake were available for more time periods, the newest data are presented in the tables and figures. In some cases, data is shown from more time periods for a country, if judged relevant. Data from Table 6.1 is shown in Figures 6.2–6.3, but in countries where data is available from several studies/sources, the sources that are considered most reliable and/or recent are shown.

In Figures 6.2 and 6.3, intake of *whole grains in g/day* are shown for children/adolescents and adults, respectively. Overall, the intake was observed to be highest in Scandinavia, Germany and Ireland, whereas it was low in Singapore, France, the Netherlands, the United Kingdom and the United States. Among adolescents and children (Figure 6.2), the intake was highest in Denmark, Ireland and Germany (>20 g/day). In France, the United Kingdom and the Unites States, the intake was observed to be approximately 15 g/day or lower. Among Danes age 4–14 years, the intake has increased from 28 g/day in 2000–2004 to 58 g/day in 2011–2013 (Table 6.1). The intake among British adolescents was calculated from national nutrition surveys, and seems to have decreased from the mid-1980s until 2000–2001 (Thane et al. 2007).

In the adult population (Figure 6.3), intake was highest in the Scandinavian countries (Denmark, Sweden and Norway), and was observed to be approximately 10 g/day in France, the United Kingdom, the United States, the Netherlands and Singapore.

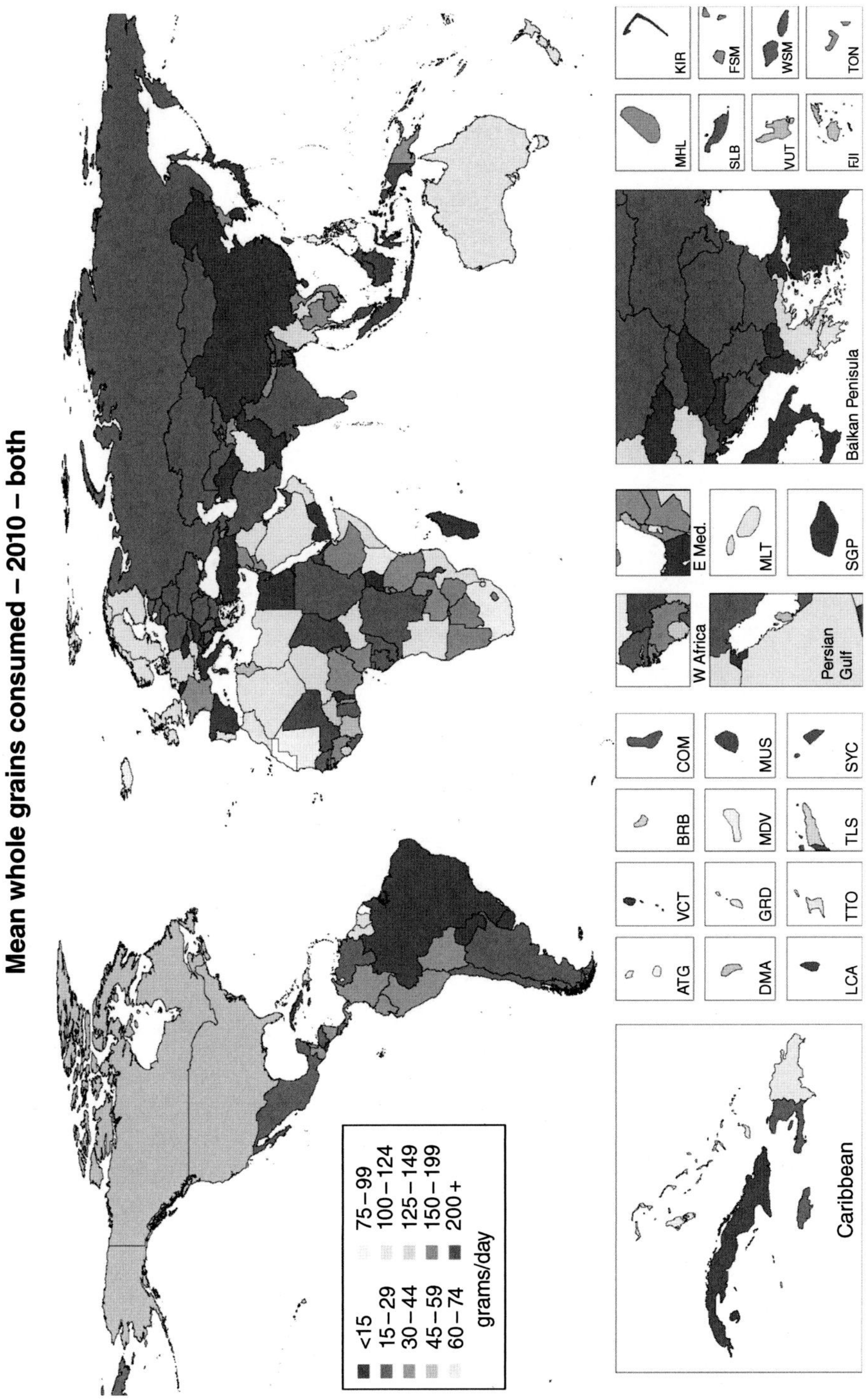

Figure 6.1 Global and regional mean whole grains consumed (g products/day) in 2010 for adults ≥20 years of age. (Source: Micha et al. [2015]). (*See color representation of this figure in the color plate section*).

Table 6.1 Whole grain intake in different countries, means with standard deviations (SD) or standard error (SE) or medians. In alphabetical order.

Country	Year – assessment	No. of subjects	Age	Sex	Intake (mean)	SD (SE[1])	Ref.
Denmark	1993–1997	1922	50–65	Men	48	42	(Kyro et al. 2012)
Denmark	1993–1997	1994	50–65	Women	37	32	
Denmark	2000–2004	1159	4–14	Both	28		(DTU Food 2008
Denmark	2000–2004	4692	15–75	Both	33		
Denmark	2011–2012	762	4–14	Both	58		(Mejborn et al. 2014)
Denmark	2011–2012	3189	15–75	Both	58		
France	2009–2010	1171	3–17	Both	4.1	0.3[1]	(Bellisle et al. 2014)
France	2009–2010	1389	18+	Both	4.7	0.3[1]	
Germany	1997–2008	262	2–5	Boys	20.3	20.3	(Alexy et al. 2010)
Germany	1997–2008	280	6–12	Boys	27.1	29.5	
Germany	1997–2008	170	13–18	Boys	33.1	43.7	
Germany	1997–2008	264	2–5	Girls	17.7	18.6	
Germany	1997–2008	275	6–12	Girls	21.5	22.9	
Germany	1997–2008	165	13–18	Girls	24.1	28.7	
Iran	1999–2001	357	18–74	Men	98.0 (whole grain products)	36.0	(Esmaillzadeh et al. 2005)
Iran	1999–2001	470	18–74	Women	90.0 (whole grain products)	24.0	
Ireland	2008–2010	1051	≥18	Both	29.4	37	(Burns et al. 2013)
Ireland	2003–2004	594	5–12	Both	18.5	18.2	(Devlin et al. 2013)
Ireland	2003–2004	441	13–17	Both	23.2	29.5	
Italy	2005–2006	193	3–9	Both	2.0	6.0	(Sette et al. 2015)
Italy	2005–2006	247	10–19	Both	2.2	6.7	
Italy	2005–2006	2313	18–64	Both	3.8	12.2	
Italy	2005–2006	517	65+	Both	3.3	12.7	

Malaysia	2011	2318	6–12	Boys	2.4		6.3	(Ak et al. 2015)
Malaysia	2011	2847	6–12	Girls	2.1		5.4	
Malaysia	2011	1419	13–17	Boys	1.6		4.6	
Malaysia	2011	1528	13–17	Girls	1.8		4.8	
Norway	1998	1797	40–55	Women	51		36	(Kyro et al. 2012)
Puerto Rico	2010–2011	796	12	Both	6.4		0.0[1]	(Torres et al. 2014)
Singapore	2010	1647	18–69	Both	12.2[2]			(Health Promotion Board Singapore, 2011)
Singapore	2014–2015	561	6–12	Both	0.0[2]		IQR: 0-9.39	(Neo et al. 2016)
Sweden	1992–1996	1372	30–60	Men	58		50	(Kyro et al. 2012)
Sweden	1992–1996	1617	30–60	Women	41		32	
UK	2008–2011	1502	1.5–17	Both	17.8		18.1	(Mann et al. 2015b)
UK	2008–2011	1571	18+	Both	26.2		27.8	
UK	1986–1987	2197	16–64	Both	29		34	(Thane et al. 2007)
UK	2000–2001	1724	19–64	Both	23		28	
UK	1997	1583	4–18	Both	13			(Thane et al. 2005)
US	2001–2002	3147	6–18	Both	9.0		0.5[1]	(Albertson et al. 2016)
US	2011–2012	2151	6–18	Both	11.8		0.5[1]	
US	2001–2002	4647	19+	Both	11.5		0.5[1]	
US	2011–2012	4878	19+	Both	15.5		0.8[1]	
US	1999	669	Adolescents	Men	9.0		0.5[1]	(Burgess-Champoux et al. 2010)
US	1999	822	Adolescents	Women	9.0		0.5[1]	
US	2004	327	Adolescents	Men	10.6		0.8[1]	
US	2004	400	Adolescents	Women	9.0		0.6[1]	
US	1994–1995	9323	≥20	Both	16			(Cleveland et al. 2000)
US	1994–1996	4802	2–18	Both	14.4			(Harnack et al. 2003)
US	1986	27082	40–75	Men	19.9		18.4	(Koh-Banerjee et al. 2004)
US	1994	27082	40–75	Men	27.2		19.2	

(continued)

Table 6.1 Whole grain intake in different countries means with standard deviations (SD) or standard error (SE) or medians. In alphabetical order. (*continued*)

Country	Year – assessment	No. of subjects	Age	Sex	Intake (mean)	SD (SE[1])	Ref.
US	2001–2002	14973	4–18	Both	9.0	0.32[1]	(McGill et al. 2015)
US	2001–2002	13268	19–50	Both	9.9	0.64[1]	
US	2001–2002	11541	51+	Both	14.1	0.80[1]	
US	2009–2010	14973	4–18	Both	8.8	0.32[1]	
US	2009–2010	13268	19–50	Both	11.5	0.64[1]	
US	2009–2010	11541	51+	Both	14.1	0.64[1]	
US	1999–2004	7039	19–50	Both	10.1		(O'Neil et al. 2011)
US	1999–2004	6237	≥51	Both	12.3		
US	1999–2004	2278	2–5	Both	7.2		
US	1999–2004	3868	6–12	Both	9.4		
US	1999–2004	4931	13–18	Both	10.1		
US	2009–2010	3124	2–18	Both	9.1	0.32[1]	(Reicks et al. 2014)
US	2009–2010	5918	≥19	Both	13.1	0.48[1]	

SD; standard deviation, SE: standard error,
[1] : standard error, [2] : median,

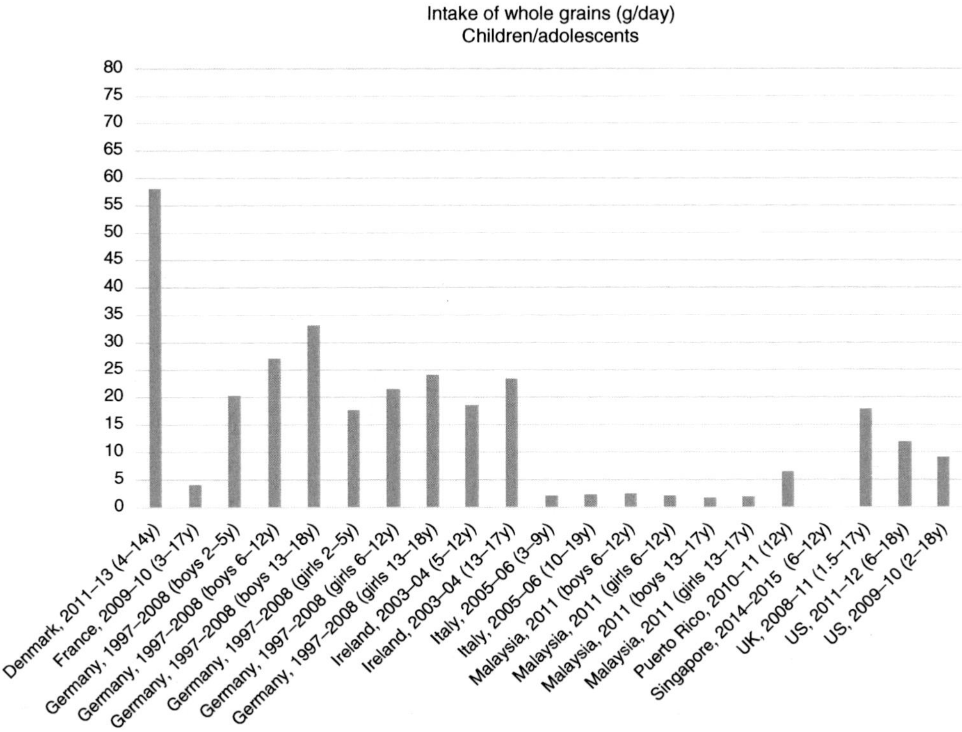

Figure 6.2 Mean whole grain daily intake in children/adolescents (g/day) presented in alphabetical order. White bars: both boys and girls, gray bars: girls, black bars: boys.

In Denmark, the intake has increased from a mean intake of 33 g in 2000–2004 to 58 g in 2011–2013. This is very likely to be an effect of the Danish Whole Grain Campaign that has focused on enlighten the Danish population of health effects of whole grain. In the other countries, no apparent change in whole grain intake was observed. However, for most of the countries this is difficult to estimate since whole grain intake is not routinely calculated.

6.5 Consumers of whole grains

In Table 6.2, the percentage of the population estimated to consume whole grains is shown. In Scandinavia and Ireland, the majority of the population consumes at least some whole grains each day. In France, Italy, Malaysia, Singapore and Germany (data available on children/adolescents only), the minority of the population were whole grain consumers.

6.6 Recommendations and compliance with recommendations

Within the last approximately ten years, the health benefits of whole grains has been recognized to an increasing extent by agencies, national authorities and nutrition societies.

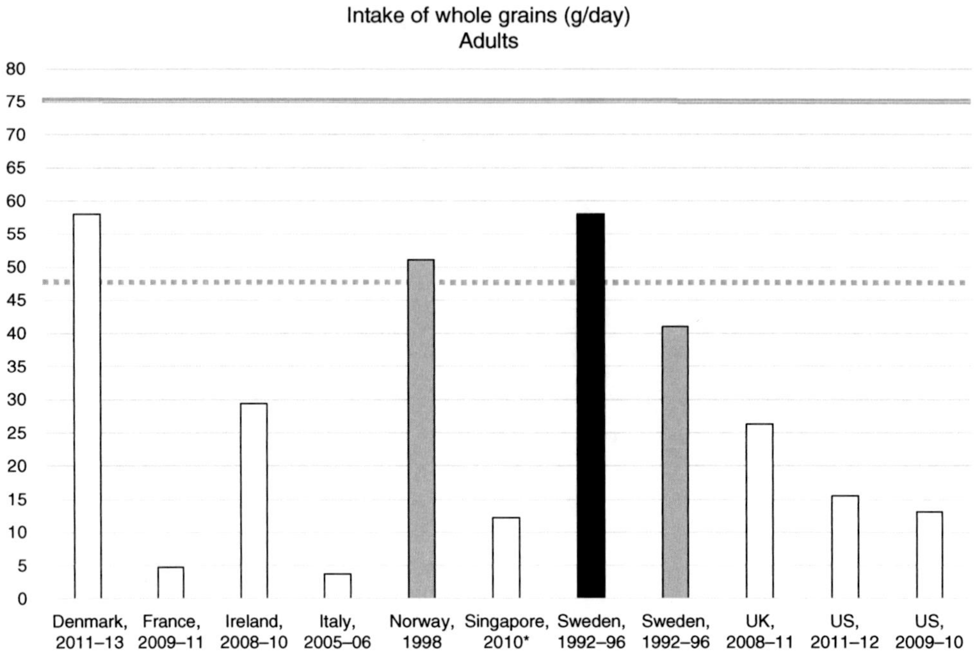

Figure 6.3 Mean whole grain intake in adults (g/day) in different populations are presented in alphabetical order. The solid line indicates the recommendation of 75 g/day and the dotted line indicates the recommendation of three servings/day (48 g/day). White bars: both men and women, gray bars: women, black bars: men.*Median intake.

In 2003, the World Health Organization (WHO) and the Food and Agricultural Organization (FAO) of the United Nations recommended that governments included whole grain in their strategy to prevent chronic diseases: "… supporting the availability and selection of nutrient dense foods (fruits, vegetables, legumes, whole grains, lean meats and low-fat dairy products" (WHO/FAO, 2003). Since then, recommendations on whole grain intake have been made in several countries. Table 6.3 shows a list of recommendations in various countries. In the Scandinavian countries, approximately 75 g of whole grains per 10 MJ are recommended each day (equal to 60 g/day for 2000 kcal) (Helsedirektoratet [The Norwegian Directorate of Health], 2016; Fødevarestyrelsen [Danish Veterinary and Food Administration] 2020; Livsmedelsverket [Swedish Food Agency] 2016). In the United States and Canada, half of the six cereal servings are recommended to be of whole grain variety (Health Canada 2014; DHHS/USDA 2015). Assuming that a portion size contains 16 g of whole grain, 48 g per day (three servings) are advised.

Few comply with the recommendations made; in Scandinavia, approximately one third complies with the recommended intake of approximately 75 g/day. Elsewhere, where the recommended intake is lower, even fewer comply with the recommended intake. In Singapore in 2010, 27% consumed at least one serving of whole grains each day. In Ireland, below 10% consumed three servings (48 g) of whole grains each day. In most countries, we have not been able to get information about compliance with recommendations, but based

Table 6.2 Estimated share of population consuming whole grains. If data were available for several assessments, only the most recent estimation are included.

Estimated share of population consuming whole grains	Countries	References
>80%	**Denmark** (children/adolescents and adults) **Ireland** (children/adolescents) **Norway** (women, 40–55y) **Sweden** (adults 30–60y) **UK** (children/adolescents and adults)	(Mejborn et al. 2014; Devlin et al. 2013; Kyro et al. 2012; Mann et al. 2015b)
>60–80%	**Ireland** (adults)	(Burns et al. 2013)
>40–60%	**France** (children/adolescents) **US** (children/adolescents and adults)	(Bellisle et al. 2014; Albertson et al. 2016)
≤40%	**France** (adults) **Germany** (children/adolescents) **Italy** (children/adolescents and adults) **Malaysia** (children/adolescents) **Singapore** (children/adolescents)	(Bellisle et al. 2014; Alexy et al. 2010; Sette et al. 2015; Ak et al. 2015; Neo et al. 2016)

on the available data, it seems plausible that intake elsewhere also are far below the recommended intake. Interestingly, the percentage of the population that meets the recommended intake has increased dramatically in Denmark and Singapore, suggesting that increased focus on whole grains has been effective.

6.7 Different cereal and product sources of whole grains

Intake of whole grains not only differs in quantity between countries, but also in regard to which product types and cereal type that are predominantly consumed. In Table 6.4, the main cereal and product sources in different populations are shown. In Singapore, the main source of whole grain is rice. This probably also applies to many other Asian countries. In Europe and the United States, the consumed cereal types are mainly wheat, rye and oats. In Denmark and Sweden, rye is the predominant whole grain source. Elsewhere in Europe and in the United States, the predominant source is by far wheat. Oats comprise around 10% of the whole grain intake in most countries in Europe and the United States. Whole grains are mainly consumed as bread or as ready-to-eat breakfast cereals (RTEBC) in most European countries and in the United States. In the United States, a large source of whole grain (7–12% of intake) is popcorn. Popcorn is not consistently regarded as whole grain in other countries. Knowledge about the preferred whole grain product and cereal types might be useful for several reasons. When conducting observational studies on whole grains and disease outcomes, it is important to keep in mind which cereal types the whole grain intake is reflected by. The different cereals have different expected health effects due to their different dietary fibre, vitamin, mineral and phytochemical contents (Frolich et al. 2013). Hence, the expected association might be different depending on which whole grain type is consumed. When making public health initiatives and recommendations, knowledge about the preferred

Table 6.3 Whole grain dietary recommendations and compliance with recommendations for different populations.

Country	Recommendation	Recommendation by (reference)	Compliance with recommendation (reference)
Arab Gulf Countries	"At least half of your daily intake of grains must be whole grain as much as possible"."	Arab Center for Nutrition (Musaiger et al. 2012)	
Australia	"Enjoy grain (cereal) foods, mostly whole grain and/or high cereal fibre varieties. 6 servings of grains food recommended for adults per day."	National authorities (2013) (National Health and Medical Research Council 2013)	
Canada	"Make at least half of your grain products whole grain each day. Adults are recommended to eat 6–8 servings of grain products each day."	National authorities (Health Canada 2013)	
Croatia	"Bread, grains and preferably whole grain products are recommended to constitute the base of the food pyramid."	National authorities (WHO Regional Office for Europe 2003)	
Denmark	"Whole grains are part of the National Dietary Recommendations 'Choose Whole Grains', and an intake of 75 g/day per 10 MJ is recommended."	National authorities (Fødevarestyrelsen [Danish Veterinary and Food Administration] 2020)	2000–2004: 6% 2011–2013: 30% (Mejborn et al. 2014)
Estonia	"Eat mostly rye bread and cereals."	National authorities (WHO Regional Office for Europe 2003)	
France	"Eat bread and starchy foods at every meal. . .. Whole grains are. . .rich in fiber. Bread should be preferably whole grain or semi-whole grain."	National authorities (Manger Bouger – Programme National Nutrition Santé 2014)	
Germany	"Plenty of cereal products – and potatoes. Bread, pasta, rice, grain flakes preferably made of whole grain, and potatoes contain nearly no fat, but plenty of vitamins, minerals, trace elements as well as dietary fiber and phytochemicals. Combine these products with low-fat food items."	German Nutrition Society (Deutsche Gesellschaft für Ernährung e.V. 2014)	
Hungary	"5–9 unit/day of cereals (mostly whole grains)."	National authorities (WHO Regional Office for Europe 2003)	
Ireland	"Bread, cereal and potatoes: 3–7 servings/day for adults depending on sex and level of physical activity. Wholemeal and whole grain products are recommended."	National authorities (Food Safety Authority of Ireland 2011)	Compliance with America recommendation (48 g/day): Children: 0% Adolescents: 3% Adults: 7% (Bellisle et al. 2014)
Malaysia	"Ensure at least half of daily cereal intake includes whole grains."	Ministry of Health, Malaysia (Seal et al. 2016)	

Mexico	"Include whole grain cereals in each meal, combined with seeds of legumes."	National authorities (Whole Grains Council 2012)	
The Netherlands	"Eat lots of fruit, vegetables and bread. Vary as much between different types of products with fiber such as potatoes, couscous, whole grains (such as whole-wheat bread, whole wheat pasta and brown rice) and legumes.... Choose within the category of bread preferably whole wheat bread and rye bread."	The Netherlands Nutrition Centre Foundation (Voedingscentrum 2014)	
Norway	"Eat whole grain products each day. 70–90 g/day."	National authorities (Helsedirektoratet [The Norwegian Directorate of Health] 2016)	75 g/day per 10 MJ Women: 35% (Kyro et al. 2012)
Oman	"It is advised to consume at least a third of daily consumption of cereals from whole grain bread and foods that contain whole grains."	Ministry of Health, Department of Nutrition (Seal et al. 2016)	
Singapore	"1 serving of whole grain products per day."	National authorities (Health Promotion Board, Singapore 2013	2004: 8% 2010: 27% (Health Promotion Board Singapore 2013)
Slovak Republic	"Increase intake of cereals and cereal products (mostly whole grains)."	National authorities (WHO Regional Office for Europe 2003)	
Sweden	"Choose whole grains when you eat bread, breakfast cereals, pasta and rice. 75 g/day per 10 MJ."	National authorities (Livsmedelsverket [Swedish Food Agency] 2016)	75 g/day pr. 10 MJ Men: 29% Women: 27% (Kyro et al. 2012)
Switzerland	"Each main meal should be served with 1 starch-rich side dish (i.e., 3 portions a day... including at least two portions of whole grain products."	Swiss Society for Nutrition (Walter et al. 2007)	
United Kingdom	"Base your meals on starchy foods. Starchy foods should make up around one third of the foods you eat. Starchy foods include potatoes, cereals, pasta, rice and bread. Choose whole grain varieties (or eat potatoes with their skins on) when you can: they contain more fibre, and can make you feel full for longer."	National authorities (NHS [National Health Service] 2016)	
United States	"Increase whole grain intake. Consume at least half of all grains as whole grains."	National authorities (DHHS/USDA 2015)	15% (U.S. Department of Agriculture and U.S. Department of Health and Human Services 2010) Adults: 8% Children: 3% (Reicks et al. 2014)

Table 6.4 Whole grain cereal and product sources in different populations. In alphabetical order.

Country	Ref. No	Preferred product type	Preferred cereal type
Denmark	(DTU Food 2008; Kyro et al. 2012)	Rye bread (≈60%), rolled oats (RTEBC), bread, muesli, etc.	Rye (≈72%), oats (≈17%), wheat (≈9%)
France	(Bellisle et al. 2014)	RTEBC, bread and toast	Wheat (≈70%), oats (8–15%) and buckwheat (7–9%)
Germany Children	(Alexy et al. 2010)	Bread, rice/pasta, grain, RTEBC and muesli	
Iran	(Esmaillzadeh et al. 2005)	Barbari, Taftoon and Sangakbreads	
Ireland adults	(Burns et al. 2013)	Bread and rolls (41%), RTEBC (33%)	Wheat
Ireland Children/ teenagers	(Devlin et al. 2013)	**Children:** RTEBC (59.3%); bread and rolls (14.4%); savory biscuits, crackers and popcorn (12.0%); other breakfast cereals (6.5%); rice, pasta and their dishes (3.9%); sweet biscuits, cereal bars and desserts (2.7%); meat, tofu and yoghurts (1.1%) **Teenagers:** RTEBC (44.3%); bread and rolls (26.5%); savory biscuits, crackers and popcorn (7.2%); other breakfast cereals (10.8%); rice, pasta and their dishes (6.6%); sweet biscuits, cereal bars and desserts (3.2%); meat, tofu and yoghurts (1.4%)	Children: wheat (65.0%), oats (16.2%), maize (12.5%), rice (3.3%), barley (1.8%), rye (0.5%) Teenagers: wheat (67.2%), oats /18.4%), maize (6.9%), rice (5.2%), barley (1.0%, rye (0.8%)
Malaysia Children/ adolescents	(Ak et al. 2015)	RTEBC (68.6%), hot cereal (18.6%), biscuits (8.7%), bread (1.8%), others (1.6%), rice (0.6%), pasta/noodles (0.1%)	Wheat (77.7%), Oats (13.7%), Maize/Corn (7.4%), Rice (1.2%)
Norway, Women only	(Kyro et al. 2012)	Bread (84%), RTEBC (8%)	Wheat (72%), rye (20%), oats (6%)
Singapore	(Health Promotion Board Singapore 2011 and 2013)	Wholemeal bread, brown/red rice	
Singapore Children/ adolescents	(Neo et al. 2016)	Rice (40.1%), breads (23.7%), pasta/noodles (19.7%), RTEBC (8.2%), sweet snacks (3.3%), savory snacks (2.9%), hot cereals (2.1%).	Rice (42.0%), wheat (39.4%), buckwheat (8.7%), oats (5.3%), maize/corn (4.7%)
Sweden	(Kyro et al. 2012)	RTEBC (≈44%), bread (≈30%), crisp bread (≈20%)	Rye (≈55%), wheat (≈18%), oats (≈15%)
UK	(Mann et al. 2015b and 2015a)	**Children/teenagers**: RTEBC (36%), whole grain breads (35%) **Adults**: whole grain breads (44%), RTEBC (27%)	Wheat (77%), oats (15%), maize (3%), rice, rye, barley, quinoa, millet (each less than 2%)
US		Children/adolescents: RTEBC (31%), yeast breads/rolls (21%), crackers and salty grain snacks (21%), cakes/cookies/pies, pastries (6%), Pancakes/waffles/French toast/crepes (6%), quick breads (2%), grain mixtures/frozen plate (2%) Adults: RTEBC (23%), yeast breads/rolls (27%), crackers and salty grain snacks (17%), cakes/cookies/pies, pastries (4%), Pancakes/waffles/French toast/crepes (3%), quick breads (3%), grain mixtures/frozen plate (1%), all other foods (1%)	
US Adults	(Reicks et al. 2014)	Yeast bread, rolls (27%), RTEBC (20%), Oatmeal (21%), popcorn (9%)	
US Children and adolescents	(Reicks et al. 2014)	Yeast bread, rolls (24%), RTEBC (25%), Oatmeal (12%), popcorn (12%)	Wheat, corn, oats

cereal types as well as product types might be helpful in attempts to increase the whole grain consumption.

6.8 Factors associated with whole grain intake

Whole grain intake has rather consistently been found to be associated with other healthy dietary habits as well as a healthy lifestyle in general. In Scandinavian cohort studies, high whole grain intake was associated with high intake of other healthy foods, including fruits and vegetables, and inversely associated with intake of red meat and refined bread. For lifestyle variables, participants with a high whole grain intake were less likely to be smokers and had lower BMI. Furthermore, socioeconomic status was associated with whole grain intake in some of the Scandinavian countries, as participants with a high whole grain intake were more likely to have a long education (Egeberg et al. 2009; Kyro et al. 2011). Based on data from the Danish national dietary survey, whole grain intake was not found to be associated with socioeconomic status, but it was found that the diet of people who ingested the recommended level of whole grains had a more favorable health profile and were less likely to be smokers (DTU Food 2008). A Norwegian cohort study investigating the association between whole grain intake and mortality also looked at differences between consumers and non-consumers of whole grains (Jacobs et al. 2001). It was found that consumers of whole grain had a healthier diet, for example, a lower intake of total and saturated fat, and were less likely to be smokers.

US and UK studies also found that whole grain consumers were of more healthy body weight/body composition and were inclined to be on healthier diets. Additionally, it was also found that whole grain consumers were less likely to be smokers and had higher education (Jacobs et al. 1998; Cleveland et al. 2000; Lang and Jebb 2003; Koh-Banerjee et al. 2004). Finally, a systematic review found that whole grain intake was associated with lower BMI and central adiposity. Furthermore, whole grain consumers were found to be less likely to smoke, more likely to be physical active, and had a lower intake of fat and a higher intake of dietary fibre (Harland and Garton 2008).

Overall, the evidence points toward that a high whole grain intake is associated with other health dietary and lifestyle factors. This is illustrated in Figure 6.4. This is important to have in mind when conducting studies on whole grains and disease risk, as these other factors can be potential confounders and thereby lead to bias of the studied associations. Furthermore, the findings also highlight a very important public health issue, namely, that healthy lifestyle factors cluster, and that the healthy part of the population might be easier to reach when making dietary recommendations. It is therefore of outmost importance to reach the population prone to unhealthy dietary habits when making health initiatives, as this group of individuals might benefit the most.

6.9 Acknowledgements

This work was supported by grants from The Danish Council for Strategic Research (project 0603-00580B "ELIN – The effects of enterolignans in chronic disease"), Wereld Kanker Onderzoek Fonds (WCRF NL; grant 2011/436), as part of the WCRF International

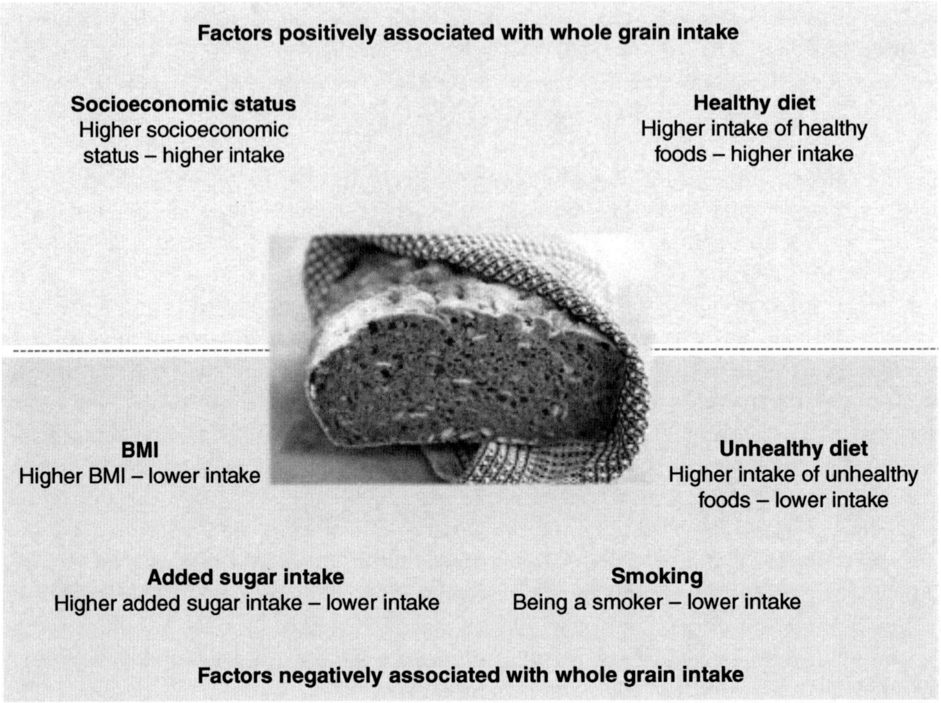

Figure 6.4 Dietary and lifestyle factors suggested to be associated with whole grain intake. BMI; body mass index. (*See color representation of this figure in the color plate section*).

grant program, NordForsk (Centre of Excellence programme HELGA; 070015), and Danish Cancer Society.

6.10 References

Ak, N., Koo, H.C., Jm, H.J., Mt, M.N., Tan, S.Y., , Appukutty, M., Ar, N. Thielecke, F., Hopkins, S., Ong, M.K., Ning, C., and Tee, E.S. (2015). Whole grain intakes in the diets of Malaysian children and adolescents – Findings from the My Breakfast Study. *PLoS One*, 10,: e0138247.

Albertson, A.M., Reicks, M., Joshi, N., and Gugger, C.K. (2016). Whole grain consumption trends and associations with body weight measures in the United States: Results from the cross sectional National Health and Nutrition Examination Survey 2001–2012. *Nutr. J.*, 15, 8.

Alexy, U., Zorn, C., and Kersting, M. (2010). Whole grain in children's diet: Intake, food sources and trends., *Eur.J.Clin.Nutr.*, 64, 745–751.

Bellisle, F., Hebel, P., Colin, J., Reye, B., and Hopkins, S. (2014). Consumption of whole grains in French children, adolescents and adults. *Br. J. Nutr.*, 1–11.

Bjørnstad, Å. (2010). *Vårt daglige brød [Our daily bread]* (Vidarforlaget: Oslo [available in Norwegian and English]).

Burgess-Champoux, T.L., Larson, N.I., Neumark-Sztainer, D.R., Hannan, P.J., and Story. M.T. (2010). Longitudinal and secular trends in adolescent whole-grain consumption, 1999–2004. *Am. J. Clin. Nutr.*, 91, 154–159.

Burns, A.M., Devlin, N.F.C., McNulty, B.A., Gibney, M.J., and Nugent, A.P. (2013). Dietary intake of whole grain in Irish adults. *Proc. Nutr. Soc.*, 72(OCE3), E135.

Cleveland, L.E., Moshfegh, A.J., Albertson, A.M., and Goldman, J.D. (2000). Dietary intake of whole grains. *J. Am. Coll. Nutr.*, 19, 331s–338s.

Deutsche Gesellschaft für Ernährung e.V. [German Nutrition Society]. *Whole-grain recommendations* Available: http://www.dge.de (accessed August 2014).

Devlin, N.F., McNulty, B.A., Gibney, M.J., Thielecke, F., Smith, H., and Nugent, A.P. (2013). Whole grain intakes in the diets of Irish children and teenagers. *Br. J. Nutr.*, 110, 354–362.

DTU Food – The National Food Institute. (2008). Fuldkorn – Definition og vidensgrundlag for anbefaling af fuldkornsindtag i Danmark [Wholegrain – definition and scientific background for recommendations], 2nd ed., November 2008, Søborg, Denmark

Livsmedelsverket [Swedish Food Agency]. (2016). *Fullkorn [whole grains].* Available: https://www.livsmedelsverket.se/matvanor-halsa--miljo/kostrad-och-matvanor/rad-om-bra-mat-hitta-ditt-satt/Fullkorn_rad/#F%C3%B6r%20h%C3%A4lsan [December, 2016]

National Health and Medical Research Council. (2013). Australian Dietary Guidelines. Available: https://www.eatforhealth.gov.au/guidelines (accessed December 2016).

Egeberg, R., Frederiksen, K., Olsen, A., Johnsen, N.F., Loft, S., Overvad, K., and Tjonneland, A. (2009). Intake of wholegrain products is associated with dietary, lifestyle, anthropometric and socio-economic factors in Denmark. *Public Health Nutr.*, 12, 1519–1530.

Esmaillzadeh, A., Mirmiran, P., and Azizi, F. (2005). Whole-grain consumption and the metabolic syndrome: A favorable association in Tehranian adults. *Eur. J. Clin. Nutr.*, 59, 353–362.

Frolich, W., Aman, P., and Tetens, I. (2013). Whole grain foods and health – A Scandinavian perspective. *Food Nutr. Res.*, 57. doi:0.3402/fnr.v57i0.18503

Fødevarestyrelsen [Danish Veterinary and Food Administration]. (2020). *The Official Dietary Guidelines*. Available: https://altomkost.dk/raad-og-anbefalinger/de-officielle-kostraad/vaelg-fuldkorn/ (accessed November 2020).

Harland, J.I., and Garton, L.E. (2008). Whole-grain intake as a marker of healthy body weight and adiposity. *Public Health Nutr.*, 11, 554–563.

Harnack, L., Walters, S.A., and Jacobs, D.R., Jr. (2003). Dietary intake and food sources of whole grains among US children and adolescents: Data from the 1994–1996 Continuing Survey of Food Intakes by Individuals. *J. Am. Diet. Assoc.*, 103, 1015–1019.

Health Canada. (2014). *Eating well with Canada's Food Guide — A resource for educators and communicators.* available at: http://www.healthcanada.gc.ca/foodguide. (Aug. 14) (accessed September, 2014).

Health Promotion Board, Singapore. (2011). *Report of the National Nutrition Survey 2010*, Singapore.

Health Promotion Board, Singapore. (2013). *Press release: more Singaporeans opting for wholegrain foods*, Singapore.

Helsedirektoratet [The Norwegian Directorate of Health]. (2016). *Kostholdsråd [Dietary Recommendations].* Available: http://helsedirektoratet.no/folkehelse/ernering/kostholdsrad/Sider/default.aspx [December, 2016]

Food Safety Authority of Ireland. (2011). *Scientific Recommendations for Healthy Eating Guidelines in Ireland* Dublin, Ireland.

Jacobs, D.R., Jr., Meyer, H.E., and Solvoll, K. (2001). Reduced mortality among whole grain bread eaters in men and women in the Norwegian County Study. *Eur .J. Clin.Nutr.*, 55. 137–143.

Jacobs, D.R., Jr., Meyer, K.A., Kushi, L.H., and Folsom, A.R. (1998). Whole-grain intake may reduce the risk of ischemic heart disease death in postmenopausal women: The Iowa Women's Health Study, *Am. J. Clin. Nutr.*, 68, 248–257.

Koh-Banerjee, P., Franz, M., Sampson, L, Liu, S., Jacobs, D.R., Jr., Spiegelman, D., Willett, W., and Rimm, E. (2004). Changes in whole-grain, bran, and cereal fiber consumption in relation to 8-y weight gain among men. *Am. J. Clin. Nutr.*, 80, 1237–1245.

Kyro, C., Skeie, G., Dragsted, L.O., Christensen, J., Overvad, K., Hallmans, G., Johansson, I., Lund, E., Slimani, N., Johnsen, N.F., Halkjaer, J., Tjonneland, A., andOlsen, A. (2011). Intake of whole grains in Scandinavia is associated with healthy lifestyle, socio-economic and dietary factors. *Public Health Nutr.*, 14, 1787–1795.

Kyro, C., Skeie, G., Dragsted, L.O., Christensen, J., Overvad, K., Hallmans, G., Johansson, I., Lund, E., Slimani, N., Johnsen, N.F., Halkjaer, J., Tjonneland, A., and Olsen, A. (2012). Intake of whole grain in Scandinavia: Intake, sources and compliance with new national recommendations. *Scand. J. Public Health*, 40, 76–84.

Lang, R., and Jebb, S.A. (2003). Who consumes whole grains, and how much? *Proc. Nutr. Soc.*, 62, 123–127.

Manger Bouger – Programme National Nutrition Santé. (2014). Cereal recommendations. Available: http://www.mangerbouger.fr/ (accessed August 2014).

Mann, K.D., Pearce, M.S., McKevith, B., Thielecke, F., and Seal, C.J. (2015a). Low whole grain intake in the UK: Results from the National Diet and Nutrition Survey rolling programme 2008–11. *Br. J. Nutr.*, 1–9.

Mann, K.D., Pearce, M.S. McKevith, B., Thielecke, F., and Seal, C.J. (2015b). Whole grain intake and its association with intakes of other foods, nutrients and markers of health in the National Diet and Nutrition Survey rolling programme 2008–11. *Br. J. Nutr.*, 1–8.

McGill, C.R., Iii, V.L., and Devareddy, L. (2015). Ten-year trends in fiber and whole grain intakes and food sources for the United States population: National health and nutrition examination survey 2001–2010. *Nutrients.*, 7, 1119-1130.

Mejborn, H., Ygil, K.H., Fagt, S., Trolle, E., Kørup, K., and Christensen, T. (2014). Danskernes fuldkornsindtag 2011-2013 [Whole-grain intake in Denmark 2011-2013]. *E-artikel fra DTU Fødevareinstitutet [E-paper from National Food Institute, Technical University of Denmark].*

Micha, R., Khatibzadeh, S., Shi, P., Andrews, K.G., Engell, R.E., and Mozaffarian, D. (2015). Global, regional and national consumption of major food groups in 1990 and 2010: A systematic analysis including 266 country-specific nutrition surveys worldwide. *BMJ Open*, 5, e008705.

Musaiger, A.O., Takruri, H.R., Hassan, A.S., and Abu-Tarboush, H. (2012). Food-based dietary guidelines for the Arab Gulf countries. *J. Nutr. Metab*, 905303.

Neo, J.E., Binte Mohamed Salleh, S., Toh, Y.X., How, K.Y., Tee, M., Mann, K., Hopkins, S., Thielecke, F., Seal, C.J., and Brownlee, I.A. (2016). Whole-grain food consumption in Singaporean children aged 6-12 years. *J. Nutr. Sci.*, 5, e33.

NHS [National Health Service]. (2016). The Eatwell Plate - Starchy foods. Available: http://www.nhs.uk/Livewell/Goodfood/Pages/starchy-foods.aspx (accessed December 2016).

O'Neil, C.E., Nicklas, T.A., Zanovec, M., Cho, S.S., and Kleinman, R. (2011). Consumption of whole grains is associated with improved diet quality and nutrient intake in children and adolescents: The National Health and Nutrition Examination Survey 1999-2004. *Public Health Nutr.*, 14, 347–355.

Reicks, M., Jonnalagadda, S., Albertson, A.M., and Joshi, N. (2014). Total dietary fiber intakes in the US population are related to whole grain consumption: results from the National Health and Nutrition Examination Survey 2009 to 2010. *Nutr. Res.*, 34, 226–234.

Rothman, K.J., and Greenland, S. (1998). Precision and validity in epidemiologic studies. In K.J. Rothman and S. Greenland (eds.), *Modern Epidemiology* (Lipponcott-Raven Publishers).

Seal, C.J., Nugent, A.P., Tee, E.S., and Thielecke, F.(2016). Whole-grain dietary recommendations: The need for a unified global approach. *Br. J. Nutr., June*, 115(11), 2031–2038.

Sette, S., D'Addezio, L., Piccinelli, R., Hopkins, S., Le Donne, C., Ferrari, M., Mistura, L., and Turrini, A. (2015). Intakes of whole grain in an Italian sample of children, adolescents and adults. *Eur. J. Nutr.*

Thane, C.W., Jones, A.R., Stephen, A.M., Seal, C.J., and Jebb, S.A. (2005). Whole-grain intake of British young people aged 4–18 years. *Br.J.Nutr.*, 94, 825–931.

Thane, C.W., Jones, A.R., Stephen, A.M., Seal, C.J., and Jebb, S.A. (2007). Comparative whole-grain intake of British adults in 1986–7 and 2000–1. *Br. J. Nutr.*, 97, 987–992.

Torres, R., Santos, E., Orraca, L., Elias, A., and Palacios, C. (2014). Diet quality, social determinants, and weight status in Puerto Rican children aged 12 years. *J. Acad. Nutr. Diet*, 114, 1230–1235.

U.S. Department of Health and Human Services and U.S. Department of Agriculture (DHHS/USDA). (2015). Report: *2015–2020 Dietary Guidelines for Americans. 8th Edition.* December 2015. Available: http://health.gov/dietaryguidelines/2015/guidelines [December, 2016]

Voedingscentrum [Netherlands Nutrition Centre]. (2014). *Eet veel groente, fruit en brood [eat lots of fruit, vegetables and bread].* Available: http://www.voedingscentrum.nl/nl/schijf-van-vijf/eet-veel-groente-fruit-en-brood.aspx (accessed September, 2014).

Walter, P., Infanger, E., and Mühlemann, P. (2007). Food Pyramid of the Swiss Society for Nutrition. *Annals of Nutrition & Metabolism*, 51, 15–2

WHO Regional Office for Europe. (2003). *Food based dietary guidelines in the WHO European Region* Copenhagen, Denmark.

WHO/FAO. (2002). *Diet, nutrition and the prevention of chronic diseases: Report of a joint WHO/FAO expert consultation,* Geneva, Switzerland.

Whole Grains Council. (2012). *Canada and Mexico promote Whole grains.* Available: http://wholegrainscouncil.org/blog/2012/11/canada-and-mexico-promote-whole-grains (accessed December 2016).

7 Alkylresorcinols and Their Metabolites as Biomarkers for Whole grain Wheat and Rye

Matti Marklund[1], Izabela Biskup[2], Afaf Kamal-Eldin[3], and Rikard Landberg[2]

[1]Gerald J. and Dorothy R. Friedman School of Nutrition Science and Policy, Jaharis Family Center for Biomedical and Nutrition Sciences, Tufts University, Boston, Massachusetts, USA
[2]Division of Food and Nutrition Science, Department of Biology and Biological Engineering, Chalmers University of Technology, Gothenburg, Sweden
[3]Department of Food Science, College of Food & Agriculture, United Arab Emirates University, Al-Ain, UAE

7.1 Introduction

Previous chapters in this book have extensively discussed the health benefits of whole grains and numerous studies have linked increased consumption of whole grains (on the expense of refined grain products) with reduced risk of several chronic diseases. A crucial part in nutritional studies investigating relationships between diet and health is the correctness of dietary assessment. The reliability of the intake estimation will have large implications for the outcomes in such studies, and inaccuracy or imprecision of the estimation may lead to mistaken conclusions (Freedman et al. 2010a, 2010b; Prentice 2010). In observational studies where associations between habitual intake and risk of disease or mortality are investigated, unreliable intake estimation may lead to misclassification of participants that, in turn, can result in over- or under-estimation of relationships between the food (or nutrient) and the health outcome (Kaaks 1997). Intake estimation is also of importance in randomized controlled trials (RCT) where participants are randomized to consume a specific nutrient, food, or diet, in parallel or in sequence, and effects on disease risk or risk factors are evaluated (Praticò et al. 2018). To allow correct interpretation of results in such studies, researchers must ensure that study participants have been compliant with the dietary instructions (Kristensen et al. 2017).

Traditionally, intake estimation has been conducted using methods based on self-reported intakes. These methods include food frequency questionnaires (FFQ), food recalls and food records. In observational studies, FFQ is usually the most advantageous of these methods as it is an inexpensive tool to reflect long-time intake (i.e., months or years), while the more detailed information of food recalls and especially food records make them suitable in RCT or for validation of FFQs (Hedrick et al. 2012; Ortega et al. 2015;

Whole Grains and Health, Second Edition. Edited by Rikard Landberg and Nathalie Scheers.

Additional materials available for download online at https://www.wiley.com/en-gb/Whole+Grains+and+Health-p-9781118939437

Penn et al. 2010; Willett 2012). However, as all these methods are based on intakes reported by study participants, they share some common sources of error. First, they are dependent on the motivation and memory of the study subjects (Fraser 2003). Second, the calculation of actual food or nutrient intake depends on the availability and quality of food databases and the coding of the dietary assessment method (Adelman et al. 1983; Slimani et al. 2000). In addition to these general obstacles related to traditional assessment tools, estimation of whole grain intake is subjected to some specific sources of error. First, participants may have difficulties in identifying whole grain products and also determining the amount of WG in such products (Kantor et al. 2001). In addition, FFQ that are regularly employed to assess habitual intake often lack detailed questions regarding Whole grain consumption (Landberg 2009; van Dam and Hu 2008). Finally, comparison of results from diverse studies may be hampered by the use of different *whole grain* definitions (Ross et al. 2015).

7.2 What is a biomarker?

To overcome some of the obstacles of the traditional assessment methods, biochemical indicators or biomarkers may be used for intake estimation. Several definitions of *biomarker* have been presented. The National Institute of Health Biomarker Definition Working Group defined a biomarker as "a characteristic that is objectively measured and evaluated as an indicator of normal biological processes, pathogenic processes, or pharmacologic responses to a therapeutic intervention" (Strimbu and Tavel 2011), and the International Programme on Chemical Safety, led by the World Health Organization, stated that a biomarker is "any substance, structure, or process that can be measured in the body or its products and influence or predict the incidence of outcome or disease" (WHO 2001). In general, biomarkers can be classified into three categories: exposure, effect and susceptibility biomarkers (Henderson et al. 1987). Exposure biomarkers include xenobiotics, their metabolites and endogenous surrogates that can be related to an exposure. In nutritional science, many biomarkers belong to this class where they are utilized to link dietary exposure and disease risk. Effect biomarkers are indicators of a change in biological function that can be related to a disease or health outcome while biomarkers of susceptibility may indicate which individuals are more sensitive to an exposure (e.g., genetics factors that influence how the body responses to the exposure) (Gao et al. 2017; Henderson et al. 1987).

7.3 Dietary biomarkers

As mentioned, biomarkers in nutritional research can be used to reflect the exposure of a food, nutrient or a dietary pattern. Due to the simple sample collection, such dietary biomarkers are commonly measured in biological liquids like blood or urine, while other biological tissues (e.g., adipose tissue, skin and nails) are more rarely utilized for biomarkers assessment. As the biomarkers represent objective measurements of intake, independent of the subjects' cognitive abilities, they can be utilized to validate traditional dietary assessment methods (Beaton et al. 1997; Bingham 2002). In addition, the biomarker may act as a ranking tool (either alone or in combination with traditional methodology) to categorize individuals based on their intake (Freedman et al. 2010a).

As some dietary biomarkers correlate with intake while other can provide absolute estimates of intake, dietary biomarkers can be classified in different categories (Gao et al. 2017; Kaaks 1997; Tasevska et al. 2006). Biomarkers for which a quantitative relationship between intake and biomarker level exists can be utilized as recovery biomarkers to provide an estimate on an absolute scale of the intake over a specific time interval (Kaaks 1997). Urinary excretion of nitrogen, sodium, potassium and doubly labeled water over 24 h are considered as recovery biomarkers of 24-h intakes of protein, sodium, potassium and energy, respectively (Bingham 2003; Livingstone and Black 2003; Tasevska et al. 2006). For concentration biomarkers, no precise quantitative relationship between intake and biomarker level exists, although the biomarker level correlates with intake and thus can be used to rank or categorize individuals. Most dietary biomarkers are concentration biomarkers as they may be affected differently by factors other than the specific intake (e.g., food matrix and genetic polymorphism of metabolizing enzymes) (Freedman et al. 2010a; Gao et al. 2017). Examples of concentration biomarkers are circulating fatty acids and plasma carotenoids as biomarkers for dietary fat composition and vegetable intake, respectively (Al-Delaimy et al. 2005; Wolk et al. 2001). A third class, prediction biomarkers, has been proposed and includes 24-h urinary excretion of sucrose and fructose as biomarkers of sugar intake. For these biomarkers, only a small fraction of the intake is recovered; however, the strong correlation between the intake and biomarker allows prediction of the absolute intake (Tasevska 2015).

Different types of dietary biomarkers may have different usability in nutritional research. The quantitative nature of recovery and prediction biomarkers makes them useful as reference instruments in calibration studies (Spiegelman et al. 2005) and they can be used as tools for compliance control in dietary intervention studies (Dragsted et al, 2018). However, until now, only a limited number of recovery biomarkers have been established and they often reflect short-term intake, which require repeated measurements or a stable intake to reflect long-term intake. Concentration biomarkers reflect a concentration at a specific time point, which prevents quantification of intake on an absolute scale. A concentration is dependent on non-dietary determinants too, such as differences in bioavailability and/or metabolism (Willett 2012).

7.3.1 Biomarker features

Two important features of dietary biomarkers are validity and reproducibility. The validity of a biomarker indicates how well the biomarker reflects what it is intended to reflect. Ideally, the validity should be assessed by evaluating the relationship between the true intake and the biomarker. As the true intake is seldomly known, the validity is usually evaluated by comparing the biomarker levels with a surrogate measure of the true intake (e.g., repeated weighed food records). Correlations between the intake estimate and biomarkers indicate the relative validity that can be considered as the lower limit of biomarker validity (Kaaks 1997).

The reproducibility indicates how stable the biomarker levels are over multiple samples (Kaaks 1997). This is an important feature, as it gives an idea of how many samples are needed to reflect the true biomarker level. The reproducibility is determined both by the pharmacokinetics of the biomarker (e.g., elimination half-life) and the frequency of intake. For example, a biomarker that is rapidly eliminated from the circulation may still have acceptable reproducibility if the intake it should reflect is both frequent and consistent in amount (van Dam and Hu 2008). The reproducibility is often estimated by calculating the intra=class correlation (ICC) (Vineis 1997).

$$ICC = \frac{\sigma_B^2}{\sigma_B^2\, \sigma_W^2},$$

where σ_B^2 is the between-person variance and σ_W^2 is the within-person variance. Thus, ICC is a measure of how big proportion of the total biomarker variance is due to between-person variations. A high ICC indicates that the biomarker level varies little within persons (as compared to between persons), which limits the number of samples needed to represent an individual's true biomarker level and thereby correctly rank individuals.

7.4 Discovery and validation of a biomarker

7.4.1 Approaches for biomarker discovery

Different approaches may be utilized in finding new potential biomarkers. First, targeted approaches are based on a priori knowledge of food composition. Compounds specific for certain foods may be hypothesized as biomarkers for food intake based on their unique presence in certain foods (Praticò et al., 2018). Thorough characterization (e.g., structure) of these compounds may help evaluate their use as biomarkers and suggest in what biological matrices they may be quantified (Wierzbicka et al. 2015). Analytical methods targeting the compounds in food material as well in body tissues or fluids should be developed.

Non-targeted methods utilizing metabolomics approaches have increased in popularity. These approaches necessitate no previous knowledge of the food composition and are based on global analysis of the metabolome resulting from a certain treatment (Scalbert et al. 2014). The major limitation of these studies is the analytical capacity to detect all metabolites of interest as well as identification of unknown compounds. However, the availability of diverse analytical techniques (e.g., GC-MS, LC-MS and NMR) allows detection of a very large number of analytes (Alonso et al. 2015). In nutritional studies, metabolomics has been used to discover biomarker candidates for a number of foods, nutrients or diets and the samples used for these analyses are usually obtained from either controlled dietary interventions or cross-sectional population studies (Gibbons and Brennan 2017). In dietary interventions, the metabolome in different biofluids (e.g., plasma, serum or urine) can be analyzed after a single dose or after repeated doses in a certain time period. Compounds that differ between treatment groups are thus identified as potential biomarkers of that specific treatment (e.g., food, nutrient or diet). It is also possible to compare the metabolome in the same individual before and after the treatment. However, candidate biomarkers identified in short-term intervention may not be specific for the food in free-living individuals due to large variations in background diets. Thus, findings from such studies should preferably be verified in cross-sectional studies. When samples from cross-sectional studies are utilized, individuals with extreme intakes of the exposure of interest are identified with traditional dietary assessment methods. The metabolome of individuals with high intakes is compared to the metabolome of non- or low-consumers and discriminating compounds may be candidates as biomarker of the exposure of interest (Brouwer-Brolsma et al. 2017; Scalbert et al. 2014).

7.4.2 Biomarker evaluation

After identification by either targeted or untargeted methods, candidate biomarkers need to be evaluated for their potential usability in nutritional research. First, a biomarker should be specific for the food or nutrient it should reflect (Marshall 2003). Although plasma concentration of vitamin C may be considerably elevated after consumption of citric fruits, this nutrient is not only present in other fruits and vegetables, but is also used as a food preservative, and thus, vitamin C may not be an exclusive biomarker of citric fruit intake (Jenab et al. 2009). Second, the biomarker should be sensitive in the sense that the biomarker level should be affected by the quantity of intake, and thus, enable the differentiation of low- and high-consumers (Marshall 2003; Spencer et al. 2008; van Dam and Hunter 2012). The sensitivity of the biomarker is affected by several factors. First, the bioavailability determines how much of the consumed biomarker that actually reaches the circulation and is dependent not only on the uptake from the intestinal lumen, but also the degree of elimination in the gut wall and liver. Several dietary and non-dietary factors affect the bioavailability, for example, food matrices impact the uptake into the gut wall, dietary fats increase absorption of fat-soluble vitamins, and metabolizing enzymes are influenced by dietary components and genetic polymorphism. Second, many endogenous and xenobiotic compounds are under strict homeostatic control, and thus, the dose-response relationship of the compound is nonexistent or very weak. Third, the temporal aspect of the biomarker determines how well it reflects intake. Biomarkers measured in adipose tissue have usually a slow turn-over, and thus, are more able to reflect long-term intakes compared to most biomarkers measured in body fluids, which often are more quickly eliminated from the body (Jenab et al. 2009; Willett 2012). However, even biomarkers with fast elimination may provide good estimates of habitual intake if the consumption is regular in both amount and time (van Dam and Hu 2008).

The pharmacokinetics of the biomarker should preferably be assessed to evaluate the time interval of intake that the biomarker reflects. Pharmacokinetic studies of nutritional biomarkers are usually conducted by repeatedly measure biomarker levels after a single-dose consumption of the food interest and can provide quantitative data regarding absorption, distribution, metabolism, and excretion (ADME). Such studies are mainly performed utilizing data from biomarkers measured in blood compartments, but different types of matrices (e.g., urine) can be used. In addition to providing basal information on maximal concentration, time to reach maximal concentration, half-life and area under the concentration curve, data from these studies can be evaluated in compartmental mathematical models that may generate or support hypotheses on different pathways involved in biomarker ADME (Marklund et al. 2014b, 2013c). As previously described, reproducibility and validity are important features of the biomarker and should be evaluated thoroughly in the population of interest (Landberg et al. 2014; Peeters et al. 2007).

7.5 Biomarkers of whole grain intake and cereal fibre

The development of a general biomarker that can reflect intake of all varieties of WG products eaten worldwide is unlikely, due to the wide range of cereals that are consumed as WG. Thus, it is more plausible that a biomarker can be used to estimate intake of WG products from a specific cereal or a group of cereals under certain conditions. For example, although avenanthramides are a group of polyphenols uniquely found selectively in oats are unlikely to function as reliable biomarkers of WG oat intake (Collins 1989; Sur et al. 2008; Zhang et al. 2017). This is because their concentration in oat grains is low (2–289 μg/g) (Skoglund 2008) and they are quickly eliminated from the human body (Ross 2012a). Similarly, the outer layers of rice contain high concentration (100–700 μg/g) of γ-oryzanols, a group of ferulic acid-phytosterol conjugates, which suggest that they could be utilized as biomarkers of WG rice. However, in vitro studies have confirmed that γ-oryzanols are extensively cleaved to ferulic acid and phytosterol, both found abundantly in different plant foods (Ross 2012a).

In populations were WG is a major source of dietary fibre, a good biomarker for WG intake may also be utilized to assess dietary fibre and especially intake of cereal fibre. Enterolactone, a mammalian lignan formed from plant lignans by the gut microbiota, have been evaluated as biomarker of fibre-rich foods (Stumpf and Adlercreutz 2003). Precursors of enterolactone are abundant in WG (especially from rye) and plasma, serum and urinary concentrations of enterolactone increase with WG intake (Juntunen et al. 2000; Kilkkinen et al. 2001). However, other plant foods are important sources of enterolactone precursors and concentrations in plasma and urine are considerably determined by the gut microbiota as well as other non-dietary determinants. Thus, enterolactone may rather reflect intake of plant foods or healthy lifestyle in general than consumptions of WG or cereal fibre per se (Horner et al. 2002; Johnsen et al. 2004; Kilkkinen et al. 2001; Linko-Parvinen et al. 2007).

7.6 Alkylresorcinols as biomarkers of whole grain wheat and rye

Alkylresorcinols (AR) are phenolic lipids abundant in the bran of wheat, rye, barley and triticale (Table 7.1). They consist of a 1,3-dihydroxy-5-*n*-alk(en)ylbenzene derivatives, thus they share a common structure of an aromatic benzene ring with two hydroxyl groups and one alkyl chain in meta-position relatively to each other (Figure 7.1). Cereal AR are homologs with odd-numbered side chains containing 15–27 carbon atoms, but homologues with saturated carbon chains with 17–25 carbon atoms are main and typically used for quantification (Figure 7.1) (Knödler et al. 2008; Kozubek and Tyman 1999).

Alkenyl-, hydroxyl- and keto derivatives have been also identified (Knödler et al. 2008; Suzuki et al. 1999) and contribute to about 20% of all AR in rye (Kozubek and Tyman 1999; Seitz 1992; Söderholm et al. 2011). The nomenclature of AR homologues is similar to fatty acids and indicates the length and degree of unsaturation of the carbon chain, for example, an AR with a saturated hydrocarbon chain of 19 carbon atoms is denoted C19:0 and its monounsaturated homolog C19:1. In general, the AR content in rye is higher compared to wheat, which in turn contains more AR than barley (Table 7.1). Several even-alkyl-chain, but also branched chain- and methylalkylresorcinol homologues, were identified in quinoa and in human plasma after eating quinoa and their absence in a diet without quinoa (Ross et al. 2017). Because quinoa is a pseudocereal and AR homologue fingerprint is unique compared to cereals, they are not within the scope of the chapter and will not be discussed in detail. The relative composition of the major AR homologues also differ between cereals; the amounts of the two homologues C17:0 and C21:0 are comparable in rye (C17:0/C21:0 ≈ 1.0), while in common and spelt wheat, the same ratio is ~0.1, for einkorn and emmer wheat the ratio is 0.04 and in durum wheat the amount of C21:0 is ~100-fold the amount of C17:0 (C17:0/C21:0 ≈ 0.01) (Andersson et al. 2008a; Chen et al. 2004; Landberg et al. 2006). The amount of AR in the cereal is not only determined by the cultivar, but is also to some extent determined by environment (Andersson et al. 2010; Shewry et al. 2010).

Table 7.1 Content of AR in cereal grains, bran and WG products of rye, wheat and barley.

	AR content (μg/g[2])	References
Rye		
Grains	568–1,441	(Kulawinek et al. 2008; Landberg et al. 2008b; Menzel et al. 2012; Nystrom et al. 2008; Pihlava et al. 2015; Ross et al. 2001; Ross and Kochhar 2009; Shewry et al. 2010)
Bran	1,266–4,108	(Chen et al. 2004; Kamal-Eldin et al. 2009; Kulawinek et al. 2008; Mattila et al. 2005; Ross and Kochhar 2009)
WG bread	197–707	(Chen et al. 2004; Kulawinek et al. 2008; Mattila et al. 2005; Ross et al. 2003b; Ross and Kochhar 2009)
Crisp bread	490–1,007	(Chen et al. 2004; Ross et al. 2003b)
Refined flour	44–286	(Chen et al. 2004; Kulawinek et al. 2008)
Wheat[4]		
Grains[3,5]	138–1,429	(Andersson et al. 2008a; Chen et al. 2004; Hengtrakul et al. 1991, 1990; Kulawinek et al. 2008; Menzel et al. 2012; Alastair B Ross et al. 2003b; Ross and Kochhar 2009)
Bran	2,211–4,178	(Chen et al. 2004; Holt et al. 2012; Kamal-Eldin et al. 2009; Kulawinek et al. 2008; Menzel et al. 2012; Ross et al. 2003b)
WG bread	142–608	(Chen et al. 2004; Kulawinek et al. 2008; McKeown et al. 2016; Alastair B Ross et al. 2003b; Ross 2012; Ross and Kochhar 2009)
Crisp bread	58–420	(Chen et al. 2004; Ross et al. 2003b)
WG crackers	161–305	(McKeown et al. 2016; Ross 2012; Ross and Kochhar 2009)
Breakfast cereals	131–1,784	(Chen et al. 2004; Kulawinek et al. 2008; Mattila et al. 2005; McKeown et al. 2016; Ross 2012)
Refined bread	ND-47	(Chen et al. 2004; Kulawinek et al. 2008; Mattila et al. 2005; Ross and Kochhar 2009)
Durum wheat		
Grains[3]	54–751	(Andersson et al. 2008a; Landberg et al. 2006; Ross et al. 2003b)
WG pasta	40–435	(Chen et al. 2004; Landberg et al. 2006; McKeown et al. 2016; Ross 2012; Ross and Kochhar 2009)
Refined pasta	32–44	(McKeown et al. 2016; Ross and Kochhar 2009)
Barley		
Grains	8–210	(Andersson et al. 2008b; Chen et al. 2004; Zarnowski et al. 2002; Zarnowski and Suzuki 2004)
WG products	ND	(Menzel et al. 2012)

[1]AR, Alkylresorcinol; WG, whole grain; ND, not detected.[2] Dry matter. [3]Includes grains and WG meal. [4]Includes common (*Triticum aestivum*), einkorn (*Triticum monococcum*), emmer (*Triticum dicoccum*), and spelt wheat (*Triticum spelta*). [5]The upper limit of the range was obtained by analyzing 125 samples of common wheat grown in different locations.

7.6.1 Occurrence

A vast majority of AR in the cereal kernel are located in a thin layer between the seed coat (testa) and fruit coat (pericarp) (Landberg et al. 2008b). Therefore, AR content in bran and products thereof is high. Similarly, WG flour made from all components of the cereal kernel also contains substantial amounts of AR. On the contrary, only the starchy endosperm is

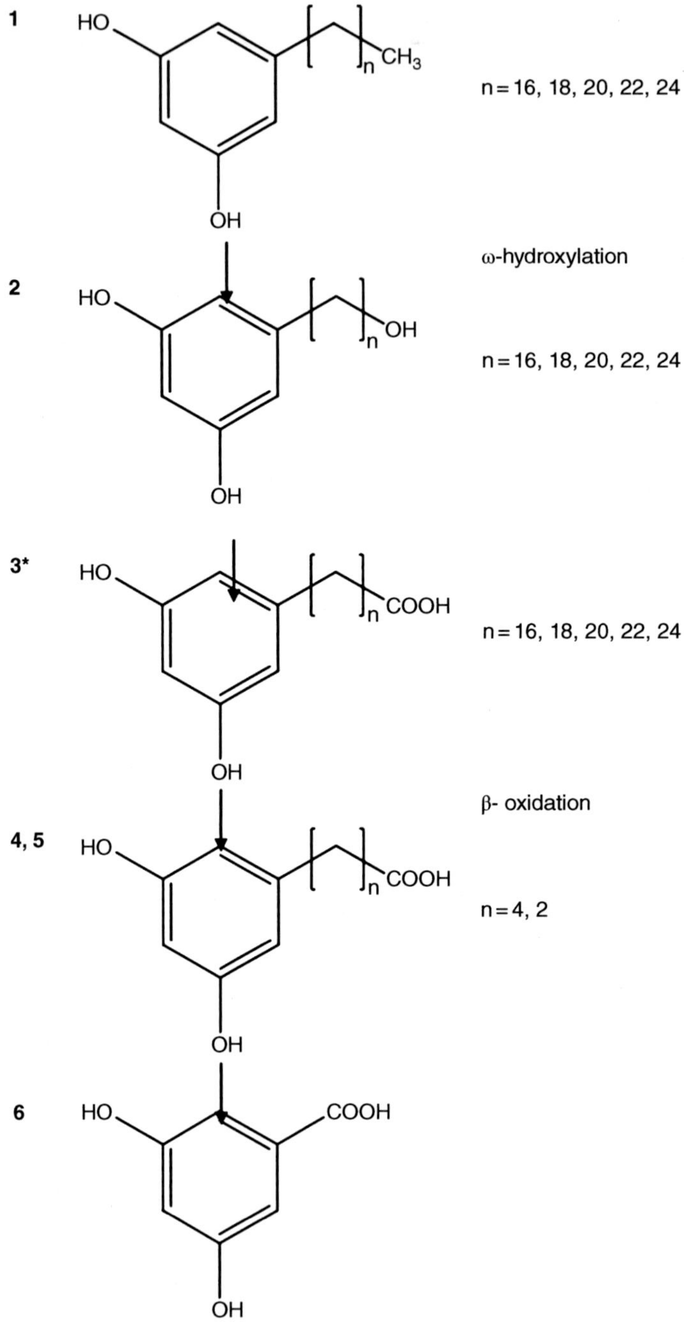

Figure 7.1 Structures and metabolism of AR. AR homologs (1) containing 17-25 carbon atoms in alkyl chain) are hydroxylated through ω-oxidation. Then, ω- hydroxyl group (2) is oxidized to a carboxyl group. The carboxylic acid (3) is further activated to an acyl-CoA ester that undergoes β-oxidation. During beta β-oxidation, the alkyl chain is gradually shortened, by two carbons at a time. Two main AR metabolites 3-(3,5-dihydroxyphenyl)-1-propanoic acid (DHPPA) (5) and 1,3- dihydroxy-benzoic acid (DHBA) (6) have been quantified in urine in free form and as a mixture of aglycones and glucuronide and sulphate conjugates (Ross et al. 2004a). Two more metabolites 5-(3,5-dihydroxyphenyl) pentanoic acid (DHPPTA) (4) and 2-(3,5- dihydroxybenzamido)acetic acid (DHHA) were suggested as metabolites from AR (Source: Wierzbicka et al. 2015; Zhu et al. 2014).

collected during the production of refined flour, and thus, AR are absent in refined flour (apart from some minor amounts resulting from bran contamination) (Table 7.1). During food processing (e.g., baking), AR form complex with starch that may lead to underestimation of AR content in cereal products unless AR are released from the complex before quantification. This release can be performed by either a hot 1-propanol:water mixture extraction (Ross et al. 2003b) or accelerated solvent extraction (Holt et al. 2012), with similar results though the latter method is more rapid. The measured AR content in foods correlates well with the AR content of the ingredients used, which thus suggest that AR are not degraded during food processing (Chen et al. 2004). Interestingly, AR have not been detected in WG products of barley (Menzel et al. 2012), although this grain contains small amounts of AR. However, as the amount of WG is highly diverse among products within the same food category, the AR content may also be substantially different in otherwise comparable products. This was displayed in comprehensive report of AR content in Swedish cereal products; for example, the AR content among 21 soft rye breads and 27 rye crisp bread ranged from 23–618, and 81–1.182 μg/g fresh weight, respectively (Menzel et al. 2012). As the homologue ratio C17:0/C21:0 differ between grains, the same ratio in cereal products may be utilized to reflect the major grain sources of the product (Kulawinek et al. 2008; Menzel et al. 2012).

7.6.2 Intake

Intake of AR is particularly high in countries where whole grain rye bread is commonly consumed (e.g., Scandinavia, Germany, Poland and the Baltic states). In Sweden and the UK, the average daily intake of AR was 18 and 12 mg/d, respectively (Ross et al. 2005).

7.6.3 Absorption

Previous animal and human studies have suggested that AR are absorbed in the small intestine after consumption. First, a study on ileal cannulated pigs fed different fractions of rye, reported that a major proportion of ingested AR were apparently absorbed in the small intestine as only minor parts of the dose were recovered in ileal effluent. Notably, diets with highest AR content resulted in the greatest recovery of AR (around 37–40%) in the ileal effluent (Ross et al. 2003a). In a rat study, 36–48% of ingested AR were collected as such in feces, while in another study (Tluscik et al. 1990), 61% of a radiolabeled AR dose was excreted in feces, mainly as intact AR, and 31% was eliminated by urinary excretion (Ross et al. 2003a). In a human study on ileostomy patients, about 32% of consumed AR were recovered as such in the ileostomal effluent, indicating that almost 70% of the dose was taken up or degraded in the small intestine. In the same study, the shorter homologues (C17:0–C21:0) were proportionally more abundant in the effluent compared to the diet, which suggest a greater absorption or degradation of longer homologues (C23:0–C25:0) (Alastair B. Ross et al. 2003).

At cellular level, the mechanism of AR absorption is still unknown, but AR in enterocytes are believed to be mainly incorporated into chylomicrons and transported in the lymph to the systemic circulation (Landberg et al. 2014). However, pharmacokinetic modeling of AR and their major metabolites in human plasma have indicated the existence of dual pathways for absorption; one prolonged and slow absorption with early onset and partial elimination of AR before reaching the systemic circulation, and one absorption pathway with delayed but rapid delivery of large amounts of AR to the central blood stream during a short time interval. Tocopherols, which share structural similarities with AR, have been suggested to be absorbed both through the lymph and by HDL-flux to the portal vein and fat intake may influence the proportions absorbed through these diverse pathways. It is possible that the quick but delayed absorption pathway suggested by pharmacokinetic modeling represents lymphatic absorption, while the other pathway represent absorption through the portal vein.

7.6.4 Distribution

In blood plasma, 70–80% of AR are present in lipoproteins whereas no AR has been detected in plasma water. Among the different lipoprotein classes, AR are most abundant in HDL and VLDL, while AR content in LDL is lower (Linko-Parvinen et al. 2007). A substantial part of AR in blood are also incorporated in erythrocytes and the ratio between plasma and erythrocytes is commonly 0.5–1.3 depending on the homologue (e.g., longer and more lipophilic homologues are more easily incorporated in erythrocytes, compared to the shorter homologues). The transfer from plasma to erythrocytes reaches equilibrium rapidly, plausibly after saturation of AR in erythrocyte membranes (Linko and Adlercreutz 2005). As suggested by studies in rats and humans, frequent AR intake may result in AR accumulation in adipose tissue (Jansson et al, 2010; Ross et al, 2004b). Adipose tissue of free-living Swedish women consuming their habitual diet contained 0–1.5 μg/g AR and long-term WG intake correlated with AR in adipose tissue (Jansson et al, 2010). AR accumulation and response to WG intervention have been confirmed in a small pilot study among men and women from the SYSDIMET intervention. AR concentration in adipose tissue in the refined diet group and the Whole grain-enriched diet group were 0.63 and 1.95 nmol/g, respectively. AR concentrations in adipose tissue were highly correlated with WG intake after a 12-wk intervention (Wu et al. 2015).

7.6.5 Metabolism

Pharmacokinetic studies have indicated rapid elimination of AR from plasma, with estimated elimination half-lives ($t_{½}$) ranging from 1.9 to 4.0 h depending on the pharmacokinetic model. If plasma AR were modeled alone, the elimination was slower ($t_{½}$=4.0 h) than the absorption and concentration of plasma AR was primarily determined by the elimination rate (Landberg et al. 2009). On the contrary, when AR and their main metabolites were modeled simultaneously, plasma concentration of AR was mainly determined by the rate of absorption, which was in general slower than the elimination, and thus, the observed elimination seldom reached the modeled elimination rate ($t_{½}$=1.9 h) due to the rate-limiting absorption (Marklund et al. 2014b). The first AR metabolites reported were discovered after comparing the chromatographic profiles of two urine samples from one individual; one sample collected after abstaining from AR-containing foods and one sample collected after consumption of whole wheat. Two phenolic acids, 3,5-dihydroxybenzoic acid (DHBA) and 3,5-dihydroxyphenyl-1-propanoic acid (DHPPA), were detected in the urine after whole-wheat intake, but were seemingly absent in the urine collected after the AR-free diet. In addition to the fact that their excretion appeared AR-dependent, the structural similarities of DHBA and DHPPA and intact AR (two hydroxyl groups in meta-positions with respect to the side chain) suggested that the two identified phenolic acids were metabolites of AR (Ross et al. 2004a). Where the major cereal AR have saturated alkyl chains, DHBA and DHPPA possess carboxylic acids suggesting that AR are metabolized in a similar manner as tocopherols (Ross et al. 2004c, 2004a). The metabolism of tocopherols is initiated by a cytochrome P450 (CYP) dependent ω-oxidation where tocopherols are hydroxylated and subsequently carboxylated. This results in a phytyl side chain with a carboxylic group at the end, which is activated by the formation of an acyl-CoA ester. The ester is a suitable substrate for β-oxidation where the side chain is gradually shortened by two carbons per cycle, until only small phenolic acids remain. These more hydrophilic acids are then easily excreted in urine (Marklund et al. 2013b; Ross et al. 2004c).

The suggested metabolic pathway of AR have been supported by the findings that AR inhibit γ-tocopherol metabolism in rats and in human Hep G2 cells, possibly through competitive inhibition (Ross et al. 2004b). Later in vitro studies have tentatively identified hydroxylated AR after incubation of AR with the enzyme catalyzing ω-hydroxylation of γ-tocopherol, CYP4F2, while incubation of AR with human liver microsomes resulted in tentative identification of both hydroxylated and carboxylated AR (Marklund et al. 2013b). The suggested metabolic pathway has since been further supported by the identification of longer-chained 3,5-dihydroxyphenolic acids in mice and human urine (Wierzbicka et al. 2015; Zhu et al. 2014). Lately, 5-(3,5- dihydroxyphenyl) pentatonic acid (DHPPTA), 2-(3,5-dihydroxybenzamido) acetic acid (DHHA=DHBA-glycine) and a sulphated conjugate of 3,5-dihydroxycinnamic acid (DHCA) have also been described as urinary metabolites derived from AR (Bondia-Pons et al. 2013; Zhu et al. 2014).

In addition to the chain-shortening phase I metabolism, AR or their metabolites may undergo phase II metabolism where they are conjugated to hydrophilic groups (e.g., glucuronate and sulphonate) in order to increase excretability (Koskela et al. 2008; Ross 2003). As enzymatic deconjugation of blood plasma does not liberate AR it is believed that AR are not present in plasma as conjugates resulting from phase II metabolism (Linko et al. 2002). However, in bile from pigs fed a high-AR rye diet, AR homologues C19:0 and C21:0 were tentatively identified, but only after enzymatic deconjugation, suggesting phase II metabolism of intact AR. This is further supported by preliminary analysis of AR and their metabolites in human fecal material (Biskup, unpublished results). About half of urinary DHBA and DHPPA were conjugated (i.e., glucuronides or sulfonides) among Swedish women and men consuming their habitual diet. While a greater proportion of DHBA was found as free aglycones, the proportion of glucuronides was comparatively greater for the less hydrophilic DHPPA, which was also suggested to be present as conjugates of both sulfonic and glucuronic acid (i.e., sulfoglucuronides). Although the absolute amount of AR metabolites in urine largely depended on AR intake, the proportions of conjugates were determined by several anthropometric and dietary factors (including age, sex, BMI and intakes of water, whole grain wheat, vitamins and minerals) (Marklund et al. 2012). Glucuronides and sulfates (or a combination thereof) are believed to be the main conjugates of AR metabolites, however other conjugates exist (e.g., glycine conjugates of DHBA have been identified in human urine) (Koskela et al. 2008; Marklund et al. 2012; Zhu et al. 2014).

The liver has been suggested as the main site of AR metabolism and incubation of HepG2 with AR resulted in the release of DHPPA to the cell medium. However, CYP4F2 and other enzymes involved in the proposed AR metabolism are expressed in other tissues, thus it is plausible that AR are metabolized at other sites (e.g., gut wall or kidneys). The initial step of AR metabolism, the ω-oxidation, is believed to be located in the endoplasmatic reticulum and the formation of hydroxylated and carboxylated AR after incubation with human microsomal S9 supports this hypothesis (Marklund et al. 2013b). Whether β-oxidation is located to the mitochondria alone or if AR metabolism also includes peroxisomal β-oxidation similar to the metabolism of very long-chained fatty acids is still unknown.

7.6.6 Excretion

As previously mentioned, conjugated AR have been tentatively identified in pig bile, suggesting this as a potential route of AR elimination (Ross et al. 2003a). Also, minute amounts of conjugated AR in human urine after wheat bran consumption presents another possible minor elimination pathway. However, the main route of AR elimination has been shown to be through hepatic metabolism followed by urinary excretion of formed AR metabolites (Ross et al. 2004a). In an intervention trial where participants consumed 33, 66 or 131 mg/d of AR, the mean proportions of ingested dose recovered as urinary DHPPA and DHBA were 89±18 (mean±SD), 59±13, and 45±15%, respectively. Hence, the urinary recovery of AR metabolites decreased with increased intakes that also were observed among Swedes consuming their habitual diet where the recovery was greatest among participants with lower AR-intake (Landberg et al. 2009).

It is still unclear if this reduced recovery is due to limitations in AR absorption, a shift in elimination route from urinary to hepatic excretion, a saturation of metabolizing enzymes and thereby increased excretion of minor longer-chained metabolites, reduced re-absorption of biliary excreted AR metabolites, or other unknown causes (Marklund et al. 2014b). In most previous studies, the DHPPA/DHBA ratio in urine is usually around 1.3–1.5 although variabilities within and between individuals and studies are large (Landberg et al. 2014). Recently, 20–25% of ingested AR were recovered as DHBA and DHPPA in human ileostomal effluent, which could be a result of microbial degradation of unabsorbed AR, AR metabolism in the gut wall or biliary excretion of hepatically formed AR metabolites. In the same study, DHBA and DHPPA were detected in pig bile, which further provide evidence of excretion of AR metabolites from the liver via the bile. The reduction of urinary AR metabolite recovery at higher doses have been hypothetically attributed to a shift in elimination from urinary to biliary excretion, and in fact, the concentration of DHPPA in pig bile increased with higher AR dose and so did the proportion of conjugated DHPPA. The presence of AR metabolites in ileostomal effluent also suggests that they are available for reabsorption and enterohepatic circulation. In addition, if plasma concentrations of AR, DHPPA, and DHBA were modeled simultaneously, the pharmacokinetic model with best fit to plasma data suggested a prolonged duration for eliminated plasma AR to re-enter the systemic circulation as metabolites (mainly DHPPA), which could indicate enterohepatic circulation. Thus, it can be hypothesized that AR metabolites formed in the liver and transported to the intestine via the bile may be excreted in urine after reabsorption (Marklund et al. 2014b). An in vitro metabolomics study, suggested that phenolic compounds identified in urine after rye consumption were potential products of hepatic AR metabolism and subsequent transformation of the gut microbiota (Hanhineva et al. 2012). However, the extent of biliary excretion, gut wall elimination, microbial transformation, reabsorption, and enterohepatic circulation is largely unknown and further research on their roles in the elimination of AR and their metabolites is warranted. Suggested AR metabolic pathway in humans has been depicted in Figure 7.2.

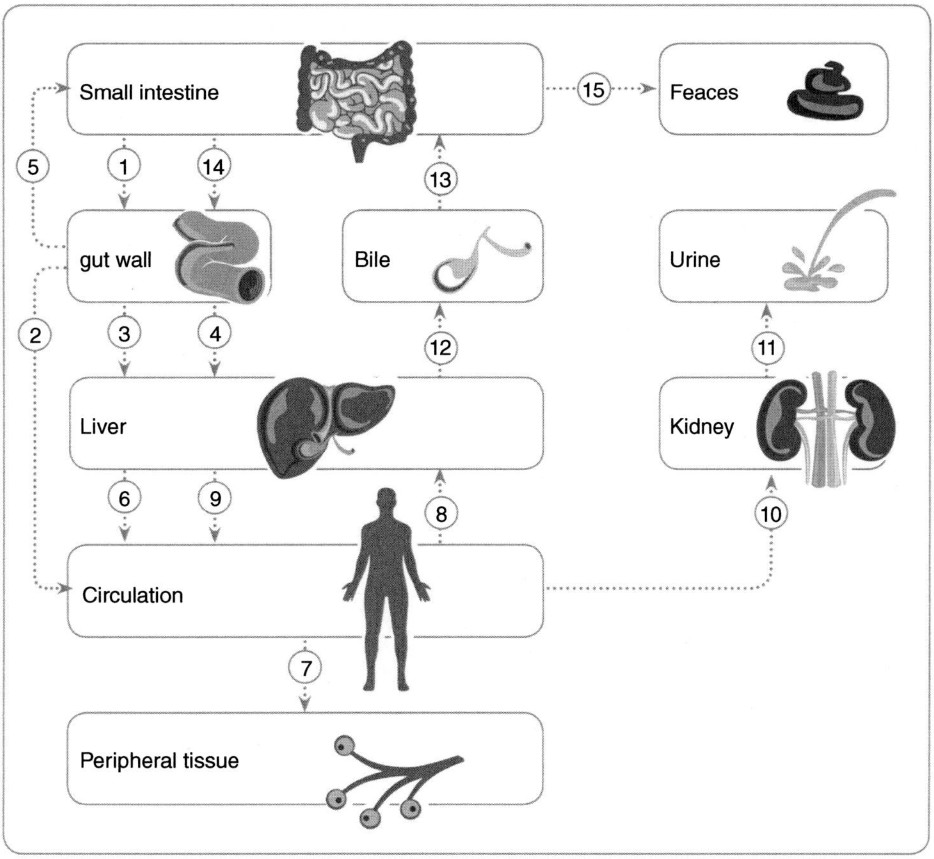

Figure 7.2 Suggested absorption, distribution, metabolism and excretion of AR. Ingested AR are absorbed to the gut wall from the small intestine (1). Intact AR are transported to the systemic circulation directly in chylomicrons via the lymphatic pathway (2) or to the liver by HDL-lipoprotein flux via the portal vein (3). AR may also be metabolized in enterocytes followed by excretion of metabolites to the portal vein (4) or the intestinal lumen (5). AR excreted to the portal vein are subjected to metabolizing enzymes in the liver, and thus, a substantial part of AR may be metabolized before reaching the systemic circulation (6). Circulating AR are distributed to peripheral tissue (7; e.g., adipocytes) or taken up by the liver (8) where they can be redistributed to different lipoprotein particles or undergo metabolism, of which the latter produces more easily excreted metabolites. These metabolites can either be released to the circulation (9) and subsequently eliminated via the kidneys (10) to the urine (11) or excreted via the bile (12) to the intestine (13). AR metabolites may be re-absorbed from the intestine (14), and thus, be available for urinary or biliary excretion. If not absorbed, AR and their metabolites eventually exit the intestine in feces (15) (Source: Based on Marklund et al. 2014b).

7.7 Analytical methods

Several analytical methods have been employed over the years to detect AR in cereal and cereal foods (e.g., fluorometry, spectrophotometry and chromatography, also coupled with mass spectrometry). A few protocols for analysis of AR and their metabolites in diverse human sample types (e.g., plasma, urine, serum and adipose tissue) have been published over the years (Table 7.2). The generally low concentrations demand sensitive and selective

Table 7.2 Analytical methods for quantification of AR and their metabolites in human samples.

Matrix	Analyte	Volume	Pre-treatment	Extraction	Purification	Derivatization	Quantification	Reference
Plasma	AR C15:0–C25:0	0.50 ml	Ionized water	Diethyl ether	Sephadex A-25	Silylation	GC-MS	(Linko et al. 2002)
	AR C17:0–C25:0	0.20 ml	None	Diethyl ether	Oasis MAX	Silylation	GC-MS	(Landberg et al. 2009b)
	AR C15:0–C25:0	0.20 ml	Deproteination	Diethyl ether	None	None	LC-MS/MS	(Ross et al. 2010)
	AR C17:0–C25:0	0.20 ml	None	Diethyl ether	Oasis MAX	Acylation	GC-MS	(Wierzbicka et al., 2015)
	AR C19:0–C23:0	0.50 ml	Deproteination	Diethyl ether	Oasis MAX	Acylation	GC-MS	(McKeown et al. 2016)
	DHBA & DHPPA	0.10 ml	Hydrolysis and pH-adjustment	Ethyl acetate	None	None	HPLC-CEAD	(Koskela et al., 2008)
	DHBA & DHPPA	0.20 ml	Hydrolysis and pH-adjustment	Diethyl ether	Oasis-MAX	Silylation	GC-MS	(Marklund et al. 2010)
Serum	AR C17:0–C25:0 AR C18:0,C20:0, C22:0, C24:0, C26:0	0.10 ml	None	Acetone	None	None	LC-MS/MS	(Choung et al. 2017)
RBC	AR C15:0–C25:0	3.00 ml	Denaturation	Heptane	DEAE- Sephadex A-25	Silylation	GC-MS	(Linko and Adlercreutz 2005)
	AR C15:0–C25:0	2.00 ml	Denaturation	Heptane	Oasis-MAX	Silylation	GC-MS/MS	(Nagy et al. 2008)
Adipose tissue	AR C17:0–C25:0	10-25 mg	None	Diethyl ether	Oasis-MAX	Silylation	GC-MS	(Jansson et al. 2010)
	AR C17:0–C25:0	10-50 mg	None	Diethyl ether	Oasis-MAX	Acylation	GC-MS	(Wierzbicka et al. 2015)
Urine	DHBA & DHPPA	0.10 ml	Hydrolysis	Ethyl acetate	DEAE- Sephadex A-25	None	HPLC-CEAD	(Koskela et al. 2007)
	DHBA & DHPPA	0.05 ml	Hydrolysis and pH-adjustment	Ethyl acetate	Oasis-MAX	Silylation	GC-MS	(Marklund et al. 2010)
	DHBA & DHPPA	0.05 ml	Hydrolysis and pH-adjustment	Ethyl acetate	None	None	HPLC-CEAD	(McKeown et al. 2016)
	DHBA & DHPPA	0.05 ml	Hydrolysis and pH-adjustment	Ethyl acetate	None	None	ELISA	(Wierzbicka et al. 2014)
	DHBA, DHPPA, DHPPTA, DHCA, DHCA-amide, DHHA	0.05 ml	Hydrolysis and pH-adjustment	Ethyl acetate	Oasis-MAX	Silylation	GC-MS	(Wierzbicka et al. 2015)

AR, alkylresorcinol; DHBA, 3,5-dihydroxybenzoic acid; DHPPA, 3,5-dihydroxyphenylpropanoic acid; RBC, red blood cell.

analytical methods, and thus, the most protocols utilize liquid- or gas-chromatography coupled to mass spectrometry detectors. To reduce the number of interfering compounds, the analyses of AR and their metabolites necessitate diverse degree of sample treatment, depending on the methodology employed. Furthermore, the same or similar methods utilized for human samples have been employed to analyze AR or their metabolites in animal studies for example, lymph, plasma, bile and intestine from pig (Marklund et al. 2013c; Ross et al. 2003a).

Although no study has reported systematic evaluation of long-term stability of AR and their metabolites, or how they are affected by repeated freeze-thaw cycles, we have not observed any statistical drift in quality control samples repeatedly analyzed for more than two years. Thus, AR content is seemingly stable over this time period when stored at -80°C. Similarly, up to five repeated freezing and thawing cycles of urine and plasma samples do not affect concentrations of AR or their metabolites, which suggest that these samples can be stored for longer time periods without introducing analytical bias due to poor stability (unpublished results). This is in line with the findings that AR are stable during food processing and not easily oxidized (Chen et al. 2004; Kamal-Eldin et al. 2001).

7.8 Dose-response

Increased intake of AR generally results in increased levels of plasma AR and their urinary metabolites, although large inter-individual differences exist (Landberg et al. 2008a; Ross et al. 2011). This was visualized by Ross, who used data from previous studies to present linear relationships (R^2>0.8) between mean AR intakes and mean plasma AR concentrations or mean urinary excretion of AR metabolites (Ross 2012b). Several controlled studies have so far examined the dose-response relationship between AR or WG intake and AR concentration in plasma (Table 7.3). Together, these studies clearly suggest that plasma AR concentration increases with increased intake. When AR intake was strictly controlled by providing participants rye bran flakes at three distinct dose levels (33, 66, 131 mg/d), there relationship between intake and plasma AR appeared linear for the majority of 16 participants (Landberg et al. 2009). Together with the data from other studies compiled by Ross, this indicates that plasma levels of AR is not saturated at higher intakes, as otherwise may have been expected given that the proportion of consumed AR apparently absorbed decreases at higher doses (Ross 2012b).

Furthermore, when AR intake is strictly controlled, that is. absolute amounts of rye bran per day (Landberg et al. 2009), plasma AR levels can distinguish different levels of intake and not only low or none versus high intakes. In other studies, investigating the effect of different doses on plasma AR, the intake of AR has not been fully controlled but rather the WG intake has been of interest. In two individual studies conducted in UK and US (Table 7.3), respectively, no significant differences in plasma AR were detected after 3 versus 6 daily servings of WG, due to a great variation between participants. However, it should be noted that that WG in these studies include non-AR cereals (e.g., rice and oats), and intake of rye (i.e., the richest AR source) was limited (Ross et al. 2012). Also, it is possible that these studies lacked power to statistically detect differences in plasma AR between the doses and in the American study, only three of the major five AR homologues were measured due to analytical complications (McKeown et al. 2016). Two of the studies in Table 7.3 have also investigated the response of urinary AR metabolites at different dose levels (Landberg et al. 2009; McKeown et al. 2016). Both studies reported significant

Table 7.3 Dose-response relationship of plasma AR in controlled intervention studies.

Study population	Study design	Intervention	AR intake [mg/d]	Total plasma AR [nmol/L]	Reference
Healthy, slightly overweight Finnish women (n=39)	2×8 wk randomized cross-over with 8-wk washout period	20% of daily energy intake from low-fibre wheat bread	n/a	36.6±4.2	(Linko et al. 2005)
		20% of daily energy intake from high-fibre rye bread	~200	352±25	
Healthy, slightly overweight Swedish men and women (n=30)	2×6 wk randomized cross-over with 6–8-wk washout period	Provided all cereal products as RG	6.8±1.9	59±57	(Landberg et al. 2008a)
		Provided all cereal products as WG	65.0±12.2	202±107	
Healthy Swedish adults (n=16)	3×1 wk randomized cross-over with 1-wk washout periods	Adding 22.5 g/d of rye bran flakes to habitual diet	33	148±60	(Landberg et al. 2009)
		Adding 45 g/d of rye bran flakes to habitual diet	66	210±81	
		Adding 90 g/d of rye bran flakes to habitual diet	131	455±189	
Swedish men with prostate cancer (n=17)	2×6 wk randomized cross-over with 2- wk washout period	Provided all cereal products as RG	8.2±2.0	72±101	(Landberg et al. 2009a)
		Provided all cereal products as WG	566 ±160	1159±1221	
Healthy Swiss men and women (n=17) with low WG intake	2×2 wk randomized cross-over with 5–7-wk washout period	Fully controlled diet: All cereal products as RG	5±1	44±4	(Ross et al. 2011)
		Fully controlled diet: All cereal products as WG	62±10	357±40	

Overweight and obese British men and women (n=266) with low WG intake	Three-arm 16-wk parallel intervention	Maintain habitual diet (control)	13 (10–16)	66 (56, 78)	(Ross et al. 2012)
		60g/d WG servings for 16 wk	30 (26–36)	95 (79, 115)	
		60g/d WG for 8 wk, followed by 8 wk with 120g/d WG	47 (40–55)	116 (93, 145)	
Overweight and obese Danish women (n=79)	Two-arm 12-wk parallel intervention	Replacing 2 MJ of habitual diet with RG products	3.1	~65	(Kristensen et al. 2012)
		Replacing 2 MJ of habitual diet with WG products	25.5	~150	
Healthy, normal weight American men and women (n=19)	2×1 wk randomized cross-over with 2-wk washout period	3 servings/d WG wheat (48 g)	23 (21, 24)	87 (60, 126)	(McKeown et al. 2016)
		6 servings/d WG wheat (96 g)	44 (41, 46)	103 (69, 154)	

differences in urinary excretion of DHBA and DHPPA. In the Swedish study, mean amounts of AR metabolites in 24 h collections were 76, 123, 189 μmol at AR intakes doses of 33, 66 and 131 mg/d, respectively, and the DHPPA/DHBA ratio of around 1.4 did not change over the doses. Although the excretion increased with increased intake, the recovery (i.e., the proportion of the ingested dose excreted as DHPPA or DHBA in urine) decreased from 89% at the lowest dose to 45% at the highest dose (Landberg et al. 2009). In the American study, the urinary excretion of metabolites increased when the dose was doubled from 3 to 6 daily servings of WG; the geometric mean excretion after 3 and 6 servings/d were 32 and 56 μmol/d, respectively. While the mean DHPPA/DHBA ratio after 3 and 6 servings differed significantly and were 3.3 and 2.8, respectively, no difference in recovery was observed between doses (McKeown et al. 2016). The inconsistencies between the two studies regarding recovery and metabolite ratios may be explain by a number of study diversities (e.g., dose amount, dose matrix, cereal origin of AR dose, study population and analytical methods).

7.9 Reproducibility

As previously mentioned in this chapter, the reproducibility is an important feature of a biomarker as it indicates how representative a single measurement is of the true biomarker status over a certain time period (i.e., the mean of infinite number of measurements in the specific time-interval) (Kaaks 1997). The higher reproducibility of the biomarker, the smaller sample size (or number of repeated measurements) is needed to enable sufficiently powered investigations of relationships between the biomarker and outcomes (Freudenheim and Marshall 1988). The relative short elimination half-life of AR and their main metabolites, suggests that their reproducibility is depended on the stability of intake (van Dam and Hu 2008). Thus, in intervention studies where AR intake is controlled, the reproducibility is expectedly higher than under free-living conditions. In a study on 17 Swedish men with prostate cancer who consumed Whole grain/bran rye products or refined wheat products during 6-wk treatment periods and three repeated blood samples were collected during the periods. Plasma AR concentration was remarkably higher during the rye period compared to the wheat period and remained stable during the treatment periods (ICC=0.88-0.90) (Landberg et al. 2009a).

Over the years, the reproducibility of AR, DHPPA and DHBA have been investigated over varying time intervals and in diverse free-living populations (Table 7.4). Short-term (3d) reproducibility of these biomarkers was assessed in Swedish men and women consuming their habitual diet. During three consecutive days at two separate occasions, blood was drawn daily from 18 participants; at one occasion after overnight fast, while at the other occasion the participants were non-fasting at the time for blood sampling. Similarly, the participants collected 24-h urine and provided spot samples of morning urine during three consecutive days. The reproducibility of total AR was considerably greater in fasting plasma (ICC: 0.60) compared to non-fasting plasma (ICC: 0.18) (Andersson et al. 2011). The participants also provided repeated 24-h urine collections and spot samples of morning urine during three repeated days at the same occasions. For the urinary AR metabolites, similar reproducibility (ICC: 0.63-0.68) as for fasting plasma AR was observed and did not apparently differ between metabolites or sample type (creatinine-adjusted morning spot vs. 24-h collection) (Marklund 2012). In the same study, the reproducibility of the same biomarkers was assessed over 2–3 mo in a larger number of Swedish men and women. At two

Table 7.4 Reproducibility of AR and their metabolites.

Time period	Study population			Matrix	Biomarker	ICC (95% CI)	Reference
	Country	N	Females (%)				
3 days	Sweden	18	61	Fasting plasma	AR	0.60 (0.36, 0.80)	(Andersson et al. 2011)
				Non-fasting plasma	AR	0.18 (0.03, 0.62)	
				24-h urine	DHPPA	0.68 (0.40, 0.85)	(Marklund 2012)
					DHBA	0.63 (0.39, 0.81)	
		16	69	Spot urine	DHPPA	0.65 (0.40, 0.83)	
					DHBA	0.67 (0.43, 0.84)	
2 weeks	Sweden	40	50	Spot urine	DHBA	0.59 (0.38, 0.77)	(Landberg et al. 2018)
					DHPPA	0.58 (0.37, 0.76)	
					DHCA	0.49 (0.27, 0.71)	
					DHPPTA	0.65 (0.44, 0.81)	
					DHHA(DHBA-gly)	0.54 (0.32, 0.74)	
2–3 months	Sweden	51	80	Fasting plasma	AR	0.47 (0.27, 0.67)	(Andersson et al. 2011)
		66	76	24-h urine	DHPPA	0.51 (0.34, 0.68)	(Marklund et al. 2013a)
					DHBA	0.46 (0.28, 0.65)	
				Spot urine	DHPPA	0.37 (0.19, 0.59)	
					DHBA	0.32 (0.15, 0.56)	
2–3 months	Sweden	69		24-h urine	DHBA	0.55 (0.11, 0.72)	(Wierzbicka et al. 2017)
					DHPPA	0.44 (0.12, 0.66)	
					DHCA	0.63 (0.49, 0.75)	
					DHPPTA	0.63 (0.49, 0.75)	
					DHHA(DHBA-gly)	0.59 (0.45, 0.73)	

(continued)

Table 7.4 Reproducibility of AR and their metabolites. (*continued*)

Time period	Study population			Matrix	Biomarker	ICC (95% CI)	Reference
	Country	N	Females (%)				
16 weeks	UK	96	49	Fasting plasma	AR	0.48 (N/A)	(Ross et al. 2012)
4 months	Germany	50	100	Fasting plasma	AR	0.55 (0.32, 0.72)	(Montonen et al. 2010)
					DHPPA	0.30 (0.02, 0.53)	(Montonen et al. 2012)
					DHBA	0.27 (-0.01, 0.51)	
		50	0	Fasting plasma	AR	0.17 (-0.11, 0.42)	(Montonen et al. 2010)
					DHPPA	0.33 (0.06, 0.56)	(Montonen et al. 2012)
					DHBA	0.23 (-0.05, 0.48)	
0–4 years	Sweden	36	100	Fasting plasma	AR	0.73 (0.56, 0.85)	(Landberg et al. 2013)
		37	0	Fasting plasma	AR	0.34 (0.13, 0.64)	
1–3 years	USA	104	100	Spot urine	DHPPA	0.31 (0.17, 0.51)	(Landberg et al. 2012)
				Spot urine	DHBA	0.17 (0. 05, 0.43)	

occasions separated by 2–3 months, these individuals had blood drawn after overnight fast and provided spot urine from the same morning and a 24-h urine collection from the day before. The reproducibility of AR in fasting plasma from 51 individuals was moderate (ICC: 0.47) and comparable to self-reported intakes of total WG (ICC: 0.44) and AR (ICC: 0.46). The shorter homologues (C17:0–C21:0) had somewhat higher ICC than the longer (Andersson et al. 2011). Similar reproducibility was observed for 24-h urinary excretion of DHBA (ICC: 0.46) and DHPPA (ICC: 0.51), while the reproducibility of creatinine-adjusted urinary AR metabolite concentrations were lower (DHBA, ICC: 0.32; DHPPA, ICC: 0.37) (Marklund et al. 2013a).

The reproducibility of fasting plasma AR over 16 weeks was evaluated in the control group of a large WG intervention study conducted in the United Kingdom. Concentration of AR was measured in fasting plasma collected from 96 overweight or obese men and women at three occasions separated by 8-wk intervals. Although the AR intake was considerably lower than among the participants in the above mentioned Swedish study, the reproducibility of fasting plasma AR in the UK population (ICC: 0.48) (Ross et al. 2012) was comparable to that of the Swedes (Andersson et al. 2011). In addition, the ICC values were slightly higher in women (ICC: 0.47) than in men (ICC: 0.43) (Ross et al. 2012). The reproducibility of fasting plasma AR, DHPPA, and DHBA over 4 months have been investigated in the 50 men and 50 women of the German EPIC-Potsdam cohort. The reproducibility of plasma AR was considerably greater among women (ICC: 0.55) compared to men (ICC: 0.17) (Montonen et al. 2010), while for AR metabolites no sex-difference was observed. However, the ICC point estimate of DHPPA was higher (0.37 in men and women together) than that of DHBA (0.32 in men and women together) (Montonen et al. 2012).

The greatest reproducibility of plasma AR during habitual diet (ICC: 0.73) has been reported among 36 Swedish women who had fasting plasma samples collected at two occasions separated by 0.1–3.9 y. However, also in this study, the reproducibility was considerably lower (ICC: 0.34) among men (n=37) (Landberg et al. 2013). The medium-term reproducibility over the 2–3 month period for four AR metabolites recently identified in 24-h urine collection was evaluated in 69 Swedish men and women known to consume WG regularly. Estimated ICC coefficients for DHPPTA, DHCA, DHCA-amide and DHHA were 0.63, 0.63, 0.78 and 0.59, respectively (Wierzbicka et al. 2017). Reproducibility of two other metabolites, DHBA and DHPPA, were 0.55 and 0.44, respectively (Wierzbicka et al. 2017) and was similar to earlier study (Marklund et al, 2013a). Good reproducibility of the new AR metabolites (DHCA, DHPPTA and DHHA) was shown in creatinine adjusted spot urine samples over a period of 2 wk from 40 Swedish men and women enrolled in the Swedish CArdioPulmonary bio- Image Study (SCAPIS) (Landberg et al, 2018). This suggest that they may be useful as biomarkers of Whole grain intake in free-living populations.

As shown in Table 7.4, most studies investigating reproducibility of AR and their metabolites have been conducted in Europe. However, one study have calculated ICC of creatinine-adjusted AR metabolite concentrations in spot urine collected 1–3 years apart from 104 women in the United States (Landberg et al. 2012). Means of self-reported WG intake and urinary DHBA excretion differed between occasions and suggested increased true WG intake, which may have affected the low reproducibility of DHBA (ICC: 0.17). DHPPA had a higher reproducibility (0.31) that was comparable to the medium-term reproducibility (2–3 months) of DHPPA in morning urine among Swedish men and women (Marklund et al. 2013a). Although the reproducibility reported in the different studies vary by biomarker, time period, study population and sample type, some general patterns can be found. First, plasma AR is seemingly more reproducible in women compared to men although the concentration is generally lower among women. Second, reproducibility of plasma AR and 24-h urinary AR metabolites are greater than those of AR metabolites in spot urine and plasma. Third, DHPPA appears to be more reproducible than DHBA in both plasma and urine. In conclusion, reproducibility of AR and their metabolites are mainly determined by consistency of AR intake.

7.10 Relative validity

Several studies have investigated relative validity of AR and their metabolites as biomarkers for intakes of WG and cereal fibre in free-living individuals in different countries (Tables 7.5 and 7.6). Correlations between self-reported WG intake and fasting plasma AR have varied between studies (Table 7.5). In a study conducted in Switzerland, 29 men and women completed a food frequency questionnaire (FFQ) at two occasions separated by 14 days. In addition, they provided a three-day weighed food record (3DWFR) in the time between the two occasions and a fasting blood was drawn within 1 week of the second FFQ. The correlation coefficients between plasma AR concentration and total WG consumption estimated by 3DWFR ($r=0.57$, $P<0.01$) and the two FFQ ($r=0.54$-0.57, $P<0.01$) were comparable (Ross et al. 2009). When relative validity was assessed in 51 Swedish men and women, total AR in fasting plasma was significantly correlated ($r=0.53$, $P<0.001$) with intake of WG wheat and rye (estimated by 3DWFR), but not to total WG ($r=0.24$) due to a large intake of WG oats (~20g/d) (Andersson et al. 2011). Also in another study, the sum of reported WG wheat and rye and WG rye separately was moderately correlated with plasma AR homologs among all Scandinavian subjects and for Danish and Swedish subjects separately, whereas WG wheat was not (Biskup et al. 2016). Among older Americans, a generally low intake of WG (median: 14g/d; estimated by FFQ) was weakly but significantly correlated to fasting plasma AR ($r=0.11$, $P<0.05$) (Ma et al. 2012). Only one study has assessed the relative validity of AR in non-fasting plasma and in that study on 360 Danish women a modest correlation ($r=0.25$, $P<0.001$) was observed between WG intake (estimated by FFQ) and intact AR in non-fasting plasma (Landberg et al. 2011).

In addition, intake of WG bread (estimated by FFQ) was correlated (0.48, $P<0.05$) with AR in adipose tissue from 20 Swedish women (Jansson et al. 2010). Plasma and adipose tissue AR concentrations were highly correlated with average WG intake estimated by food records ($r= 0.60$–0.72 ($P< 0.05$, $n= 16$) for total and individual AR homolog concentrations in the plasma; $r= 0.60$—0.84, ($P< 0.05$, $n= 16$) for total and individual AR homolog concentrations in the adipose tissue after 12w intervention (Wu et al. 2015). Wu et al. recently showed also that AR in adipose tissue were correlated with long-term WG intake estimated by FFQ, but that it did not seem to reflect long-term intake to a greater extent than plasma in free-living Swedish women (Wu et al. 2018). The relative validity of plasma AR as biomarkers for intake of cereal fibre have also been investigated in different populations (Table 7.6). In the previously mentioned Swiss validation study, plasma AR was correlated to cereal fibre when estimated by FFQ ($r=0.44$-0.60, $P<0.05$), but not when assessed by 3DWFR ($r=0.13$), suggesting a greater contribution of non-WG sources to the latter estimate of cereal fibre intake (Ross et al. 2009). Among the already mentioned 51 Swedish men and women, plasma AR were more strongly correlated to intake of cereal fibre (0.32, $P<0.05$) than to total WG (Andersson et al. 2011). Cereal fibre intake, estimated by 5-day

Table 7.5 Relationships between reported intake of WG or rye products and AR or their metabolites in free-living individuals.

	Intake						
Study population	Method	Food	g/d	Biomarker	Sample	Correlation	Reference
Healthy Swiss men and women (n=29)	3DWFR	Total WG	26±22	AR	Fasting plasma	0.57	(Ross et al. 2009)
	FFQ$^{(on\ day1)}$	Total WG	28±25			0.54	
Danish women (n=360)	FFQ	Bread	133±38	AR	Non-fasting plasma	-	(Landberg et al. 2011)
		Rye bread	62.5			0.25***	
Healthy Swedish women (n=20)	FFQ	WG bread	30–200 (range)	AR	Adipose tissue	0.48*	(Jansson et al. 2010)
Healthy Finnish women (n=60)	5DWFR	Rye intake	45±12	DHBA+DHPPA[1]	Fasting plasma	0.33*	(Aubertin-Leheudre et al. 2010b)
				DHBA+DHPPA[2]	72-h urine	0.48***	
Healthy Swedish men and women (n=51)	3DWFR	Total WG	71±52	AR	Fasting plasma	0.24	(Andersson et al. 2011)
		WG wheat and rye	47±36			0.53***	
American women (n=95)	FFQ	Total WG	16 (14, 18)	DHBA+DHPPA	Spot urine	0.41***	(Landberg et al.2012)
			23 (20, 27)			0.32**	
Older American men and women (n=407)	FFQ	Total WG	14 (median)	AR	Fasting plasma	0.11*	(Ma et al. 2012)

(continued)

Table 7.5 Relationships between reported intake of WG or rye products and AR or their metabolites in free-living individuals. (*continued*)

	Intake						
Study population	Method	Food	g/d	Biomarker	Sample	Correlation	Reference
Healthy Swedish men and women (n=66)	3DWFR	Total WG	70±52	DHBA+DHPPA	24-h urine	0.47***	(Marklund et al. 2013a)
					Spot urine	0.39**	
		WG wheat and rye	45±34	DHBA+DHPPA	24-h urine	0.61***	
					Spot urine	0.52***	
Healthy Swedish men and women (n=258)	FFQ	WG wheat and rye	74±44 (men) 53±26 (women)	AR	Plasma	0.19**-0.36***	(Wu et al. 2018)
					Adipose tissue	0.26***-0.35***	
		WG wheat	27±16 (men) 21±11 (women)	AR	Plasma	0.06-0.15*	
					Adipose tissue	0.12-0.18***	
		WG rye	47±34 (men) 32±19 (women)	AR	Plasma	0.23***-0.40***	
					Adipose tissue	0.29***-0.40***	

Table 7.6 Relationships between reported intake of cereal fibre and AR or their metabolites in free-living individuals.

		Cereal fibre intake					
Study population	N	Method	Amount (g/day)	Sample	Biomarker	Correlation	Reference
Healthy, Finnish women	56	5DWFR	10±3	Fasting plasma[1]	AR	0.38**	(Aubertin-Leheudre et al. 2008)
				72-h urine	DHPPA[2]	0.41**	
				72-h urine	DHBA	0.37**	
Healthy Swiss men and women	29	3DWFR	9±5	Fasting plasma	AR	0.13	(Ross et al. 2009)
		FFQ$^{\text{on day 1}}$	7±4			0.60	
		FFQ$^{\text{on day 14}}$	9±6			0.44	
Danish women	360	FFQ	N/A	Non-fasting plasma	AR	0.19***	(Landberg et al. 2011)
Healthy, Finnish women	56	5DWFR	10±3	Fasting plasma[1]	DHBA+DHPPA[1]	0.42***	(Aubertin-Leheudre et al. 2010a)
Healthy Swedish men and women	51	3DWFR	11±12	Fasting plasma	AR	0.32*	(Andersson et al. 2011)
American women	95	FFQ (1995)	5.8 (5.3, 6.3)	Spot urine	DHBA+DHPPA	0.40***	(Landberg et al. 2012)
		FFQ (1999)	6.4 (5.8, 7.0)			0.29**	
Healthy Swedish men and women	66	3DWFR	13±9	24-h urine	DHBA+DHPPA	0.57***	(Marklund et al. 2013a)
				Spot urine	DHBA+DHPPA	0.44***	
European men and women	810	FFQ	8 (median)[4]	Fasting plasma	AR	0.30***	(Kyrø et al. 2014a)
	1354	FFQ	8 (median)	Non-fasting plasma	AR	0.30***	

[4]Median of all participants (n=2845).

weighed food records (5DWFR), in 56 postmenopausal Finnish women was correlated with concentrations of AR ($r=0.38$, $P<0.01$) in fasting plasma pooled from 3 consecutive days (Aubertin-Leheudre et al., 2010a). Surprisingly, AR concentrations in fasting (>6 h postprandial), semi-fasting (3–6 postprandial), and non-fasting (<3 h postprandial) plasma were comparably correlated (0.30–0.32, $P<0.001$) to intake of cereal fibre (estimated by FFQ) in a multicenter study of 2845 Europeans (Kyrø et al. 2014a). Non-fasting plasma AR was also weakly correlated to cereal fibre intake in the 360 Danish women, but the correlation coefficient was numerically lower (0.19, $P<0.001$) compared to that of plasma AR and rye bread intake (Landberg et al. 2011).

Urinary excretion of AR metabolites DHBA and DHPPA has been correlated to intakes of WG in diverse populations with varying intakes (Table 7.5). Rye intake estimated by 5DWFR among 60 Finnish women was moderately correlated with DHBA ($r=0.52$, $P<0.001$) and DHPPA ($r=0.44$, $P<0.001$) in 72-h urine collections (Aubertin-Leheudre et al. 2010b). Total WG intake, estimated by FFQ at two occasions (1995 and 1999, respectively), in 104 American women was weakly correlated (FFQ_{1995}: $r=0.39$ and FFQ_{1999}: $r=0.30$) to mean creatinine-adjusted DHPPA concentration in spot urine samples collected 1–3 years in between. As expected, adjustment for intra-individual variation in biomarker concentration resulted in increased correlation coefficients (FFQ_{1995}: $r=0.60$ and FFQ_{1999}: $r=0.45$) (Landberg et al. 2012). The relative validity of creatinine-adjusted concentrations of DHBA and DHPPA in spot urine was also assessed among Swedish men and women. Daily intakes of WG (total and cereal specific) were assessed by 3DWFR in 66 men and women. The participants also provided one spot sample of morning urine and a 24-h urine collection. Both DHPPA and DHBA in morning urine were moderately correlated with intakes of total WG, WG rye, and the sum of WG wheat and rye. No significant correlation was observed to WG wheat alone, probably due to the lower intakes of WG wheat compared to WG rye (19±22 and 29±27 g/d, respectively). Similar but stronger correlations were observed between WG intakes and 24-h excretion of the two AR metabolites. The strength of correlations was similar for DHBA and DHPPA, in line with comparability regarding their reproducibility in the study population (Marklund et al. 2013a). In 69 Swedish adults, intakes of total WG intake (rye, wheat, oat, barley, maize and rice) as well as whole grain based on AR containing cereals (wheat and rye), estimated by 3-day weighed food records (3DWFR), were correlated with excretion of total six AR metabolites ($r=0.45$, $P<0.001$) and all metabolites separately: DHBA ($r=0.61$, $P<0.001$), DHPPA ($r=0.51$, $P<0.001$), DHCA ($r=0.53$, $P<0.001$), DHPPTA ($r=0.44$, $P<0.001$) in 24-urine samples from two occasions 2–3 months apart. Reported total WG intake was not correlated with DHCA-amide neither DHHA (DHBA-gly). The strongest correlations were observed for WG rye intake and DHCA, DHPPA, DHBA and DHPPTA (r = 0.53-0.70, $P<0.001$) (Wierzbicka et al. 2017).

Relative validity of AR metabolites DHBA and DHPPA as biomarkers of cereal fibre was investigated in studies in Table 7.6. In American women (n=104), urinary DHPPA was correlated to intakes of cereal fibre estimated in 1995 ($r_{crude}=0.40$; $r_{adjusted}=0.61$) and 1999 ($r_{crude}=0.25$; $r_{adjusted}=0.38$). Urinary DHBA was less strongly correlated to intakes of cereal fibre, probably due to its lower reproducibility compared to DHPPA (Landberg et al. 2012). In the Swedish population (n=66), the creatinine-adjusted concentrations of DHBA and DHPPA in morning spot urine were moderately correlated with intakes of cereal fibre. Similar but stronger correlations were observed between cereal fibre intakes and 24-h urine excretion of these two AR metabolites (Marklund et al. 2013a). Comparable correlations were observed between cereal fibre intake and DHPPA ($r=0.41$, $P<0.01$) and DHBA ($r=0.37$, $P<0.01$) in 72-h urine samples from Finnish women (Aubertin-Leheudre et al. 2008). Only one study evaluated relative validity of plasma AR metabolites as biomarker of cereal fibre intake. Correlation between cereal fibre intake and metabolites in fasting plasma pooled from three consecutive days was higher for DHPPA ($r=0.46$, $P<0.001$) than for DHBA ($r=0.41$, $P<0.01$) (Aubertin-Leheudre et al. 2010a).

The strength of the correlations between self-reported intake and biomarkers depends on several factors. First, different dietary assessment tools are designed to estimate intakes over varying time intervals. While food records allow highly detailed estimation of short-term intake, FFQ are designed to assess habitual diets over longer time periods (e.g., several months or years) (Willett 2012). As previously discussed, AR and their metabolites are quickly eliminated from the circulation, and thus, their ability to reflect long-term intake is dependent on the stability of AR intake (van Dam and Hu 2008). Second, although AR and their metabolites may be utilized to reflect intake of different dietary components (e.g., intakes of total WG, cereal-specific WG, and cereal fibre), this usability is determined by the covariance between such intakes and AR intake, which is the strongest determinant of the biomarker levels. For example, in a hypothetical population where WG rye is the major sources of dietary fibre, plasma AR may be a valid biomarker for intakes of AR, WG rye, total WG, and dietary fibre (Landberg et al. 2013). While in a different population where intake of AR is low and not correlated with total WG, cereal fibre, and total fibre, AR or their metabolites are unlikely to function as good biomarkers of WG intake or dietary fibre (McKeown et al. 2015). Also, in populations with wide ranges of AR intake, the validity of the biomarkers is usually greater as the impact of analytical error diminishes with greater between-person variation in intake (Andersson et al. 2011; Landberg et al. 2012; McKeown et al. 2015; Montonen et al. 2010).

7.11 Applications

To date, AR or their metabolites have been utilized as plasma biomarkers to investigate relationships between WG intake and disease or risk factors thereof (Table 7.7). In a cross-sectional study of 407 American men and women, plasma AR was inversely associated with BMI, trunk fat, and insulin resistance, even after adjustments for potential confounders (Ma et al. 2012). So far, plasma AR has been utilized as surrogate estimate for WG intake in prospective nested case-control studies to investigate associations to different cancers (3 studies) and type 2 diabetes (1 study). In the first study, non-fasting plasma AR was not significantly associated with incident endometrial cancer among Danish women (177 cases and 152 controls) (Olsen et al. 2010). In a nested case-control study of the European Prospective Investigation into Cancer and Nutrition (EPIC), plasma AR in European men and women was significantly associated with a reduced risk of distal colon cancer; 47% lower risk in the highest versus lowest plasma AR quartile (Kyrø et al. 2014b). No significant associations between plasma AR and incident of total colorectal cancer was observed. Later, both plasma AR alone and a combined score of plasma AR and self-reported intake of WG products were strongly associated with a reduced risk of distal colon cancer in a Nordic subsample of the EPIC cohort, while no risk reduction was observed for self-reported intake alone. The relative risks per 1 interquartile range increment of the self-reported intake, plasma AR, and the combined score were 0.84 (95% CI: 0.59, 1.19), 0.59 (95% CI: 0.41, 0.83) and 0.55 (95% CI: 0.35, 0.87) (Knudsen et al. 2014). The total AR

Table 7.7 Observational studies utilizing AR as surrogate measures of whole grain intake.

Population	N (cases/total)	Design	Outcome		Reference
Danish women	177/329	NCC	Incident endometrial cancer	No significant risk reduction.	(Olsen et al. 2010)
American men and women	-/407	CS	BMI	0.9 kg/m^2 lower geometric mean in the highest versus lowest plasma AR quartile, after adjustment for potential confounders.	(Ma et al. 2012)
			Trunk fat	1.7 % (of total fat) lower geometric mean in the highest versus lowest plasma AR quartile, after adjustment for potential confounders.	
			Insulin resistance	0.3 HOMA-IR units lower geometric mean in the highest versus lowest plasma AR quartile, after adjustment for potential confounders.	
European men and women	1372/2744	NCC	Incident total colorectal cancer	No significant risk reduction.	(Kyrø et al. 2014b)
	427/854		Incident distal colon cancer	47% lower risk in the highest versus the lowest quartile of plasma AR, after adjusting for potential confounders.	
Men and women from Denmark, Norway, Sweden	287/574	NCC	Incident total colon cancer	No significant risk reduction.	(Knudsen et al. 2014)
	198/396		Incident distal colon cancer	66% lower risk in the highest versus the lowest quartile plasma AR, after adjusting for potential confounders.	
Men and women from Sweden and Denmark	975/1950	NCC	Risk of T2D	Total plasma AR was not associated with a lower risk of T2D. In contrast, the plasma C17:0/C21:0 ratio was inversely associated with T2D.	(Biskup et al. 2016)
Chinese men and women	1060/1443	CC	Type 2 diabetes	43% lower risk in the highest versus the lowest quartile of plasma DHPPA, after adjustment for age, sex, BMI and family history of diabetes.	(Sun et al. 2018)
	736/1443		Impaired glucose regulation	34% lower risk in the highest versus the lowest quartile of plasma DHPPA, after adjustment for age, sex, BMI and family history of diabetes.	
Men and women from Denmark	-/516	cohort	Body weight Waist circumference	Plasma AR concentration was associated with reduced WC, but not body weight, for women (ΔWC per 50 nmol/l increment: – 0.69 cm, 95% CI: – 1.26 cm; – 0.13 cm), but no association was found for men.	(Kyrø et al. 2017)
Men from Sweden	1016/1817	NCC	Risk of prostate cancer	The increased risk of prostate cancer among men with high plasma AR metabolites.	(Drake et al. 2014)

AR, Alkylresorcinols; BMI, body mass index; CS, Cross-sectional study; NCC, Nested case control study; CC case control study.

concentration was not associated with a lower risk of type 2 diabetes (T2D) in a nested case-control study established within the Northern Sweden Health and Disease Study and the Danish Diet, Cancer and Health cohort. However, the C17:/ C21:0 ratio was inversely associated with T2D risk (odds ratio OR: 0.54; 95% CI: 0.37, 0.78) for the highest compared with the lowest quartiles in multivariable adjusted models. Analyses with WG wheat and rye intake estimated from FFQs yielded similar results (Biskup et al. 2016).

Two observational studies utilized plasma AR metabolites in a nested case–control studies (Table 7.7). In the first study, association between plasma AR metabolites and prostate cancer was examined for 1016 cases and 1817 controls in the Malmö Diet and Cancer Study. The sum of DHBA and DHPPA concentrations was positively associated with prostate cancer risk but the relationship was not linear. The lowest risk was observed among Swedish men with moderate plasma AR metabolites concentrations. The OR for high compared with moderate plasma AR metabolites was 1.41 (95% CI: 1.10, 1.80) (Drake et al. 2014). The second observational study evaluated plasma DHPPA as biomarker of WG intake in relation to type 2 diabetes (T2D) and impaired glucose regulation (IGR) in Chinese population (n=1443). The odds ratios of T2D and IGR were 0.57 (95% CI: 0.45, 0.73) and 0.66 (95% CI: 0.50, 0.85), respectively, comparing the lowest with the highest quartile of plasma DHPPA concentrations (Sun et al, 2018).

7.12 Interventions

Another potential use of AR and their metabolites is as tools to assess compliance during dietary interventions. An increasing number of studies have used AR as biomarkers of compliance in dietary interventions in recent years. In a Danish study where participants consumed whole wheat or refined wheat bread, both total plasma AR concentration and the C17:0/C21:0 ratio were utilized to confirm compliance on group level. In addition, pre-specified thresholds (<80 nmol/L and >100 nmol/L fasting plasma AR in the refined and whole wheat groups, respectively) were used to define compliance on an individual level. According to these thresholds, 40% of the participants (45% and 35% in whole and refined wheat groups, respectively) were identified as non-compliant. Exclusion of non-compliant participants did not substantially change the results or conclusions of the intervention, however a greater and more significant difference between the groups in fat mass reduction (i.e., the primary outcome) was observed in spite of the smaller sample size (Kristensen et al. 2012).

Plasma AR has also been suggested as biomarkers for a healthy Nordic diet (HND); apart from WG also rich in fatty fish, root vegetables, cabbage, canola oil, apples and berries. In a Nordic multi-center trial, 201 men and women with the metabolic syndrome were randomized to either a HND or a control diet for 18–24 wk. The groups did not differ in plasma AR at baseline (median [IQR]: 72 [73]) nmol/L), but the AR concentration in the HND group was significantly higher (106 [105] nmol/L) compared to the control group (61 [40] nmol/L). Plasma AR concentrations displayed moderate to good reproducibility (ICC: 0.44-0.72) during the last 6–12 wks of the intervention. Plasma AR was suggested as a biomarker of the HND, due to the great contribution of WG wheat and rye to this specific diet (Magnusdottir et al. 2013). Plasma AR was combined with other potential biomarkers of the healthy Nordic diet, to assess compliance in the above-mentioned intervention. Participants in each group were ranked based on their concentrations of plasma AR and β-carotene (rich in certain vegetables) as well as their plasma phospholipid proportions of fatty acids reflecting intakes of fatty fish, vegetable oils and dairy fats. Subsequently, the ranks for each biomarker were combined to a single score, which was utilized to define compliance to control or healthy Nordic diet. When the least compliant participants were excluded, differences in treatment effects increased between the groups compared to when the total study population was analyzed (Marklund et al. 2014a). A recent WG intervention study used plasma AR concentration to monitor the compliance of participants and observed that >60% of participants in the whole grain group did not follow the study design, as defined by their plasma AR concentrations <70 nmol/L, which was applied as a conservative cutoff for compliance. Therefore it was impossible to conclude any effect of WG on studied outcome (Kristensen et al. 2017).

In contrast, subject compliance to the protocol was confirmed by a difference in plasma AR in another intervention trial where WG diet reduced body weight and systemic low-grade inflammation without inducing major changes of the gut microbiome among 60 Danish adults at risk of developing metabolic syndrome. Fasting plasma AR concentrations were increased by WG diet compared with the refined grain diet ($p<0.0001$) and were positively correlated with consumption of WG ($r=0.69$, $p<0.0001$) and total dietary fibre ($r=0.52$, $p<0.0001$) (Roager et al. 2017). Absolute threshold concentrations may not be suitable to identify non-compliers, due to large between-person variation in plasma AR. Especially so in trials where differences in AR intake between treatments are small (e.g., if background intake of WG rye and wheat is not under strict control) (Kristensen et al. 2017). It is possible that urinary AR metabolites may be useful to assess compliance, however, so far this has not been investigated and their reproducibility under interventional settings is unknown. Alkylresorcinols could also be used as biomarker to monitor compliance to a gluten-free diet (Lind et al. 2016; Ross 2012b). This aspect is of special importance for patients with coeliac disease (CD) but also may help investigations on possible effects of gluten on the wider population. Preliminary results from a Finnish study, where only very small amounts of alkylresorcinols were present in a plasma sample drawn from a person following a gluten-free diet (Linko et al. 2002), have been recently confirmed in a study among Danes. A classification tree was built on the basis of plasma AR concentration to objectively determine compliance to gluten-poor diet in an 8-wk RCT with a 6-wk wash-out period. An overall participant misclassification error was 3.9% (Lind et al. 2016). Alkylresorcinols are mainly found with cereal food products containing gluten and therefore may be an alternative as biomarkers of compliance to a gluten-free diet.

New methodologies should be employed in the development of novel and existing biomarkers of WG intake, especially for grain specific biomarkers as health benefits of consumption may differ between cereals and also because the diversity of cereals consumed as WG is likely to prevent the usability of one single universal biomarker of total WG intake. With improved laboratory infrastructure and decreased analysis cost, metabolomics studies can prove useful in identifying biomarker candidates. Higher analytical through-put and lower costs enable metabolomics studies of large sample sets from cross-sectional studies which may better suited for identification of potential biomarkers for habitual intakes than samples from dietary interventions. When identified candidates have been fully validated with satisfactory validity and reproducibility, they may be utilized as surrogates of their respective intake in prospective studies, either alone or in combination with traditional assessment methods. As previously mentioned, different biomarkers may be combined to assess compliance to complex foods or diets, and it can be speculated that an array of cereal-specific biomarkers may be utilized to reflect intake of total WG.

7.13 References

Adelman, M.O., Dwyer, J.T., Woods, M., Bohn, E., and Otradovec, C.L. (1983). Computerized dietary analysis systems: a comparative view. *J. Am. Diet. Assoc.*, 83, 421—429.

Al-Delaimy, W.K., Ferrari, P., Slimani, N., Pala, V., Johansson, I., Nilsson, S., Mattisson, I., Wirfalt, E., Galasso, R., Palli, D., Víneis, P., Tumino, R., Dorronsoro, M., Pera, G., Ocké, M.C., Bueno-De-Mesquita, H.B., Overvad, K., Chirlaque, M.D., Trichopoulou, A., Naska, A., Tjønneland, A., Olsen, A., Lund, E., Alsaker, E.H.R., Barricarte, A., Kesse, E., Boutron-Ruault, M.C., Clavel-Chapelon, F., Key, T.J., Spencer, E., Bingham, S., Welch, A.A., Sanchez-Perez, M.J., Nagel, G., Linseisen, J., Quirós, J.R., Peeters, P.H.M., van Gils, C.H., Boeing, H., van Kappel, A.L., Steghens, J.P., and Riboli, E. (2005). Plasma carotenoids as biomarkers of intake of fruits and vegetables: Individual-level correlations in the European Prospective Investigation into Cancer and Nutrition (EPIC). *Eur. J. Clin. Nutr.*, 59, 1387–1396.

Alonso, A., Marsal, S., and JuliÃ , A. (2015). Analytical methods in untargeted metabolomics: State of the Art in 2015. *Front. Bioeng. Biotechnol.*, 3, 1–20.

Andersson, A., Kamal-Eldin, A., and Åman, P. (2010). Effects of environment and variety on alkylresorcinols in wheat in the HEALTHGRAIN Diversity Screen. *J. Agric. Food Chem.*, 58, 9299–9305.

Andersson, A., Kamal-Eldin, A., Fras, A., Boros, D., and Aman, P. (2008a). Alkylresorcinols in wheat varieties in the HEALTHGRAIN Diversity Screen. *J. Agric. Food Chem.*, 56, 9722–9725.

Andersson, A., Lampi, A., Nystro, L., Piironen, V., Li, L., L, J., Gebruers, K., Courtin, C.M., Delcour, J. A, Boros, D., Fras, A., Dynkowska, W., Rakszegi, M., Bedo, Z., Shewry, P.R., and Åman, P. (2008b). Phytochemical and dietary fibre components in barley varieties in the HEALTHGRAIN Diversity ScreenFibre. *J. Agric. Food Chem.*, 9767–9776.

Andersson, A., Marklund, M., Diana, M., and Landberg, R. (2011). Plasma alkylresorcinol concentrations correlate with whole grain wheat and rye intake and show moderate reproducibility over a 2- to 3-month period in free-living Swedish adults 1 – 3. *J. Nutr.*, 141, 1712–1718.

Aubertin-Leheudre, M., Koskela, A., Marjamaa, A., and Adlercreutz, H, (2008). Plasma alkylresorcinols and urinary alkylresorcinol metabolites as biomarkers of cereal fibre intake in finnish women. *Cancer Epidemiol. Biomarkers Prev.*, 17, 2244–2248.

Aubertin-Leheudre, M., Koskela, A., Samaletdin, A., and Adlercreutz, H. (2010a). Plasma alkylresorcinol metabolites as potential biomarkers of whole-grain wheat and rye cereal fibre intakes in women. *Br. J. Nutr.*, 103, 339–343.

Aubertin-Leheudre, M., Koskela, A., Samaletdin, A., and Adlercreutz, H. (2010b). Responsiveness of urinary and plasma alkylresorcinol metabolites to rye intake in finnish women. *Cancers (Basel).* 2, 513–522.

Beaton, G.H., Burema, J., and Ritenbaugh, C. (1997). Errors in the interpretation of dietary assessments. *Am. J. Clin. Nutr.* 65, 1100–1107.

Bingham, S. A. (2002). Biomarkers in nutritional epidemiology. *Public Health Nutr.*, 5, 821–827.

Bingham, S.A. (2003). Urine nitrogen as a biomarker for the validation of dietary protein intake. *J. Nutr.*, 133, 921–924.

Biskup, I., Kyrø, C., Marklund, M., Olsen, A., Dam, R.M. Van, Tjønneland, A., Overvad, K., Lindahl, B., Johansson, I., and Landberg, R. (2016). Plasma alkylresorcinols, biomarkers of whole-grain wheat and rye intake , and risk of type 2 diabetes in Scandinavian men and women. *Am. J. Clin. Nutr.*, 104, 88–96.

Bondia-Pons, I., Barri, T., Hanhineva, K., Juntunen, K., Dragsted, L.O., Mykkänen, H., and Poutanen, K. (2013). UPLC-QTOF/MS metabolic profiling unveils urinary changes in humans after a whole grain rye versus refined wheat bread intervention. *Mol. Nutr. Food Res.*, 57, 412–422.

Brouwer-Brolsma, E.M., Brennan, L., Drevon, C.A., Van Kranen, H., Manach, C., Dragsted, L.O., Roche, H.M., Andres-Lacueva, C., Bakker, S.J.L., Bouwman, J., Capozzi, F., De Saeger, S., Gundersen, T.E., Kolehmainen, M., Kulling, S.E., Landberg, R., Linseisen, J., Mattivi, F., Mensink, R.P., Scaccini, C., Skurk, T., Tetens, I., Vergeres, G., Wishart, D.S., Scalbert, A., and Feskens, E.J.M. (2017). Combining traditional dietary assessment methods with novel metabolomics techniques: Present efforts by the Food Biomarker Alliance. *Proc. Nutr. Soc.*, 76, 619–627.

Chen, Y., Ross, A.B., Aman, P., and Kamal-Eldin, A. (2004). Alkylresorcinols as markers of whole grain wheat and rye in cereal products. *J. Agric. Food Chem.*, 52, 8242–8246.

Choung, R.S., Murray, J.A., Marietta, E. V., Van Dyke, C.T., and Ross, A.B. (2017). Serum alkylresorcinols as biomarkers of dietary gluten exposure in coeliac disease. *Aliment. Pharmacol. Ther.*, 45, 643–652.

Collins, F.W. (1989). Oat phenolics: avenanthramides, novel substituted N-cinnamoylanthranilate alkaloids from oat groats and hulls. *J. Agric. Food Chem.*, 37, 60–66.

Dragsted, L.O., Gao, Q., Scalbert, A., Vergères, G., Kolehmainen, M., Manach, C., Brennan, L., Afman, L.A., Wishart, D.S., Andres Lacueva, C., Garcia-Aloy, M., Verhagen, H., Feskens, E.J.M., and Praticò, G. (2018). Validation of biomarkers of food intake – Critical assessment of candidate biomarkers. *Genes Nutr.*, 13, 1–14.

Drake, I., Sonestedt, E., Gullberg, B., Bjartell, A., Olsson, H., Adlercreutz, H., Tikkanen, M.J., Wirfält, E., and Wallström, P. (2014). Plasma alkylresorcinol metabolites as biomarkers for whole-grain intake and their association with prostate cancer: A Swedish nested case-control study. *Cancer Epidemiol. biomarkers Prev.*, 23, 73–83.

Fraser, G.E. (2003). A search for truth in dietary epidemiology. *Am. J. Clin. Nutr.*, 78, 521–525.

Freedman, L.S., Kipnis, V., Schatzkin, A., and Tasevska, N. (2010a). Can we use biomarkers in combination with self-reports to strengthen the analysis of nutritional epidemiological studies? *Epidemiol. Perspect. Innov.*, 7, 2.

Freedman, L.S., Tasevska, N., Kipnis, V., Schatzkin, A., Mares, J., Tinker, L., and Potischman, N. (2010b). Gains in statistical power from using a dietary biomarker in combination with self-reported intake to strengthen the analysis of a diet-disease association: An example from CAREDS. *Am. J. Epidemiol.*, 172, 836–842.

Freudenheim, J.L., and Marshall, J.R. (1988). The problem of profound mismeasurement and the power of epidemiological studies of diet and cancer. *Nutr. Cancer*, 11, 243–250.

Gao, Q., Praticò, G., Scalbert, A., Vergères, G., Kolehmainen, M., Manach, C., Brennan, L., Afman, L.A., Wishart, D.S., Andres-Lacueva, C., Garcia-Aloy, M., Verhagen, H., Feskens, E.J.M., and Dragsted, L.O. (2017). A scheme for a flexible classification of dietary and health biomarkers. *Genes Nutr.*, 12, 1–15.

Gibbons, H., and Brennan, L. (2017). Irish Section Postgraduate Meeting Metabolomics as a tool in the identification of dietary biomarkers. *Proc. Nutr. Soc.*, 76, 42–53.

Hanhineva, K., Aura, A.M., Rogachev, I., Matero, S., Skov, T., Aharoni, A., Poutanen, K., and Mykkänen, H. (2012). In vitro microbiotic fermentation causes an extensive metabolite turnover of rye bran phytochemicals. *PLoS One*, 7, e39322.

Hedrick, V.E., Dietrich, A.M., Estabrooks, P.A., Savla, J., Serrano, E., and Davy, B.M. (2012). Dietary biomarkers: advances, limitations and future directions. *Nutr. J.*, 11, 109.

Henderson, R., Hobbie, J., Landrigan, P., Mattisoti, D., Perera, F., Pfttaer, E., Silbergeld, E., and Wogan, G. (1987). Biological markers in environmental health research. *Environ. Health Perspect.*, 7, 3–9.

Hengtrakul, P., Lorenz, K., and Mathias, M. (1990). Alkylresorcinols in U.S. and Canadian wheats and flours. *Cereal Chem.*, 67, 413–417.

Hengtrakul, P., Lorenz, K., and Mathias, M. (1991). Alkylresorcinol homologs in cereal grains. *J. Food Compos. Anal.*, 4, 52–57.

Holt, M.D., Moreau, R.A., Dermarderosian, A., Mckeown, N., and Jacques, P.F. (2012). Accelerated solvent extraction of alkylresorcinols in food products. *J. Agric. Food Chem.*, 60, 4799–4802.

Horner, N.K., Kristal, A.R., Prunty, J.A., Skor, H.E., Potter, J.D., and Lampe, J.W. (2002). Dietary determinants of plasma enterolactone. *Cancer Epidemiol. Biomarkers Prev.*, 11, 121–126.

Jansson, E., Landberg, R., Kamal-Eldin, A., Wolk, A., Vessby, B., and Aman, P. (2010). Presence of alkylresorcinols, potential whole grain biomarkers, in human adipose tissue. *Br. J. Nutr.*, 104, 633–636.

Jenab, M., Slimani, N., Bictash, M., Ferrari, P., and Bingham, S.A. (2009). Biomarkers in nutritional epidemiology: Applications, needs and new horizons. *Hum. Genet.*, 125, 507–525.

Johnsen, N.F., Hausner, H., Olsen, A., Tetens, I., Christensen, J., Knudsen, K.E.B., Overvad, K., and Tjønneland, A. (2004). Intake of whole grains and vegetables determines the plasma enterolactone concentration of Danish women. *J. Nutr.*, 134, 2691–2697.

Juntunen, K.S., Mazur, W.M., Liukkonen, K.H., Uehara, M., Poutanen, K.S., Adlercreutz, H.C., and Mykkänen, H.M. (2000). Consumption of wholemeal rye bread increases serum concentrations and urinary excretion of enterolactone compared with consumption of white wheat bread in healthy Finnish men and women. *Br. J. Nutr.*, 84, 839–846.

Kaaks, R.J. (1997). Biochemical markers as additional measurements in studies of the accuracy of dietary questionnaire measurements: Conceptual issues. *Am. J. Clin. Nutr.*, 65, 1232–1239.

Kamal-Eldin, A., Lærke, H.N., Knudsen, K.-E.B., Lampi, A.-M., Piironen, V., Adlercreutz, H., Katina, K., Poutanen, K., and Åman, P. (2009). Physical, microscopic and chemical character of industrial rye and wheat brans from the Nordic countries. *Food Nutr. Res., 53,* (There are no page numbers for citation purpose: see: https://www.ncbi.nlm.nih.gov/pmc/articles/PMC2675562/pdf/FNR-53-1912.pdf

Kamal-Eldin, A., Pouru, A., Eliasson, C., and Åman, P. (2001). Alkylresorcinols as antioxidants: Hydrogen donation and peroxyl radical-scavenging effects. *J. Sci. Food Agric.*, 81, 353–356.

Kantor, L.S., Variyam, J.N., Allshouse, J.E., Putnam, J.J., and Lin, B.H. (2001). Choose a variety of grains daily, especially whole grains: A challenge for consumers. *J. Nutr.*, 131, 473S–486S.

Kilkkinen, A., Stumpf, K., Pietinen, P., Valsta, L.M., Tapanainen, H., and Adlercreutz, H. (2001). Determinants of serum enterolactone concentration. *Am. J. Clin. Nutr.*, 73, 1094–1100.

Knödler, M., Kaiser, A., Carle, R., and Schieber, A. (2008). Profiling of alk(en)ylresorcinols in cereals by HPLC-DAD-APcI-MSn. *Anal. Bioanal. Chem.*, 391, 221–228.

Knudsen, M.D., Kyrø, C., Olsen, A., Dragsted, L.O., Skeie, G., Lund, E., Aman, P., Nilsson, L.M., Bueno-de-Mesquita, H.B., Tjønneland, A., and Landberg, R. (2014). Self-reported whole-grain intake and plasma alkylresorcinol concentrations in combination in relation to the incidence of colorectal cancer. *Am. J. Epidemiol.*, 179, 1188–1196.

Koskela, A., Linko-Parvinen, A.-M., Vuori, P.H., Samaletdin, A., Kamal-Eldin, A., Tikkanen, M.J., and Adlercreutz, H. (2007). Quantification of alkylresorcinol metabolites in urine by HPLC with coulometric electrode array detection. *Clin. Chem.*, 53, 1380–1383.

Koskela, A., Samaletdin, A., Aubertin-Leheudre, M., and Adlercreutz, H. (2008). Quantification of alkylresorcinol metabolites in plasma by high-performance liquid chromatography with coulometric electrode array detection. *J. Agric. Food Chem.*, 56, 7678–7681.

Kozubek, A., and Tyman, J.H.P. (1999). Resorcinolic lipids, the natural non-isoprenoid phenolic amphiphiles and their biological activity. *Chem. Rev.*, 99, 1–26.

Kristensen, M., Pelletier, X., Ross, A.B., and Thielecke, F. (2017). A high rate of non-compliance confounds the study of whole grains and weight maintenance in a randomised intervention trial-the case for greater use of dietary biomarkers in nutrition intervention studies. *Nutrients*, 9, 55.

Kristensen, M., Toubro, S., Jensen, M.G., Ross, A.B., Riboldi, G., Petronio, M., Bugel, S., Tetens, I., and Astrup, A. (2012). Whole grain compared with refined wheat decreases the percentage of body fat following a 12-week, energy-restricted dietary intervention in postmenopausal women. *J. Nutr.*, 142, 710–716.

Kulawinek, M., Jaromin, A., Kozubek, A., and Zarnowski, R. (2008). Alkylresorcinols in selected polish rye and wheat cereals and whole-grain cereal products. *J. Agric. Food Chem.*, 56, 7236–7242.

Kyrø, C., Kristensen, M., Jakobsen, M.U., Halkjær, J., Landberg, R., Bueno-de-Mesquita, H., Christensen, J., Romieu, I., Tjønneland, A., and Olsen, A. (2017). Dietary intake of whole grains and plasma alkylresorcinol concentrations in relation to changes in anthropometry: The Danish diet, cancer and health cohort study. *Eur. J. Clin. Nutr.*, 1–9.

Kyrø, C., Olsen, A., Bueno-de-Mesquita, H.B.A., Skeie, G., Loft, S., Åman, P., Leenders, M., Dik, V.K., Siersema, P.D., Pischon, T., Christensen, J., Overvad, K., Boutron-Ruault, M.-C., Fagherazzi, G., Cottet, V., Kühn, T., Chang-Claude, J., Boeing, H., Trichopoulou, A., Naska, A., Oikonomidou, D., Masala, G., Pala, V., Tumino, R., Vineis, P., Mattiello, A., Peeters, P.H., Bakken, T., Weiderpass, E., Asli, L.A., Sánchez, S., Jakszyn, P., Sánchez, M.-J., Amiano, P., Huerta, J.M., Barricarte, A., Ljuslinder, I., Palmqvist, R., Khaw, K.-T., Wareham, N., Key, T.J., Travis, R.C., Slimani, N., Freisling, H., Ferrari, P., Gunter, M.J., Murphy, N., Riboli, E., Tjønneland, A., and Landberg, R. (2014a). Plasma alkylresorcinol concentrations, biomarkers of whole-grain wheat and rye intake, in the European Prospective Investigation into Cancer and Nutrition (EPIC) cohort. *Br. J. Nutr.*, 111, 1881–1890.

Kyrø, C., Olsen, A., Landberg, R., Skeie, G., Loft, S., Åman, P., Leenders, M., Dik, V.K., Siersema, P.D., Pischon, T., Christensen, J., Overvad, K., Fagherazzi, G., Cottet, V., Kühn, T., Chang-Claude, J., Boeing, H., Trichopoulou, A., Bamia, C., Trichopoulos, D., Palli, D., Krogh, V., Tumino, R., Vineis, P., Panico, S., Peeters, P.H., Weiderpass, E., Bakken, T., Åsli, A., Argüelles, M., Jakszyn, P., Sánchez, M.-J., Amiano, P., Huerta, J.M., Barricarte, A., Ljuslinder, I., Palmqvist, R., Khaw, K.-T.T., Wareham, N., Key, T.J., Travis, R.C., Ferrari, P., Freisling, H., Jenab, M., Gunter, M.J., Murphy, N., Riboli, E., Tjønneland, A., Bueno-de-mesquita, H.B.A., Boutron-Ruault, M.-C.C., Åsli, L.A., Fagherazzi, G., Cottet, V., Kühn, T., Chang-Claude, J., Boeing, H., Trichopoulou, A., Bamia, C., Trichopoulos, D., Palli, D., Krogh, V., Tumino, R., Vineis, P., Panico, S., Peeters, P.H., Weiderpass, E., Bakken, T., Åsli, L.A., Argüelles, M., Jakszyn, P., Sánchez, M.-J., Amiano, P., Huerta, J.M., Barricarte, A., Ljuslinder, I., Palmqvist, R., Khaw, K.-T.T., Wareham, N., Key, T.J., Travis, R.C., Ferrari, P., Freisling, H., Jenab, M., Gunter, M.J., Murphy, N., Riboli, E., Tjønneland, A., Bueno-de-mesquita, H.B.A., Kyro, C., Olsen, A., Landberg, R., Skeie, G., Loft, S., Aman, P., Leenders, M., Dik, V.K., Siersema, P.D., Pischon, T., Christensen, J., Overvad, K., Boutron-Ruault, M.-C.C., Fagherazzi, G., Cottet, V., Kuhn, T., Chang-Claude, J., Boeing, H., Trichopoulou, A., Bamia, C., Trichopoulos, D., Palli, D., Krogh, V., Tumino, R., Vineis, P., Panico, S., Peeters, P.H., Weiderpass, E., Bakken, T., Asli, L.A., Arguelles, M., Jakszyn, P., Sanchez, M.J., Amiano, P., Huerta, J.M., Barricarte, A., Ljuslinder, I., Palmqvist, R., Khaw, K.-T.T., Wareham, N., Key, T.J., Travis, R.C., Ferrari, P., Freisling, H., Jenab, M., Gunter, M.J., Murphy, N., Riboli, E., Tjonneland, A., and Bueno-de-mesquita, H.B.A. (2014b). Plasma alkylresorcinols, biomarkers of whole-grain wheat and rye intake, and incidence of colorectal cancer. *J. Natl. Cancer Inst.*, 106, 1–9.

Landberg, R. (2009). Alkylresorcinols as biomarkers of whole grain wheat and rye intake. Swedish University of Agricultrural Sciences.

Landberg, R., Åman, P., Friberg, L.E., Vessby, B., Adlercreutz, H., and Kamal-Eldin, A. (2009). Dose response of whole-grain biomarkers: Alkylresorcinols in human plasma and their metabolites in urine in relation to intake. *Am. J. Clin. Nutr.*, 89, 1478.

Landberg, R., Aman, P., Hallmans, G., and Johansson, I. (2013). Long-term reproducibility of plasma alkylresorcinols as biomarkers of whole-grain wheat and rye intake within Northern Sweden Health and Disease Study Cohort. *Eur. J. Clin. Nutr.*, 67, 259–263.

Landberg, R., Kamal-Eldin, a, Aman, P., Christensen, J., Overvad, K., Tjønneland, A, and Olsen, A. (2011). Determinants of plasma alkylresorcinol concentration in Danish post-menopausal women. *Eur. J. Clin. Nutr.*, 65, 94–101.

Landberg, R., Kamal-Eldin, A., Andersson, A., Vessby, B., and Aman, P. (2008a). Alkylresorcinols as biomarkers of whole-grain wheat and rye intake: plasma concentration and intake estimated from dietary records. *Am J Clin Nutr.*, 87, 832–838.

Landberg, R., Kamal-Eldin, A., Andersson, R., and Åman, P. (2006). Alkylresorcinol content and homologue composition in durum wheat (Triticum durum) kernels and pasta products. *J. Agric. Food Chem.*, 54, 3012–3014.

Landberg, R., Kamal-Eldin, A., Andersson, S.-O., Johansson, J.-E., Zhang, J.-X., Hallmans, G., and Aman, P. (2009a). Reproducibility of plasma alkylresorcinols during a 6-week rye intervention study in men with prostate cancer. *J. Nutr.*, 139, 975–980.

Landberg, R., Kamal-Eldin, A., Salmenkallio-Marttila, M., Rouau, X., and Åman, P. (2008b). Localization of alkylresorcinols in wheat, rye and barley kernels. *J. Cereal Sci.*, 48, 401–406.

Landberg, R., Man, P., and Kamal-Eldin, A. (2009b). A rapid gas chromatography-mass spectrometry method for quantification of alkylresorcinols in human plasma. *Anal. Biochem.*, 385, 7–12.

Landberg, R., Marklund, M., Kamal-Eldin, A., and Åman, P. (2014). An update on alkylresorcinols – Occurrence, bioavailability, bioactivity and utility as biomarkers. *J. Funct. Foods*, 7, 77–89.

Landberg, R., Townsend, M.K., Neelakantan, N., Sun, Q., Sampson, L., Spiegelman, D., and van Dam, R.M. (2012). Alkylresorcinol metabolite concentrations in spot urine samples correlated with whole grain and cereal fibre intake but showed low to modest reproducibility over one to three years in U.S. women. *J. Nutr.*, 142, 872–877.

Landberg, R., Wierzbicka, R., Shi, L., Nybacka, S., Kamal-Eldin, A., Hedblad, B., Lindroos, A.K., Winkvist, A., and Forslund, H.B. (2018). New alkylresorcinol metabolites in spot urine as biomarkers of whole grain wheat and rye intake in a Swedish middle-aged population. *Eur. J. Clin. Nutr.*, 1–8.

Lind, M. V., Madsen, M.L., Rumessen, J.J., Vestergaard, H., Gobel, R.J., Hansen, T., Lauritzen, L., Pedersen, O.B., Kristensen, M., and Ross, A.B. (2016). Plasma alkylresorcinols reflect gluten intake and distinguish between gluten-rich and gluten-poor diets in a population at risk of metabolic syndrome. *J. Nutr.*, 146, 1991–1998.

Linko-Parvinen, A.-M., Landberg, R., Tikkanen, M.J., Adlercreutz, H., and Penalvo, J.L. (2007). Alkylresorcinols from whole-grain wheat and rye are transported in human plasma lipoproteins. *J. Nutr.*, 137, 1137–1142.

Linko, A.-M., and Adlercreutz, H. (2005). Whole-grain rye and wheat alkylresorcinols are incorporated into human erythrocyte membranes. *Br. J. Nutr.*, 93, 11.

Linko, A.-M., Juntunen, K.S., Mykkanen, H.M., and Adlercreutz, H. (2005). Whole-grain rye bread consumption by women correlates with plasma alkylresorcinols and increases their concentration compared with low-fibre wheat bread. *J. Nutr.*, 135, 580–583.

Linko, A.-M., Parikka, K., Wähälä, K., and Adlercreutz, H. (2002). Gas chromatographic-mass spectrometric method for the determination of alkylresorcinols in human plasma. *Anal. Biochem.*, 308, 307–313.

Livingstone, M., and Black, A.E. (2003). Biomarkers of nutritional exposure and bnutritional status. *J. Nutr.*, 133, 895–920.

Ma, J., Ross, A.B., Shea, M.K., Bruce, S.J., Jacques, P.F., Saltzman, E., Lichtenstein, A.H., Booth, S.L., and McKeown, N.M. (2012). Plasma alkylresorcinols, biomarkers of whole-grain intake, are related to lower BMI in older adults. *J. Nutr.*, 142, 1859–1864.

Magnusdottir, O.K., Landberg, R., Gunnarsdottir, I., Cloetens, L., Åkesson, B., Önning, G., Jonsdottir, S.E., Rosqvist, F., Schwab, U., Herzig, K.-H., Savolainen, M.J., Brader, L., Hermansen, K., Kolehmainen, M., Poutanen, K., Uusitupa, M., Thorsdottir, I., and Risérus, U. (2013). Plasma alkylresorcinols reflect important whole-grain components of a healthy Nordic diet. *J. Nutr*,. 143, 1383–90.

Marklund, M. (2012). Alkylresorcinol metabolites. Swedish University of Agricultural Sciences.

Marklund, M., Landberg, R., Aman, P., and Kamal-Eldin, A. (2010). Determination of alkylresorcinol metabolites in human urine by gas chromatography-mass spectrometry. *J. Chromatogr. B. Analyt. Technol. Biomed. Life Sci.*, 878, 888–894.

Marklund, M., Landberg, R., Andersson, A., Åman, P., and Kamal-Eldin, A. (2013a). Alkylresorcinol metabolites in urine correlate with the intake of whole grains and cereal fibre in free-living Swedish adults. *Br. J. Nutr.*, 109, 129–136.

Marklund, M., Landberg, R., Andersson, R., Aman, P., and Kamal-Eldin, A. (2012). Alkylresorcinol metabolism in Swedish adults is affected by factors other than intake of whole-grain wheat and rye. *J. Nutr.*, 142, 1479–1486.

Marklund, M., Magnusdottir, O.K., Rosqvist, F., Cloetens, L., Landberg, R., Kolehmainen, M., Brader, L., Hermansen, K., Poutanen, K.S., Herzig, K.-H., Hukkanen, J., Savolainen, M.J., Dragsted, L.O., Schwab, U., Paananen, J., Uusitupa, M., Akesson, B., Thorsdottir, I., and Risérus, U. (2014a). A dietary biomarker approach captures compliance and cardiometabolic effects of a healthy nordic diet in individuals with metabolic syndrome. *J. Nutr.*, 144, 1642–1649.

Marklund, M., McKeown, N.M., Blumberg, J.B., and Chen, C.-Y.O. (2013b). Hepatic biotransformation of alkylresorcinols is mediated via cytochrome P450 and β-oxidation:A a proof of concept study. *Food Chem.*, 139, 925–930.

Marklund, M., Stromberg, E.A., Hooker, A.C., Hammarlund-Udenaes, M., Aman, P., Landberg, R., and Kamal-Eldin, A. (2013c). Chain length of dietary alkylresorcinols affects their in vivo elimination kinetics in rats. *J. Nutr.*, 143, 1573–1578.

Marklund, M., Stromberg, E.A., Lærke, H.N., Knudsen, K.E.B., and Kamal-Eldin, A. (2014b). Simultaneous pharmacokinetic modeling of alkylresorcinols and their main metabolites indicates dual absorption mechanisms and enterohepatic elimination in humans 1 – 3. *J. Nutr.*, 144, 1674–1680.

Marshall, J.R. (2003). Methodologic and statistical considerations regarding use of biomarkers of nutritional exposure in epidemiology. *J. Nutr.*, 881S–887S.

Mattila, P., Pihlava, J.M., and Hellström, J. (2005). Contents of phenolic acids, alkyl- and alkenylresorcinols, and avenanthramides in commercial grain products. *J. Agric. Food Chem.*, 53, 8290–8295.

McKeown, N.M., Hruby, A., Landberg, R., Herrington, D.M., and Lichtenstein, A.H. (2015). Plasma alkylresorcinols, biomarkers of whole-grain intake, are not associated with progression of coronary artery atherosclerosis in postmenopausal women with coronary artery disease. *Public Health Nutr.*, 1–6.

McKeown, N.M., Marklund, M., Ma, J., Ross, A.B., Lichtenstein, A.H., Livingston, K. a., Jacques, P.F., Rasmussen, H.M., Blumberg, J.B., and Chen, C.-Y.O. (2016). Comparison of plasma alkylresorcinols (AR) and urinary AR metabolites as biomarkers of compliance in a short-term, whole-grain intervention study. *Eur. J. Nutr.*, 55, 1235–1244.

Menzel, C., Kamal-Eldin, A., Marklund, M., Andersson, A., Åman, P., and Landberg, R. (2012). Alkylresorcinols in Swedish cereal food products. *J. Food Compos. Anal.*, 28, 119–125.

Montonen, J., Landberg, R., Kamal-Eldin, a, Åman, P., Boeing, H., Steffen, A., and Pischon, T. (2012). Reliability of fasting plasma alkylresorcinol metabolites concentrations measured 4 months apart. *Eur. J. Clin. Nutr.*, 66, 968–970.

Montonen, J., Landberg, R., Kamal-Eldin, A., Aman, P., Knueppel, S., Boeing, H., and Pischon, T. (2010). Reliability of fasting plasma alkylresorcinol concentrations measured 4 months apart. *Eur. J. Clin. Nutr.*, 64, 698–703.

Nagy, K., Ross, A., Fay, L., Bourgeois, A., and Kussmann, M. (2008). Gas chromatography/tandem mass spectrometry analysis of alkylresorcinols in red blood cells. *Rapid Commun. Mass Spectrom.*, 22, 4098–4104.

Nystrom, L., Lampi, A.-M., Andersson, A.A.M., Kamal-Eldin, A., Gebruers, K., Courtin, C.M., Delcour, J.A., Li, L., Ward, J.L., Fras, A., Boros, D., Rakszeg, M., Bedo, Z., Shewry, P.R., and Piironen, V. (2008). Phytochemicals and dietary fibre components in rye varieties in the HEALTHGRAIN Diversity Screen. *J. Agric. Food Chem.*, 56, 9758–9766.

Olsen, A., Landberg, R., Aman, P., Kamal-Eldin, A., Christensen, J., Johnsen, N.F., Overvad, K., and Tjønneland, A. (2010). Plasma levels of alkylresorcinols and incidence of endometrial cancer. *Eur. J. Cancer Prev.*, 19, 73–77.

Ortega, R.M., Perez-Rodrigo, C., and Lopez-Sobaler, A.M. (2015). Dietary assessment methods: dietary records. *Nutr. Hosp.*, 31, 38–45.

Peeters, P.H., Slimani, N., van der Schouw, Y.T., Grace, P.B., Navarro, C., Tjonneland, A., Olsen, A., Clavel-Chapelon, F., Touillaud, M., Boutron-Ruault, M.C., Jenab, M., Kaaks, R., Linseisen, J., Trichopoulou, A., Trichopoulos, D., Dilis, V., Boeing, H., Weikert, C., Overvad, K., Pala, V., Palli, D., Panico, S., Tumino, R.,

Vineis, P., Bueno-de-Mesquita, H.B., van Gils, C.H., Skeie, G., Jakszyn, P., Hallmans, G., Berglund, G., Key, T.J., Travis, R., Riboli, E., and Bingham, S.A. (2007). Variations in plasma phytoestrogen concentrations in European adults. *J. Nutr.*, 137, 1294–1300.

Penn, L., Boeing, H., Boushey, C.J., Dragsted, L.O., Kaput, J., Scalbert, A., Welch, A.A., and Mathers, J.C. (2010). Assessment of dietary intake: NuGO symposium report. *Genes Nutr.*, 5, 205–213.

Pihlava, J.-M., Nordlund, E., Heiniö, R.-L., Hietaniemi, V., Lehtinen, P., and Poutanen, K. (2015). Phenolic compounds in wholegrain rye and its fractions. *J. Food Compos. Anal.*, 38, 89–97.

Praticò, G., Gao, Q., Scalbert, A., Vergères, G., Kolehmainen, M., Manach, C., Brennan, L., Pedapati, S.H., Afman, L.A., Wishart, D.S., Vázquez-Fresno, R., Lacueva, C.A., Garcia-Aloy, M., Verhagen, H., Feskens, E.J.M., and Dragsted, L.O. (2018). Guidelines for Biomarker of Food Intake Reviews (BFIRev): How to conduct an extensive literature search for biomarker of food intake discovery. *Genes Nutr.*, 13, 1–14.

Prentice, R.L. (2010). Dietary assessment and the reliability of nutritional epidemiology research reports. *J. Natl. Cancer Inst.*, 102, 583–585.

Roager, H.M., Vogt, J.K., Kristensen, M., Hansen, L.B.S., Ibrügger, S., Mærkedahl, R.B., Bahl, M.I., Lind, M.V., Nielsen, R.L., Frøkiær, H., Gøbel, R.J., Landberg, R., Ross, A.B., Brix, S., Holck, J., Meyer, A.S., Sparholt, M.H., Christensen, A.F., Carvalho, V., Holst, J.J., Rumessen, J.J., Linneberg, A., Sicheritz-pontén, T., Dalgaard, M.D., Blennow, A., Frandsen, H.L., Villas-bôas, S., Kristiansen, K., Vestergaard, H., Hansen, T., Ekstrøm, C.T., Ritz, C., Nielsen, H.B., Pedersen, O.B., Gupta, R., Lauritzen, L., and Licht, T.R. (2017). Whole grain-rich diet reduces body weight and systemic low-grade inflammation without inducing major changes of the gut microbiome : A randomised cross-over trial. *Gut*, 1–11.

Ross, A.B. (2003). Alkylresorcinols in cereal grains. Swedish University of Agricultural Sciences.

Ross, A.B. (2012a). Biomarkers of whole grain Intake. In Whole Grains Summit 2012, 4–5.

Ross, A.B. (2012b). Present status and perspectives on the use of alkylresorcinols as biomarkers of whole grain wheat and rye intake. *J. Nutr. Metab.*, 1–12.

Ross, A.B. (2012). Analysis of alkylresorcinols in cereal grains and products using ultrahigh-pressure liquid chromatography with fluorescence, ultraviolet, and coulArray electrochemical detection. *J. Agric. Food Chem.*, 60, 8954–8962.

Ross, A.B., Åman, P., and Kamal-Eldin, A. (2004a). Identification of cereal alkylresorcinol metabolites in human urine - Potential biomarkers of wholegrain wheat and rye intake. *J. Chromatogr. B Anal. Technol. Biomed. Life Sci.*, 809, 125–130.

Ross, A.B., Becker, W., Chen, Y., Kamal-Eldin, A., and Aman, P. (2005). Intake of alkylresorcinols from wheat and rye in the United Kingdom and Sweden. *Br. J. Nutr.*, 496–499.

Ross, A.B., Bourgeois, A., Ndung, H., Kochhar, S., Jebb, S.A., Brownlee, I.A., and Seal, C.J. (2012). Plasma alkylresorcinols as a biomarker of whole-grain food consumption in a large population: Results from the WHOLEheart Intervention Study. *Am. J. Clin. Nutr.*, 95, 204–211.

Ross, A.B., Bruce, S.J., Blondel-Lubrano, A., Oguey-Araymon, S., Beaumont, M., Bourgeois, A., Nielsen-Moennoz, C., Vigo, M., Fay, L.-B., Kochhar, S., Bibiloni, R., Pittet, A.-C., Emady-Azar, S., Grathwohl, D., and Rezzi, S. (2011). A whole-grain cereal-rich diet increases plasma betaine, and tends to decrease total and LDL-cholesterol compared with a refined-grain diet in healthy subjects. *Br. J. Nutr.*, 105, 1492–1502.

Ross, A.B., Chen, Y., Frank, J., Swanson, J.E., Parker, R.S., Kozubek, A., Lundh, T., Vessby, B., Åman, P., and Kamal-Eldin, A. (2004b). Cereal alkylresorcinols elevate γ-tocopherol levels in rats and inhibit γ-tocopherol metabolism in vitro. *J. Nutr.*, 134, 506–510.

Ross, A.B., Kamal-Eldin, A., and Åman, P. (2004c). Dietary alkylresorcinols: Absorption, bioactivities, and possible use as biomarkers of whole-grain wheat- and rye-rich foods. *Nutr. Rev.*, 62, 81–95.

Ross, A.B., Kamal-Eldin, A., Jung, C., Shepherd, M.J., and Åman, P. (2001). Gas chromatographic analysis of alkylresorcinols in rye (Secale cereale L) grains. *J. Sci. Food Agric.*, 81, 1405–1411.

Ross, A.B., Kamal-Eldin, A., Lundin, E.A., Zhang, J.-X., Hallmans, G., and Aman, P. (2003). Cereal alkylresorcinols are absorbed by humans. *J. Nutr.*, 133, 2222–2224.

Ross, A.B., and Kochhar, S. 2009). Rapid and sensitive analysis of alkylresorcinols from cereal grains and products using HPLC-Coularray-based electrochemical detection. *J. Agric. Food Chem.*, 57, 5187–5193.

Ross, A.B., Kristensen, M., Seal, C.J., Jacques, P., and McKeown, N.M. (2015). Recommendations for reporting whole-grain intake in observational and intervention studies. *Am. J. Clin. Nutr.*, 101, 903–907.

Ross, A.B., Pineau, N., Kochhar, S., Bourgeois, A., Beaumont, M., and Decarli, B. (2009). Validation of a FFQ for estimating whole-grain cereal food intake. *Br. J. Nutr.*, 102, 1547–1551.

Ross, A.B., Redeuil, K., Vigo, M., Rezzi, S., and Nagy, K. (2010). Quantification of alkylresorcinols in human plasma by liquid chromatography/tandem mass spectrometry. *Rapid Commun. Mass Spectrom.*, 24, 1554–1560.

Ross, A.B., Shepherd, M.J., Bach Knudsen, K.E., Vibe Glitsø, L., Bowey, E., Phillips, J., Rowland, I., Guo, Z.-X., Massy, D.J.R., Åman, P., and Kamal-Eldin, A. (2003a). Absorption of dietary alkylresorcinols in ileal-cannulated pigs and rats. *Br J Nutr.* 90, 787-794.

Ross, A.B., Shepherd, M.J., Schüpphaus, M., Sinclair, V., Alfaro, B., Kamal-Eldin, A., and Aman, P. (2003b). Alkylresorcinols in cereals and cereal products. *J. Agric. Food Chem.*, 51, 4111–8.

Ross, A.B., Svelander, C., Karlsson, G., and Savolainen, O.I. (2017). Identification and quantification of even and odd chained 5-n alkylresorcinols, branched chain-alkylresorcinols and methylalkylresorcinols in Quinoa (Chenopodium quinoa). *Food Chem.*, 220, 344–351.

Scalbert, A., Brennan, L., Manach, C., Andres-Lacueva, C., Dragsted, L.O., Draper, J., Rappaport, S.M., Hooft, J.J. van der, and Wishart, D.S. (2014). The food metabolome: A window over dietary exposure. *Am. J. Clin. Nutr.*, 99, 1286–1308.

Seitz, L.M. (1992). Identification of 5-(2-oxoalkyl)resorcinols and 5-(2-oxoalkenyl)resorcinols in wheat and rye grains. *J. Agric. Food Chem.*, 40, 1541–1546.

Shewry, P.R., Piironen, V., Lampi, A.M., Edelmann, M., Kariluoto, S., Nurmi, T., Fernandez-Orozco, R., Andersson, A.M., Åman, P., Fraś, A., Boros, D., Gebruers, K., Dornez, E., Courtin, C.M., Delcour, J. A., Ravel, C., Charmet, G., Rakszegi, M., Bedo, Z., and Ward, J.L. (2010). Effects of genotype and environment on the content and composition of phytochemicals and dietary fibre components in rye in the HEALTHGRAIN diversity screen. *J. Agric. Food Chem.*, 58, 9372–9383.

Skoglund, M. (2008). Phenolic compounds in oats effects of steeping, germination and related enzymes. PhD thesis, Swedish Univ. Agric. Sci. Uppsala. Swedish University of Agricultural Sciences.

Slimani, N., Charrondière, U.R., Van Staveren, W., and Riboli, E. (2000). Standardization of food composition databases for the European prospective investigation into cancer and nutrition (EPIC): General theoretical concept. *J. Food Compos. Anal.*, 13, 567–584.

Söderholm, P.P., Lundin, J.E., Koskela, A.H., Tikkanen, M.J., and Adlercreutz, H.C. (2011). Pharmacokinetics of alkylresorcinol metabolites in human urine. *Br. J. Nutr.*, 106, 1040–1044.

Spencer, J.P.E., Abd El Mohsen, M.M., Minihane, A.M., and Mathers, J.C. (2008). Biomarkers of the intake of dietary polyphenols: Strengths, limitations and application in nutrition research. *Br. J. Nutr.*, 99, 12–22.

Spiegelman, D., Zhao, B., and Kim, J. (2005). Correlated errors in biased surrogates: Study designs and methods for measurement error correction. *Stat. Med.*, 24, 1657–1682.

Strimbu, K., and Tavel, J.A. (2011). What are biomarkers? *Curr. Opin. HIV AIDS*, 5, 463–466.

Stumpf, K., and Adlercreutz, H. (2003). Short-term variations in enterolactone in serum, 24-hour urine, and spot urine and relationship with enterolactone concentrations. *Clin. Chem.*, 49, 178–181.

Sun, T., Rong, Y., Hu, X., Zhu, Y., Huang, H., Chen, L., Li, P., Li, S., Yang, W., Cheng, J., Yang, X., Yao, P., Hu, F.B., and Liu, L. (2018). Plasma alkylresorcinol metabolite, a biomarker of whole-grain wheat and rye intake, and risk of type 2 diabetes and impaired glucose regulation in a Chinese population. *Diabetes Care*, 1–6.

Sur, R., Nigam, A., Grote, D., Liebel, F., and Southall, M.D. (2008). Avenanthramides, polyphenols from oats, exhibit anti-inflammatory and anti-itch activity. *Arch. Dermatol. Res.*, 300, 569.

Suzuki, Y., Esumi, Y., and Yamaguchi, I. (1999). Structures of 5-alkylresorcinol-related analogues in rye. *Phytochemistry*, 52, 281–289.

Tasevska, N. (2015). Urinary sugars — A biomarker of total sugars intake. *Nutrients*, 7, 5816–5833.

Tasevska, N., Runswick, S.A., Bingham, S.A. (2006). Urinary potassium is as reliable as urinary nitrogen for use as a recovery biomarker in dietary studies of free living individuals. *J. Nutr.*, 136, 1334–1340.

Tluscik, F., Kupiec, R., and Rakowska, M. (1990). Studies on antinutritive components of the rye grain. Pt. 2. Balance and metabolism of 5-N-alkylresorcinols in rats. *Acta Aliment. Pol.*, 16, 119-128.

van Dam, R.M., and Hu, F.B. (2008). Are alkylresorcinols accurate biomarkers for whole grain intake? *Am. J. Clin. Nutr.*, 87, 797–798.

van Dam, R.M., and Hunter, D. (2012). Biochemical indicators of dietary intake. In Nutritional Epidemiology. Oxford University Press.

Vineis, P. (1997). Sources of variation in biomarkers. *IARC Sci. Publ.* 59—71.

WHO. (2001). Biomarkers in risk assessment: Validity and validation [WWW Document]. http://www.inchem.org/documents/ehc/ehc/ehc222.htm (accessed August 12, 2018).

Wierzbicka, R., Eyer, L., Landberg, R., Kamal-Eldin, A., and Franek, M. (2014). Development of antibodies for *Immunol. Methods*, 413, 12–24.

Wierzbicka, R., Wu, H., Franek, M., Kamal-Eldin, A., and Landberg, R. (2015). Determination of alkylresorcinols and their metabolites in biological samples by gas chromatography–mass spectrometry. *J. Chromatogr. B* 1000, 120–129.

Wierzbicka, R., Zamaratskaia, G., Kamal-Eldin, A., and Landberg, R. (2017). Novel urinary alkylresorcinol metabolites as biomarkers of whole grain intake in free-living Swedish adults. *Mol. Nutr. Food Res.*, 61, 1–8.

Willett, W. (2012). Nutritional Epidemiology, 3d ed., Toxicological Sciences. Oxford University Press, US.

Wolk, A., Furuheim, M., and Vessby, B. (2001). Nutritional methodology fatty acid composition of adipose tissue and serum lipids are valid biological markers of dairy fat intake in men 1. *J. Nutr.*, 131, 828–833.

Wu, H., Kolehmainen, M., Mykkanen, H., Poutanen, K., Uusitupa, M., Schwab, U., Wolk, A., and Landberg, R. (2015). Alkylresorcinols in adipose tissue biopsies as biomarkers of whole-grain intake: an exploratory study of responsiveness to advised intake over 12 weeks. *Eur. J. Clin. Nutr.*, 69, 1244–1248.

Wu, H., Mhd Omar, N.A., Håkansson, N., Wolk, A., Michaëlsson, K., and Landberg, R. (2018). Evaluation of alkylresorcinols in adipose tissue biopsies as a long-term biomarker of whole-grain wheat and rye intake in free-living Swedish men and women. *Public Health Nutr.*, 21, 1933–1942.

Zarnowski, R., and Suzuki, Y. (2004). 5-n-alkylresorcinols from grains of winter barley (Hordeum vulgare L.). *Phytochemistry*, 4, 4–6.

Zarnowski, R., Suzuki, Y., Yamaguchi, I., and Pietr, S.J. (2002). Alkylresorcinols in barley (Hordeum vulgare L. distichon) grains. Zeitschrift fur Naturforsch. – Sect. *C J. Biosci.*, 57, 57–62.

Zhang, T., Shao, J., Gao, Y., Chen, C., Yao, D., Chu, Y.F., Johnson, J., Kang, C., Yeo, D., and Ji, L.L. (2017). Absorption and elimination of oat avenanthramides in humans after acute consumption of oat cookies. *Oxid. Med. Cell. Longev.* (NO pages for publication see : https://www.ncbi.nlm.nih.gov/pmc/articles/PMC5752969/pdf/OMCL2017-2056705.pdfs

Zhu, Y., Shurlknight, K.L., Chen, X., and Sang, S. (2014). Identification and pharmacokinetics of novel alkylresorcinol metabolites in human urine, new candidate biomarkers for whole-grain wheat and rye intake. *J. Nutr.*, 144, 114–122.

8 Body Composition and Weight Management

Nicola McKeown[1] and Mette Bredal Kristensen[2]

[1]Jean Mayer USDA Human Nutrition Research Center on Aging, Tufts University, Boston, Massachusetts, USA
[2]Department of Nutrition, Exercise and Sports, Faculty of Science, University of Copenhagen, Frederiksberg, Denmark

8.1 Introduction

Overweight and obesity are key features of the metabolic syndrome (MS) and closely linked to risk of developing chronic diseases (1). With the rising prevalence of overweight and obesity, fibre-rich foods such as whole grains have received increased attention for their potential role in weight regulation. This chapter reviews evidence from both observational and dietary intervention studies to provide a comprehensive picture of the relationship between whole grains and body weight management.

8.2 Obesity prevalence around the globe

The rising prevalence of overweight and obesity across the different regions of the world has been described as a global pandemic (2). Between 1980 and 2013, the combined prevalence of overweight and obesity rose by 27.5% for adults and 47.1% for children worldwide, with the number of overweight and obese individuals increasing from 857 million in 1980 to 2.1 billion in 2013 (3). This obesity pandemic is associated with multiple comorbidities including diabetes, cardiovascular diseases, several types of cancers, and decreased quality of life reflecting both diminished physical and mental health. Worldwide, the proportion of overweight men increased from 28.8% in 1980 to 36.9% in 2013, while the proportion of overweight women increased from 29.8% to 38.0% over the same period (3). The prevalence has increased in both developed and developing countries (3); however, interestingly, different sex patterns have been observed with a greater number of overweight and obese men in developed countries, and a greater number of overweight and obese women in developing countries. Rates of overweight and obesity peaked between 1992 and 2002 and have slowed down over the last decade, especially in developed countries. Alarmingly, childhood obesity has increased substantially in developed countries where 23.8% of boys and 22.6% of girls were overweight or obese in 2013 (3). Obesity among children and adolescents has also increased in developing countries, from 8.1% in 1980 to 12.9% in 2013 for boys, and

Whole Grains and Health, Second Edition. Edited by Rikard Landberg and Nathalie Scheers.

Additional materials available for download online at https://www.wiley.com/en-gb/Whole+Grains+and+Health-p-9781118939437

from 8.4% to 13.4% in girls (3). Although the rates differ across countries and there appears to be a plateauing off, the rates of obesity remain alarmingly high in this segment of the population (4).

8.3 Abdominal adiposity and cardiometabolic risk

There is consensus among medical professionals that greater abdominal obesity predisposes individuals to greater cardiometabolic risk through a myriad of potential mechanisms, including dyslipidemia, increasing insulin resistance, greater inflammation and increasing blood pressure (5). Two surrogate measures of abdominal adiposity, waist circumference (WC) measured at the iliac crest and waist-hip ratio, have been used for decades to capture central adiposity in epidemiological studies. Elevated WC is one of five criteria used in the clinical diagnosis of the metabolic syndrome (MS), with a WC of ≥102 cm for men and ≥88 cm for women categorizing individuals as abdominally obese (6). Over the past couple of decades, the prevalence of abdominal obesity has increased in adults, paralleling the increased prevalence of obesity (7). Although the prevalence of abdominal obesity has leveled off in US children and adolescents (8), a large proportion remain abdominally obese. Using gender- and age- specific 90th percentiles based on data from a representative sample of children from 1988 to 1994, it is estimated that 18% of children aged 2 to 18 years in 2011–2012 were abdominally obese as defined by a WC equal to or above the 90th percentile cut-point (8). Imaging techniques, such as magnetic resonance imaging (MRI) and computed tomography (CT), provide objective measures of abdominal adipose tissue, allowing researchers to distinguish fat from muscle, bone, and other tissues in the abdominal cavity. It is due to advancement in this field, using more sophisticated methods to identify fat depots, that researchers have recognized that excess visceral adipose tissue (VAT), rather than subcutaneous abdominal tissue (SAT), is the key correlate of metabolic abnormalities. As such, the increased availability of methods offering more precise measures of adiposity has helped to expand our understanding of relationships between whole grain intake and abdominal adiposity in nutrition research.

8.4 Studies investigating the link between body weight and whole grain consumption

A cohort study is a non-randomized investigation of individuals, in which, for example, those who consume the greatest amount of whole grains, in this case typically 2 to 3 servings per day, are compared to those who consume very little, if any, whole grain foods. The association between whole grain intake and measures of weight is then typically compared between these two extreme groups. Prospective cohort designs have an advantage over cross-sectional study designs because the measurement of the exposure, whole grain intake, is evaluated before weight status may change, thus providing a temporal sequence between whole grain intake and outcome. In contrast to observational studies, randomized controlled trials (RCTs) are studies whereby individuals are randomly allocated to a treatment arm to receive, for example, whole grain foods, the exposure of interest. The other group is allocated to receive a placebo or control treatment, which in the arena of whole grain research typically means that these individuals would receive the equivalent serving amount of refined grains and/or be instructed to avoid whole grain foods altogether. The effect of the whole grain intake on changes in adiposity is then compared between the treatment and control groups. Both prospective cohort studies and randomized controlled trials have strengths and limitations. In randomized studies, potential confounding from other lifestyle factors, which is an inherent problem with observational studies, can be avoided to a great extent. However, RCTs, as opposed to cohort studies, are typically small in sample size and short in duration.

A meta-analysis is a particular type of systematic review that applies a quantitative statistical technique to synthesize data from relevant studies; however, the quality and comprehensiveness of the meta-analysis is highly dependent on the criteria used during the systematic literature review. There have been some meta-analyses performed examining all the relevant studies linking higher whole grain intake to measures of adiposity or weight gain based both on observational studies and randomized controlled studies. Harland and colleagues used data from 15 cross-sectional studies to determine that the weighted mean difference in body mass index (BMI) was 0.63 kg/m^2 less in high whole grain consumers when compared with low or non-consumers of whole grains (9). This result may be more meaningful than the results from each of the 15 individual studies alone. Recently, a comprehensive meta-analysis examining effects of whole grain intake on body weight was published (10). This analysis included data from 26 intervention studies with 2060 total study participants. The majority of these studies incorporated mixed whole grain diets, although wheat was the predominant whole grain in most studies, which likely reflects the consumption pattern in most Western countries. Overall, whole grains did not show any effect on body weight compared to control diets (weighted difference: 0.06 kg; 95% CI: 20.09, 0.20 kg; P = 0.45); whereas a small, but significant, effect on body fat percentage in favor of whole grain was observed (weighted difference: -0.48%; 95% CI: -0.95; -0.01%; P = 0.04). However, these pooled estimates cover a heterogeneous group of studies with and without a weight-loss program, on both mixed grain diets and single-grain diets using daily doses of whole grain ranging from 18.2–150 g/d. Some of the studies published after this meta-analysis used doses of whole grain up to 213 g/d (11, 12).

It is important to recognize that evidence from both observational and dietary intervention studies contribute to our interpretation of the role of whole grains in weight management; however, plausible biological mechanisms as well as proven dose-response relationships should be included when evaluating the evidence to determine a cause-and-effect relationship.

8.5 Defining grain ingredients and foods in observational studies

As with estimates of other aspects of diet, most estimates of whole grain intake in observational studies have been captured using food frequency questionnaires (FFQ), 24-hour recalls, or multiple day food intake records (Table 8.1). In some cases, comparisons between observational studies examining the relationship between whole grains and health have been complicated by the fact that definitions of *whole grains* have varied from study to study. In early studies, for instance, whole grains were classified based on the Jacobs definition (13), a classification that includes whole grain breakfast cereals (containing ≥25% whole grain content), dark bread, brown rice, oatmeal and other FFQ-specific foods such as wild rice, bran muffins and whole-wheat crackers. This broader definition of *whole grains* includes added bran and added germ (components of whole grains) and, thus, does not conform to the FDA definition of *whole grains*. Most studies estimating whole grain intake have expressed intake in servings per day, thereby failing to consider that the amount

Table 8.1 Cross-sectional evidence: Relationship between higher intakes of whole grains and measures of adiposity in adults.

Reference	Country	Study Population	Dietary Method	Measures of Adiposity			
				BMI	WC	BW	WHR
Jacobs et al. (1998) (13)	USA	34 492 (F)	FFQ	-			-
Jacobs et al. (2001) (52)	Norway	33 848 (16 933 M/ 16 915 F)	FFQ	-†			
McKeown et al. (2002) (53)	USA	2941 (1338 M/1603 F)	FFQ	X			-
Montonen et al. (2003) (54)	Finland	4316 (2286 M/2030 F)	Dietary History Interview	-			
Esmaillzadeh et al. (2005) (55)	Iran	827 (357 M/470 F)	FFQ	-	X		-
Sahyoun et al. (2006) (56)	USA	535 (179 M/356 F)	3-d food record	-			
Lutsey et al. (2007) (57)	USA	5496 (2594 M/2902 F)	FFQ	-			
Newby et al. (2007) (58)	USA	1516 (M/F)	7-d dietary record	-	-	-	
Rose et al. (2007) (59)	USA	159 (42 M/117 F)	7-d food record (x2)	-			
Good et al. (2008) (60)	USA	2091 (F)	24-h dietary recall	-	-		
McKeown et al. (2009) (61)	USA	434 (177 M/257 F)	FFQ	X			
Thane et al. (2009) (62)	UK	3778 (1799 M/ 1979 F)	7-d food diary	-‡	X	X	
van de Vijver et al. (2009) (63)	Netherlands	4237 (2078 M/2159 F)	FFQ	-			
Masters et al. (2010) (64)	USA	1015 (M/F)	FFQ	X	X		
McKeown et al. (2010) (65)	USA	2834 (1434 M/1400 F)	FFQ	-	-		

O'Neil et al. (2010) (66)	USA	13,276	24-hour dietary recall	-	-	
Kyro et al. (2011) (67)	Norway, Sweden and Denmark	8,702	24-hour dietary recall	-		
Montonen et al. (2013) (68)	Germany	2198 (836 M//1362 F)	FFQ	X	X	
Mostad et al. (2014) (69)	Norway	50 339 (~22 880 M/27459 F)	Quantitative Questionnaire (HUNT3)			-

4/4

(-) indicates there was a significant inverse association between whole grain consumption and the measure of adiposity; X indicates there was no significant association between whole grain consumption and the measure of adiposity; cells were left blank if the study did not evaluate that measure of adiposity; significant relationships were based on $p<0.05$.

†Stratified by sex. Associations between whole grain consumption and measures of adiposity were only significant for men ($p<0.05$).

‡Two national surveys were conducted (1986–1987 and 2000–2001) and results were stratified by sex. Associations between whole grain consumption and measures of adiposity were only significant for men from the 1986–1987 national survey.

of whole grain in each serving can vary substantially; for example, one serving of whole-wheat bread typically contains 16 g of whole grain, while ready-to-eat breakfast cereal may contain a substantially greater amount. Some observational studies (14, 15) have used a more quantitative database that contains data on the grams of whole grains per food to estimate whole grain intake. This database provides researchers with the opportunity to estimate not only the grams of whole grain but, additionally, to separate out the contribution of bran and germ in the whole grain and examine the independent relationship with health outcomes.

8.6 Defining grain ingredients and foods in intervention studies

In most intervention studies, some proportion of the intervention foods are provided to participants (11, 12, 16-48). However, other studies may only provide participants with instructions on which products to choose when shopping for groceries, leaving participants to supply their own intervention diet (49). Directly providing participants with intervention foods increases the certainty by which we can determine what types of products were actually consumed in the different studies; however, even with studies providing foods, investigators may not always provide a detailed description (e.g., whole grain content, particle size, method of preparation) of the intervention products used in their presentations or manuscripts. The majority of the intervention studies have used either wheat, predominantly wheat in a mixed whole grain diet or oats, whereas studies using exclusively whole grain rice, rye, barley and corn are fewer in number (50). In two recent meta-analyses on whole grains, the first examining body weight (10) and the second examining blood lipids (51), efforts were made to identify the whole grain doses administered in the intervention. These meta-analyses excluded studies in which there was uncertainty around whether products were truly whole grain. Generally, no lower limit was set with respect to percentage of whole grain (i.e., ≥25% WG per weight) in intervention foods, although most use products with a large proportion of whole grain such as breads, breakfast cereals and pastas. Thus, in these meta-analyses, whole grain intake has been estimated in absolute amounts (grams/day) rather than in servings of whole grain foods to ease comparison between studies.

8.7 Evidence from observational studies

8.7.1 Cross-sectional studies

Several cross-sectional studies have examined the association between whole grain intake (13, 52-74), cereal fibre intake (15, 54, 58, 61, 63, 66, 72), and measures of adiposity in Table 8.1. The vast majority of these studies have been conducted in adults using estimates of whole grain intake derived mainly from FFQs. A summary of these studies, including detailed information on study population, dietary assessment method and measures of adiposity, are presented in Table 8.1. The majority of cross-sectional studies (15 of 21) reported a significant inverse association between higher intakes of whole grain and BMI (13, 52, 54-63, 65-67) or WC (58, 60, 65). Of the studies that stratified by sex (52, 62, 63), two observed significant inverse associations between whole grain intake and BMI among men (52, 62). In one study, McKeown and colleagues (61) examined associations between measures of adiposity and intakes of grain (whole and refined), dietary fibre and food group sources of fibre (fruit, vegetable and cereal fibre) using FFQs in a sample of 434 older adults (60–80 years). After adjustment for potential confounding variables (age, sex, total energy intake, percent energy from fat, physical activity, smoking, alcohol intake and multivitamin use), whole grain intake and cereal fibre were associated with lower percent body fat and trunk fat mass. In contrast, total fibre, fruit fibre, vegetable fibre and refined-grain intakes were not associated with any measures of body composition, suggesting that dietary fibre from cereal sources may be important in improving body composition. Using a biomarker of whole grain wheat intake, plasma alkylresorcinols, Ma and colleagues (75) confirmed the observed inverse relationship between whole grain wheat intake and BMI reported by McKeown and colleagues (61).

A subsequent study conducted by McKeown and colleagues (65) examined associations between whole- and refined-grain intakes and WC measures, abdominal subcutaneous adipose tissue (SAT) and visceral adipose tissue (VAT) in 2834 adults enrolled in the Framingham Heart Study Cohorts (32–83 years). After adjustment for age, sex, smoking status, total energy and alcohol intake, whole grain intake was inversely associated with WC (97.0 vs. with 93.7 cm in the lowest vs. the highest quintile, P for trend<0.001), SAT (2895 vs. with 2552 cm^3 in the lowest vs. the highest quintile, p for trend<0.001) and VAT (1883 vs. with 1563 cm^3 in the lowest vs. the highest quintile, p for trend<0.001). In contrast, higher intakes of refined grains were positively associated with SAT and VAT. There was only a moderate positive association between refined-grain intake and WC (p for trend=0.06). One important observation from this research is that in the presence of high refined-grain intake, the observed benefits of high whole grains on visceral adiposity are no longer present. This observation highlights the need to emphasize substituting refined grains with whole grains, rather than merely adding whole grains to an existing diet high in refined grains.

To date, few studies have examined whole- and refined-grain intake, estimated from dietary recalls, in relation to body weight in children (72, 74) or adolescents (70–73). Four cross-sectional studies have assessed the association between whole grain intake and measures of adiposity, three of which were conducted in the United States (70, 72, 73). In contrast to adults, much of the data on whole grain intake in adolescents and children is based on dietary recalls (72, 73). Details of the population, dietary assessment method, and measures of adiposity for studies assessing the association between whole grain intake and measures of adiposity among children and adolescents are presented in Table 8.2. Of the 5 cross-sectional analyses conducted in children and adolescents, all reported significant inverse associations between higher intakes of whole grain and BMI (70, 73), BMI z-score (72-74), and/or WC (70, 72).

Dietary pattern analysis captures other aspects of diet that may be attributed to improved body weight or measures of adiposity. Cross-sectional studies with grain-related dietary patterns and measures of adiposity in adults (76-79) have reported inconsistent findings on the relationship between these dietary patterns, often characterized by high fibre intake and measures of adiposity. While some have found that dietary patterns characterized by a high fibre intake are associated with a smaller WC (76, 78, 79) or lower BMI, particularly among men, others have not (77).

8.7.2 Prospective cohort studies

To date, seven prospective cohort studies have examined the extent to which higher WG intake may prevent or reduce long-term (≥1 year) weight gain or fat accumulation in adults (Table 8.3) (15, 80-85). Originally, researchers considered the impact of diets high in whole

Table 8.2 Cross-sectional evidence: Relationship between higher intakes of whole grains and measures of adiposity in adolescents and children.*

Reference	Country	Study Population	Dietary Method	Measure of Adiposity	Result
Adolescents					
Steffen (2003) (70)	USA	357 (155 M/130 F)	FFQ	BMI	-
				WC	-
Cheng et al. (2009) (71)	Germany	215 (M/F)	3-d dietary records	BMI	X
Zanovec et al. (2010) (72)	USA	4,931 (M/F)	24-h dietary recall	BMI z-score	-
				BMI percentile	-
				WC	-
Hur et al. (2012) (73)	USA	4,928 adolescents	24-h dietary recall	BMI	-
				BMI z-score	-
Children					
Zanovec et al. (2010) (72)	USA	3,868 (M/F)	24-h dietary recall	BMI z-score	-
				BMI percentile	-
				WC	-
Choumenkovitch et al. (2013) (74)	USA	792 (M/F)	Block Food Screener (2007 version)	BMI z-score	-

(-) indicates there was a significant inverse association between whole grain consumption and the measure of adiposity; X indicates there was no significant association between whole grain consumption and the measure of adiposity; significant relationships were based on $p<0.05$.

grains on weight gain in several large US cohorts of health professional men (15, 82) or women (80). In these studies, whole grain intake captured over several years, ranging from 8 to 13 years, was related to changes in self-reported body weight, BMI or WC. Dr. Liu and colleagues (80) were the first to examine the prospective relationship between whole grain intake and weight gain in 74,091 women participating in the Nurses' Health Study. In this study, whole grain intake was estimated as servings per day from an FFQ and included ready-to-eat breakfast cereals (RTEBC) with ≥25% WG by weight as well as added bran and added germ (added to the diet or obtained from fortified-grain foods). In this study, Liu and colleagues observed that those women with the greatest increase in whole grain intake gained 1.07 kg over two 4-year intervals, while women with a minimal increase in whole grain intake gained 1.58 kg. This observed benefit of increasing whole grain intake was more striking among women who were already overweight at enrollment into the study. On the other hand, women who increased refined-grain intake had a 26% increased risk of major weight gain (>25 kg) over 12 years while, in contrast, shifting from low to high whole grain intake over the same time period reduced risk of major weight gain by 23%. These findings may suggest that dietary substitution of refined with whole grains may contribute to less weight gain. Using a more precise estimate of whole grain intake (grams/day), Koh-Banerjee et al. (15) estimated that men who increased their whole grain intake by 23.8 g/d gained less weight over 8 years compared to men who decreased their whole grain intake by 14.2 g/d. In this study of 27,082 men, the authors noted that for every 40 gram increment increase in whole grains, weight gain was reduced by 0.49 kg over 8 years.

Table 8.3 Longitudinal cohorts examining the relationship between whole grain intake, cereal fibre and change in measure of adiposity in adults.

Author, Year, Country	Subjects	Outcome	Dietary Method/Exposure	Methodology	Results and Conclusions
Liu et al. 2003, USA (80)	74 091 US female nurses (38–63 y) taking part in the NHS; 12 y of followup (1984–1996)	Changes in weight from 2–4 y intervals between 1984 and 1986 and from 1984 to 1996	Four 126-item, semi-quantitative FFQs; quintiles of WG intake (median: 0.07-1.62 servings/1000 kcal/d) and RG intake (median: 0.40-2.27 servings/1000 kcal/d) WG foods: dark bread, brown rice, WG breakfast cereal popcorn, cooked oatmeal, wheat germ, bran and other grains RG foods: sweet rolls and cakes/desserts, white bread, pasta, English muffins, muffins/biscuits, RG breakfast cereal, white rice, pancakes/waffles and pizza	Examined changes in WG or RG intake in relation to changes in weight at 2–4 y intervals; calculated odds of developing obesity and major weight gain over 12 y; stratified analyses using BMI in 1984 Confounders: age; changes in exercise; change in smoking status; change in hormone replacement therapy status; changes in intake of alcohol, caffeine and total energy; changes in intakes of saturated fat, polyunsaturated fat, monounsaturated fat, trans fat and protein; BMI at baseline	Increases in the intake of WG were associated with less weight gain (mean weight gain of 1.58 kg in 2–4 y in the lowest quintile vs. 1.07 kg in the highest quintile; P for trend<0.0001). Increases in the intake of RG were associated with greater weight gain (mean weight gain of 0.99 kg in 2–4 y in the lowest quintile vs. 1.65 kg in the highest quintile; P for trend <0.0001). Over 12 y (1984–1996), increases in the intake of WG were associated with less weight gain (mean weight gain of 4.51 kg in the lowest quintile vs. 4.12 kg in the highest quintile; P for trend <0.0001). Increases in the intake of RG were associated with greater weight gain (mean weight gain of 4.25 kg in the lowest quintile vs. 4.68 kg in the highest quintile; P for trend <0.0001). Compared with women who were in the lowest quintile of WG intake, those who increased their WG intake to the highest quintile reduced their risk of major weight gain by 23% (OR=0.77; 95% CI: 0.59, 1.01; P for trend=0.03) and reduced their risk of developing obesity by 29% (OR=0.81; 95% CI: 0.73, 0.91; P for trend 0.0002).

(continued)

Table 8.3 Longitudinal cohorts examining the relationship between whole grain intake, cereal fibre and change in measure of adiposity in adults. (*continued*)

Author, Year, Country	Subjects	Outcome	Dietary Method/Exposure	Methodology	Results and Conclusions
					Compared with women who were in the lowest quintile of RG intake, those who increased their RG intake to the highest quintile increased their risk of major weight gain by 26% (OR=1.26; 95% CI: 0.97, 1.64; P for trend 0.04) and increased their risk of developing obesity by 18% (OR=1.18; 95% CI: 1.08, 1.28; P for trend <0.0001).
Halkjaer et al. 2004, Denmark (81)	2300 middle-aged men and women participating in the MONICA1 study; 6 y of followup; data collected in 1982, 1987, 1993	Change in WC between the second and third followup; adjusted for changes in BMI	Two 26-item FFQs; analyzed diet information in two ways Food item groups: 24 food items grouped into 10 groups of items (1 group for WG and 1 group for RG) Factors scores; three food factors ("traditional," "green," and "sweet") were identified for men; two food factors ("traditional/ sweet" and "green") were identified for women	Examined changes in diet (1987–1993) in relation to WC; analyzed with and without adjustments for concurrent changes in BMI; stratified analyses by sex Confounders: age at baseline; WC at baseline; each food group; BMI; change in diet; educational level; physical activity; smoking status; alcohol habits	For females, a high intake of RG bread (white wheat bread and rye bread without WG) was associated with increased WC (persisted after adjustment for concurrent BMI changes; β=0.29; 95% CI: 0.7, 0.51; p<0.05). There were no significant associations between RG bread intake and WC (p>0.05) for men. There were no significant associations between WG bread intake and WC (p>0.05) for men and women. None of the food factors were associated with changes in WC (p>0.05).
Koh-Banerjee et al. 2004, USA (15)	27 082 healthy US men (40-75 y) participating in the HPFS; 8 y of followup (1986–1994)	Change in body weight at 8 y followup	Three semi-quantitative FFQs; quintiles of WG intake (1.4–54.7 g/d) WG and RG foods: cooked and cold breakfast cereals, white and dark bread, white and brown rice, and pasta (partitioned all foods on FFQ into WG vs. RG food ingredients)	Examined changes in consumption of WG, RG, added bran and germ, cereal fibre, vegetable fibre and fruit fibre in relation to change in weight Confounders: age; baseline exposure; smoking; baseline weight; baseline values and changes in RG intake; calories; total	An increase in WG intake was inversely associated with long-term weight gain (P for trend <0.0001). For every 40 g/d increment in WG intake from all foods, weight gain was reduced by 0.49 kg. Bran that was added to the diet or obtained from fortified-grain foods further reduced the risk of weight gain (P for trend=0.01). For every 20 g/d increase in intake, weight gain was reduced by 0.36 kg.

				physical activity; alcohol; protein; trans, saturated, monounsaturated, and polyunsaturated fat	Changes in cereal (0.91 kg in the highest quintile vs. 1.30 kg in the lowest quintile; P for trend=0.0004) and fruit fibre (0.64 kg in the highest quintile vs. 1.59 kg in the lowest quintile; P for trend <0.0001) were inversely related to weight gain. No associations were observed for vegetable fibre and weight. No associations were observed between changes in RG or added germ consumption and body weight.
Bazzano et al. 2005, USA (82)	17 881 male physicians (40–84 y) participating in the Physicians' Health Study; 13 y of followup	Changes in BMI and body weight at 8 y and 13 y followup	61-item abbreviated semi-quantitative FFQ at baseline; included two questions on breakfast cereal consumption; quartiles of WG and RG intake (none, 1 serving/week, 2-6 serving/week, and ≥6 servings/week) Classification of breakfast cereals into WG and RG: breakfast cereals were evaluated for WG and bran content (≥25% WG or bran by weight)	Average changes in BMI and weight calculated for 8 y followup (1982–1990) and 13 y followup (1982–1995) according to quartiles of WG, RG and total breakfast cereals Risk of BMI≥25 kg/m^2 and weight gain≥10 kg or ≥15 kg calculated for 8 y followup (1982–1990) and 13 y followup (1982–1995) according to quartiles of WG, RG and total breakfast cereals Confounders: age; baseline BMI; smoking alcohol intake; physical activity; history of hypertension; history of high cholesterol; use of multivitamins	After 8 y, mean weight gain was significantly lower among participants consuming WG cereals (1.13 kg vs. 1.55 kg; P for trend=0.003), RG cereals (0.94 kg vs. 1.46 kg; P for trend=0.005) and total breakfast cereals (1.07 kg vs. 1.66 kg; P for trend<0.0001) at least 1 serving/d compared with those who rarely or never consumed these cereals. After 13 y, weight gain did not significantly differ by WG cereal consumption (P for trend=0.08) or RG cereal consumption (P for trend=0.33). Weight gain was significantly lower among participants consuming total breakfast cereals at least 1 serving/d compared with those who rarely or never consumed cereal (1.81 kg vs. 2.27 kg; P for trend=0.007). Compared with men who rarely or never consumed breakfast cereals, those who consumed ≥1serving/d were 22% (P for trend=0.001) and 12% (P for trend=0.01) less likely to become overweight at 8 y and 13 y followup, respectively. There were no significant differences in risk of becoming overweight according to WG cereal at 8 y and 13 y followup. Compared with those who rarely or never consumed RG cereals, those who consumed ≥1 serving/d were 19% less likely to become overweight (P for trend=0.03).

(*continued*)

Table 8.3 Longitudinal cohorts examining the relationship between whole grain intake, cereal fibre and change in measure of adiposity in adults. (*continued*)

Author, Year, Country	Subjects	Outcome	Dietary Method/Exposure	Methodology	Results and Conclusions
					Compared with men who rarely or never consumed breakfast cereals, those who consumed ≥1 serving breakfast cereals/d were 30% less likely to gain ≥10 kg at 13 y followup (P for trend=0.0003), and those who consumed ≥1 serving WG cereal/d were 22% less likely to gain ≥10 kg of weight (P for trend=0.01). All other associations between WG, RG and total breakfast cereals and risk of body weight gain were insignificant (P for trend ≥0.05).
Du et al. 2010, Netherlands (83)	89 432 European men and women (20–78 y) from 8 countries participating in the EPIC study; average followup time of 6.5 y	~6.5 year changes in WC and body weight	Country-specific validated FFQs at baseline; cereal fibre as marker for WG intake; quintiles of cereal fibre intake (10.7–17.5 g/d) Total dietary fibre: fibre intake from all foods and beverages Cereal fibre: cereals and cereal products (rice, pasta, breads, biscuits, crackers, breakfast cereals and other products made of flour)	Examined the associations between total and cereal fibre intake and changes in weight and WC Confounders: baseline age; weight and height; sex; smoking; education; physical activity; followup duration; alcohol consumption; intake of fat, carbohydrate, and protein; glycemic index; menopausal status and use of hormone replacement therapy; baseline WC	Total dietary fibre intake was inversely associated with changes in body weight. 10 g/d total dietary fibre intake was associated with an annual weight change of -39 g/y (95% CI: -71, -7 g/y; P for heterogeneity=0.01) and a BMI change of ~0.013. The heterogeneity across study centers for change in WC was not significant (P for heterogeneity=0.2). Cereal fibre was inversely associated with weight and WC change. On average, a 10 g/d cereal fibre was associated with an annual weight change of -77 g/y (95% CI: -127, -26 g/y; P for heterogeneity=0.01) and an annual WC of -0.10 cm/y (95% CI: -0.18, -0.02 cm/y; P for heterogeneity<0.001).

Mozaffarian et al. 2011, USA (84)	120 877 US men and women free of obesity and chronic disease taking part in the HPFS (1986–2006), NHS (1986–2006), and NHS II (1991–2003); 12-20 y of followup	Change in body weight evaluated every 4 y	Biennial validated diet questionnaires; quintiles of WG and RG intake	Examined the independent relationships between changes in WG and RG intake and weight changes within 4 y periods over a period of 12 y and 20 y for NHS I&II and HPFS, respectively Confounders: age; baseline BMI at the beginning of each 4 y period; sleep duration; changes in physical activity, alcohol use, television watching, smoking and all dietary factors	Weight gain was associated with increased consumption of refined grains (0.39 lb per serving per day, $P<0.001$). Inverse associations with weight gain, per serving per day, were seen for increased consumption of whole grains (-0.37 lb; $P<0.001$)
Mirmiran 2012 (85)	1938 adults (19–70 y); 3 y of follow up (2006–2008 to 2009–2011)	Changes in weight, WC and BAI	Semi-quantitative 168-item FFQ; quartiles of WG intake (median: 7.5 g–177g/d). Other dietary exposures reported (Vegetables, legumes, fruits, soy, nuts, olive and olive oils)	Baseline WG intake in relation to changes in weight, WC, and BAI Confounders: sex, age, BMI, education, smoking, physical activity, total energy intake, % EI from carbohydrates, fat and protein	Highest quartile of WG intake gained less weight (-1.0 kg) and WC gain (-1.43 cm), and less change in BAI (-0.46) compared to those in lowest quartile of WG intake over 3 years. Higher WG intake is one attribute of diet that could have favorable effects on prevention of weight gain and reduction of body adiposity.

NHS, Nurses' Health Study; FFQ, Food Frequency Questionnaire; WG, whole grain; RG, refined grain; BAI, body adiposity index; BMI, body mass index; WC, waist circumference; MONICA1, MONItoring of trends and determinants in CArdiovascular diseases; HPFS, Health Professional Follow-Up Study; EPIC, European Prospective Investigation into Cancer and Nutrition; CVD, Cardiovascular Disease; PREDIMED, PREvencion con DIeta MEDiterranean.

Table 8.4 Intervention studies investigating the effect of whole grain intake on measures of body weight and/or composition. Data are presented as mean ± SD. Where data were not accessible the mean or the range is presented.

Reference	Design and subjects[1]	Age BMI[2]	Intervention groups, type of whole grain and intervention products	WG intake (g/d)	Results
Non-calorie-restricted studies					
Ampatzoglou 2014 (12) (UK)	CO, 6 wk N: 33 ♂: 36%	49 ± 6 27.9±0.7	RG and mixed WG. Bread, pasta, rice, snacks and breakfast cereals. Test foods were provided for both groups.	159	Changes in both BW (0.2 vs. -0.2kg) and BMI (0.1 vs. -0.1kg/m^2) tended to differ between RG and WG groups (p=0.10 and p=0.08, respectively). No difference in BF% was seen.
Andersson 2007 (21) (Sweden)	CO, 6wk N=30 ♂: 27%	59 ± 5 28.3 ± 2.0	RG and mixed WG. Bread, crisp bread, muesli and pasta. Test foods were provided for both groups.	112	BMI increased more during WG consumption compared to RG (0.3 vs. 0.2 kg/m^2; p=0.046).
Bird 2008 (22) (Australia)	CO, 4 wk N = 17 ♂: 56%	56 ± 9 27.2 ± 5.1	RG wheat, WG wheat and WG barley. Bread, crackers, muffins and RTE-cereal. Test foods were provided for all groups.	90	BW were similar at the end of each of the three dietary interventions (RG: 80.1; WG wheat: 80.5 and WG barley: 79.3 kg; p>0.05) and were not different from baseline. Baseline BW were not reported.
Bodinham 2011 (23) (UK)	CO, 3 wk N = 14 ♂: 36%	26 ± 5 21.8 ± 3.0	RG wheat and WG wheat. Bread rolls. Test foods were provided for both groups.	48	There was no effect of WG compared with RG on BW, BF% or WC. Data were not reported.
Brownlee 2010 (17) (UK)	P, 16 wk N = 266 ♂: 50%	46 ± 10 30.1 ± 4.1	Control, mixed WG (low/ high dose) Bread, cereals, rice, pasta, cereal bar, crisps. Test foods were only provided for WG groups.	Control: 19 WG low: 74 WG high: 115	Changes in BW (0.0 vs. 0.7 vs. 0.2kg) and BF% (0.3 vs. 1.0 vs. 0.3%) did not differ between control and low and high dose WG groups.
Chang 2013 (16) (Taiwan)	P, 12 wk N: 34 ♂: ?	39 ± 12	RG and WG oat. Oat cereal. Test foods were provided for both groups.	75	Consumption of oat reduced body weight, BMI, body fat and the waist-to-hip ratio.
Davidson 1991 (24) (United States)	P, 6 wk N:76♂: 53	52.8	Control and WG oat (3 doses). Dry oat meal (hot cereal, muffins, shakes as recipe) and dry farina. Test foods were provided for both groups.	28 56 84	There was no effect of WG compared with RG on BW or WC. Data were not reported.

De Mello 2011 (18) (Finland)	P, 12 wk N = 68 ♂: 51%	59 ± 7 31.2 ± 3.5	RG and mixed WG. Snack bars, breads and pasta. Test foods were provided only for WG group.	N.A.	Changes in BW and BMI did not differ between RG and WG groups (p>0.05). Data were not reported.
Giacco 2010 (25) (Italy)	CO, 3 wk N = 15 ♂: 80%	55 ± 8 27.4 ± 3.0	RG wheat and WG wheat. Bread, pasta, rusks and crackers. Test foods were provided for both groups.	N.A.	Changes in BW (-0.1 vs. -0.2kg) did not differ between WG and RG groups (p=0.36).
Johnston 1998 (27) (USA)	P, 6 wk N = 124 ♂: 63%	57 N.A.	RG corn and WG oat. RTE cereal (cornflakes and Cheerios). Test foods were provided for both groups.	74	Changes in BW (0.3 vs. 0.5kg) did not differ between WG and RG groups.
Karmally 2005 (28) (USA)	P, 6 wk N = 152 ♂: 32%	49 ± 11 29.2 ± 3.8	RG corn and WG oat. RTE cereal (cornflakes and Cheerios). Test foods were provided for both groups.	74	Changes in BW (0.1 vs. 0.2kg) did not differ between WG and RG groups.
Kirwan 2016 (48) (USA)	CO, 8 wk N:33 ♂: 18%	40 ± 7	RG and mixed WG. Bread, pasta, rice, snacks and breakfast cereals. All foods were provided for both groups	108	No significant difference in weight loss between WG or RG (3% vs. 6%). There was no effect of WG compared with RG on reductions in BMI, BF%, WC, or FFM.
Kristensen 2017 (France) (47)	P, 12 wk N = 178 ♂: 0%	35 ± 9 30.1 ± 2.0	RG and mixed WG. Commercially available pasta, rice, bread, couscous, cereal bars, snacks and breakfast cereals foods were provided for both groups.	80	No significant difference in body weight and total fat mass between WG and RG intervention. Increase in abdominal fat (%) greater on WG compared to refined grain (0.7% compared to -0.3%), but only marginally significant (p=0.052).
Leinonen 2000 (29) (Finland)	CO, 4 wk N = 40 ♂: 45%	43 ± 8 24.5 ± 2.8	RG and WG rye. Bread and crisp bread. Test foods were provided for both groups.	N.A.	Changes in BW among men (0.1 vs. -0.4kg) and women (-0.3 vs. -0.4kg) did not differ between WG and RG groups.
Li 2016 (88) (China)	P, 1 year N=298 ♂: 52%	60 ± 6.1 26.8 ± 2.5	Control and WG oat (low/high dose). All foods were provided for WG oat groups for 30 days, then just oats provided for 1 year of followup.	WG Low: 50 WG High: 100	No significant differences in BW, BMI, WC, WHR, body fat (%) or visceral fat index between groups after 30 day intervention. After 1 year, those provided with 100g oat/day reduced BW by 1.86kg compared to control (usual diet).

(continued)

Table 8.4 Intervention studies investigating the effect of whole grain intake on measures of body weight and/or composition. Data are presented as mean ± SD. Where data were not accessible the mean or the range is presented. (*continued*)

Reference	Design and subjects[1]	Age BMI[2]	Intervention groups, type of whole grain and intervention products	WG intake (g/d)	Results
Li 2003 (26) (Japan)	CO, 4 wk N = 10 ♂: 0%	20 ± 1 19.2 ± 2.0	RG rice (white) and WG barley. Barley kernels and rice. All food was provided for both groups.	89	There was no effect of WG compared with RG on BW or BMI. Data were not reported.
McIntosh 2003 (30) (Australia)	CO, 4 wk N = 28 ♂: 100%	40-65 30.0 ± 4.8	RG wheat, WG wheat and WG rye. Bread, crisp bread and RTE cereal. Test foods were provided for all groups.	88	There was no effect of WG wheat or rye compared with RG on BW or BMI. Data were not reported.
Pereira 2002 (32) (USA)	CO, 6 wk N = 11 ♂: 45%	42 ± 9 30.2 ± 3.3	RG and mixed WG. RTE cereal, muffin, bread, chips, pasta and cookies. All food was provided for both groups.	N.A.	Changes in BW (0.0 vs. 0.1kg) did not differ between WG and RG diets.
Reynolds 2000 (34) (USA)	CO, 4 wk N = 43 ♂: 49%	52 24.4 ± 3.9	RG corn and WG oat. RTE cereals (cornflakes and Cheerios). Test foods were provided for both groups.	70	There was no effect of WG wheat or rye compared with RG on BW or BMI. Data were not reported.
Ross 2011 (35) (Switzerland)	CO, 2 wk N = 17 ♂: 35%	35 ± 4 23.7 ± 2.2	RG and mixed WG. RTE cereals, pasta, crackers, bread, cereal bars, frozen meals, couscous, risotto, noodles, pizza. All food was provided for both groups.	150	BW was 0.5kg lower after the WG compared with the RG diet (P=0·19).
Suhr 2017 (87) (Denmark)	P, 6 wk N= 70 ♂: 46%	51 ± 9.5 27.8 ± 1.9	RG wheat, WG wheat and WG rye RTE cereals, pasta, kernels, crisp bread and two choices of bread. Test foods were provided for both groups.	Wheat: 145 Rye: 124	BW and FM decreased more in the WG rye compared to the RG group (−1.06 vs 0.15kg and −0.75 vs. -0.04 kg, respectively; P<0.01 and P<0.05, respectively). The decrease in FM in the WG rye group tended to exceed that in the WG wheat group (P=0.07).
Tighe 2010 (19) (UK)	P, 16 wk N = 206 ♂: 50%	52 ± 7 27.7 ± 3.9	RG wheat, WG wheat and WG wheat/oat. Bread and RTE cereals. Test foods were provided for both groups.	N.A.	There was no effect of WG wheat or wheat/oat compared to RG on BW. Data were not reported.

Tucker 2010 (20) (Canada)	CO, 6 wk N = 28 ♂: 71%	55 ± 7 31.1 ± 4.3	RG and mixed WG. Bread. Test foods were provided for both groups	53	Changes in BW among NGI (-0.5 vs. -0.1kg) and women (-0.6 vs. -0.5kg) did not differ between WG and RG groups.
Turpeinen 2000 (36) (Finland)	CO, 4 wk N: 40 ♂: 45%	43 ± 12.6	RG wheat and WG rye Four different WG rye breads and 6 different RG wheat breads. Test foods was provided for both groups.	N.A.	There was no effect of WG compared to RG on BW. Data were not reported.
Van Horn 1988 (37) (USA)	P, 8 wk N = 236 ♂: 36%	42 N.A.	Control and WG oat. Oatmeal. Test food was only provided for WG group.	56	There was no effect of WG compared to RG on BW. Data were not reported.
Van Horn 1991 (38) (USA)	P, 8 wk N = 80 ♂: 50%	42 ± 13 26.2 ± 3.6	Control and WG oat. Instant oat. Test food was provided only for WG group.	54	There was no effect of WG compared to RG on BW. Data were not reported.
Vitaglione 2015 (89) (Italy)	P, 8 wk N = 68 ♂: 34%	39 ± 2.5 29.8 ± 0.5	RG and WG wheat. Commercially available WG RTE cereal and RG crackers and sliced bread. Test food was provided for both groups.	N.A.	There were no significant changes in body composition.
Zhang 2011 (33) (China)	P, 16 wk N = 193 ♂: 53%	50 ± 7 25.7 ± 3.0	RG rice (white) and WG rice (brown). Test food was provided for both groups.	100	Changes in BMI (-0.17 vs. -0.08kg/m^2) did not differ between WG and RG groups (p=0.23), although the decrease from baseline was significant in the WG group (p=0.02).
Calorie-restricted studies					
Gilhooly 2008 (41) (USA)	P, 6 wk N = 33 ♂: 24%	35 ± 5 27.5 ± 1.4	RG and WG wheat. RTE cereal (FiberOne or no extra fibre). All food was provided for both groups.	18.2	Changes in BW (-2.7 vs. -2.6kg) did not differ between WG and RG groups.
Harris Jackson (11) 2014 (United States)	P, 12 wk N: 50 ♂: 50%	46.1 ± 6	RG and mixed WG. Breads, crackers, chips, breakfast cereals, pasta, cookies, pancakes, rice. Test foods were provided for both groups.	213	No difference between WG and RG groups in changes in BW (-5.0 vs. -4.4kg), BF% (-1.0 vs. -0.8%), SAT (-44 vs. -51g) or VAT (-63 vs. -51g).

(continued)

Table 8.4 Intervention studies investigating the effect of whole grain intake on measures of body weight and/or composition. Data are presented as mean ± SD. Where data were not accessible the mean or the range is presented. (*continued*)

Reference	Design and subjects[1]	Age BMI[2]	Intervention groups, type of whole grain and intervention products	WG intake (g/d)	Results
Katcher 2008 (49) (USA)	P, 12 wk N = 47 ♂: 51%	46 ± 9 35.8 ± 4.5	Control (avoid WG) and mixed WG. Bread, rolls, RTE cereals, rice, pasta, snacks. Test foods were not provided for any group.	N.A.	Changes in BW (-3.7 vs. -5.3kg), WC (-2.5 vs. -4.7cm) or total BF% (-1.2 vs. -1.0%) did not differ between WG and RG groups; but abdominal BF% loss was greater with WG compared to RG (-2.2 vs. -0.9%; p=0.03 for time×group interaction).
Kim 2008 (44) (South Korea)	P, 6 wk N = 40 ♂: 0%	20-35 27.4 ± 2.5	RG rice (white) and WG rice (brown and black). MR powders. Test foods were provided for both groups.	N.A.	A greater weight loss was observed in WG (-6.75kg) than in RG (-5.4kg) group (p<0.05), as well as a greater reduction in BF% (-5.5 vs. -4.3%; p<0.05). Change in WC did not differ between groups.
Kristensen 2012 (40) (Denmark)	P, 12 wk N = 72 ♂: 0%	60 ± 5 30.2 ± 3.0	RG wheat and WG wheat. Bread, pasta and biscuits. Test foods were provided for both groups.	105	Weight loss in WG (-3.6kg) tended to be greater than in RG (-2.7kg) group (p=0.11). Decrease in BF% was greater in WG (-3.0%) than in RG (-2.1%) (p=0.04). Change in WC did not differ between groups.
Maki 2010 (42) (USA)	P, 12 wk N = 144 ♂: 22%	49 ± 1 32.1 ± 0.5	RG corn and WG oat. RTE cereals (cornflakes and Cheerios), white toast, bagels, muffins, rice, cakes and snacks. Test foods were provided for both groups	66	Change in BW (-2.2 vs.-1.7kg) did not differ between WG and RG groups (p=0.33), whereas WC decreased more in the WG compared to RG group (-3.3 vs. -.1.9cm; p=0.012).
Melanson 2006 (39) (USA)	P, 12 wk N = 91 ♂: 21%	42 ± 9 30.8 ± 16.0	Control and mixed WG. RTE cereals. Test foods were provided for both groups.	N.A.	Weight loss in WG (-4.7kg) and control (-5.0kg) groups did not differ.
Saltzman 2001 (46) (USA)	P, 6 wk N = 43 ♂: 47%	45 ± 22 26.4 ± 3.3	Control and WG oat. Quick oat as hot cereal, bread, casseroles. All food was provided for both groups.	82	Weight loss in WG (-3.9kg) and control (-4.0kg) groups did not differ (p=0.80). Also, changes in BF did not differ between WG (-2.5kg) and control (-2.7kg) groups (p=0.65).

BF: body fat; BMI: body mass index; BW: body weight; CO: crossover study design; MR: meal replacement; P: parallel study design; RG: refined grain; RTE: ready-to-eat; SAT: subcutaneous adipose tissue; WC: waist circumference; FM: Fat Mass; FFM: Fat Free Mass; WG: whole grain; VAT: visceral adipose tissue.

In addition, the authors also considered dietary fibre intake by food source, including fibre from cereal, fruits and vegetables, and examined whether other attributes of whole grains, such as bran and germ, were associated with weight gain. Added bran further reduced the risk of weight gain, and the authors reported that for every 20 g/d increase in bran intake, weight gain was reduced by 0.36 kg. A higher intake of fruit and cereal fibres, but not vegetable fibre, was associated with less weight gain over the 8-year period. In contrast to the previous studies (80), a higher intake or an increase in refined-grain intake did not lead to greater weight gain. Bazzano and colleagues (82), using data from the Physicians' Health Study cohort, examined the relationship between breakfast cereal consumption and weight gain. Over a period of 8 and 13 years of followup, men who consumed breakfast cereal consistently weighed less than those who consumed breakfast cereals less often, regardless of whether the cereal was whole or refined gain. Compared with men who rarely or never consumed breakfast cereals, those who consumed ≥1 serving/d of breakfast cereals were 22% and 12% less likely to become overweight during follow-up periods of 8 and 13 years.

In a subsequent meta-analysis using data from Nurses' Health Study and Health Professionals Follow-up cohorts and including additional data from the Nurses' Health Study II cohort, Mozaffarian et al. (84) found that multiple lifestyle changes were independently associated with long-term weight gain, including changes in whole- and refined-grain intakes. Based on dietary data collected between 1986 and 2006 in two cohorts, and between 1991 and 2003 in one cohort, it was estimated that every 1 serving/d increase in whole grain intake could be attributed to an annual weight loss of 0.04 kg, while each increase in serving of refined-grain intake could be attributed to a similar magnitude of weight gain. In a sample of Danish adults, Halkjaer and colleagues (81) examined dietary factors and food groups, including refined- and whole grain bread intake in relation to change in WC over a 6-year period. Independent of overall weight gain, a positive relationship was found between increased consumption of refined-grain bread and abdominal adiposity in females, but not males. A higher intake of whole grains was not associated with changes in adiposity in neither men nor women. More recently, using data from the PREvención con Dieta MEDiterránea (PREDIMED) trial, the first large randomized controlled trial for the primary prevention of CVD, Bautista-Castano et al. examined change in bread consumption (total, whole and refined grain) on changes in adiposity over 4 years (86). For the primary study, 2213 participants were randomized to one of three dietary patterns, namely, two Mediterranean-type diets (Med-diet) with different fat sources, mixed nuts or virgin olive oil and one low-fat diet (control group). However, because no significant interactions between the trial intervention and changes in total white or whole grain bread consumption were identified in the statistical analysis, Bautista-Castano and colleagues included data on all participants in a secondary analysis to examine the prospective relationship between bread intake and weight gain (data not presented in Table 8.3). They observed that an increase in white bread consumption was associated with greater gains in both WC and body weight. Conversely, losing weight and lower WC were associated with a decrease in white bread consumption. In contrast, no significant dose–response relationship was observed for change in whole grain bread consumption and overall or abdominal adiposity.

For most individuals, whole grain foods are the major contributors to dietary fibre in cereals. Using data from 89,432 men and women in the large European Prospective Investigation into Cancer (EPIC) study, Du and colleagues (83) observed a 77 g annual decrease in body weight and a 0.10 cm annual decrease in WC for each 10 grams of cereal fibre consumed per day. Of the seven prospective studies investigating whole grain consumption and risk of weight gain, whole grain intake was associated with a significant reduction in weight gain in 4 out of the 5 studies (15, 80, 83–85). Though effects of whole grains on body weight appear considerably small, both avoidance of weight gain as well as relatively small reductions in body weight are thought to significantly reduce chronic disease risk in the proportion of the population that is overweight or obese (31).

8.8 Intervention studies

During the last decade, an increasing number of randomized controlled intervention studies on whole grains has been published (n=33), which included measures of body weight and/or composition (Table 8.4). These studies do, however, vary considerably in terms of study length, study design and type and dose of whole grain administered in the intervention. Such variations in study design may be important to consider when interpreting results. A summary of these studies, including information on study population, dietary intervention, whole grain dose and type, and main results are presented in Table 8.4.

8.9 Studies without calorie-restriction

To date, 28 whole grain intervention studies (12, 16-30, 32-38, 47, 48, 87-89) have been published that also include some measure of body weight and/or composition (Table 8.4, of which 19 (17-23, 25-30, 32-35, 37, 38) were included in the aforementioned meta-analysis (10). Of the 28 studies included here, 10 used a mixed whole grain diet (12, 17-21, 32, 35, 47, 48), 6 used whole grain wheat (19, 22, 23, 25, 30, 87), 8 used whole grain oat (16, 24, 27, 28, 34, 37, 38, 88), 4 used rye (29, 30, 36, 87) and two or fewer studies used barley and rice. Whole grain doses varied greatly between studies, ranging from 28–159 g/d, and study length varied greatly with durations from 2 weeks (35) to 16 weeks (17, 19, 33). The majority of these studies focused on investigating the effect of increasing whole grain consumption on CVD risk markers such as blood lipids or glucose metabolism; body weight and composition were not the primary endpoints. Nonetheless, most of these studies provided measures of body weight and/or composition, yet results should be interpreted with caution due to the lack of detail on whether actions were taken to ensure weight stability during the study. Ampatzoglou and colleagues (12) recently conducted a randomized crossover study in which 33 overweight middle-aged adults completed two dietary intervention periods of 6 weeks duration. Study volunteers consumed a variety of mixed whole grain or refined-grain products during the intervention periods, and the average whole grain dose was 159 g/d (range: 85-338 g/d) during the whole grain period; thus, a relatively high dose compared to most other studies. After 6 weeks, a small decrease in body weight of -0.2 ± 0.2 kg was observed during the whole grain period, while body weight increased slightly (0.2 ± 0.2 kg) during the refined-grain period ($p = 0.10$ for difference), whereas no difference was observed in change in percent body fat. During each intervention, dietary intake was estimated using a 3-day food diary, and energy intake did not differ between the two periods (2,076 ± 82 vs. 2,045 ± 88 kcal/d in the refined- and whole grain periods, respectively). In contrast, a similarly designed study in 30 overweight/obese adults, randomized to mixed refined- or whole grain diets, reported a small but significant increase in BMI after a 6 week whole grain intervention (0.3 ± vs. 0.2 in the whole grain and refined-grain periods, respectively; $p=0.046$) (21). One difference in the dietary intervention was the amount of intervention foods was fixed, independent of sex and energy requirements. This may have resulted in overconsumption among some participants; however, such overconsumption is anticipated to be similar during the refined- and whole grain periods. Similar to the study by Ampatzoglou and colleagues (12), no difference in energy consumed during the two dietary periods was observed. It is important to note that the differences in body weight were very modest in both of these studies.

In summary, the incorporation of whole grains into a weight maintenance diet appears to have little or no effect on body weight reduction. As previously mentioned, it is not clear whether the different studies included measures to keep weight stable during the dietary interventions in order not to confound potential effects of changes in body weight on CVD risk markers. Also, in evaluating the evidence, the circumstances around how intervention foods were supplied and consumed must be considered. First, foods may have been supplied in some studies and recommended in others. Second, foods may have been added to the participants' habitual diets, as opposed to replacing other foods, either because the participants lacked instructions on how to substitute grain-based foods or because products were provided only for the participants in the whole grain group. For example, in the UK WHOLEHEART study (17), where habitual whole grain consumption is low, products were only provided for the participants in the two whole grain intervention groups, whereas the control group was instructed to maintain their habitual diet low in whole grain. As a consequence, the intervention lead to an increase in overall energy intake in participants consuming the high dose of whole grain (120 g/d for 16 weeks) compared to the control group ($p=0.005$). The frequency of fruit consumption among the intervention group decreased, which may reflect a change in dietary pattern in order to incorporate the large dose of whole grain into the diet. Such a change, in light of the fact that fruit has low energy density, may explain the overall increase in energy intake among participants. From these studies it cannot, however, be concluded whether long-term weight maintenance may be improved with whole grain as indicated by the prospective cohort studies reviewed above. However, in the prospective cohorts, the average difference in weight gain over a period of ~10 years was ~0.5kg. This very subtle difference would be difficult to reproduce in an intervention study due to lack of statistical power, as this would correspond to <0.1kg difference in body weight.

8.10 Studies with calorie-restriction

Whole grains contribute considerably more dietary fibre than their refined-grain counterparts, which may contribute to suppression of hunger. This may ease adherence to a calorie-restricted diet. For this reason, it may be speculated that during weight loss, a greater change in body weight may occur on a whole- versus refined-grain diet. A total of 8 studies have applied a calorie-restricted, whole grain intervention lasting from 6 to 12 weeks with interventions including mixed whole grains (11, 39, 49), whole grain wheat (40, 41), whole grain oat (42, 43) or whole grain rice (44). Only one of the eight studies found a significantly greater reduction in body weight with whole grain compared to refined grain intake (44). This study was conducted in 40 South-Korean overweight and obese younger women, randomized to consume a meal replacement product containing either a white rice or brown/black rice mixture as powders. Over the 6-week study period, the women eating the brown/black rice mixture lost 6.75 ± 0.40 kg, and the control group lost 5.37 ± 0.40 kg ($p<0.05$ for difference between groups). In addition, women eating the rice mixture had a significantly greater reduction in body fat percentage (-5.50 ± 0.51 vs. -4.30 ± 0.30 %; $p<0.05$). While this study reports an exceptionally low daily energy intake of approximately 260 kJ/d among the intervention and control group, such a low reported level of energy intake is likely an error and does not reflect a normal diet, even under calorie-restricted conditions. In light of this, the results of this study must be interpreted with caution.

Another study found a beneficial effect of whole grain intake on body composition, despite no effect on body weight, in 72 overweight and obese postmenopausal women in Denmark (40), a country where habitual whole grain intake is relatively high (90). In this study, women were randomized to consume either whole grain or refined-grain wheat products (breads, pasta and biscuits) for 12 weeks following a 2-week run-in period on refined-grain wheat products. Changes in body weight reduction only tended to differ between groups (-2.7 ± 1.9 vs. -3.6 ± 3.2 kg in the refined- and whole grain groups, respectively, $p=0.11$), whereas the difference in percentage body fat, measured by Dual energy X-ray Absorptiometry (DEXA) scans, was reduced significantly more in those consuming whole grain compared to refined grain (-2.1 vs. -3.0 % in the refined- and whole grain groups, respectively, $p=0.04$). Katcher and colleagues (49) completed a 12-week, open-labeled randomized weight loss study in 50 obese individuals, randomized to either consume or avoid whole grain products. However, intervention products were not provided for the study participants. After 12 weeks, central abdominal fat mass, assessed by DEXA scanning, decreased significantly more in those eating whole grain foods compared to those who were instructed to avoid whole grain foods, whereas no group difference was observed in body weight. In this study, the authors also found that C-reactive protein (CRP) decreased more in those consuming whole grain foods perhaps suggesting that an anti-inflammatory driven effect of whole grain may be mediated by a reduction in abdominal fat mass (49). To follow up on this, the same group recently completed a highly controlled study, where 50 participants followed either a whole grain or refined-grain diet for 12 weeks using an isocaloric approach for the first 6 weeks followed by a 6-week calorie-restricted intervention (11). In contrast to the earlier study, all foods were provided for the participants in a highly controlled manner, eliminating differences in energy intake, which could result in differences in weight loss between groups. In this more recent intervention, however, they were unable to replicate the changes in body weight observed in the previous study, and no significant differences were observed in total abdominal fat mass, SAT or VAT as assessed by MRI in a subgroup of participants. In summary, the evidence appears to be slightly more promising in terms of the benefits of whole grain intake under conditions of weight loss. As previously mentioned, adherence to a calorie-restricted diet is facilitated by a whole grain diet high in dietary fibre, which may diminish hunger between meals. Also, studies of whole grains in the context of weight loss focused more on body weight regulation and, therefore, were designed to detect differences in body weight.

Overall, evidence from randomized controlled intervention studies provide only limited evidence supporting a benefit of whole grain intake on body weight regulation. Although randomized controlled intervention designs have a number of advantages over observational designs, most importantly the elimination of considerable confounding and a high level of control over dietary intake, they also suffer from some drawbacks. Such drawbacks include short study durations that render it impossible to draw conclusions on long-term effects of whole grain consumption. Also, the sometimes unrealistically high dose of whole grain consumed decreases the validity of the results to some degree, although a complete substitution of refined for whole grain products would result in a daily intake similar to intakes reported in some intervention studies. Finally, the inability to blind the participants to their diet (whole grain vs. control) is likely a major disadvantage in light of the fact that whole grain consumption in most countries is associated with a more healthy lifestyle; thus, participants randomized to a whole grain diet may act differently than those randomized to a refined-grain diet (e.g., complying better with consumption of intervention products risking overconsumption or a change in other lifestyle patterns such as physical activity or intake of other foods). Such differences in behavior between groups are difficult to identify and, therefore, difficult to take into account when interpreting results.

8.11 Proposed mechanism of action by which whole grains influence weight gain

A number of potential mechanisms have been proposed to explain the effect of whole grains on body weight. Some of these mechanisms include the satiating effect of whole grains resulting from their high fibre content, the potential role of magnesium and fibre in lowering post-prandial glucose and insulin response, improved insulin sensitivity and, more recently, the impact of fermentable fibres and prebiotics on modulating the gut microbiota (91).

8.12 Conclusion

8.12.1 Summary of the evidence

Although evidence from prospective studies suggests that higher whole grain intakes may modestly attenuate weight gain after controlling for other lifestyle and dietary factors, while increasing refined-grain intake may contribute to weight gain, too few studies have specifically addressed this hypothesis to draw firm conclusions. There is limited evidence linking higher whole grain consumption to long-term changes in abdominal adiposity, and a lack of observational studies using more precise methods to measure body fat deposition, such as CT or MRI, and body fat distribution. Most prospective studies have estimated total whole grain intake by individual food groups, rather than quantifying as grams of whole grain per day; therefore, observed associations may be attenuated by non-differential misclassification of whole grain intake.

A relatively large number of randomized controlled whole grain intervention studies have been conducted to date, although only a few studies focus primarily on measures of body weight and composition. Of the 23 studies reviewed here that did not apply a weight-loss regimen, only one study reported a significant reduction in body weight from a whole grain diet compared to control. Among the eight whole grain weight loss studies, only one reported significantly greater weight loss with whole grain rice compared to white rice, and only one other study reported a significantly greater reduction in body fat percentage with a whole grain wheat diet compared to refined wheat. Thus, overall, randomized controlled whole grain intervention studies provide only very limited support of a benefit of whole grain on body weight regulation in the short-term and, thus far, it is unclear why some studies report benefits whereas others do not, as neither whole grain dose nor type, or study duration appear to explain these differences.

8.12.2 Future directions

Currently existing observational data largely reflects whole grain intake more than a decade ago, with estimated intakes largely derived from FFQ with fixed food categories. Given the increase in availability of a wider variety of whole grain foods, incorporating more quantitative methods into diet surveys, such as recalls or food records, will capture this diversity in whole grain intake. Most of the current evidence from observational studies of higher whole grain intake being linked to lower body weight is from cross-sectional studies. Furthermore, the majority of large observational cohorts originate in the United States, whereas less data is available from other countries, where both the type and amount of whole grain intake may be different. This may provide greater insight into whether regions where whole grain foods are staple foods exhibit different patterns and make differentiating between whole grain varieties possible. The number of well-conducted randomized whole grain intervention studies has increased dramatically over the last decade. However, interventions are all relatively small in size, short in study duration and, as such, a large long-term study lasting >1 year is lacking (50). A study designed to increase whole grain consumption would contribute data on long-term weight maintenance in a randomized, real-life setting. The evidence is also lacking on a side-by-side comparison of different grain varieties, as well as the importance of particle size and other food characteristics on body weight regulation, as there are some indications that these factors may be of importance for appetite control, glucose metabolism and fermentation patterns of whole grain foods.

8.13 Acknowledgements

NMM would like to thank Caitlin Blakley, MS, for her help in preparing the tables, and Caleigh M. Sawicki, MS, MPH, for her help with editing.

This study was supported by a grant from the USDA Agricultural Research Service (agreement 58-1950-0-014).

List of abbreviations: FFQ. Food Frequency Questionnaire; BMI, Body Mass Index; WC, Waist Circumference; NHS, Nurses' Health Study; FFQ, Food Frequency Questionnaire; WG, whole grain; RG, refined grain.

8.14 References

1 Grundy, S.M. (2004). Obesity, metabolic syndrome, and Cardiovascular disease. *The Journal of Clinical Endocrinology & Metabolism*, 89(6), 2595–2600.

2 Popkin, B.M., Adair, L.S., and Ng, S.W. (2012). Global nutrition transition and the pandemic of obesity in developing countries. *Nutrition Reviews*, 70(1), 3–21.

3 Ng, M., Fleming, T., Robinson, M., Thomson, B., Graetz, N., Margono, C., et al. (2014). Global, regional, and national prevalence of overweight and obesity in children and adults during 1980–2013: A systematic analysis for the Global Burden of Disease Study 2013. *Lancet*, 384(9945), 766–781.

4 Abarca-Gómez, L., Abdeen, Z.A., Hamid, Z.A., Abu-Rmeileh, N.M., Acosta-Cazares, B., Acuin, C., et al. (2017). Worldwide trends in body-mass index, underweight, overweight, and obesity from 1975 to 2016: A pooled analysis of 2416 population-based measurement studies in 128·9 million children, adolescents, and adults. *The Lancet*, 390(10113), 2627–2642.

5 Despres, J.P. (2012). Body fat distribution and risk of cardiovascular disease: An update. *Circulation*, 126(10), 1301–1313.

6 Executive Summary of The Third Report of The National Cholesterol Education Program (NCEP) Expert Panel on Detection, Evaluation, and Treatment of High Blood Cholesterol In Adults (Adult Treatment Panel III). (2001). *JAMA, 285*(19), 2486–2497.

7 Ford, E.S., Li, C., Zhao, G., and Tsai, J. (2005). Trends in obesity and abdominal obesity among adults in the United States from 1999–2008. *International Journal of Obesity*, 35(5), 736–743.

8 Xi, B., Mi, J., Zhao, M., Zhang, T., Jia, C., Li, J., et al. (2014). Trends in abdominal obesity among U.S. children and adolescents. *Pediatrics*, 134(2), e334–e339.

9 Harland, J.I., and Garton, L.E. (2008). Whole-grain intake as a marker of healthy body weight and adiposity. *Public Health Nutrition*, 11(6), 554–563.

10 Pol, K., Christensen, R., Bartels, E.M., Raben, A., Tetens, I., and Kristensen, M. (2013). Whole grain and body weight changes in apparently healthy adults: A systematic review and meta-analysis of randomized controlled studies. *Am. J. Clin. Nutr.*, 98(4), 872–884.

11 Harris Jackson, K., West, S.G., Vanden Heuvel, J.P., Jonnalagadda, S.S., Ross, A.B., Hill, A.M., et al. (2014). Effects of whole and refined grains in a weight-loss diet on markers of metabolic syndrome in individuals with increased waist circumference: A randomized controlled-feeding trial. *Am. J. Clin. Nutr.*, 100(2), 577–586.

12 Ampatzoglou, A., Atwal, K.K., Maidens, C.M., Williams, C.L., Ross, A.B., Thielecke, F., et al. (2015, in press). Increased whole grain consumption does not affect blood biochemistry, body composition, or gut microbiology in healthy, low-habitual whole grain consumers. *Journal of Nutrition.*

13 Jacobs, D.R., Meyer, K.A., Kushi, L.H., and Folsom, A.R. (1998). Whole-grain intake may reduce the risk of ischemic heart disease death in postmenopausal women: The Iowa Women's Health Study. *Am. J. Clin. Nutr.*, 68(2), 248–257.

14 Jensen, M.K., Koh-Banerjee, P., Hu, F.B., Franz, M., Sampson, L., Gronbaek, M., et al. (2004). Intakes of whole grains, bran, and germ and the risk of coronary heart disease in men. *Am. J. Clin. Nutr.*, 80(6), 1492–1499.

15 Koh-Banerjee, P., Franz, M., Sampson, L., Liu, S., Jacobs, D.R., Spiegelman, D., et al. (2004). Changes in whole-grain, bran, and cereal fiber consumption in relation to 8-y weight gain among men. *Am. J. Clin. Nutr.*, 80(5), 1237–1245.

16 Chang, H.C., Huang, C.N., Yeh, D.M., Wang, S.J., Peng, C.H., and Wang, C.J. (2013). Oat prevents obesity and abdominal fat distribution, and improves liver function in humans. *Plant Foods for Human Nutrition (Dordrecht, Netherlands)*, 68(1), 18–23.

17 Brownlee, I.A., Moore, C., Chatfield, M., Richardson, D.P., Ashby, P., Kuznesof, S.A., et al. (2010). Markers of cardiovascular risk are not changed by increased whole-grain intake: The WHOLEheart study, a randomised, controlled dietary intervention. *Br. J. Nutr.*, 104(1), 125–134.

18 de Mello, V.D., Schwab, U., Kolehmainen, M., Koenig, W., Siloaho, M., Poutanen, K., et al. (2011). A diet high in fatty fish, bilberries and wholegrain products improves markers of endothelial function and inflammation in individuals with impaired glucose metabolism in a randomised controlled trial: The Sysdimet study. *Diabetologia*, 54(11), 2755–2767.

19 Tighe, P., Duthie, G., Vaughan, N., Brittenden, J., Simpson, W.G., Duthie, S., et al. (2010). Effect of increased consumption of whole-grain foods on blood pressure and other cardiovascular risk markers in healthy middle-aged persons: A randomized controlled trial. *Am. J. Clin. Nutr.*, 92(4), 733–740.

20 Tucker, A.J., Mackay, K.A., Robinson, L.E., Graham, T.E., Bakovic, M., and Duncan, A.M. (2010). The effect of whole grain wheat sourdough bread consumption on serum lipids in healthy normoglycemic/normoinsulinemic and hyperglycemic/hyperinsulinemic adults depends on presence of the APOE E3/E3 genotype: A randomized controlled trial. *Nutrition & Metabolism*, 7, 7.

21 Andersson, A., Tengblad, S., Karlstrom, B., Kamal-Eldin, A., Landberg, R., Basu, S., et al. (2007). Whole-grain foods do not affect insulin sensitivity or markers of lipid peroxidation and inflammation in healthy, moderately overweight subjects. *J. Nutr.*, 137(6), 1401–1407.

22 Bird, A.R., Vuaran, M.S., King, R.A., Noakes, M., Keogh, J., Morell, M.K., et al. (2008). Wholegrain foods made from a novel high-amylose barley variety (Himalaya 292) improve indices of bowel health in human subjects. *Br. J. Nutr.*, 99(5), 1032–1040.

23 Bodinham, C.L., Hitchen, K.L., Youngman, P.J., Frost, G.S., and Robertson, M.D. (2011). Short-term effects of whole-grain wheat on appetite and food intake in healthy adults: A pilot study. *British Journal of Nutrition*, 1(1), 1–4.

24 Davidson, M.H., Dugan, L.D., Burns, J.H., Bova, J., Story, K., and Drennan, K.B. (1991). The hypocholesterolemic effects of beta-glucan in oatmeal and oat bran. A dose-controlled study. *JAMA*, 265(14), 1833–1839.

25 Giacco, R., Clemente, G., Cipriano, D., Luongo, D., Viscovo, D., Patti, L., et al. (2010). Effects of the regular consumption of wholemeal wheat foods on cardiovascular risk factors in healthy people. Nutrition, metabolism, and cardiovascular diseases. *NMCD*, 20(3), 186–194.
26 Li, J., Kaneko, T., Qin, L.Q., Wang, J., and Wang, Y. (2003). Effects of barley intake on glucose tolerance, lipid metabolism, and bowel function in women. *Nutrition*, 19(11–12), 926–929.
27 Johnston, L.R.H., Hunninghake, D.B., Schultz, K., and Westereng, B. (1998). Cholesterol-lowering benefits of a whole grain oat ready-to-eat cereal. *Nutrition in Clinical Care*, 1, 6–12.
28 Karmally, W., Montez, M.G., Palmas, W., Martinez, W., Branstetter, A., Ramakrishnan, R., et al. (2005). Cholesterol-lowering benefits of oat-containing cereal in Hispanic americans. *Journal of the American Dietetic Association*, 105(6), 967–970.
29 Leinonen, K.S., Poutanen, K.S., and Mykkanen, H.M. (2000). Rye bread decreases serum total and LDL cholesterol in men with moderately elevated serum cholesterol. *J. Nutr.*, 130(2), 164–170.
30 McIntosh, G.H., Noakes, M., Royle, P.J., and Foster, P.R. (2003). Whole-grain rye and wheat foods and markers of bowel health in overweight middle-aged men. *Am. J. Clin. Nutr.*, 77(4), 967–974.
31 Clinical Guidelines on the Identification, Evaluation, and Treatment of Overweight and Obesity in Adults – The Evidence Report. (1998). National Institutes of Health. *Obes Res.*, 6(Suppl. 2), 51S–209S.
32 Pereira, M.A., Jacobs, D.R., Jr., Pins, J.J., Raatz, S.K., Gross, M.D., Slavin, J.L., et al. (2002). Effect of whole grains on insulin sensitivity in overweight hyperinsulinemic adults. *Am. J. Clin. Nutr.*, 75(5), 848–855.
33 Zhang, G., Pan, A., Zong, G., Yu, Z., Wu, H., Chen, X., et al. (2011). Substituting white rice with brown rice for 16 weeks does not substantially affect metabolic risk factors in middle-aged Chinese men and women with diabetes or a high risk for diabetes. *J. Nutr.*, 141(9), 1685–1690.
34 Reynolds, H.R. Quiter, E., and Hunninghake, D.B. (2000). Whole grain oat cereal lowers serum lipids. *Topics in Clinical Nutrition*, 15, 74–83.
35 Ross, A.B., Bruce, S.J., Blondel-Lubrano, A., Oguey-Araymon, S., Beaumont, M., Bourgeois, A. et al (2011). A whole-grain cereal-rich diet increases plasma betaine, and tends to decrease total and LDL-cholesterol compared with a refined-grain diet in healthy subjects. Br. J. Nutr.,105(10), 1492–1502.
36 Turpeinen, A.M., Juntunen, K., Mutanen, M., and Mykkanen, H. (2000). Similar responses in hemostatic factors after consumption of wholemeal rye bread and low-fiber wheat bread. *Eur. J. Clin. Nutr.*, 54(5), 418–423.
37 Van Horn, L., Emidy, L.A., Liu, K.A., Liao, Y.L., Ballew, C., King, J., et al. (1988). Serum lipid response to a fat-modified, oatmeal-enhanced diet. *Preventive Medicine*, 17(3), 377–386.
38 Van Horn, L., Moag-Stahlberg, A., Liu, K.A., Ballew, C., Ruth, K., Hughes, R., et al. Effects on serum lipids of adding instant oats to usual American diets. *American Journal of Public Health*, 81(2), 183–188.
39 Melanson, K.J., Angelopoulos, T.J., Nguyen, V.T., Martini, M., Zukley, L., Lowndes, J., et al. (2006). Consumption of whole-grain cereals during weight loss: effects on dietary quality, dietary fiber, magnesium, vitamin B-6, and obesity. *Journal of the American Dietetic Association*, 106(9), 1380–1388; quiz 9-90.
40 Kristensen, M., Toubro, S., Jensen, M.G., Ross, A.B., Riboldi, G., Petronio, M., et al. (2012). Whole grain compared with refined wheat decreases the percentage of body fat following a 12-week, energy-restricted dietary intervention in postmenopausal women. *J. Nutr.*, 142(4), 710–716.
41 Gilhooly, C.H., Das, S.K., Golden, J.K., McCrory, M.A., Rochon, J., DeLany, J.P., et al. (2008). Use of cereal fiber to facilitate adherence to a human caloric restriction program. *Aging Clinical and Experimental Research*, 20(6), 513–520.
42 Maki, K.C., Beiseigel, J.M., Jonnalagadda, S.S., Gugger, C.K., Reeves, M.S., Farmer, M.V., et al. (2010). Whole-grain ready-to-eat oat cereal, as part of a dietary program for weight loss, reduces low-density lipoprotein cholesterol in adults with overweight and obesity more than a dietary program including low-fiber control foods. *Journal of the American Dietetic Association*, 110(2), 205–214.
43 Saltzman, E., Moriguti, J.C., Das, S.K., Corrales, A., Fuss, P., Greenberg, A.S., et al. (2001). Effects of a cereal rich in soluble fiber on body composition and dietary compliance during consumption of a hypocaloric diet. *J. Am. Col.l Nutr.*, 20(1), 50–57.
44 Kim, J.Y., Kim, J.H., Lee, da H., Kim, S.H., and Lee, S.S. (2008). Meal replacement with mixed rice is more effective than white rice in weight control, while improving antioxidant enzyme activity in obese women. *Nutrition Research (New York;)*, 28(2), 66–71.
45 Kristensen, M., Jensen, M.G., Riboldi, G., Petronio, M., Bugel, S., Toubro, S., et al. (2010). Wholegrain vs. refined wheat bread and pasta: Effect on postprandial glycemia, appetite, and subsequent ad libitum energy intake in young healthy adults. *Appetite*, 54(1), 163–169.

46 Saltzman, E., Das, S.K., Lichtenstein, A.H., Dallal, G.E., Corrales, A., Schaefer, E.J., et al. (2001). An oat-containing hypocaloric diet reduces systolic blood pressure and improves lipid profile beyond effects of weight loss in men and women. *J. Nutr,*. 131(5), 1465–1470.
47 Kristensen, M., Pelletier, X., Ross, A.B., and Thielecke, F. (2017). A high rate of non-compliance confounds the study of whole grains and weight maintenance in a randomised intervention trial—The case for greater use of dietary biomarkers in nutrition intervention studies. *Nutrients*, 9(1).
48 Kirwan, J.P., Malin, S.K., Scelsi, A.R., Kullman, E.L., Navaneethan, S.D., Pagadala, M.R., et al. (2016). A whole-grain diet reduces cardiovascular risk factors in overweight and obese adults: A randomized controlled trial. *J. Nutr.*, 146(11), 2244–2251.
49 Katcher, H.I., Legro, R.S., Kunselman, A.R., Gillies, P.J., Demers, L.M., Bagshaw, D.M., et al. (2008). The effects of a whole grain-enriched hypocaloric diet on cardiovascular disease risk factors in men and women with metabolic syndrome. *Am. J. Clin. Nutr.*, 87(1), 79–90.
50 Sawicki, C., Livingston, K., Ross, A., Jacques, P., Koecher, K., McKeown, N., et al. (2018). Evaluating whole grain intervention study designs and reporting practices using evidence mapping methodology. *Nutrients*, 10(8), 1052.
51 Hollænder, P.L.B., Ross, A.B., and Kristensen, M. (2015). Whole-grain and blood lipid changes in apparently healthy adults: A systematic review and meta-analysis of randomized controlled studies. *Am. J. Clin. Nutr.*, 102(3), 556–572.
52 Jacobs, D.R., Meyer, H.E., and Solvoll, K. (2001). Reduced mortality among whole grain bread eaters in men and women in the Norwegian County Study. *Eur. J. Clin. Nutr.*, 55(2), 137–143.
53 McKeown, N.M., Meigs, J.B., Liu, S., Wilson, P.W.F., and Jacques, P.F. (2002). Whole-grain intake is favorably associated with metabolic risk factors for type 2 diabetes and cardiovascular disease in the Framingham Offspring Study. *Am. J. Clin. Nutr.*, 76(2), 390–398.
54 Montonen, J., Knekt, P., Järvinen, R., Aromaa, A., and Reunanen, A. (2003). Whole-grain and fiber intake and the incidence of type 2 diabetes. *Am. J. Clin. Nutr.*, 77(3), 622–629.
55 Esmaillzadeh, A., Mirmiran, P., and Azizi, F. (2005). Whole-grain consumption and the metabolic syndrome: A favorable association in Tehranian adults. *Eur. J. Clin. Nutr.*, 59(3), 353–362.
56 Sahyoun, N.R., Jacques, P.F., Zhang, X.L., Juan, W., and McKeown, N.M. (2006). Whole-grain intake is inversely associated with the metabolic syndrome and mortality in older adults. *Am. J. Clin. Nutr.*, 83(1), 124–131.
57 Lutsey, P.L., Jacobs, D.R., Kori, S., Mayer-Davis, E., Shea, S., Steffen, L.M., et al. (2007). Whole grain intake and its cross-sectional association with obesity, insulin resistance, inflammation, diabetes and subclinical CVD: The MESA Study. *Br. J. Nutr.*, 98(2), 397–405.
58 Newby, P.K., Maras, J., Bakun, P., Muller, D., Ferrucci, L., and Tucker, K.L. (2007). Intake of whole grains, refined grains, and cereal fiber measured with 7-d diet records and associations with risk factors for chronic disease. *Am. J. Clin. Nutr.*, 86(6), 1745–1753.
59 Rose, N., Hosig, K., Davy, B., Serrano, E., and Davis, L. (2007). Whole-grain intake is associated with body mass index in college students. *J. Nutr. Educ. Behav.*, 39(2), 90–94.
60 Good, C.K., Holschuh, N., Albertson, A.M., and Eldridge, A.L. (2008). Whole grain consumption and body mass index in adult women: An analysis of NHANES 1999–2000 and the USDA pyramid servings database. *J. Am. Coll. Nutr.*, 27(1), 80–87.
61 McKeown, N.M., Yoshida, M., Shea, M.K., Jacques, P.F., Lichtenstein, A.H., Rogers, G., et al. (2009). Whole-grain intake and cereal fiber are associated with lower abdominal adiposity in older adults. *J. Nutr.*, 139(10), 1950–1955.
62 Thane, C.W., Stephen, A.M., and Jebb, S.A. (2009). Whole grains and adiposity: Little association among British adults. *Eur. J. Clin. Nutr.*, 63(2), 229–237.
63 van de Vijver, L.P.L., van den Bosch, L.M.C., van den Brandt, P.A., and Goldbohm, R.A. (2009). Whole-grain consumption, dietary fibre intake and body mass index in the Netherlands cohort study. *Eur. J. Clin. Nutr.*, 63(1), 31–38.
64 Masters, R.C., Liese, A.D., Haffner, S.M., Wagenknecht, L.E., and Hanley, A.J. (2010). Whole and refined grain intakes are related to inflammatory protein concentrations in human plasma. *J. Nutr.*, 140(3), 587–594.
65 McKeown, N.M., Troy, L.M., Jacques, P.F., Hoffmann, U., O'Donnell, C.J., and Fox, C.S. (2010). Whole- and refined-grain intakes are differentially associated with abdominal visceral and subcutaneous adiposity in healthy adults: The Framingham Heart Study. *Am. J. Clin. Nutr.*, 92(5), 1165–1171.
66 O'Neil, C.E., Zanovec, M., Cho, S.S., and Nicklas, T.A. (2010). Whole grain and fiber consumption are associated with lower body weight measures in US adults: National Health and Nutrition Examination Survey 1999–2004. *Nutrition Research*, 30(12), 815–822.

67 Kyrø, C., Skeie, G., Dragsted, L.O., Christensen, J., Overvad, K., Hallmans, G., et al. (2011). Intake of whole grains in Scandinavia is associated with healthy lifestyle, socio-economic and dietary factors. *Public Health Nutrition*, 14(10), 1787–1795.

68 Montonen, J., Boeing, H., Fritsche, A., Schleicher, E., Joost, H.-G., Schulze, M.B., et al. (2013). Consumption of red meat and whole-grain bread in relation to biomarkers of obesity, inflammation, glucose metabolism and oxidative stress. *Eur. J. Nutr.*, 52(1), 337–345.

69 Mostad, I.L., Langaas, M., and Grill, V. (2014). Central obesity is associated with lower intake of whole-grain bread and less frequent breakfast and lunch: Results from the HUNT Study, an adult all-population survey. *Appl. Physiol Nutr. Metab.*, 39(7), 819–828.

70 Steffen, L.M., Jacobs, D.R., Murtaugh, M.A., Moran, A., Steinberger, J., Hong, C.-P., et al. (2003). Whole grain intake is associated with lower body mass and greater insulin sensitivity among adolescents. *Am. J. Epidemiol.*, 158(3), 243–250.

71 Cheng, G., Karaolis-Danckert, N., Libuda, L., Bolzenius, K., Remer, T., and Buyken, A.E. (2009). Relation of dietary glycemic index, glycemic load, and fiber and whole-grain intakes during puberty to the concurrent development of percent body fat and body mass index. *Am. J. Epidemiol.*, 169(6), 667–677.

72 Zanovec, M., O'Neil, C.E., Cho, S.S., Kleinman, R.E., and Nicklas, T.A. (2010). Relationship between whole grain and fiber consumption and body weight measures among 6- to 18-year-olds. *J. Pediatr.*, 157(4), 578–583.

73 Hur, I.Y., and Reicks, M. (2012). Relationship between whole-grain intake, chronic disease risk indicators, and weight status among adolescents in the National Health and Nutrition Examination Survey, 1999–2004. *Journal of the Academy of Nutrition and Dietetics*, 112(1), 46–55.

74 Choumenkovitch,, S.F., McKeown, N.M., Tovar, A., Hyatt, R.R., Kraak, V.I., Hastings, A.V., et al. (2013). Whole grain consumption is inversely associated with BMI Z-score in rural school-aged children. *Public Health Nutrition*, 16(02), 212–218.

75 Ma, J., Ross, A.B., Shea, M.K., Bruce, S.J., Jacques, P.F., Saltzman, E., et al. (2012). Plasma alkylresorcinols, biomarkers of whole-grain intake, are related to lower BMI in older adults. *The Journal of Nutrition.* 142(10), 1859–1864.

76 Wirfält, E., Hedblad, B., Gullberg, B., Mattisson, I., Andrén, C., Rosander, U., et al. (2001). Food patterns and components of the metabolic syndrome in men and women: A cross-sectional study within the Malmö Diet and Cancer cohort. *Am. J. Epidemiol.*, 154(12), 1150–1159.

77 Ledikwe, J.H., Smiciklas-Wright, H., Mitchell, D.C., Miller, C.K., and Jensen, G.L. (2004). Dietary patterns of rural older adults are associated with weight and nutritional status. *J. Am. Geriatr. Soc.*, 52(4), 589–595.

78 Azadbakht L, Mirmiran P, Shiva N, and Azizi F. General obesity and central adiposity in a representative sample of Tehranian adults: prevalence and determinants. *Int J Vitam Nutr Res.* 2005;75(4):297–304.

79 Byrd-Williams, C.E., Strother, M.L., Kelly, L.A., and Huang, T.T.K. (2009). Dietary fiber and associations with adiposity and fasting insulin among college students with plausible dietary reports. *Nutrition*, 25(9), 896–904.

80 Liu, S., Willett, W.C., Manson, J.E., Hu, F.B., Rosner, B., and Colditz, G. (2003). Relation between changes in intakes of dietary fiber and grain products and changes in weight and development of obesity among middle-aged women. *Am. J. Clin. Nutr.*, 78(5), 920–927.

81 Halkjaer, J., Sørensen, T.I.A., Tjønneland, A., Togo, P., Holst, C., and Heitmann, B.L. (2004). Food and drinking patterns as predictors of 6-year BMI-adjusted changes in waist circumference. *Br. J. Nutr.*, 92(4), 735–748.

82 Bazzano, L.A., Song, Y., Bubes, V., Good, C.K., Manson, J.E., and Liu, S. (2005). Dietary intake of whole and refined grain breakfast cereals and weight gain in men. *Obes. Res.*, 13(11), 1952–1960.

83 Du, H., van der, A.D., Boshuizen, H.C., Forouhi, N.G., Wareham, N.J., Halkjaer, J., et al. (2010). Dietary fiber and subsequent changes in body weight and waist circumference in European men and women. *Am. J. Clin. Nutr.*, 91(2), 329–336.

84 Mozaffarian, D., Hao, T., Rimm, E.B., Willett, W.C., and Hu, F.B. (2011). Changes in diet and lifestyle and long-term weight gain in women and men. *N. Engl. J. Med.*, 364(25), 2392–2404.

85 Mirmiran, P., Bahadoran, Z., Golzarand, M., Shiva, N., and Azizi, F. (2012). Association between dietary phytochemical index and 3-year changes in weight, waist circumference and body adiposity index in adults: Tehran Lipid and Glucose study. *Nutrition & Metabolism*, 9(1), 108.

86 Bautista-Castaño, I., Sánchez-Villegas, A., Estruch, R., Martínez-González, M.A., Corella, D., Salas-Salvadó, J., et al. (2013). Changes in bread consumption and 4-year changes in adiposity in Spanish subjects at high cardiovascular risk. *Br. J. Nutr.*, 110(2), 337–346.

87 Suhr, J., Vuholm, S., Iversen, K.N., Landberg, R., and Kristensen, M. (2017). Wholegrain rye, but not wholegrain wheat, lowers body weight and fat mass compared with refined wheat: A 6-week randomized study. *Eur. J. Clin. Nutr.*, 71(8), 959–967.
88 Li, X., Cai, X., Ma, X., Jing, L., Gu, J., Bao, L., et al. (2016). Short- and long-term effects of wholegrain oat intake on weight management and glucolipid metabolism in overweight type-2 diabetics: A randomized control trial. *Nutrients*, 8(9).
89 Vitaglione, P., Mennella, I., Ferracane, R., Rivellese, A.A., Giacco, R., Ercolini, D., et al. (2015). Whole-grain wheat consumption reduces inflammation in a randomized controlled trial on overweight and obese subjects with unhealthy dietary and lifestyle behaviors: Role of polyphenols bound to cereal dietary fiber. *Am. J. Clin. Nutr.*, 101(2), 251–261.
90 National Food Institutute. (2008). Wholegrain: Definition and scientific background for recommendations of wholegrain intake in Denmark. Danish Technical University.
91 Karl, J.P., and Saltzman, E. (2012). The role of whole grains in body weight regulation. *Advances in Nutrition*, 3(5), 697–707.

9 Whole Grains and Type 2 Diabetes

Shilpa N. Bhupathiraju[1] and Frank B. Hu[2]

[1]Department of Nutrition, Harvard T. Chan School of Public Health, Boston, Massachusetts, USA
[2]Department of Nutrition and Department of Epidemiology, Harvard T. Chan School of Public Health, Boston, Massachusetts, USA

9.1 Introduction

Type 2 diabetes (T2D) continues to remain a significant public health burden with an increasing trend towards younger adults. Currently, an estimated 422 million adults around the world are living with diabetes in 2014, compared to 108 million in 1980 (Organization, 2016). The burden of T2D is reflected not only in the growing prevalence in every country but in the increasing number of deaths. It is estimated that every six seconds a person dies from T2D, and in 2015 alone, diabetes caused 5.0 million deaths (Federation, 2015). Last year, the disease caused at least $673 billion US dollars, equivalent to 12% of the total spending on adults, in health care costs (Federation, 2015). The rapid increases in the prevalence of T2D has partly been attributed to rapid economic and nutrition transitions that have been further accelerated by increases in global free trade. With swift urbanization, traditional diets abundant in whole grains (WGs), fruits and vegetables are now being replaced by diets rich in refined carbohydrates, added sugars and devoid of dietary fibre (Popkin et al., 2012). Although it has been common knowledge that a healthy diet and adequate exercise are the foundations for preventing T2D, only in the past few decades has evidence emerged from well-conducted long-term prospective cohort studies and randomized controlled trials about the role of dietary factors, such as WGs, on T2D risk. In this chapter, we review the historical evidence surrounding the role of WG in T2D, while considering both epidemiological data and results from randomized controlled trials.

9.2 Evidence from epidemiological studies

The earliest evidence for a protective effect of WGs on T2D came from the works of Trowell in the United Kingdom. Using an ecological study design, Trowell (1974) noted that death rates from diabetes mellitus started falling dramatically from 1940–1954 when the less processed fibre-rich "National flour" replaced white flour. Most importantly, death rates among those aged 45 and older started rising again when production of the "National flour" ceased (Trowell, 1974). Subsequently, Trowell reviewed data from rural and urban Africa and noted that blood glucose concentrations were much higher in urban children who consumed Western diets while those who ate much lightly refined corn meal had lower

Whole Grains and Health, Second Edition. Edited by Rikard Landberg and Nathalie Scheers.

Additional materials available for download online at https://www.wiley.com/en-gb/Whole+Grains+and+Health-p-9781118939437

glucose concentrations. In light of these data, the authors proposed the dietary-fibre hypothesis that states that dietary-fibre depleted starchy foods are conducive to the development of diabetes mellitus in susceptible human genotypes (Trowell, 1975). Following these observations, several basic, clinical, and observational studies have examined the associations between WGs and chronic diseases, including T2D.

9.2.1 Prospective studies

Several well-established prospective cohort studies have examined the association between consumption of WG and incidence of T2D (Table 9.1). However, the definition of *WG* varied across studies. Most studies employed the definition suggested by Jacobs et al. (Jacobs et al., 1998), which includes dark bread, WG breakfast cereal (≥25% bran or WG) and other WGs such as brown rice, popcorn, wheat germ, bran, cooked oatmeal, bulgur, kasha and couscous. On the other hand, the Food and Drug Administration defines foods as WG if they contain ≥51% WG ingredients by weight per reference amount customarily consumed (Food and Drug Administration 1999; Food and Drug Administration 2003), but does not include bran-rich foods as done by Jacobs et al. In the United States, seven prospective cohorts have identified a significantly lower risk of T2D with higher intakes of WG, although only a few used the FDA definition. Using repeated measures of diet, Sun et al. (Sun et al., 2010) examined the prospective associations of WG, defined as any intact or milled form of grain that consists of the expected proportions of bran, germ and endosperm, with incident T2D. In this large study with 39 765 male health professionals and 157 463 female nurses with 14–22 years of followup, the authors found a monotonically lower risk of T2D associated with higher consumption of WG, including brown rice. In pooled multivariable analysis, compared to those with the lowest WG intake (median in 3 cohorts=3.6–6.2 g/day), those with the highest intakes of WG (median in 3 cohorts=31.3–47.1 g/day) had a 27% lower risk (95% CI: 22%–32%) for T2D. When examining brown rice alone, participants consuming more than 2 servings/week had an 11% (95% CI: 3%–19%) lower T2D risk. Because ethnicity is an important confounder of the association between rice and T2D, when analyses were restricted to white participants, the RR was 13% (95% CI: 4%–21%) for 2 or more servings/week. Most importantly, the authors found that substituting 1/3 of a serving (50 g) of white rice with the same amount of brown rice was associated with 16% lower (95% CI: 9%–21%) T2D risk. On the other hand, if this substitution included the same amount of any WG, the risk was lower by 36% (95% CI: 30%–42%). The protective effect of WG on T2D risk is also evident among African American women. In the Black Women's Health Study (van Dam et al., 2006), consumption of at least one serving of WG per day was associated with a lower risk of T2D (HR=0.69; 95% CI: 0.60–0.79) compared to women who rarely consumed WG. Most importantly, this association remained even after adjustment for magnesium, a component of WG. In the Iowa Women's Health Study, after accounting for differences in cereal fibre and dietary magnesium, associations between WG breakfast cereals and T2D were attenuated and were no longer significant (Meyer et al., 2000). Inclusion of these variables in a statistical model may represent an over-adjustment as both cereal fibre and dietary magnesium are components of WG and are partly responsible for the lower risk seen with T2D (Yao et al., 2014, Dong et al., 2011). Like Meyer et al. (2000), Kochar and colleagues (2007) also examined the association of WG breakfast cereals with T2D risk in 21 152 male health professionals. Men who consumed one or more servings/day of WG breakfast cereals were found to have a 40% (95% CI: 29%–50%) lower T2D risk compared to never consumers, but this is likely an overestimate of the true relative risk due to residual confounding. For example, the study did not account for variations in total

Table 9.1 Prospective studies on the association of whole grains with type 2 diabetes.

Citation	Cohort/Participants	Dietary instrument	Exposure	WG definition	WG intake in extreme categories	Outcome assessment	Confounders	Results
Meyer et al 2000, USA	Iowa Women's Health Study n=35,988 Age=55-69 y Cases=1141 F/up=6 y	127 item FFQ	WG	Breakfast cereals were considered WG if they contained ≥25% whole grain or bran by weight. Bran cereals were included in the WG category.	Q5 vs. Q1: 20.5 vs. 1 serving/week	T2D; Self report of physician diagnosis	Age, total EI, BMI, WHR, education, pack-years of smoking, alcohol intake, physical activity	WG were inversely associated with T2D risk. Adjustment for cereal fibre attenuated the association and the RR was 0.93 (95% CI: 0.75–1.16), P-trend=0.46 Results (Q5 vs. Q1) 0.79 (0.65–0.96), P-trend=0.0089
Montonen et al 2003, Finland	Finnish Mobile Clinic Health Examination Survey n=4316 Age=40-69 y Cases=154 F/up=23 y	Diet history	WG	WG foods included rye bread, rye crisp bread, WG flours, rye, whole wheat, wheat germ, rolled oats, barley, millet, buckwheat. Foods derived from different grain foods [e.g., porridge, gruel and Karelian pie (a national food of rice pudding baked in rye pastry and greased by butter)]. 3Breads containing at least 25% WG were considered WG.	238-1321 g/d vs. 0–109 g/d	T2D; Nationwide medical registry	Age, sex, geographic area, EI, smoking, BMI, intakes of fruits, berries and vegetables	Results (Q5 vs. Q1) RR=0.65 (95% CI: 0.36–1.18; P-trend=0.02 Further adjustment for intake of saturated fat, vitamins E, C, β-carotene, B-6, folic acid, flavonoids and magnesium attenuated the association (RR=0.67; 95% CI: 0.32–1.38; P=0.09). Inclusion of cereal fibre further attenuated the association (RR=1.14; 95% CI: 0.49–2.66; P=0.63).

(continued)

Table 9.1 Prospective studies on the association of whole grains with type 2 diabetes. (*continued*)

Citation	Cohort/Participants	Dietary instrument	Exposure	WG definition	WG intake in extreme categories	Outcome assessment	Confounders	Results
Hodge et al 2004, Australia	Melbourne Collaborative Cohort Study n=31,641 Age=40-69 y Cases=365 F/up=4 y	121 item FFQ	Wholemeal bread	Whole wheat or rye bread, rolls, or toast	≥17.5 vs. <0.5 times/week	T2D; Self-report and doctor confirmation of diagnosis	Age, sex, country of birth, physical activity, family history of diabetes, alcohol intake, education level, weight change in the last 5 years, total EI, BMI, WHR	Intake of wholemeal bread was not associated with T2D risk. Adjustment for BMI attenuated the association. For every one serving consumed per week, the HR was 0.99 (95% CI: 0.88–1.11). Results (Q4 vs. Q1) 0.86 (0.63–1.18), P-trend=0.80
Van Dam et al, 2006 USA	Black Women's Health Study n=41,186 Age=21-69 y Cases=1964 F/up=8 y	68 item FFQ	WG	Daily number of servings of dark breads such as wheat, rye, pumpernickel [2 slices] and high fibre bran or granola cereals, shredded wheat [1 medium bowl]	≥1 serving per week vs. < 1 serving per week	T2D; Self-report	Age, total EI, BMI, smoking status, strenuous physical activity, alcohol consumption, parental history of T2D, education, intakes of coffee, sugar-sweetened beverages, processed meat and other red meat	Daily consumption of one or more servings of WG was associated with a lower risk of T2D (HR=0.69; 95% CI: 0.60–0.79; P-trend<0.0001). This inverse association remained after adjustment for magnesium (HR=0.73; 95% CI: 0.63–0.85; P-trend<0.0001)

Schulze et al, 2007, Germany	European Prospective Investigation into Cancer and Nutrition - Potsdam study n=25,067 Age=35-65 y Cases=844 F/up=7 y	148 item FFQ	WG bread	Not specified	≥80.2 vs. <4.4 g/d	T2D; Self report, diabetes relevant medication, diet treatment owing to diabetes	Age, sex, BMI, sports activities, education, cycling, occupational activity, smoking, alcohol, total EI, waist circumference, PUFA:SFA and MUFA:SFA	Similar to the finding for cereal fibre, higher WG bread intake was inversely associated with T2D risk (RR=0.78; 95% CI: 0.62–0.97). Further adjustment for carbohydrates and magnesium did not change the association (RR=0.78; 95% CI: 0.61–0.99).
Fisher et al, 2009, Germany	European Prospective Investigation into Cancer and Nutrition - Potsdam study n=2318 Age=35-65 y Cases=798 F/up=7.1 y	148 item FFQ	WG, rs7903146 CC genotype WG, rs7903146 CT + TT genotype	Sum of whole grain bread, whole grain bread rolls and whole grain cereals	Per 50 g increment	T2D; Self report, use of medications, reasons reported for a change in diet, record linkages with registries and databases	Age, sex, BMI, waist circumference, educational attainment, occupational activity, sports activity, smoking, alcohol, red meat, processed meat, low-fat dairy, butter, margarine, vegetable fat, coffee, total EI	The beneficial effect of WG intake on T2D risk is modified by TCF7L2 rs7903146. <u>Results: HR (95% CI)</u> rs7903146 CC genotype : 0.86 (0.75-0.99) rs7903146 CT + TT genotype: 1.08 (0.96–1.23)
Von Ruesten et al, 2013, Germany	European Prospective Investigation into Cancer and Nutrition - Potsdam study n=23,531 Age=35-65 y Cases=837 F/up=8 y	148 item FFQ	WG bread	Sum of whole grain bread, whole grain bread rolls and whole grain cereals	Per 50 g increment	T2D- self report, use of medication, reasons reported for a change in diet, record linkages with registries and databases	Age, sex, smoking status, pack-years of smoking, alcohol consumption, WHR, BMI, leisure-time physical activity, education, use of vitamin supplements, non-consumption of WG, total EI, prevalent hypertension at baseline, history of high blood pressure	Each serving (50 g) of WG intake was associated with a lower T2D risk (HR=0.98; 95% CI: 0.85–1.00). However, after adjustment for 44 other food groups, the association was no longer significant (HR=0.92; 95% CI: 0.82–1.03)

(continued)

Table 9.1 Prospective studies on the association of whole grains with type 2 diabetes. (*continued*)

Citation	Cohort/Participants	Dietary instrument	Exposure	WG definition	WG intake in extreme categories	Outcome assessment	Confounders	Results
Simmons et al, 2007, UK	European Prospective Investigation into Cancer and Nutrition - Norfolk study n=25,633 Age=40–79 y Cases=417 F/up=4.6 y	FFQ	Wholemeal bread	Not specified	≥1 vs. <1 portion/d	T2D - follow-up health checks in EPIC, hospital and general practice registers, prescription of hyperglycemic medicine, HbA1c>7% at baseline or follow-up	unadjusted	Consumption of one or more daily portions of wholemeal bread was associated with a lower T2D risk compared to those consuming less than one portion per day (RR=0.72; 95% CI: 0.53–0.97)
Kochar et al, 2007, USA	Physicians' Health Study 1 n=21,152 Age=53 y Cases=1958 F/up=19.1 y	FFQ	WG cereals	Breakfast cereals that contain at least 25% of oat or bran	≥7 vs. 0 servings/ week	T2D; Self-report	Age, smoking, vitamin intake, alcohol consumption, vegetable consumption, physical activity, BMI	After adjustment for BMI, consumption of one or more servings of whole grain cereals per day was associated with a lower risk of T2D (HR=0.60; 95% CI: 0.50–0.71; P-trend<0.0001). This association was present in those with normal BMI (HR=0.65; 95% CI: 0.50–0.84) and those who were overweight (HR=0.57; 95% CI: 0.45–0.73) but not among obese individuals (HR=0.75; 95% CI: 0.41–1.40).

Sun Q et al, 2010, USA	Health Professionals Follow-up Study n=39,765 Age=32-87 y Cases=2648 F/up=20 y	131 item FFQ	WG, bran, germ, brown rice	Any intact or milled form of grain that consisted of the expected proportions of bran, germ, and endosperm were considered WG. Breakfast cereals were considered to be WG if the product contained ≥25% whole grain or bran by weight.	WG: 47.1 vs. 5.1 g/d Bran: 14.3 vs. 0.6 g/d Germ: 2.3 vs. 0.2 g/d Brown rice: ≥2/wk vs. <1/mo	T2D; Self-report and confirmation from medical records.	Age, ethnicity, BMI, family history of diabetes, smoking, alcohol, multivitamin use, physical activity, total EI, intakes of red meat, fruit and vegetables, and white rice. Bran and germ were mutually adjusted for each other.	<u>Results:</u> WG: 0.72 (0.63–0.83) Bran: 0.69 (0.60–0.81) Germ: 1.04 (0.89–1.21) Brown--1.12) Substituting 50 g/d of white rice with brown rice (RR=0.93, 95% CI: 0.83–1.05) or WG (RR=0.74, 95% CI: 0.64–0.86) was associated with a lower T2D risk
Sun Q et al, 2010, USA	Nurses' Health Study n=69,120 Age=37-65 y Cases=5500 F/up=22 y	131 item FFQ	WG, bran, germ, brown rice	Any intact or milled form of grain that consisted of the expected proportions of bran, germ and endosperm were considered WG. Breakfast cereals were considered to be WG if the product contained ≥25% whole grain or bran by weight.	WG: 31.3 vs. 3.6 g/d Bran: 9.5 vs. 0.6 g/d Germ: 1.5 vs. 0.2 g/d Brown rice: ≥2/wk vs. <1/mo	T2D; Self-report and confirmation from medical records.	Age, ethnicity, BMI, family history of diabetes, smoking, alcohol, multivitamin use, physical activity, total EI, intakes of red meat, fruit and vegetables, and white rice, postmenopausal status, hormone use. Bran and germ were mutually adjusted for each other.	<u>Results:</u> WG: 0.70 (0.64–0.77) Bran: 0.77 (0.69–0.86) Germ: 0.88 (0.79–0.97) Brown rice: 0.83 (0.72–0.96) Substituting 50 g/d of white rice with brown rice (RR=0.75, 95% CI: 0.66–0.85) or WG (RR=0.51, 95% CI: 0.44–0.60) was associated with a lower T2D risk

(continued)

Table 9.1 Prospective studies on the association of whole grains with type 2 diabetes. (*continued*)

Citation	Cohort/Participants	Dietary instrument	Exposure	WG definition	WG intake in extreme categories	Outcome assessment	Confounders	Results
Sun Q et al, 2010, USA	Nurses' Health Study II n=88,343 Age=26-45 y Cases=2359 F/up=14 y	131 item FFQ	WG, bran, germ, brown rice	Any intact or milled form of grain that consisted of the expected proportions of bran, germ and endosperm were considered WG. Breakfast cereals were considered to be WG if the product contained ≥ 25% whole grain or bran by weight.	WG: 40.0 vs. 6.2 g/d Bran: 12.1 vs. 1.0 g/d Germ: 2.0 vs. 0.3 g/d Brown rice: ≥2/wk vs. <1/mo	T2D; Self-report and confirmation from medical records.	Age, ethnicity, BMI, family history of diabetes, smoking, alcohol, multivitamin use, physical activity, total EI, intakes of red meat, fruit and vegetables, and white rice, and oral contraceptive use. Bran and germ were mutually adjusted for each other.	Results: WG: 0.81 (0.70–0.94) Bran: 0.83 (0.71–0.97) Germ: 1.04 (0.90–1.21) Brown rice: 0.89 (0.75–1.07) Substituting 50 g/d of white rice with brown rice (RR=0.84, 95% CI: 0.79–0.1) or WG (RR=0.64, 95% CI: 0.58–0.70) was associated with a lower T2D risk
Parker et al, 2013, USA	Women's Health Initiative Observational Study n=72,215 Age=50-79 y Cases=3465 F/up=7.9 y	122 item FFQ	WG	Whole grain bread and cereals	>=2 vs. 0 servings/d	T2D; Self report of physician diagnosis treated with oral hypoglycemic drugs or insulin	Baseline age, total EI, race/ethnicity, smoking, pack years, alcohol consumption, hormone therapy use, education, family history of diabetes, BMI, dairy, fruits, vegetables	Results: 0.79 (0.66–0.94; P-trend=0.07) Adjustment for energy adjusted folic acid, magnesium, potassium and vitamin D attenuated the associations but was still significant (RR for extreme categories=0.81, 95% CI: 0.67–0.97). Further adjustment for total fibre resulted in a RR of 078 (95% CI: 0.64–0.95). Among women who gained fewer than 5 lbs there was a strong inverse association that was not seen in women who gained more than 5 lbs between baseline and year-3 followup

Ericson et al, 2013, Sweden	Malmo Diet and Cancer Cohort n=27,140 Age=45-74 y Cases=1709 F/up=12 y	Modified diet history, 168 item FFQ, interview	WG	Fibre-rich bread (soft bread=50 g/portion; crisp bread=30g/ portion) and breakfast cereals (25 g/portion)	Women: 2.0 vs. 0.1 portions/d Men: 2.3 vs. 0.01 portions/d*	T2D; Regional Diabetes 2000 Register of Scania, Malmo HbA1c register, Swedish National Diabetes Register	Age, diet method version, season, total EI, education, smoking, alcohol intake, leisure time physical activity, BMI	A protective association was observed between intakes of fibre-rich bread and cereals and T2D (HR=0.84; 95% CI: 0.73–0.98; P-trend=0.004). Among women, the HR (95% CI) was 0.85 (0.68–1.06). Among men, the corresponding HR (95% CI) was 0.84 (0.68–1.04).
Wirstrom et al 2013, Sweden	Prospective study of Swedish middle-aged men and women n=5477 Age=35-56 y Cases=701 F/up=8-10 y	7-d weighed diet records	WG	Foods that contain ≥50% of WG on a dry-matter basis	>59.1 vs. <30.6 g/d	Prediabetes and T2D; Oral glucose tolerance test	Age, sex, family history of diabetes, BMI, leisure-time physical activity, smoking, education and blood pressure	In the overall sample, a higher intake of WG was associated with a 22% (95% CI: 4%–37%) lower risk to deteriorate in glucose tolerance (to prediabetes or T2D). This protective effect was not observed in those who harbored polymorphisms in the TCF7L2 gene.
AlEssa et al 2015, USA	Nurses Health Study, n=70,025 Age=30-55 y Cases=6934 F/up=24 y	FFQ	Cereal fibre	Cereal fibre measured from nutrient database	Dark bread: 1.7 vs. 7.0 servings/wk	T2D; Self-report and confirmation from medical records.	Age, BMI, race, family history of diabetes, postmenopausal status, smoking, alcohol, multivitamin use, physical activity, total EI, intakes of red meat, coffee, magnesium, ratio of polyunsaturated to saturated fat, trans fat, glycemic load, fruit fibre, vegetable fibre.	Cereal fibre was associated with a 29% (95% CI: 22%–35%) lower risk of T2D.

(continued)

Table 9.1 Prospective studies on the association of whole grains with type 2 diabetes. (*continued*)

Citation	Cohort/Participants	Dietary instrument	Exposure	WG definition	WG intake in extreme categories	Outcome assessment	Confounders	Results
Biskup et al 2016	Nested case control study within the Northern Sweden Health and Disease Study and Danish Diet, Cancer, and Health Study n=931 case control pairs Age 40–62 y	Plasma alkylresorcinols and FFQ	Plasma alkylresorcinols, WG wheat and rye	WG wheat and rye	WG wheat intake: Cases= 3g/d Controls=3 g/d; WG rye intake: Cases=24 g/day, Controls=25 g/d; Plasma alkylresorcinol Q1=0-19 nmol/L Q4=>58 nmol/L	T2D cases identified from diabetes register in Northern Sweden and from the National Diabetes Registry	Cases and controls were matched on year of birth, sex, age, fasting status, country. Models were adjusted for BMI, smoking status, education, physical activity, alcohol intake, coffee intake and energy intake.	Total plasma alkylresorcinol concentrations was not associated with T2D risk (OR=1.34, 95% CI: 0.95–1.88). No associations were seen with WG wheat and rye intake (RR per 20 g increase=0.92, 95% CI: 0.80–1.06).

Abbreviations: BMI, body mass index; CI, confidence interval; EI, energy intake; FFQ, Food frequency questionnaire; F/up, follow-up; HR, hazard ratio; MUFA, monounsaturated fatty acids; PUFA, polyunsaturated fatty acids; Q, quintile; RR, relative risk; SFA, saturated fatty acids; T2D, type 2 diabetes; WG, whole grains; WHR, waist-to-hip ratio.

*From Aune et al. (2013), who obtained this information via direct correspondence from the authors.

energy, coffee and overall dietary pattern, although an adjustment was made for vegetable intake (Kochar et al., 2007).

Using the Women's Health Initiative-Observational Study data with nearly 8 years of followup, Parker et al. (Parker et al., 2013) found that per each increasing categories of consumption of WG breads and cereals were associated with a statistically significant lower risk of incident T2D (RR=0.79; 95% CI: 0.66-0.94). When stratified by smoking status, inverse associations were much stronger among never smokers (RR for 2 servings/day vs. none=0.57, 95% CI: 0.44–0.73) than in ever smokers (RR for 2 servings/day vs. none=0.98, 95% CI: 0.77–1.25). Likewise, the inverse association was stronger among women who maintained their weight within 5 pounds during follow-up (RR for 2 servings/day vs. none=0.67, 95% CI: 0.54–0.82) compared to women who gained more than 5 pounds (RR for 2 servings/day vs. none=0.86, 95% CI: 0.52–1.43).

Several prospective cohort studies conducted outside the United States have examined similar associations of WG foods with T2D risk. In the European Prospective Investigation into Cancer and Nutrition (EPIC)-Potsdam study, every 50 g of WG bread or rolls, which is equivalent to 1 slice of bread or one roll in this population, was not associated with a lower risk of T2D after mutual adjustment for 44 other major food groups (HR=0.92, 95% CI: 0.82–1.03) (von Ruesten et al., 2013). However, in an earlier analysis of the same cohort that examined extreme quintiles of WG bread (80.2 vs. 4.4 g/day), the HRs (95% CI) were 0.78 (0.61–0.99) after adjustment for age, sex, BMI, education, physical activities, lifestyle, waist circumference, polyunsaturated fatty acids to saturated fatty acid ratio, monounsaturated fatty acids to saturated fatty acids ratio and intakes of magnesium and carbohydrate (Schulze et al., 2007). The discrepancies in these results may be due to differences in the covariates included in the statistical model.

While Schulze et al. (2007) only included nutrients and did not consider potential confounding due to intakes of coffee, red meat, fruits, vegetables and dairy, the analysis by von Ruesten et al. (2013) mutually adjusted WG bread intake for other food groups, including other breads, dairy, fish, red and processed meat and various fruit and vegetables all of that are known to be associated with both WG consumption and T2D risk. Using the same cohort, Fisher et al. (Fisher et al., 2009) employed a case-cohort design to examine if the purported associations between WG bread and T2D are modified by polymorphisms in the transcription factor 7-like 2 (TCF7L2) gene. Polymorphisms in this gene are suggested to lead to T2D by promoting early insulin secretory defects. While WG intake was inversely associated with T2D risk among C homozygotes at rs7903146 of the TCF7L2 gene (HR for 50 g portion per day=0.86, 95% CI: 0.75–0.99), the T allele negated the protective association (HR=1.08, 95% CI: 0.96–1.23). In the Norfolk component of EPIC, Simmons et al. (Simmons et al., 2007) followed 25 633 men and women for a mean of 4.6 years and developed a diabetes risk prediction model using simple measures of physical activity and diet. In univariate analysis, they found that compared to those consuming less than one portion per day of wholemeal or brown bread, those consuming at least one portion had a 28% lower odds (95% CI: 3%–47%) of T2D, although addition of wholemeal or brown bread to the risk prediction model did not improve prediction beyond those of known risk factors. In the Melbourne Collaborative Cohort Study that included 36 787 men and women, aged 40–69 years, at baseline, whole meal bread consumption (≥17.5 times/week vs. <0.5 times/week) was not associated with T2D incidence (OR=0.86, 95% CI: 0.60–1.23) possibly due to the short duration of follow-up (4–years) (Hodge et al., 2004). On the other hand, using a combination of both 7-day diet histories and validated FFQ in the Malmo Diet and Cancer cohort, Ericson et al. (2013) noted that consumption of fibre rich bread and cereals were inversely associated with T2D when comparing extreme categories of intake

(HR=0.84, 95% CI: 0.73–0.98). However, like Hodge et al. (2004), the authors failed to account for potential confounding due to other dietary factors. In another smaller study of 5477 men and women in Sweden, a higher intake of WG (>59.1 compared with <30.6 g/d) was associated with a 34% lower risk (95% CI: 4%–37%) to deteriorate in glucose tolerance (to pre-diabetes or T2D). At the same time, WG intake correlated inversely with HOMA-IR, a measure of insulin resistance (Wirstrom et al., 2013). Similar to the findings of Fisher et al. (2009), the impact of WG consumption was not detectable in men who carried the T-allele at rs7903146 and rs4506565 of the TCF7L2 gene. However, an important limitation of this study is that there was no adjustment for total energy intake. It is well known that adjustment for total energy not only controls for confounding, but also reduces extraneous variation in food that is due to variation in energy intake and not related to disease risk (Willett et al., 1997).

In a smaller study of 2286 men and 2030 women in Finland, there were no differences in the incidence of T2D among consumers of extreme quintiles of WG (238–1321 g/d vs. 0–109 g/d) although a significant trend was observed for a protective effect (RR for extreme quintiles=0.65, 95% CI: 0.36–1.18, P-trend=0.02) (Montonen et al., 2003). While the small sample size may have limited statistical power in this cohort, Montonen et al. (2003) used a definition of WG that was limited to products that contained WG, but not bran and included breads, whole grain flours and minimally disrupted food products such as porridge, gruel and Karelian pie, a national food of rice pudding baked in a rye crust. Most recently, Aune et al. (2013) summarized data from the prospective cohort studies previously described and noted that the summary RR per 3 servings of WG per day was 0.68 (95% CI: 0.58–0.81) with similar inverse associations being observed for each type of WG. Interestingly, the authors found no association between overall refined grain intake and T2D risk. Since the publication of the meta-analysis by Aune et al. (2013), there were two additional reports on the association of markers of WG with T2D risk. In the Nurses' Health Study, during 1 484 213 person-years of followup, we found that carbohydrate quality as assessed by cereal fibre intake was inversely associated with T2D risk (RR comparing extreme quintiles=0.71, 95% CI: 0.65–0.78, P-trend<0.0001). However, starch-to-cereal-fibre ratio that indicates a greater amount of refined grain to WG intake was associated with a higher risk of T2D (RR comparing extreme quintiles=1.39, 95% CI: 1.27–1.53) (AlEssa et al., 2015). Unlike our findings, total WG wheat and rye intake, reflected by alkyl resorcinols in plasma, were not associated with a lower risk of T2D (OR=1.34, 95% CI: 0.95–1.88) in a population of Scandinavian men and women with high WG intake (Biskup et al., 2016). In addition to T2D incidence, Aune et al. summarized evidence from 3 prospective studies that examined the association between WG intake and mortality from T2D. The authors found that per 90 g/day increase in WG intake (equivalent to 3 servings – 2 slices of bread and one bowl of cereal or one and half pieces of WG pita bread), the risk of T2D mortality was lower by 26% (95% CI: 4%–44%) (Aune et al., 2016).

9.2.2 Cross-sectional studies

Several cross-sectional studies that have examined the relationship between WG intake, metabolic syndrome and measures of glycaemia have provided mechanistic insights into the role of WG on glycemic control (Table 9.2). Two of the earliest

Table 9.2 Cross-sectional studies on the association of whole grain intakes and measures of glycaemia and insulin sensitivity.

Author	Cohort	Participants	Diet instrument	WG foods/ definition	WG intake	Outcome	Covariates	Results
McKeown 2002	Framingham Offspring Study	1338 men and 1603 women Mean age: 54 y	126 item FFQ	≥25% WG or bran by weight	Men: 8.3 servings/ wkWomen: 8.8 servings/ wkQ5 vs. Q1: 20.5 vs. 0.90 servings/wk	Fasting glucose, 2-h glucose, fasting insulin, 2-h insulin, HbA1c	Age, sex, EI, treatment of hypertension, smoking, alcohol intake, multivitamin use, estrogen use, physical activity, BMI	Higher WG intake is associated with lower fasting insulin concentrations. Associations were independent of vitamin E, folate and vitamin B6 but were attenuated after adjustment for dietary fibre and magnesium Results (Q5 v.s Q1) (P-trend) Fasting glucose (mmol/L): 5.24 vs. 5.30 (P=0.24)2-h glucose (mmol/L): 5.82 vs. 5.84 (P=0.87)Fasting insulin (pmol/L): 198 vs. 207 (P=0.002)2-h insulin (pmol/L): 568 vs. 592 (P=0.16)HbA1c (%): 5.24 vs. 5.26 (P =0.63)
Liese 2003	Insulin Resistance Atherosclerosis Study	978 men and women with normal or impaired glucose tolerance Age: 54.8±8.5 y	114 item FFQ	WG foods included dark bread (whole wheat, rye, pumpernickel, other high-fibre bread), high-fibre bran/granola cereals, shredded wheat and cooked cereal (oatmeal, cream of wheat, grits)	Study mean=0.8 servings/d	Fasting insulin, insulin sensitivity measured using frequently sampled intravenous-glucose tolerance test	Age, sex, ethnicity, clinic, total EI, total energy expenditure, smoking, family hx of diabetes, BMI, waist circumference	Insulin sensitivity was 13.5% higher with each extra serving of WG, independent of BMI and waist circumference. Insulin sensitivity was significantly lower with higher WG intakes but was not independent of BMI and waist circumference. Associations attenuated after adjustment for dietary fibre and magnesium intake Results: Insulin sensitivity: β=0.043±0.020 (P=0.03)Fasting insulin: β=-0.024±0.024 (P=0.32)

(*continued*)

Table 9.2 Cross-sectional studies on the association of whole grain intakes and measures of glycaemia and insulin sensitivity. (*continued*)

Author	Cohort	Participants	Diet instrument	WG foods/ definition	WG intake	Outcome	Covariates	Results
McKeown 2004	Framingham Offspring Study	1290 men and 1544 women Mean age: 54±9.8 y	126 item FFQ	≥25% WG or bran by weight	Study mean: 6.4 servings/wk *Q5 vs. Q1: 20.4 vs. 0.90 servings/wk	HOMA-IR Insulin resistance syndrome	Age, sex, BMI, WHR, cigarette dose, EI, alcohol intake, % saturated fat, % polyunsaturated fat, multivitamin use, physical activity and treatment for blood pressure	WG intake is inversely associated with HOMA-IR and a lower prevalence of MS. These associations were largely attributed to cereal fibre. Results (Q5 vs. Q1) (P-trend) Mean HOMA-IR: 6.6 vs. 6.8 (P=0.05) OR for MS: 0.67 (0.48–0.91) (P=0.01)
Esmaillzadeh 2005	Tehran population based cross-sectional study	357 men and 470 women Age: 18–74 y	FFQ	≥25% whole grain or bran content by weight	Study mean ± SE=93±29 g/dQ4 vs. Q1: 229 vs. 6 g/d	Fasting blood glucose (mg/dL), 2-h blood glucose (mg/dL), diabetes mellitus, MS	Age, sex, smoking, physical activity, BMI, WHR, EI, % energy from fat, consumption of meats, fish, fruits, vegetables, use of blood pressure medication, use of estrogen	WG intake is inversely associated with a lower odds of diabetes and MS Results Q4 vs. Q1 Fasting glucose: 91±2 vs. 96±2 (P>0.05)2-h blood glucose: 108±4 vs. 117±4 (P<0.05) OR for diabetes: 0.88 (0.80–0.94)OR for MS: OR=0.68 (0.60–0.78)
Sahyoun 2006	Boston	535 men and women Age: 60–98 y	3-d food record	WG servings defined based on proportion of grain ingredients that were WG	Men: 1.6 servings/ dWomen: 1.3 servings/dQ4 vs. Q1: 2.9 vs. 0.31 servings/d	Glucose, MS	Age, sex, race, education, marital status, smoking, alcohol intake, exercise, BMI, EI, % saturated fat, use of anti-hypertensive medication or lipid-lowering medication	Higher intakes of WG were associated with lower fasting glucose concentrations and lower odds of MS. Results (Q4 vs. Q1) (P-trend) Glucose (mg/dL): 108.5 vs. 114.9 (P=0.01)OR for MS: 0.46 (0.27–0.79) (P=0.005)

Jensen 2006	Nurses' Health Study II, Health Professionals Follow-Up Study	938 men and women Men: 40–75 y Women: 25–42 y	131 item FFQ	>25% WG or bran by weight	Study mean: 22.3 g/d* Q5 vs Q1: 43.8 g/d vs. 8.2 g/d	HbA1C, plasma insulin, leptin and C-peptide	Age, sex, EI, alcohol intake, smoking, BMI, physical activity, hypercholesterolemia, intakes of fruit, vegetable, sucrose, fructose	WG intake was inversely associated with insulin, C-peptide and leptin. % difference between Q5 and Q1 (P-trend)HbA1C: -0.18 (P=0.83)Insulin: -14.4 (P=0.13)C-peptide: -13.6 (P=0.03)Leptin: -11.0 (P=0.03)
Lutsey et al 2007	Multi-Ethnic Study of Atherosclerosis	5496 men and women free of CHD and diabetes Age: 45–84 y	127 item FFQ	WG breakfast cereal, oatmeal, dark or WG bread and rolls, bran muffins, brown or wild rice	Study mean: 0.5 servings/d Q5 vs. Q1: 1.39 vs. 0.02 servings/d	Insulin resistance, type 2 diabetes	Age, sex, race, education, survey center, EI, current smoking, current alcohol use, dietary intakes of fruit, vegetables, refined grains, dairy, fish and poultry, meat, leisure physical activity, and sedentariness score, BMI and insulin. Insulin and HOMA-IR models were not adjusted for BMI and insulin.	WG intake inversely associated with insulin resistance, elevated fasting glucose or newly diagnosed diabetes. Results (Q5 vs. Q1) (P-trend) Mean insulin (mU/l): 5.16 vs. 5.37 (P=0.002)Mean HOMA-IR (mU/I*mmol/L): 1.53 vs. 1.68 (P- =0.002) Glucose (mg/dL): 97.6 vs. 99.0 (P=0.08)IFG or newly diagnosed diabetes (%): 33.8 vs. 37.7 (P =0.23)Newly diagnosed diabetes (%): 4.1 vs. 3.8 (P =0.63)

Abbreviations: BMI, body mass index; CHD, coronary heart disease; CI, confidence interval; EI, energy intake; FFQ, Food frequency questionnaire; HbA1c, glycated hemoglobin; HR, hazard ratio; HOMA-IR, homeostasis model of insulin resistance; IFG, impaired fasting glucose; MS, metabolic syndrome; Q, quantile; RR, relative risk; SFA, saturated fatty acids; T2D, type 2 diabetes; WG, whole grains; WHR, waist-to-hip ratio.

cross-sectional reports originated from the fifth examination cycle of the Framingham Offspring Study. In 2002, McKeown et al. (2002) demonstrated that higher WG consumption was inversely associated with fasting insulin concentrations, a surrogate measure of insulin sensitivity. Associations with fasting insulin were attenuated, but remained significant even after accounting for dietary patterns associated with diets high in WG such as percentage of polyunsaturated fatty acids, intakes of meat, fish, fruit and vegetables. Most importantly, the authors found BMI to modify the association between WG intake and fasting insulin such that the association was much stronger among overweight participants. Interestingly, no associations were found for HbA1c or fasting glucose possibly because the Framingham Offspring Study participants are middle-aged (mean age=54 years) in whom glucose control is more tightly regulated. In the same cohort, the authors noted that those consuming more than 20 servings of WG per week (or ~3 servings/day, the amount recommended by the Dietary Guidelines Advisory Committee) had a 33% lower odds (95% CI: 9%–52%) of insulin resistance syndrome compared to those with consumption levels less than 1.5 servings/week (McKeown et al., 2004).

In a more ethnically diverse cohort, Liese and colleagues (2003) noted that WG consumption among 978 middle-aged adults (40% non-Hispanic white, 35% Hispanic and 26% African American) in the Insulin Resistance Atherosclerosis Study was much less than national recommendation (<1 serving of WG/day). Yet, even within such low intakes, each serving/day (β) of WG were significantly associated with better insulin sensitivity ($min^{-1} \cdot \mu U^{-1} \cdot mL^{-1} \cdot 10^{-4}$) (β= 0.082, P = 0.0005) and fasting insulin (pmol/L) (β= -0.0646, P = 0.019) after adjustment for demographics, lifestyle, and total energy intake and expenditure. The addition of BMI and waist circumference attenuated but did not explain the association with insulin sensitivity. However, after accounting for differences in fibre and magnesium, two components of WG, there was a non-significant association that is consistent with the hypothesis that these constituents account for some of the effect of WG on insulin sensitivity. In another multi-ethnic sample of 5496 men and women who were free of CVD and diabetes, Lutsey et al. (2007) found a significant inverse trend between higher WG intakes and serum insulin, HOMA-IR, serum glucose, and impaired fasting glucose or newly diagnosed diabetes after adjustment for important confounders. However, some associations were attenuated after adjustment for BMI and insulin, two factors that are thought to be in the causal pathway. In an urban population of Tehran, compared to those with the lowest intakes (~6 g/d), those with very high WG intakes (~229 g/d) had a more favorable response to a 75-g oral glucose tolerance test and were less likely to have diabetes (OR=0.88, 95% CI: 0.80–0.94). Similar to the Framingham Offspring study, the odds of having metabolic syndrome were about 32% lower (95% CI: 22%—-40%) than those with very low intakes (Esmaillzadeh et al., 2005).

In a combined analysis of healthy men and women from the HPFS and NHS II, Jensen et al. (2006) found that intakes of WG were modestly associated in the inverse direction with markers of glycemic control, including insulin, C-peptide and serum leptin. However, in line with the Framingham Offspring findings, the authors found no associations with HbA1c, possibly because of the younger age range of the study participants. While most of these studies were conducted in middle-aged adults, associations in older adults who have a greater degree of metabolic abnormalities are less well understood. Using a cohort of 538 older adults, aged 60–98 years, in Boston, Sahyoun et al. (2006) noted that fasting glucose concentrations were lower across higher quartile categories of WG intake (P-trend=0.01) even after accounting for differences in several demographic, lifestyle and dietary factors. Concomitantly, higher intakes of refined grains were associated with higher glucose concentrations (P-trend=0.04). Taken together, the evidence from cross-sectional studies consistently shows that higher intakes of WG are associated with lower insulin concentrations and better insulin sensitivity, key factors that influence the risk of developing T2D. Among older adults, WG intake also appears to be associated with lower glucose concentrations.

9.3 Evidence from randomized controlled trials

While current dietary recommendations to consume WG are primarily based on evidence from large, well-designed, prospective cohort studies, a true causal association can only be established with randomized, double-blind, placebo-controlled studies. However, it is extremely difficult, if not impossible, to conduct double-blinded trials of foods or eating patterns due to several factors: 1) lack of compliance, 2) potential cross-contaminations between the groups, 3) long duration of follow-up needed for assessing T2D, 4) possible attrition over time, 5) uncertainties surrounding the ideal intervention period, 6) difficulties with blinding and placebo control and 7) incomplete control of other factors in free-living conditions. Therefore, several randomized controlled trials have directly investigated the effects of WG on metabolic intermediates including fasting glucose, insulin secretion and sensitivity, and urinary C-peptides (Table 9.3). Most randomized trials were conducted in "high risk" groups such as overweight and obese participants as effects of dietary intervention are more pronounced in those with poor habitual diets and in those with pronounced metabolic abnormalities. Test diets usually contained the same amount of carbohydrate as the control diet but varied in the type and structure of carbohydrate.

In one of the earliest studies, Saltzman et al. (2001) compared the effect of a hypocaloric diet containing oats to a usual diet on glycemic measures, including fasting glucose, insulin and HOMA-IR, a measure of insulin resistance in 43 healthy weight-stable men and women. At the end of 9 weeks, improvements were seen in all measures but these were not significant. However, in another study (Pins et al., 2002), consumption of a daily serving of 60 g (~3/4 cup) of whole oats cereal for 12 weeks significantly improved blood glucose concentrations in 88 hypertensive men and women. The mean (SE) difference between post- and pre-study values between the oats cereal group and the wheat group (control) was -16.2 mg/dL (± 4.4). Pereira et al. (2002) examined the effect of WG consumption for 6 weeks on insulin sensitivity in 11 overweight and obese adults. In this cross-over study, participants consumed a diet that contained foods made with refined grains that contained no bran or germ and little fibre or a whole grain diet that was created by substitution of an equal volume of whole grain food items for the refined-grain products. At the end of the 6-week period, fasting insulin was found to be significantly lower during the follow-up with the WG diet than with refined grain diet (141 ± 3.9 pmol/L vs. 156 ± 3.9 pmol/L). Fasting glucose tended to be lower with the WG diet than with the refined grain diet, although these differences were not significant (5.2 ± 0.08 mmol/L versus 5.3 ± 0.08 mmol/L). At the same time, the homeostasis model indicated that insulin resistance was lower with WG than with refined grains (5.4 ± 0.18 IU vs. 6.2 ± 0.18 IU). In contrast to these findings, consumption of a diet rich in WG for 6 weeks did not change peripheral insulin sensitivity that was measured using the same methodology in overweight men and women. Although the BMI of these participants was similar to those in the Pereira et al.

Table 9.3 Randomized controlled trials on the effect of whole grain intake on measures of glycaemia and insulin sensitivity.

Author	Design	Participants	Duration, weeks	Comparator (C)	Treatment (T)	Endpoint	Results
Saltzman 2001	Parallel	43 healthy weight-stable men and women	8	Usual food items	Hypocaloric diet containing oats	Fasting glucose, insulin, HOMA-IR	Improvements in fasting glucose and insulin were observed but were not significant. Δ fasting glucose mmol/L (T vs. C): -0.21±0.29 vs. -0.005±0.9 Δ fasting insulin pmol/L (T vs. C): -28.7±26.5 vs. -9.3±46.7 Δ HOMA-IR (T vs. C): -1.1±1.2 vs. -0.5±2.1.
Pereira 2002	Crossover	11 overweight or obese men and women	6	Refined grains	Whole grains	Fasting glucose and insulin	Fasting insulin was 10% lower during consumption of WG than consumption of refined grains (mean difference=-15±5.5 pmol/L, P=0.03). Insulin sensitivity was higher after a WG diet.
Pins 2002	Parallel	88 hypertensive men and women	12	Wheat cereal	Whole oats cereal	Fasting glucose	Blood glucose levels in the oats group improved significantly (P<0.01). The mean differences between post study and pre-study values (±SE) between the 2 groups were -16.2 mg/dl (±4.4).
Juntunen 2003	Crossover	20 postmenopausal women	8	White wheat bread	High fibre rye bread	Fasting glucose, insulin and acute insulin response	No significant changes in plasma glucose (P=0.96) or insulin concentrations (P=0.99) during the study. However, rye bread increased the acute insulin response suggesting that it may have favorable long-term effects on the maintenance of normal β-cell secretion or the improvement of pancreatic β-cell dysfunction.

McIntosh 2003	Crossover	28 overweight men	4	Low fibre cereal grain	High fibre wheat/rye	Plasma glucose and insulin	Postprandial insulin response with high-fibre rye and high-fibre wheat breads were 46% and 49% lower than with low-fibre cereal grain (P=0.0001). Glucose response with high-fibre rye bread was 15% lower with rye and 20% lower with wheat than with the low-fibre product (P=0.0005).
Andersson 2007	Crossover	30 overweight men and women	6	Refined grain	Whole grain	Fasting glucose, insulin and peripheral insulin sensitivity	No changes in fasting glucose or insulin concentrations. Peripheral insulin sensitivity (measured by the euglycemic-hyperinsulinemic insulin clamp) did not improve when subjects consumed whole grain products.
Katcher 2008	Parallel	30 obese men and women with metabolic syndrome	12	Refined grain	Whole grain	Fasting glucose, insulin and insulin sensitivity index	No significant effects were seen on the outcome measures. However, weight loss was observed in both treatment groups and subjects in both groups significantly improved their diet quality.
Brownlee 2010	Parallel	316 overweight men and women	16	Refined grain	Whole grain	Fasting glucose, insulin and quantitative insulin sensitivity check index	No effect of whole grains on measures of fasting glucose and insulin. Likewise, insulin sensitivity was not different between the groups.
Landberg 2010	Crossover	17 men with prostate cancer	6	Refined wheat	Whole grain rye and bran	Fasting glucose and insulin	Fasting glucose was lower but not significant (Mean treatment effect=-0.14 (95% CI: -0.37, 0.09). Fasting insulin was significantly lower (Mean treatment effect=-8.3 (95% CI: -13.9, -2.8) Urinary C-peptide excretion was 28% lower with WG.

(*continued*)

Table 9.3 Randomized controlled trials on the effect of whole grain intake on measures of glycaemia and insulin sensitivity. (*continued*)

Author	Design	Participants	Duration, weeks	Comparator (C)	Treatment (T)	Endpoint	Results
Tighe 2010	Parallel	206 healthy men and women	12	Refined diet	Wheat and wheat+oats	Fasting glucose, insulin, HOMA-IR, insulin sensitivity	None of the treatments significantly affected glucose and insulin concentrations or markers of insulin resistance (HOMA-IR) and sensitivity (revised Quantitative Insulin Sensitivity Check Index).
Lankinen 2011	Parallel	106 men and women with impaired glucose metabolism and at least 2 other features of MS	12	Refined products	Whole grain and low postprandial insulin response grain products (fatty fish and bilberries) – Healthy Diet group/ WG enriched diet	Fasting glucose and insulin, HOMA-IR, Disposition index, insulinogenic index, quantitative insulin sensitivity check index	There were no statistical differences in changes of glucose and insulin metabolism between the groups. In the Healthy Diet group, there were decreases in the 2h glucose concentration and the area under the curve for glucose. There was a trend towards improved insulinogenic index and disposition index within the Healthy Diet group.
Ross 2011	Crossover	17 healthy men and women	2	Refined grain	Whole grain	Fasting glucose	Average recorded WG intake =151 g/d. Fasting glucose was lower but not significant (Mean difference=-0.03 mmol/L (95% CI: -0.19, 0.14).
Jackson 2014	Parallel	50 overweight and obese men and women with increased waist circumference and one or more MS criteria	12	Refined grain	Whole grain	Fasting glucose and insulin	At the end of 12 weeks, fasting glucose was much lower in the WG group (-4.3±1.1) than the RG group (-1.0±1.1; P=0.02). Fasting insulin was not significantly different between the two groups.

Abbreviations: CI, confidence interval; HOMA-IR, homeostasis model of insulin resistance; MS, metabolic syndrome; SE, standard error; T2D, type 2 diabetes; WG, whole grains.

study, participants in the Pereira study were hyperinsulinemic with fasting insulin concentrations that were about 3 times that of participants in the current study (Andersson et al., 2007). In another randomized crossover study, Juntunen et al. (2003) modified the intake of carbohydrates from cereals by substituting cereals consumed by healthy post-menopausal women with either high fibre rye bread (17% dietary fibre) or white wheat bread (2.8% dietary fibre). At the end of 8 weeks, there were no significant changes in plasma glucose and insulin concentrations and in insulin sensitivity. However, rye bread increased the acute insulin response suggesting that, in the long term, it may have favorable effects on the maintenance of normal β-cell secretion or the improvement of pancreatic β-cell dysfunction. In another study, consumption of high-fibre rye or wheat (each providing 32 g/d of dietary fibre) for 4 weeks was found to significantly improve the postprandial insulin response in overweight men. Similarly, glucose response was 15% lower with rye bread and 20% lower with wheat bread than with the low-fibre product (McIntosh et al., 2003).

WG as part of a hypocaloric diet did not improve fasting measures of glucose, insulin and insulin sensitivity in a group of 30 obese men and women with metabolic syndrome. Although weight loss occurred in both the treatment and control groups, there was a significant lowering of C-reactive protein in the WG group that was independent of weight loss (Katcher et al., 2008). In two large-scale intervention studies of over 200 participants, there was no effect of WG on measures of glycaemia (Brownlee et al., 2010; Tighe et al., 2010). In the WHOLEheart study, 316 overweight men and women were randomized to either maintain their current diet or substitute refined grains for WG (60 g/d for 16 weeks or 60 g/d for 8 weeks and 120 g/d for 8 weeks). The lack of a significant effect on insulin sensitivity may be due to a concomitant increase in total energy intake, specifically from carbohydrates and other food accompaniments such as spreads, milk and so on in the intervention group. Therefore, participants appeared to include WG foods as a dietary addition instead of substitution. Further, at the highest level of WG intake (120 g/d), fruit intake reduced by ~1/2 serving per day, suggesting that there were changes in dietary pattern to accommodate the higher intakes of WG (Brownlee et al., 2010). Ross et al. (2011) performed a randomized crossover intervention with an average WG of 150 g/d, which is higher than the intervention by Brownlee et al. (2010). While fasting glucose was lower at the end of the study period, the differences between the groups were not significant (mean difference=-0.03 mmol/L (95% CI: -0.19, 0.14) potentially due to the short duration (2 weeks) and the small study size (17 healthy men and women). However, in another large study of 106 men and women with impaired glucose metabolism and at least 2 other features of metabolic syndrome, there was a trend towards improvement in 2-h glucose among participants randomized to a WG enriched diet. Similar improvements were not noted for disposition index, a product of insulin sensitivity and first-phase insulin secretion that is predictive of conversion to diabetes (Lankinen et al., 2011). On the other hand, Landberg et al. (2010) examined the effects of very high (485 g) rye WG and bran intakes in 17 men with prostate cancer and found lower fasting insulin concentrations at the end of 6 weeks. While no differences were seen for fasting glucose, urinary C-peptide concentrations were lower by 28% in the WG group. It remains unknown if more normal intake levels would have similar effects that are of clinical significance. In a more recent randomized, controlled, open-label parallel study, 50 overweight and obese individuals with increased waist circumference and one or more of the metabolic syndrome criteria consumed a weight-loss diet containing either WG or refined grain products for 12 weeks. WG intakes were tailored to individual energy requirements and ranged from 163–01 g/d. Compliance was measured using plasma alkylresorcinols, an objective measure of WG wheat and rye intake. In an intent-to-treat analysis, fasting glucose was lower with the consumption of WG (-4.3 ± 1.1 mg/dL vs. -1.0 ± 1.1 mg/dL, P=0.02). WG consumption had no effect on fasting insulin concentrations or HOMA-IR, a measure of insulin resistance (P>0.90) (Harris Jackson et al., 2014). Altogether, the evidence from randomized controlled trials is less consistent given the wide duration of study periods, smaller sample sizes, amount of intervention, and the differences in WG foods and control diets. In general, there were protective effects of WG on glycemic measures when studies were conducted in high risk groups with sufficient follow-up (>12 weeks).

9.4 Potential biological mechanisms

The insulin sensitizing effect of WG and its protective effect on T2D, in part, may be attributed to the nutrients that are lost during the milling process, including dietary fibre, magnesium, vitamin E and several B-vitamins. For example, in a recent dose-response analysis of 17 prospective cohort studies involving 19 033 cases and 488 293 participants, the combined RR (95% CI) of type 2 diabetes comparing high versus low intakes of cereal fibre was 0.77 (0.69-0.85). Further, for every 2 g/day increment in cereal fibre intake, the risk of T2D decreased by 6% (RR=0.94, 95% CI: 0.93–0.96) (Yao et al., 2014). In line with these findings, several prospective studies found that the association between WG and T2D was attenuated after inclusion of cereal fibre in the statistical model (Meyer et al., 2000; Montonen et al., 2003; Parker et al., 2013). Another important nutrient that is purported to mediate the effects of WG on T2D is magnesium, a nutrient that is found in the outer bran of WG. Magnesium is an essential mineral that acts as a cofactor for several enzymes involved in glucose metabolism and insulin secretion (Belin and He, 2007). In animal models, magnesium supplementation was found to delay the development of T2D (Nagai and Ito, 2013) primarily through increased in vitro glucose uptake (Chaudhary et al., 2007) and improved insulin sensitivity in rats (Chaudhary et al., 2004; Olatunji and Soladoye, 2007). In a recent meta-analysis of 13 prospective cohort studies comprising of 536 318 participants and 24 516 T2D cases, when comparing highest versus lowest category of magnesium intake, there was a significant inverse association between magnesium intake and risk of T2D (RR=0.78, 95% CI: 0.73–0.84) (Dong et al., 2011). In the dose-response analysis, for every 100 mg/day increment in magnesium intake, the risk of T2D was lower by 14% (95% CI: 11%–18%). In a randomized, crossover, pilot trial in 14 healthy, overweight volunteers, supplementation with 500 mg elemental magnesium per day for 4 weeks appeared to decrease fasting insulin concentrations (change=-2.2 μU/mL) compared to a placebo and led to distinct changes in gene expression and proteomic profiling that is consistent with favorable effects on several metabolic pathways (Chacko et al., 2011).

Another important mechanism through which WG are protective against T2D is through avoiding weight gain. In a prospective cohort study of 74,091 US female nurses, women who increased their WG intake by a median of 0.90 servings/1000 kcal/day had a lower weight gain (4.12 ± 0.09 kg) compared to women who reduced their WG intake by ½ serving for every 1000 kcal (4.51 ± 0.10 kg) even after accounting for differences in changes in diet, lifestyle, and baseline BMI. On the other hand, women who increased their refined grain intake over a 4-year period weighed more (~1/2 kg) than women who reduced intakes over the same time frame (Liu et al., 2003). Likewise, in the all-male US Health Professionals Follow-Up Study, for every 40 g/day increment in WG intake from all foods, weight gain over an 8-year period was lower by nearly ½ kg. Bran that was either added to the diet or obtained from fortification further lowered the risk of weight gain such that for every 20 g/ day higher intake, weight gain was lower by 0.36 kg (Koh-Banerjee et al., 2004). In the same cohort, a dietary pattern characterized by higher intakes of fruit, vegetables, WG and poultry was inversely associated with plasma biomarkers of obesity, including insulin, C-peptide, and leptin suggesting that the effect of a WG rich diet on type 2 diabetes may be mediated through these biomarkers (Fung et al., 2001).In another cohort of US male physicians, men who consumed 1 or more servings of WG breakfast cereals gained an average of 1.83 ± 0.13 kg over a 13-year followup, while men who rarely consumed WG breakfast cereals gained much more (2.18 ± 0.06 kg) (Bazzano et al., 2005).

In addition to its effects on body weight, WG exert their protective effects on T2D through their glycemic response. It is well known that the disruption of the intact structure of the grain during the milling process alters the glycemic index, a measure of a food's ability to raise blood glucose concentrations. WG foods, in general, have a lower GI index, than refined grains due to greater particle size and the presence of dietary fibre, and therefore may favorably influence blood glucose and insulin responses. Recently, in an updated meta-analysis of prospective cohort studies, we demonstrated that high glycemic index and glycemic load were associated with a 19% (95% CI: 14%–24%) and 13% (95% CI: 8%–17%) higher risk of T2D, respectively (Bhupathiraju et al., 2014). In another meta-analysis of 14 randomized controlled trials, low glycemic index diets reduced HbA1c by 0.43% points (95% CI: 0.72–0.13) over and above that produced by high GI diets. After accounting for baseline differences, glycated proteins (HbA1c and fructosamine) were reduced by 7.4% (95% CI: 8.8–6.0) more on the low GI diets than on the high GI diets (Brand-Miller et al., 2003). The evidence from observational cohorts and randomized controlled trials conclusively show that substituting low glycemic index WG foods for high glycemic index refined grains lowers the risk of T2D. While no mechanism alone is responsible for the lower T2D risk seen with WG consumption, WG likely act through multiple mechanisms in synergy to lower T2D risk.

9.5 Conclusions and future directions

When data from observational studies and randomized controlled trials are considered together, there is a preponderance of evidence for a protective effect of WG on T2D risk even after accounting for differences in a participant's demographic, lifestyle and dietary factors. However, it is important to note that many of these studies did not employ the definition of WG put forth by the FDA (≥51% WG ingredients by weight per reference amount customarily consumed) but instead considered WG as any foods containing 25% or more of WG or bran by weight. In light of this limitation, the Life Sciences Research Office concluded that the evidence surrounding WG intake and T2D risk is inconclusive when the definition for WG does not include bran (Office, 2008). Recently, the American Society for Nutrition considered the literature published up until December 2010 on consumption of cereal fibre, mixtures of WG and bran, and concluded that consumption of mixtures of WGs and bran is modestly associated with a reduced risk of T2D (Cho et al., 2013). Despite this conclusive evidence, WG consumption in the United States and around the world continues to be substantially lower than current dietary guidelines. In this context, it is essential to emphasize the concept of substitution. Instead of simply adding WGs to one's diet, it is important to replace refined grains and added sugars with WG products. Although whole wheat bread and brown rice are the most frequently consumed WG products, there are a plethora of other WG options that also contain higher amounts of protein that consumers can choose from, including barley, buckwheat, rye and quinoa. While consumers understand the health benefits of eating WG, there is often confusion on identifying WG products due to the presence of multiple definitions. It is, therefore, imperative to have a concerted effort on the part of the food industry, health organizations and policy makers to approve a uniform and clear strategy to identify healthy WG products.

Although there is substantial evidence on WG and T2D, much remains to be learned. First, future studies should consider adopting a consistent definition of WG to allow for comparability across studies and to provide the necessary evidence base for policy formulations. Second, given that the effects of different WG foods have different glycemic and metabolic effects, it is often difficult to reach conclusions about WG by examining only one type of grain. Therefore, it is imperative that studies also examine total WG intake. Third, while several large randomized controlled trials have examined the effects of WG on intermediate endpoints such as glycemic measures, there are no long-term (>1 year) randomized controlled trials on the effects of WG on T2D, although the feasibility of conducting such trials is uncertain due to practical considerations especially long-term compliance. Finally, the application of nutritional metabolomics to both observational studies and randomized controlled trials is a useful tool to elucidate the complex physiological effects of WG on T2D risk. Future studies need to address how changes in these metabolites mediate the association between changes in diet and subsequent disease risk.

References

FOOD AND DRUG ADMINISTRATION. 1999. Health Claim Notification for Whole Grain Foods. *In:* SERVICES, U. S. D. O. H. A. H. (ed.). Silver Spring, MD.

FOOD AND DRUG ADMINISTRATION, F. A. D. 2003. Health Claim Notification for Whole Grain Foods with Moderate Fat Content. In: SERVICES, U. D. O. H. A. H. (ed.). Silver Spring, *MD.*

ALESSA, H. B., BHUPATHIRAJU, S. N., MALIK, V. S., WEDICK, N. M., CAMPOS, H., ROSNER, B., WILLETT, W. C. & HU, F. B. 2015. Carbohydrate quality and quantity and risk of type 2 diabetes in US women. *Am J Clin Nutr*, 102, 1543–53.

ANDERSSON, A., TENGBLAD, S., KARLSTROM, B., KAMAL-ELDIN, A., LANDBERG, R., BASU, S., AMAN, P. & VESSBY, B. 2007. Whole-grain foods do not affect insulin sensitivity or markers of lipid peroxidation and inflammation in healthy, moderately overweight subjects. *J Nutr*, 137, 1401–7.

AUNE, D., KEUM, N., GIOVANNUCCI, E., FADNES, L. T., BOFFETTA, P., GREENWOOD, D. C., TONSTAD, S., VATTEN, L. J., RIBOLI, E. & NORAT, T. 2016. Whole grain consumption and risk of cardiovascular disease, cancer, and all cause and cause specific mortality: systematic review and dose-response meta-analysis of prospective studies. *BMJ*, 353, i2716.

AUNE, D., NORAT, T., ROMUNDSTAD, P. & VATTEN, L. J. 2013. Whole grain and refined grain consumption and the risk of type 2 diabetes: A systematic review and dose-response meta-analysis of cohort studies. *Eur J Epidemiol*, 28, 845–58.

BAZZANO, L. A., SONG, Y., BUBES, V., GOOD, C. K., MANSON, J. E. & LIU, S. 2005. Dietary intake of whole and refined grain breakfast cereals and weight gain in men. *Obes Res*, 13, 1952–60.

BELIN, R. J. & HE, K. 2007. Magnesium physiology and pathogenic mechanisms that contribute to the development of the metabolic syndrome. *Magnes Res*, 20, 107–29.

BHUPATHIRAJU, S. N., TOBIAS, D. K., MALIK, V. S., PAN, A., HRUBY, A., MANSON, J. E., WILLETT, W. C. & HU, F. B. 2014. Glycemic index, glycemic load, and risk of type 2 diabetes: Results from 3 large US cohorts and an updated meta-analysis. *Am J Clin Nutr*, 100, 218–32.

BISKUP, I., KYRO, C., MARKLUND, M., OLSEN, A., VAN DAM, R. M., TJONNELAND, A., OVERVAD, K., LINDAHL, B., JOHANSSON, I. & LANDBERG, R. 2016. Plasma alkylresorcinols, biomarkers of whole-grain wheat and rye intake, and risk of type 2 diabetes in Scandinavian men and women. *Am J Clin Nutr*, 104, 88–96.

BRAND-MILLER, J., HAYNE, S., PETOCZ, P. & COLAGIURI, S. 2003. Low-glycemic index diets in the management of diabetes: A meta-analysis of randomized controlled trials. *Diabetes Care*, 26, 2261–7.

BROWNLEE, I. A., MOORE, C., CHATFIELD, M., RICHARDSON, D. P., ASHBY, P., KUZNESOF, S. A., JEBB, S. A. & SEAL, C. J. 2010. Markers of cardiovascular risk are not changed by increased whole-grain intake: The WHOLEheart study, a randomised, controlled dietary intervention. *Br J Nutr*, 104, 125–34.

CHACKO, S. A., SUL, J., SONG, Y., LI, X., LEBLANC, J., YOU, Y., BUTCH, A. & LIU, S. 2011. Magnesium supplementation, metabolic and inflammatory markers, and global genomic and proteomic profiling: A randomized, double-blind, controlled, crossover trial in overweight individuals. *Am J Clin Nutr*, 93, 463–73.

CHAUDHARY, D. P., BOPARAI, R. K. & BANSAL, D. D. 2007. Effect of a low magnesium diet on in vitro glucose uptake in sucrose fed rats. *Magnes Res*, 20, 187–95.

CHAUDHARY, D. P., BOPARAI, R. K., SHARMA, R. & BANSAL, D. D. 2004. Studies on the development of an insulin resistant rat model by chronic feeding of low magnesium high sucrose diet. *Magnes Res*, 17, 293–300.

CHO, S. S., QI, L., FAHEY, G. C., JR. & KLURFELD, D. M. 2013. Consumption of cereal fiber, mixtures of whole grains and bran, and whole grains and risk reduction in type 2 diabetes, obesity, and cardiovascular disease. *Am J Clin Nutr*, 98, 594–619.

DONG, J. Y., XUN, P., HE, K. & QIN, L. Q. 2011. Magnesium intake and risk of type 2 diabetes: Meta-analysis of prospective cohort studies. *Diabetes Care*, 34, 2116–22.

ERICSON, U., SONESTEDT, E., GULLBERG, B., HELLSTRAND, S., HINDY, G., WIRFALT, E. & ORHO-MELANDER, M. 2013. High intakes of protein and processed meat associate with increased incidence of type 2 diabetes. *Br J Nutr*, 109, 1143–53.

ESMAILLZADEH, A., MIRMIRAN, P. & AZIZI, F. 2005. Whole-grain consumption and the metabolic syndrome: A favorable association in Tehranian adults. *Eur J Clin Nutr*, 59, 353–62.

FEDERATION, I. D. 2015. Diabetes Atlas [Online]. Brussels, Belgium. Available: http://www.idf.org/diabetesatlas/ [Accessed 31 October 2016].

FISHER, E., BOEING, H., FRITSCHE, A., DOERING, F., JOOST, H. G. & SCHULZE, M. B. 2009. Whole-grain consumption and transcription factor-7-like 2 (TCF7L2) rs7903146: Gene-diet interaction in modulating type 2 diabetes risk. *Br J Nutr*, 101, 478–81.

FUNG, T. T., RIMM, E. B., SPIEGELMAN, D., RIFAI, N., TOFLER, G. H., WILLETT, W. C. & HU, F. B. 2001. Association between dietary patterns and plasma biomarkers of obesity and cardiovascular disease risk. *Am J Clin Nutr*, 73, 61–67.

HARRIS JACKSON, K., WEST, S. G., VANDEN HEUVEL, J. P., JONNALAGADDA, S. S., ROSS, A. B., HILL, A. M., GRIEGER, J. A., LEMIEUX, S. K. & KRIS-ETHERTON, P. M. 2014. Effects of whole and refined grains in a weight-loss diet on markers of metabolic syndrome in individuals with increased waist circumference: Arandomized controlled-feeding trial. *Am J Clin Nutr*, 100, 577–86.

HODGE, A. M., ENGLISH, D. R., O'DEA, K. & GILES, G. G. 2004. Glycemic index and dietary fiber and the risk of type 2 diabetes. *Diabetes Care*, 27, 2701–6.

JACOBS, D. R., JR., MEYER, K. A., KUSHI, L. H. & FOLSOM, A. R. 1998. Whole-grain intake may reduce the risk of ischemic heart disease death in postmenopausal women: The Iowa Women's Health Study. *Am J Clin Nutr*, 68, 248–57.

JENSEN, M. K., KOH-BANERJEE, P., FRANZ, M., SAMPSON, L., GRONBAEK, M. & RIMM, E. B. 2006. Whole grains, bran, and germ in relation to homocysteine and markers of glycemic control, lipids, and inflammation 1. *Am J Clin Nutr*, 83, 275–83.

JUNTUNEN, K. S., LAAKSONEN, D. E., POUTANEN, K. S., NISKANEN, L. K. & MYKKANEN, H. M. 2003. High-fiber rye bread and insulin secretion and sensitivity in healthy postmenopausal women. *Am J Clin Nutr*, 77, 385–91.

KATCHER, H. I., LEGRO, R. S., KUNSELMAN, A. R., GILLIES, P. J., DEMERS, L. M., BAGSHAW, D. M. & KRIS-ETHERTON, P. M. 2008. The effects of a whole grain-enriched hypocaloric diet on cardiovascular disease risk factors in men and women with metabolic syndrome. *Am J Clin Nutr*, 87, 79–90.

KOCHAR, J., DJOUSSE, L. & GAZIANO, J. M. 2007. Breakfast cereals and risk of type 2 diabetes in the Physicians' Health Study I. *Obesity (Silver Spring)*, 15, 3039–44.

KOH-BANERJEE, P., FRANZ, M., SAMPSON, L., LIU, S., JACOBS, D. R., JR., SPIEGELMAN, D., WILLETT, W. & RIMM, E. 2004. Changes in whole-grain, bran, and cereal fiberfibre consumption in relation to 8-y weight gain among men. *Am J Clin Nutr*, 80, 1237–45.

LANDBERG, R., ANDERSSON, S. O., ZHANG, J. X., JOHANSSON, J. E., STENMAN, U. H., ADLERCREUTZ, H., KAMAL-ELDIN, A., AMAN, P. & HALLMANS, G. 2010. Rye whole grain and bran intake compared with refined wheat decreases urinary C-peptide, plasma insulin, and prostate specific antigen in men with prostate cancer. *J Nutr*, 140, 2180–6.

LANKINEN, M., SCHWAB, U., KOLEHMAINEN, M., PAANANEN, J., POUTANEN, K., MYKKANEN, H., SEPPANEN-LAAKSO, T., GYLLING, H., UUSITUPA, M. & ORESIC, M. 2011. Whole grain products, fish and bilberries alter glucose and lipid metabolism in a randomized, controlled trial: The Sysdimet study. *PLoS One*, 6, e22646.

LIESE, A. D., ROACH, A. K., SPARKS, K. C., MARQUART, L., D'AGOSTINO, R. B., JR. & MAYER-DAVIS, E. J. 2003. Whole-grain intake and insulin sensitivity: The Insulin Resistance Atherosclerosis Study. *Am J Clin Nutr*, 78, 965–71.

LIU, S., WILLETT, W. C., MANSON, J. E., HU, F. B., ROSNER, B. & Colditz, G. 2003. Relation between changes in intakes of dietary fiber and grain products and changes in weight and development of obesity among middle-aged women. *Am J Clin Nutr*, 78, 920–7.

LUTSEY, P. L., JACOBS, D. R., JR., Kori, S., Mayer-davis, E., Shea, S., Steffen, L. M., Szklo, M. & Tracy, R. 2007. Whole grain intake and its cross-sectional association with obesity, insulin resistance, inflammation, diabetes and subclinical CVD: The MESA Study. *Br J Nutr*, 98, 397–405.

MCINTOSH, G. H., NOAKES, M., ROYLE, P. J. & FOSTER, P. R. 2003. Whole-grain rye and wheat foods and markers of bowel health in overweight middle-aged men. *Am J Clin Nutr*, 77, 967–74.

MCKEOWN, N. M., MEIGS, J. B., LIU, S., SALTZMAN, E., WILSON, P. W. & JACQUES, P. F. 2004. Carbohydrate nutrition, insulin resistance, and the prevalence of the metabolic syndrome in the Framingham Offspring Cohort. *Diabetes Care*, 27, 538–46.

MCKEOWN, N. M., MEIGS, J. B., LIU, S., WILSON, P. W. & JACQUES, P. F. 2002. Whole-grain intake is favorably associated with metabolic risk factors for type 2 diabetes and cardiovascular disease in the Framingham Offspring Study. *Am J Clin Nutr*, 76, 390–8.

MEYER, K. A., KUSHI, L. H., JACOBS, D. R., JR., Slavin, J., Sellers, T. A. & Folsom, A. R. 2000. Carbohydrates, dietary fiber, and incident type 2 diabetes in older women. *Am J Clin Nutr*, 71, 921–30.

MONTONEN, J., KNEKT, P., JARVINEN, R., AROMAA, A. & REUNANEN, A. 2003. Whole-grain and fiber intake and the incidence of type 2 diabetes. *Am J Clin Nutr*, 77, 622-9.

NAGAI, N. & ITO, Y. 2013. Effect of magnesium ion supplementation on obesity and diabetes mellitus in Otsuka Long-Evans Tokushima Fatty (OLETF) rats under excessive food intake. *J Oleo Sci*, 62, 403–8.

Office, L. S. R. 2008. Whole grain intake and cardiovascular disease and whole grain intake and T2D. A review. Bethesda, MD: Life Sciences Research Office.

OLATUNJI, L. A. & SOLADOYE, A. O. 2007. Increased magnesium intake prevents hyperlipidemia and insulin resistance and reduces lipid peroxidation in fructose-fed rats. *Pathophysiology*, 14, 11–15.

Organization, W. H. 2016. Global report on diabetes. In: ORGANIZATION, W. H. (ed.). Geneva, Switzerland.

PARKER, E. D., LIU, S., VAN HORN, L., TINKER, L. F., SHIKANY, J. M., EATON, C. B. & MARGOLIS, K. L. 2013. The association of whole grain consumption with incident type 2 diabetes: The Women's Health Initiative Observational Study. *Ann Epidemiol*, 23, 321–7.

PEREIRA, M. A., JACOBS, D. R., JR., Pins, J. J., Raatz, S. K., Gross, M. D., Slavin, J. L. & Seaquist, E. R. 2002. Effect of whole grains on insulin sensitivity in overweight hyperinsulinemic adults. *Am J Clin Nutr*, 75, 848–55.

PINS, J. J., GELEVA, D., KEENAN, J. M., FRAZEL, C., O'CONNOR, P. J. & CHERNEY, L. M. 2002. Do whole-grain oat cereals reduce the need for antihypertensive medications and improve blood pressure control? *J Fam Pract*, 51, 353–9.

POPKIN, B. M., ADAIR, L. S. & NG, S. W. 2012. Global nutrition transition and the pandemic of obesity in developing countries. *Nutr Rev*, 70, 3–21.

ROSS, A. B., BRUCE, S. J., BLONDEL-LUBRANO, A., OGUEY-ARAYMON, S., BEAUMONT, M., BOURGEOIS, A., NIELSEN-MOENNOZ, C., VIGO, M., FAY, L. B., KOCHHAR, S., BIBILONI, R., PITTET, A. C., EMADY-AZAR, S., GRATHWOHL, D. & REZZI, S. 2011. A whole-grain cereal-rich diet increases plasma betaine, and tends to decrease total and LDL-cholesterol compared with a refined-grain diet in healthy subjects. *Br J Nutr*, 105, 1492–502.

SAHYOUN, N. R., JACQUES, P. F., ZHANG, X. L., JUAN, W. & MCKEOWN, N. M. 2006. Whole-grain intake is inversely associated with the metabolic syndrome and mortality in older adults. *Am J Clin Nutr*, 83, 124–31.

SALTZMAN, E., DAS, S. K., LICHTENSTEIN, A. H., DALLAL, G. E., CORRALES, A., SCHAEFER, E. J., GREENBERG, A. S. & ROBERTS, S. B. 2001. An oat-containing hypocaloric diet reduces systolic blood pressure and improves lipid profile beyond effects of weight loss in men and women. *J Nutr*, 131, 1465–70.

SCHULZE, M. B., SCHULZ, M., HEIDEMANN, C., SCHIENKIEWITZ, A., HOFFMANN, K. & BOEING, H. 2007. Fiber and magnesium intake and incidence of type 2 diabetes: A prospective study and meta-analysis. *Arch Intern Med*, 167, 956–65.

SIMMONS, R. K., HARDING, A. H., WAREHAM, N. J. & GRIFFIN, S. J. 2007. Do simple questions about diet and physical activity help to identify those at risk of Type 2 diabetes? *Diabet Med*, 24, 830–5.

SUN, Q., SPIEGELMAN, D., VAN DAM, R. M., HOLMES, M. D., MALIK, V. S., WILLETT, W. C. & HU, F. B. 2010. White rice, brown rice, and risk of type 2 diabetes in US men and women. *Arch Intern Med*, 170, 961–9.

TIGHE, P., DUTHIE, G., VAUGHAN, N., BRITTENDEN, J., SIMPSON, W. G., DUTHIE, S., MUTCH, W., WAHLE, K., HORGAN, G. & THIES, F. 2010. Effect of increased consumption of whole-grain foods on blood pressure and other cardiovascular risk markers in healthy middle-aged persons: A randomized controlled trial. *Am J Clin Nutr*, 92, 733–40.

TROWELL, H. 1974. Diabetes mellitus death-rates in England and Wales 1920–70 and food supplies. *Lancet*, 2, 998–1002.

Trowell, H. C. 1975. Dietary-fiber hypothesis of the etiology of diabetes mellitus. *Diabetes*, 24, 762–5.

VAN DAM, R. M., Hu, F. B., Rosenberg, L., Krishnan, S. & Palmer, J. R. 2006. Dietary calcium and magnesium, major food sources, and risk of type 2 diabetes in U.S. black women. *Diabetes Care*, 29, 2238–43.

VON RUESTEN, A., FELLER, S., BERGMANN, M. M. & BOEING, H. 2013. Diet and risk of chronic diseases: Results from the first 8 years of follow-up in the EPIC-Potsdam study. *Eur J Clin Nutr*, 67, 412–9.

WILLETT, W. C., HOWE, G. R. & KUSHI, L. H. 1997. Adjustment for total energy intake in epidemiologic studies. *Am J Clin Nutr*, 65, 1220S-1228S; discussion 1229S–1231S.

WIRSTROM, T., HILDING, A., Gu, H. F., Ostenson, C. G. & Bjorklund, A. 2013. Consumption of whole grain reduces risk of deteriorating glucose tolerance, including progression to prediabetes. *Am J Clin Nutr*, 97, 179–87.

YAO, B., FANG, H., Xu, W., Yan, Y., Xu, H., Liu, Y., Mo, M., Zhang, H. & Zhao, Y. 2014. Dietary fiber intake and risk of type 2 diabetes: A dose-response analysis of prospective studies. *Eur J Epidemiol*, 29, 79–88.

10 Whole Grains and Cardiovascular Disease

Chris J. Seal[1] and Iain A. Brownlee[2]

[1]Human Nutrition Research Centre, Public Health Sciences Institute, Newcastle University, Newcastle upon Tyne, UK
[2]Applied Sciences, Northumbria University, Newcastle upon Tyne, UK

10.1 Introduction

Cardiovascular disease (CVD) includes a variety of conditions affecting the heart and vascular system resulting in a range of morbidities and, if untreated, increases the risk of premature death. CVD causes reduced blood flow to the heart, peripheral tissues and vital organs such as the brain and arises in four distinct forms: coronary heart disease, stroke, peripheral arterial disease and aortic disease. In each case, the disease (or death) is caused either by release of a blood clot (thrombosis) into the vascular system or by accumulation of fatty deposits and stiffening of arterial vessel walls (atherosclerosis). CVDs are the major cause of death globally, for example, accounting for an estimated 43% of all deaths in the United States in 2018 [1] CVDs are considered modifiable by environmental factors, including dietary intake, levels of physical activity, smoking and excessive alcohol intake.

10.2 Whole grains and CVD

Observational studies have consistently shown an inverse relationship between increased whole grain intake and reduced risk and incidence of CVDs; typically in the range of 20–30% reductions for the highest whole grain consumers compared with the lowest whole grain consumers for all forms of CVD investigated. These observational studies involve large numbers of subjects, mostly from North America and Northern European populations, and have been subjected to systematic review and meta-analysis. The most recent of these [2] included 10 prospective cohort studies representing more than 4.3 million person-years of followup for 408 605 US persons. Adjusting for known CVD risk factors, the data showed a 21% reduction in relative risk for all CVD outcomes [RR=0.79 (95% CI 0.74, 0.85)]. There was some evidence of publication bias in their analysis, but nevertheless the results are very convincing and in line with earlier publications [3]. Interestingly, the reduction in relative risk due to cereal fibre intake was almost identical [RR=0.80 (95% CI 0.73, 0.88)] to that for whole grain intake (although there was much more heterogeneity in the data), suggesting that this may be the principle driver of the response. Since this publication, analysis of the largest single prospective cohort study available in the US, the National Institutes of Health AARP (formerly American Association of Retired Persons) Diet and Health Study (NIH-AARP) has been completed [4]. The data were based on 367 442

Whole Grains and Health, Second Edition. Edited by Rikard Landberg and Nathalie Scheers.

Additional materials available for download online at https://www.wiley.com/en-gb/Whole+Grains+and+Health-p-9781118939437

at-risk individuals with a total of 12.3 million person-years of followup. Numbers of deaths from CVD were reduced by 17% in the highest quintile compared with the lowest quintile of whole grain intake [HR 0.83 (95% CI 0.78, 0.88) P<0.0001] after multiple adjustments for age, gender, smoking habits, race or ethnicity, alcohol intake, education level, marital status, health status, obesity, physical activity, red meat consumption, fruit and total vegetables consumption, total energy intake and hormone usage. When the data were further adjusted for cereal fibre intake, the effect of whole grain intake was no longer significant [HR 0.95 (95% CI 0.88, 1.03) P=0.188], once again suggesting that the protective effects of whole grains may be largely attributed to their fibre content. Although this is a large study, limitations include that it does not differentiate between different types of whole grain, and the range of whole grain intakes is very small (0.13 oz equivalents in quintile 1 compared with 1.2 oz equivalents in quintile 5), and these were self-reported using a 124-item food frequency questionnaire at a single time point at the start of the 14-year follow-up period.

The beneficial effects of whole grains have been attributed to their nutritional composition, including an array of dietary fibres, vitamins, minerals and phytochemicals. The complexity of this composition makes identifying potential mechanisms for the impact of diets rich in whole grains on CVD risk difficult. Many have been suggested (see Table 10.1), but these are not fully understood, and it is likely that a combination of factors is involved, not just one single response. Each of these proposed mechanisms has been tested in a number of intervention studies but the results have been very inconsistent. Table 10.2 presents the most recent intervention studies carried out with headline results from them. As expected, the results are somewhat equivocal with some, but not all, studies showing beneficial effects on a minority of the biomarkers of CVD risk tested. Further scrutiny of these papers highlights the breadth of study design, comparisons among different varieties of whole grain, the doses of whole grain consumed, the duration of the interventions, and the age, gender and health status of the study participants. This makes comparison between studies difficult and identifying mechanisms underlying the possible effects of consuming whole grains almost impossible. One of the most commonly reported biomarker of CVD risk is blood lipid profile, and the impact of whole grain on blood lipids has been subjected to a thorough systematic review and meta-analysis by Hollænder et al. [5]. After screening 6069 articles, the authors extracted data from 24 studies published between 1988 and 2015 that met their inclusion criteria. These included both parallel and cross-over intervention studies with apparently healthy male and female adults >18 years old not taking statins. Studies were only included if they investigated the effects of consuming either specific whole grain foods (e.g., whole grain bread, brown rice) or mixed diets high in whole grain in comparison with refined grain alternatives (e.g., white bread, white rice) or mixed diets devoid or low in whole grain foods. Changes in the lipid biomarkers total, LDL and HDL cholesterol, and triglycerides were recorded in most studies whether they were primary or secondary outcome measures. This generated a large and comprehensive data set that demonstrated considerable heterogeneity across the up to 2275 subjects included. The results showed that, averaged across intake of all whole grains, there was a small but significant reduction in LDL cholesterol, with a weighted mean difference of -0.09 mM (95% CI -0.15, -0.03 mM, p<0.01) and total-cholesterol (-0.12 mM, 95% CI -0.19, -0.05 mM, p<0.001) compared with refined grain control. The effect was greater for oats (which contributed about 50% to the "weight" of the analysis) when considered alone with a mean difference of -0.17 mM (95% CI -0.25, -0.10 mM, p<0.001) compared with refined grain

Table 10.1 Suggested beneficial components and potential mechanisms for benefits of whole grains on cardiometabolic health.

Component, compared with refined grain option:
• Higher levels of soluble and insoluble fibre, non-digestible oligosaccharides and resistant starch • Higher macro- and micronutrient content, e.g., fat-soluble vitamins, magnesium, selenium [note in some countries mandatory fortification may replace some macro and micronutrients lost during processing] • Higher non-nutrient and phytochemical content. e.g., phenolic acids, phytic acid, "antioxidants", lignans • May have a lower glycaemic index [depends on cereal type and degree of processing, especially particle size]
Benefits:
• Modulate absorption of nutrients either by affecting digesta flow rate or by direct interaction between cereal components and individual nutrients • Reduced inflammatory status; exact mechanism unclear • Improved blood pressure and vascular function; exact mechanism unclear • Affect enterohepatic circulation of bile and lower cholesterol by sequestration of bile salts with soluble fibre preventing reabsorption • Possible effects on satiety/gastric emptying affecting hunger mechanisms • Reduces energy density of foods and lower total energy intake, possibly linked to satiety effects • Reduced body weight and body weight gain over time, possibly linked to satiety effects • Altered gut microbiota and fermentation products, increase faecal bulk; exact mechanism unclear

control. No effects on HDL cholesterol were observed for whole grains combined or oats alone. Triglycerides concentrations tended to be lower with whole grain intake with a mean difference of -0.04 mM (95% CI -0.08, 0.01 mM $p<0.10$). Despite the heterogeneity in the database, starting cholesterol concentration, gender, ethnicity and dose did not affect the outcome measures, although an energy-restricted diet appeared to augment the results. In a regression analysis, duration of the study appeared to be negatively correlated with change in plasma cholesterol concentration (i.e., longer study duration was associated with a smaller change from control), although this may be confounded because many of the oat studies included in that analysis were of shorter duration and resulted in the greatest reduction in plasma cholesterol concentration. The effects reported in this study for changes in cholesterol concentration are smaller than the weighted mean differences reported by Ye et al. [2], which may be related to the methods of estimating the effect size in the latter study that nevertheless demonstrate a significant benefit of consuming whole grains on fasting lipid profile and fasting glucose concentrations.

All of the preceding studies have been carried out in adults. To our knowledge, there has only been one intervention study that has investigated the effects of increased whole grain intake in children. Hajihashemi et al. [6] conducted a 6-week cross-over intervention in overweight or obese girls aged 8–15 years who had previously failed to lose weight through weight-reduction programmes. Advice on types and amounts of whole grain to consume were delivered by a dietitian, with a target to consume half of their grain intake as whole grain for the whole grain period. During this period, whole grain intake averaged 98 g/d compared with 11 g/d during the refined-grain period. There were no significant differences in changes in anthropometric measures between the two treatment periods. However, serum hsCRP concentrations were significantly reduced by whole grain compared with the control period (-21.8 vs. +12.1%, $P=0.03$); sICAM-1 (-28.4 vs. +6.3%, $p=0.02$) and serum amyloid A (-17.4 vs. +9.9%, $P=0.02$) were also significantly reduced by whole grain,

Table 10.2 Whole grain (WG) dietary intervention studies completed since 2010 that include outcomes related to cardiovascular health.

Source	Whole grain intake	Comparator Groups	Outcome measures
[7, 8]	Given advice to achieve target >80g/d, actual 168g/d; based on WG pasta, brown rice, WG snacks and WG breakfast cereals.	Refined grain equivalents to WG products.	*No change* in anthropometrics (BMI, body fat %, waist circumference), BP, blood lipid profiles (total, LDL and HDL-cholesterol), immune (lymphocyte sub-populations) and inflammatory markers (cytokines, CRP sIgA) or fasting blood glucose was noted.
[9]	2 x WG bread rolls providing 48g WG/d.	2 x Refined grain bread rolls/d.	Weight, % body fat, waist and hip circumference, DBP *unaffected by treatment*.SBP *decreased* in WG group and *increased* in Control group (P=0.015 between groups).
[10]	Mix of WG foods, including WG wheat bread, WG wheat pasta, WG oat porridge, brown rice, WG breakfast cereals providing 60 or 120 g WG/d.	No intervention, non-WG consumers' habitual diet.	Anthropometrics, SBP, DBP, glucose, insulin, TG, Total-Chol, LDL-Chol, HDL-Chol, NEFA, Insulin sensitivity by modified QUICKI, and inflammatory markers (hsCRP, Sialic acid, IL-6, ICAM-1, VACM-1, E-selectin) were *all unaffected by treatment.*
[11]	37.5 g oat breakfast cereal/d.	37.5 g non-oat breakfast cereal.	Weight (P<0.001), BMI (P<0.001) *significantly decreased* in oat group compared with control; body fat % (P=0.045) *significantly lower* in oat group; Total Chol (P=0.011) and LDL Chol (0.017) *significantly lower* in oat groupHDL Chol, TG, Free FA *unaffected by treatment*.ALT (0.009) *significantly lower* in oat group.
[12]	45 g of oat-based granola/d.	45 g of non-WG cereal	Total (P<0.001) and LDL cholesterol (P=0.009) were *reduced* in the WG cereal group. *No effect* was noted on HDL chol, or fasting glucose and TAG.
[13]	A shopping basket of mixed WG wheat corn and rice products. On average, participants consumed around half of the products given	A mixed basket of similar refined grain products.	Total (P=0.018), LDL (P=0.035) and non-HDL (P=0.047) cholesterol were *significantly lower* in the WG treatment. *No changes* to BMI, fat mass or fasting glucose were observed between treatments.
[14]	WG wheat bread, pasta, rusks and crackers included as main CHO for each meal.	Same products but in refined form.	Weight, SBP, DBP, glucose, insulin, C-peptide, free FA, hsCRP, insulin resistance by HOMA, acetate, leptin, adiponectin, total ghrelin, GIP, magnesium were *all unaffected* by treatment.Total Chol (P=0.03) , LDL Chol (P=0.04) was *significantly lower* and LDL-Tg (P=0.04) *significantly higher* on WG treatment.

[15]	Cereal products 60–80% of total CHO intake.Italy: WG wheat bread, WG wheat pasta, barley kernels, WG oat biscuits, breakfast cereals.Finland: WG rye bread, endosperm rye bread, sourdough WG wheat bread, WG wheat pasta, WG oat biscuits.	Italy: refined cereal products, including wheat bread, rice, pizza, cornmeal porridge, breakfast cereals.Finland: refined wheat breads, allowed 1–2 small portions of rye products per day.	Weight, BMI, waist, SBP, DBP, glucose, insulin, TG, Total Chol, LDL Chol, HDL Chol, Peripheral insulin sensitivity by FSIGT, hsCRP, IL-6, IL-1ra, TNF-α *all unaffected by treatment.*
[16]	Given list of WG foods and asked to consume half grains as WG. Achieved average of 98g/d during WG intervention period.	Asked to avoid all WG foods.	*No difference* in change in anthropometric measures between WG and control periods. *Significant reduction* in hs-CRP in WG period; *greater reductions* in sICAM and serum amyloid A in WG period. *Significant difference* in leptin that fell in WG period but rose in control period.
[17]	WG wheat, rice and oats top 3 grains. Intake based on energy intake, ranging from 163 g/d (1600 kcal diet) to 301 g/d (3600 kcal diet).	Comparable refined counterparts to WG foods. Wheat, rice and corn were the top 3 grains.	Both groups lost weight and BP fell during the intervention. *No difference* in anthropometric changes between groups or changes in abdominal adipose tissue loss. *Modest higher* reduction in glucose on WG diet.
[18]	62 g WG wheat bread, 60 g WG wheat pasta, 28 g WG wheat biscuits providing 105 g WG/d.	62 g refined wheat bread, 60 g refined wheat pasta, 28 g refined wheat biscuits /d.	Reduction in body weight, SBP, DBP, glucose, insulin, TG, Total Chol, LDL Chol, HDL Chol, insulin resistance by HOMA, hsCRP, IL-6, HbA1c *all unaffected by treatment.*% of initial weight loss *tended to be greater* for WG group (P=0.07), reduction in total fat mass % *greater* in WG group (P=0.04), reduction in central fat mass tended to be greater in WG group (P=0.07).
[19]	c. 88 g of whole-wheat bread/d.	C. 88 g of refined wheat bread/d.	*Significant reduction* in viscereal fat. *No significant change* to other anthropometrics, TAG, total, LDL and HDL cholesterol, glucose, insulin, SBP and DBP, and adiponectin.
[20]	Mixed WGs (50 g/1000 kcal) included in study foods.	Comparable refined grains (50 g/1000 kcal) in similar study foods.	*Significant decreases* in DBP (P=0.01) and adiponectin (p=0.05) in WG treatment. *No impact* on anthropometrics, measures of glycaemic control (HbA1c %, fasting glucose and inulin, HOMA-IR, blood lipids (TAG, Total Chol, LDL Chol, HDL Chol, VLDL Chol) and liver enzymes (ALT and AST)
[21]	Mixed WG food intervention of 3 servings/d (equivalent to 48 g/d of WG).	Mixed refined grains foods (equivalent to 48 g/d RG).	TNF-α and Lipolysaccharide-binding protein *were significantly reduced* in the WG treatment. *No significant difference* was noted for other inflammatory markers (hsCRP and IL-6).

(continued)

Table 10.2 Whole grain (WG) dietary intervention studies completed since 2010 that include outcomes related to cardiovascular health. (*continued*)

Source	Whole grain intake	Comparator Groups	Outcome measures
[22]	Replace cereal foods with 300g/d WG soft bread, 100g/d WG crisp bread, 50g/d WG breakfast cereals, 35 g/d WG porridge (uncooked).	Replace cereal foods with 300g/d soft bread, 100g/d crisp bread, 50g/d breakfast cereals, 35 g/d porridge (uncooked), plus wheat cellulose to balance fibre with WG group.	Plasma insulin and hsCRP concentrations and urinary C-peptide excretion *significantly lower during WG treatment* (P<0.05);Glucose concentration *not affected by treatment.*
[23]	Average 7.7 portions/d breads in Healthy Diet group; 7.9 portions/d in WG group.	Average 6.8 portions/d refined wheat breads.	*No significant differences* in clinical measures between groups. *Significant changes* in PUFA profiles in Healthy Diet group compared with control (likely due to fish intake).
Malin	Mixed whole grains (50 g/1000 kcal) included in study foods.	Comparable refined grains (50 g/1000 kcal) in similar study foods.	Postprandial glucose tolerance (P<0.02) and peripiheral insulin sensitivity (P>0.03) *were significantly improved with the WG treatment. There was no impact of the WG treatment* on body composition (body weight, body fat %) and fasting insulin and glucose.
[24]	6 slices sourdough WG bread/d for women, 7 slices WG bread/d for men.	4 slices bread/d for women, 5 slices bread/d for men.	*No impact of WG treatment* on PAI-1, fasting inulin, glucose or HOMA-IR.
[25]	2 portions WG RTE Oat cereal providing 3g/d β-glucan.	Low fibre breakfast/snack foods providing similar energy and macronutrient content.	*No significant reduction* in body weight, SBP between groups.Waist circumference *decreased significantly more* in WG group (P=0.012); Total Chol, LDL Chol *reduced significantly more in WG group* (P=0.038, P=0.005, respectively).
[26]	7-day menus repeated twice in each intervention period; range of WG foods providing 150 g WG/d 64% wheat, 13% oats, 9% brown rice remainder barley and rye. 277 g total cereal intake/d.	Menus with refined grain matched to WG wherever possible; 66% wheat, 27% white rice, 8% refined maize. 277g total cereal intake/d.	Plasma TAG (P=0.05) *significantly higher* on WG diet after 1 week only; trend (P=0.09) for reduction in Total Chol and LDL Chol after 2 weeks. Glucose, HDL Chol, CRP homocysteine *were all unaffected by treatment.*
[27, 28]	WG rye average intake (124 g WG/d) and whole wheat (145 g WG/d) in various products.	Similar refined grain products (<6 g of WG/d consumed on average).	*The WG rye treatment significantly reduced* body weight (P=0.013), but *WG wheat treatment did not. There was no impact of either WG treatment* on a wide variety of cytokines and the immune cell sub-classifications.

[29, 30]	3 servings /d WG (48 g/d) as: 70–80 g WG wheat bread, 30–40 g WG RTE cereals/d. For wheat + oat group, 1 serving of WG wheat, 2 servings WG oats.	3 servings/d refined cereals and white bread.	SBP *decreased significantly more than control in wheat + oat group at 6 weeks of intervention and in both groups at 12 weeks*; pulse pressure *significantly lower* in WG groups than control group.Glucose, insulin, Total-Chol, LDL-Chol, HDL-Chol, TG, Insulin resistance by HOMA, insulin sensitivity by modified QUICKI, hsCRP, IL-6, size and distribution of lipoprotein sub-classes *all unaffected by treatment.*
[31]	6 (F)–7 (M) slices WG Wheat sourdough bread/d.	4 (F)–5 (M) slices white bread/d.	Weight, BMI, %body fat, waist circumference, SBP and DBP, glucose, insulin, HOMA, glucagon, TG Total Chol, LDL Chol, HDL Chol *were all unaffected by treatment.* When *APOE* E3/E3 genotype was present, LDL Chol *significantly higher* in RG group after WG consumption (P=0.02); TAG and TAG:HDL ratio *significantly higher* in HG group after WG consumption (P=0.03 and P=0.04).
[32]	*Ad libitum* brown rice, provided in portions equivalent to 100 g of WG.	*Ad libitum* white rice (polished from same batch of brown rice used in the intervention – 100 g of refined grains per portion).	Weight *fell significantly* in WG group (P=0.002), but no difference between groups; SBP and DBP *fell significantly* (P<0.001) in both groups, but no difference between groups; Glucose, insulin and HOMA-IR *all unaffected by treatment.*Total-Chol (P=0.001), LDL Chol (P=0.001) and HDL Chol (P<0.001) all fell in RG group but not the WG group. TAG *tended to be lower* (P=0.06) in WG group.
[33]	A selection of whole-wheat products aiming to deliver 70g of WG/d.	Comparable refined wheat products,	IL-6 (p=0.03) was *significantly reduced* at the end of the study in the WG group, but not IL-10, PAI-1 and TNF-α.

ALT – alanine transaminase, AST – aspartate aminotransferase, BMI – body mass index, (S/D)BP – (systolic/diastolic) blood pressure, Chol – cholesterol (associated with HDLP – high-density lipoproteins, LDL – low-density lipoproteins or VLDL – very low density lipoproteins), hsCRP – high sensitivity assay for C-reactive protein, HOMA – homeostasis model assessment (for insulin resistance) IL – interleukin, PAI-1 - plasminogen activator inhibitor-1, RG – refined grains, sICAM-1 – soluble intercellular adhesion molecule-1, sIgA, salivary immunoglobulin-A, TAG – triacylglycerols, TNF-α – tumour necrosis factor-α, WG – whole grain.

whereas leptin concentrations were elevated in the control period compared with the whole grain period where they appeared to fall slightly (-9.7 vs. +39.2%, P=0.02). These results suggest a benefit to consuming whole grains in the young that could have implications linked to "healthy ageing" and the long-term prevention of CVD.

10.3 Summary

In summary, observational evidence would strongly point to whole grains being part of an ideal, lifelong dietary habit to reduce the risk of cardiovascular diseases. While evidence from intervention studies does not necessarily confirm a causal relationship between the intake of whole grains and health, no studies (to our knowledge) have ever indicated a negative impact of increased whole grain consumption; at best, studies show either neutral or modest effects on selected outcomes. The lack of mechanistic data to support the observational studies should not invalidate population-level dietary recommendations to replace consumption of refined grains with whole grain foods.

10.4 References

1 Benjamin, E.J., et al., *Heart Disease and Stroke Statistics – 2018 Update: A Report From the American Heart Association. Circulation*, 2018. 137(12): pp. e67–e492.

2 Ye, E.Q., et al., *Greater whole-grain intake is associated with lower risk of type 2 diabetes, cardiovascular disease, and weight gain. J Nutr*, 2012. 142(7): pp. 1304–13.

3 Seal, C.J. and I.A. Brownlee, *Whole Grains and Health, Evidence from Observational and Intervention Studies. Cereal Chemistry*, 2010. 87(2): pp. 167–74.

4 Huang, T., et al., *Consumption of whole grains and cereal fiber and total and cause-specific mortality: Prospective analysis of 367,442 individuals. BMC Med*, 2015. 13: p. 59.

5 Hollaender, P.L., A.B. Ross, and M. Kristensen, *Whole-grain and blood lipid changes in apparently healthy adults: a systematic review and meta-analysis of randomized controlled studies. Am J Clin Nutr*, 2015. 102(3): pp. 556–72.

6 Scheers, N., et al., *Vitamin B12 as a potential compliance marker for fish intake. Eur J Nutr*, 2014. 53(6): pp. 1327–33.

7 Ampatzoglou, A., et al., *Increased whole grain consumption does not affect blood biochemistry, body composition, or gut microbiology in healthy, low-habitual whole grain consumers. J Nutr*, 2015. 145(2): pp. 215–21.

8 Ampatzoglou, A., et al., *Effects of increased wholegrain consumption on immune and inflammatory markers in healthy low habitual wholegrain consumers. Eur J Nutr*, 2016. 55(1): pp. 183–95.

9 Bodinham, C.L., et al., *Short-term effects of whole-grain wheat on appetite and food intake in healthy adults: A pilot study. Br J Nutr*, 2011. 106(3): pp. 327–30.

10 Brownlee, I.A., et al., *Markers of cardiovascular risk are not changed by increased whole-grain intake: The WHOLEheart study, a randomised, controlled dietary intervention. Br J Nutr*, 2010. 104(1): pp. 125–34.

11 Chang, H.C., et al., *Oat prevents obesity and abdominal fat distribution, and improves liver function in humans. Plant Foods Hum Nutr*, 2013. 68(1): pp. 18–23.

12 Connolly, M.L., et al., *Hypocholesterolemic and prebiotic effects of a whole-grain oat-based granola breakfast Cereal in a cardio-metabolic "at risk" population. Front Microbiol*, 2016. 7: p. 1675.

13 Cooper, D.N., et al., *The effects of moderate whole grain consumption on fasting glucose and lipids, gastrointestinal symptoms, and microbiota. Nutrients*, 2017. 9(2).

14 Giacco, R., et al., *Effects of the regular consumption of wholemeal wheat foods on cardiovascular risk factors in healthy people. Nutr Metab Cardiovasc Dis*, 2010. 20(3): p. 186–94.

15 Giacco, R., et al., *A whole-grain cereal-based diet lowers postprandial plasma insulin and triglyceride levels in individuals with metabolic syndrome. Nutr Metab Cardiovasc Dis*, 2014. 24(8): pp. 837–44.

16 Hajihashemi, P., et al., *Whole-grain intake favorably affects markers of systemic inflammation in obese children: A randomized controlled crossover clinical trial. Mol Nutr Food Res*, 2014. 58(6): pp. 1301–8.

17 Harris Jackson, K., et al., *Effects of whole and refined grains in a weight-loss diet on markers of metabolic syndrome in individuals with increased waist circumference: A randomized controlled-feeding trial. Am J Clin Nutr*, 2014. 100(2): pp. 577–86.

18 Kristensen, M., et al., *Whole grain compared with refined wheat decreases the percentage of body fat following a 12-week, energy-restricted dietary intervention in postmenopausal women. J Nutr*, 2012. 142(4): pp. 710–6.

19 Kikuchi, Y., et al., *Effects of Whole grain wheat bread on visceral fat obesity in Japanese subjects: A randomized double-blind study. Plant Foods Hum Nutr*, 2018. 73(3): pp. 161–65.

20 Kirwan, J.P., et al., *A whole-grain diet reduces cardiovascular risk factors in overweight and obese adults: A randomized controlled trial. J Nutr*, 2016. 146(11): pp. 2244–2251.

21 Kopf, J.C., et al., *Role of whole grains versus fruits and vegetables in reducing subclinical inflammation and promoting gastrointestinal health in individuals affected by overweight and obesity: A randomized controlled trial. Nutr J*, 2018. 17(1): p. 72.

22 Landberg, R., et al., *Rye whole grain and bran intake compared with refined wheat decreases urinary C-peptide, plasma insulin, and prostate specific antigen in men with prostate cancer. J Nutr*, 2010. 140(12): pp. 2180–6.

23 Lankinen, M., et al., *Effects of whole grain, fish and bilberries on serum metabolic profile and lipid transfer protein activities: A randomized trial (Sysdimet). PLoS One*, 2014. 9(2): p. e90352.

24 MacKay, K.A., et al., *Whole grain wheat sourdough bread does not affect plasminogen activator inhibitor-1 in adults with normal or impaired carbohydrate metabolism. Nutr Metab Cardiovasc Dis*, 2012. 22(9): pp. 704–11.

25 Maki, K.C., et al., *Digestive and physiologic effects of a wheat bran extract, arabino-xylan-oligosaccharide, in breakfast cereal. Nutrition*, 2012. 28(11–12): pp. 1115–21.

26 Ross, A.B., et al., *A whole-grain cereal-rich diet increases plasma betaine, and tends to decrease total and LDL-cholesterol compared with a refined-grain diet in healthy subjects. Br J Nutr*, 2011. 105(10): pp. 1492–502.

27 Suhr, J., et al., *Wholegrain rye, but not wholegrain wheat, lowers body weight and fat mass compared with refined wheat: A 6-week randomized study. Eur J Clin Nutr*, 2017. 71(8): pp. 959–67.

28 Vanegas, S.M., et al., *Substituting whole grains for refined grains in a 6-wk randomized trial has a modest effect on gut microbiota and immune and inflammatory markers of healthy adults. Am J Clin Nutr*, 2017. 105(3): pp. 635–50.

29 Tighe, P., et al., *Effects of wheat and oat-based whole grain foods on serum lipoprotein size and distribution in overweight middle aged people: A randomised controlled trial. PLoS One*, 2013. 8(8): p. e70436.

30 Tighe, P., et al., *Effect of increased consumption of whole-grain foods on blood pressure and other cardiovascular risk markers in healthy middle-aged persons: A randomized controlled trial. Am J Clin Nutr*, 2010. 92(4): pp. 733–40.

31 Tucker, A.J., et al., *The effect of whole grain wheat sourdough bread consumption on serum lipids in healthy normoglycemic/normoinsulinemic and hyperglycemic/hyperinsulinemic adults depends on presence of the APOE E3/E3 genotype: A randomized controlled trial. Nutr Metab (Lond)*, 2010. 7: p. 37.

32 Zhang, G., et al., *Substituting white rice with brown rice for 16 weeks does not substantially affect metabolic risk factors in middle-aged Chinese men and women with diabetes or a high risk for diabetes. J Nutr*, 2011. 141(9): pp. 1685–90.

33 Vitaglione, P., et al., *Whole-grain wheat consumption reduces inflammation in a randomized controlled trial on overweight and obese subjects with unhealthy dietary and lifestyle behaviors: Role of polyphenols bound to cereal dietary fiber. Am J Clin Nutr*, 2015. 101(2): pp. 251–61.

11 Whole Grains and Cancer Risk

Anja Olsen and Cecilie Kyrø

Danish Cancer Society Research Center, Strandboulevarden, Copenhagen, Denmark

11.1 Introduction

In 2012, 14 million persons worldwide were diagnosed with cancer and 8 million deaths were related to cancer, making this disease one of the most important disease burdens. The preceding estimates correspond to age-standardized incidence rates of 182 per 100 000, meaning that each year 182 persons are diagnosed with cancer for each 100 000 persons alive worldwide (Ferlay et al., 2013). The sites of cancer most frequently diagnosed among men and women, respectively, in 2012 are presented in Table 11.1, showing both worldwide numbers and numbers for Europe and Asia (Ferlay et al., 2013). Compared to the worldwide age-standardized cancer incidence of 182/100 000 per year, the age-standardized incidence in Europe is higher (255/100 000 per year) and the age-standardized incidence in Asia is lower (152/100 000 per year) (Ferlay et al., 2013) , exemplifying a general pattern of higher cancer incidence in Western than in non-Western populations.

A large fraction of the differences in cancer incidence among different parts of the world are attributable to lifestyle and environmental factors. In 2010, it was estimated that 42.7% of eight frequently occurring cancers were attributable to non-optimal exposure to one or more of 14 factors: tobacco; alcohol; consumption of meat, fruits and vegetables, dietary fibre or salt; overweight; lack of physical exercise; occupation; infections; ionizing radiation; solar radiation; use of hormones and reproductive history. Of these factors, tobacco smoking, dietary factors (meat, fruits and vegetables, dietary fibre and salt), alcohol intake and overweight, alone were estimated to account for 34% of the cancers (Parkin, 2011). Though these fractions are based on exposure estimation and cancer occurrence in the population of the United Kingdom, the numbers can be regarded as a qualified estimated for most of the Western world.

11.2 Diet and cancer

Dietary patterns, and the related risk factor body weight, are among the cancer risk factors showing the most obvious differences among different parts of the world. Cancers of the breast, colorectum and endometrium are mostly related to overweight and obesity, and colorectal cancer further to high intake of red meat and low intake of fibre-rich foods, especially whole grains (World Cancer Research Fund/American Institute for Cancer Research, 2017). Looking at Table 11.1, these cancers are clearly more frequent in Europe

Whole Grains and Health, Second Edition. Edited by Rikard Landberg and Nathalie Scheers.

Additional materials available for download online at https://www.wiley.com/en-gb/Whole+Grains+and+Health-p-9781118939437

Table 11.1 Percentage of different cancer types worldwide and in Europe and Asia for men and women, respectively.

Men		Women	
Worldwide		**Worldwide**	
Lung (16.7%)		Breast (25.2%)	
Prostate (15.0%)		Colorectum (9.2%)	
Colorectum (10.0%)		Lung (8.7%)	
Stomach (8.5%)		Cervix (7.9%)	
Liver (7.5%)		Stomach (4.8%)	
Europe	**Asia**	**Europe**	**Asia**
Prostate (22.8%)	Lung (20.1%)	Breast (28.8%)	Breast (21.2%)
Lung (15.9%)	Stomach (13.1%)	Colorectum (12.7%)	Lung (9.9%)
Colorectum (13.2%)	Liver (11.7%)	Lung (7.4%)	Cervix uteri (9.3%)
Bladder (6.5%)	Colorectum (9.4%)	Corpus uteri (6.1%)	Colorectum (8.5%)
Stomach (4.6%)	Oesophagus (6.5%)	Ovary (4.1%)	Stomach (7.2%)

than in Asia. Contrary, a high intake of salt (together with *Helicobacter Pylori* infection) is related to cancer of the stomach, a disease more frequent in Asia than Europe. Other cancers more frequent in Asia are liver cancer and cervix uteri cancer; liver cancer being associated to exposure to aflatoxins (Liu et al., 2012) and cervix uteri cancer strongly associated to infection with the sexually transmitted Human Papilloma virus (HPV) (Zur Hausen, 2000). The type of cancer that is most convincingly associated with a Western-style diet is colorectal cancer (World Cancer Research Fund/American Institute for Cancer Research, 2009). The evidence for that a high intake of red and processed meat and a low intake of whole grains and other foods containing dietary fibre is related to increased risk of colorectal cancer is considered strong (i.e., highest evidence level) (World Cancer Research Fund/American Institute for Cancer Research, 2017).

11.3 Dietary fibre and colorectal cancer risk

The hypothesis that a high intake of dietary fibre reduces the risk of colorectal cancer was first presented by Sir Dennis Burkitt in the 1970s (1978). He observed that the incidence of colorectal cancer was considerably lower among "non-Westernized" African populations than in modern Western populations. The registration of cancer occurrence in the 1970s is to be interpreted with great caution, especially in non-Western countries, but the official statistics from the World Health Organization for the period 1968–1972 report colorectal cancer incidence rates of 2.9/100 000 persons per year among men and 1.1/100 000 persons per year among women in Rhodesia (now Zimbabwe). The corresponding numbers for Oxford, United Kingdom, were 36.6/100 000 persons per year for men and 39.6/100 000 persons per year for women (1976). Burkitt (1978) put forward that the most striking difference between dietary patterns in rural African and urban Western populations are that "Westernization" generally leads to a diet with a higher intake of fat and a reduced intake of fibre. He further approximated that a typical rural African diet contained 25 grams of crude fibre daily, whereas Western diets were expected to provide less than 5 grams of fibre per day (Burkitt, 1978). The potential association between intake of dietary fibre and especially colorectal cancer has been considered with diverse interest during the last 40 years, from a very specific interest in the cancer preventive effects of fibre as such to a broader interest in fibre containing foods such as vegetables, fruits, berries, legumes and cereals (Aune et al., 2011). During recent years, whole grains have attracted especial attention as an important contributor to dietary fibre, but also as a source of many other substances with potential relevance in cancer prevention (Fardet, 2010).

11.4 Possible cancer protective mechanisms

A number of mechanisms underlying the possible association between whole grain intake and cancer risk have been suggested. Some have been investigated in many studies and are considered plausible mechanisms, whereas other are suggested mechanisms based on very few studies. Colorectal cancer is the cancer form that has received the most attention. The first part of this section therefore focuses on mechanisms related to colorectal cancer followed by specific mechanisms related to cancer of the breast and prostate as well as other relevant cancer sites. Finally, suggestions for whole grain related beneficial effect in prognosis of cancer patients are discussed.

11.5 Colorectal cancer

The complex carbohydrates in whole grains have a number of beneficial effects on the large intestine. When undigested carbohydrates reach the colon, they are fermented by the microflora to short-chain fatty acids (SCFA), including acetate, butyrate and propionate (Slavin, 2004). Butyrate is the largest source of energy for colonocytes, and several mechanisms for cancer prevention have been suggested for butyrate including inhibition of cell proliferation and promotion of apoptosis (Fung et al., 2012). Furthermore, butyrate lowers the pH in the colon (Topping and Clifton, 2001), which reduces the conversion of primary bile acids to secondary bile acids (Bingham, 1990). In humans, the fermentation of fibre especially takes place in the proximal colon (Wong et al., 2006). However, a study indicated that butyrate is a more important energy source in the colonic mucosa in the distal than in the proximal colon (Roediger, 1980). It is therefore possible that butyrate especially has an effect in the distal part of the colon. Complex carbohydrates also have further "mechanical" effects on the colon. Whole grains increase fecal bulk and decrease the transit time, which allows less opportunity for harmful compounds, including secondary bile acids, to interact with the colonic epithelium because of binding of harmful compounds (Slavin, 2000). Furthermore, the complex carbohydrates have a beneficial effect on the microbiota (Roberfroid et al., 2010).There are very interesting implications for that the colonic microbiota is a significant factor in colon cancer prevention. Recently, it has been shown that both quality and diversity of the colonic microbiota differs considerably between patients diagnosed with colorectal cancer and healthy controls (Ahn et al., 2013).

Oxidative stress has been related to increased risk for colorectal cancer (Leufkens et al., 2012). Antioxidants can neutralize free radicals and stop chain reactions that lead to the production of radical oxidative species. Among the antioxidants present in whole grains are polyphenols, carotenoids and vitamin E. Whole grains are one of the richest sources of vitamin E (tocotrienols and tocopherols). Vitamin E is an antioxidant and may thereby be cancer preventive through its neutralization of free radicals (Bartlomiej et al., 2012). Furthermore, vitamin E possibly helps to maintain selenium in reduced state and inhibit the formation of nitrosamines (Slavin, 2003). However, a RCT did not find that vitamin E was associated with colorectal cancer incidence or mortality (Lippman et al., 2009), and vitamin E is, therefore, not likely to be the main substance responsible for the potential colorectal cancer prevention of whole grain. The list of compounds found in whole grains that may have potential antioxidative effects is much longer (Fardet, 2010). A high intake of whole grain foods has been related to biomarkers indicating lower levels of both oxidative stress and inflammation (Montonen et al., 2012). Whole grains are a source of lignans that are converted by the human microbiota to the mammalian lignans enterolactone and enterodiol (Slavin, 2003). Several mechanisms have been suggested as responsible for a preventive effect of the mammalian lignans on colorectal cancer. In a study using colon cancer cells, enterolactone and enterodiol inhibited growth of the tumor cells (Sung et al., 1998). Furthermore, enterolactone has antioxidant activity (Prasad, 2000) and estrogen-like properties (Adlercreutz, 1995). B-vitamins function mainly as co-enzymes in metabolic pathways. Whole grains are especially rich in thiamin, niacin, pantothenic acid and biotin. Whole grains also contain folic acid. In some countries fortification of cereal grains with folic acid is mandatory (US Food and Drug Administration, 1996), and folic acids are therefore also found in considerable amounts in refined-cereals. Especially folate has been associated with lower risk of colorectal cancer (Kennedy et al., 2011). Folic acid deficiency has been suggested as one of the risk factors of colorectal cancer because deficiency can lead to DNA strand breaks, impaired DNA methylation and thereby possible colorectal cancer initiation (Kennedy et al., 2011). In countries where folic acid fortification is not mandatory, whole grains are an important source of folate (Papas et al., 2004).

11.5.1 Alkylresorcinols and colorectal cancer

Alkylresorcinols, a polyphenol found in whole grain wheat and rye, may also have health effects per se (in addition to being used as a biomarker of intake), and its proposed biological activity is multifactorial (Fardet, 2010). Most of the studies conducted have been in vitro experiments, in which the tested doses of alkylresorcinols are much higher than what is possible to obtain from the humans diet (Ross, 2012). Alkylresorcinols are very weak antioxidants due to the location of the two hydroxyl groups in the meta-position of the phenolic ring (Kamal-Eldin et al., 2000). Nevertheless, they have been shown to have antioxidative properties, which may be attributed to their ability to become incorporated in biological membranes (Kozubek and Nienartowicz, 1995). Alkylresorcinols have antibacterial and antifungal activity, especially against gram-positive bacteria (Ross et al., 2004). Anticancer properties have also been suggested and alkylresorcinols in wheat bran have shown an inhibitory effect on human colon cancer cells in vitro (Zhu et al., 2011), possibly through increased apoptosis (Barbini et al., 2006). Furthermore, structural analogues of alkylresorcinols have been shown to interact with several enzymes (Kozubek and Tyman, 1999). Alkylresorcinols from rye and wheat inhibit glycerol-3-phosphate dehydrogenase (GPDH), and thereby possibly prevent accumulation of excessive triglycerides in adipocytes (Rejman and Kozubek, 2004; Rejman and Kozubek, 1997), which may possibly be associated with lower risk of obesity. Alkylresorcinols can furthermore interact with membranes (Kozubek and Tyman, 1999), and can incorporate into human erythrocytes

(Linko and Adlercreutz, 2005). As approximately 60% of alkylresorcinols are absorbed in the ileum (Ross et al., 2003), its local effect on the colon might be limited. However, since most water absorption takes place in the proximal colon (Sandle, 1998), the concentration of alkylresorcinols might be considerable in the distal part of the colon. Other mechanisms might also indirectly affect colorectal cancer risk. Many of the previously described mechanisms are of general "cancer relevance" due to systemic influence like antioxidant effects and insulin/glucose homeostasis. Other factors are suspected to be more directly related to colon cancer, like the butyrate production and "mechanical" effects of dietary fibre in the intestine. In the following, mechanisms of specific relevance for breast cancer and other cancers, respectively, are described.

11.6 Breast cancer

High levels of circulating estrogen are among the strongest risk factors for breast cancer (Colditz, 1998), therefore, factors influencing estrogen levels are often in focus when breast cancer prevention is studied. Especially the high fibre content of whole grains may be of relevance for estrogen balance and thereby breast cancer prevention. It has been suggested that dietary fibre may reduce endogenous estrogen levels by interrupting the enterohepatic circulation. Among the proposed mechanisms are binding of estrogens and thereby facilitation of their fecal excretion (Arts et al., 1991). Inhibition of intestinal reabsorption of estrogens through reduction or intestinal β-gluronidase activity is another mechanism potentially diminishing estrogen levels (Gerber, 1998).

As described previously, whole grains are a rich source of plant lignans that are converted to the mammalian lignans enterolactone and enterodiol by the intestinal microbiota. The lignan content of cereals varies, with rye being a particularly rich source (Tetens et al., 2013). The mammalian lignans are classified as phytoestrogens due to their estrogen-like structures (Adlercreutz, 2002). The estrogen-like structure has raised the theory that enterolactone and enterodiol can interact with estrogen receptors in competition with endogenous estrogens and thereby decrease the impact of the endogenous estrogens (Adlercreutz, 2002). In addition, especially enterolactone may also modulate the concentration of endogenous sex hormones by binding or inhibiting enzymes involved in steroid hormone biosynthesis and metabolism (Brooks and Thompson, 2005; Adlercreutz, 2002). These mechanisms are all plausible ways by which the mammalian lignans can play a role in breast cancer prevention.

11.7 Other cancers

Mechanisms linking whole grains to other cancers than colorectal and breast cancers have been studied less intensively. Both prostate and endometrial cancers are related to endogenous hormone levels, and consequently the effects of whole grains on hormone metabolism are also considered relevant for these cancers. For prostate cancer, the content of selenium in whole grains may be of particularly relevance in the parts of the world with low to intermediate selenium status levels (Christensen, 2014). Whole grains might also indirectly affect the risk of several cancers. Whole grains have been shown to have beneficial effects on weight regulation (Giacco et al., 2011) and insulin/glucose homeostasis (McKeown et al., 2002). Both overweight (Ma et al., 2013) and type 2 diabetes (Larsson et al., 2005b) are related to increased risk of colorectal cancer, endometrial cancer and breast cancer risk (among postmenopausal women). Whole grains may therefore also contribute to lower risk of these cancers through its beneficial effects in relation to body weight regulation and insulin/glucose homeostasis.

11.8 Cancer patients and prognosis

Recently, theories on beneficial effects of whole grains in cancer prognosis have been out forward, especially with regard to prostate and breast cancer. Prostate cancer mice models have shown reduced levels of prostate specific antigen (PSA), reduced tumor volumes and slower tumor growth in mice fed high amounts of whole grain rye (Landstrom et al., 1998; Bylund et al., 2000), and clinical studies on men diagnosed with prostate cancer have indicated that a diet with a high content of whole grain rye may actually slow disease progression (Bylund et al., 2003;Landberg et al., 2010). For breast cancer prognosis, the interest has primarily been aimed at the lignan derived plant estrogen enterolactone that has been shown to inhibit growth and metastasis of breast cancer in mice models (Wang et al., 2005; Chen et al., 2006).

11.9 Epidemiological evidence – colorectal cancer

Only during the recent years has the association between whole grain intake and risk of colorectal cancer been investigated in cohort studies. As seen in Table 11.2, the first study was published in 1999 and a total of 10 publications have been identified. All the studies mentioned in Table 11.2, with the exception of the studies by Pietinen et al. (1999), and Bakken et al. (2016) were included in a meta-analysis as part of the WCRF/AICR Continuous Update Project (World Cancer Research Fund/American Institute for Cancer Research (WCRF/AICR), 2017). In the meta-analysis, an inverse association between whole grains and colorectal cancer was found; an increment of three servings of whole grains per day (one serving equals 16 g of whole grain [Kyro and Tjonneland 2016]) was associated with a 17% lower risk of colorectal cancer (relative risk [RR], 0.83, 95% CI, 0.78–0.89). One of the main reasons for the somewhat limited number of studies evaluating the association between whole grain intake and colorectal cancer is probably that whole grains has not been a prioritized food group when food frequency questionnaires have been developed for dietary assessment in prospective cohort studies. This may especially be the case in populations where whole grain intake contributes to a limited fraction of the energy intake. As shown elsewhere (Chapter 6), intake of whole grains varies considerably between populations.

The problem with insufficient quality in measurement of whole grain intake, especially among low-consumption populations, may be solved by using a biomarker for intake assessment. Recently, alkylresorcinols measured in biofluids has been validated as a biomarker for intake of whole grain wheat and rye. The association between alkylresorcinol concentrations measured in plasma samples and incidence of colorectal cancer has been reported in a single study. Kyrø et al. (2014) evaluated alkylresorcinol concentrations among 1372 case-control pairs originating from the European-wide European investigation into Cancer and Nutrition (EPIC) cohort, showing a statistically significant lower incidence of distal colon cancer with higher alkylresorcinol concentrations, but no overall association with colorectal cancer (Kyro et al., 2014). As described in the introduction of this chapter, one of the expected health promoting effects of whole grains most likely goes through it

Table 11.2 Cohort studies on whole grains and colorectal cancer (in chronological order).

Reference	Country	Population	Follow-up	Participants, cases	Whole grain assessment	Comparison, intake	RR (96% CI)	Effect on risk
(Pietinen et al., 1999)	FI	Alpha-Tocopherol, Beta-Carotene Cancer Prevention study (ATBC)	8 years	27 111 male smokers, 185 CRC cases	Whole grain cereals and rye products	Whole grain cereals: Q4 (374 g/day) vs. Q1 (96 g/day) Rye products: Q4: (157 g/day) vs. Q1: (23 g/day)	CRC:Whole grain cereals: 1.0 (0.7–1.6) Rye products: 0.7 (0.5–1.1)	→ →
(McCullough et al., 2003)	US	The Cancer Prevention Study (CPS) II Nutrition Cohort	5 years	187 192 men and women, 508 colon cases	Whole grain products	Qu5: (>11.2 servings/ week) vs. Qu1: (<2.5 servings/week)	Colon cancer: ♂: 0.95 (0.64–1.42) ♀: 1.17 (0.73–1.87)	→ →
(Wu et al., 2004)*	US	The Health Professionals Follow-Up Study	14 years	120 678 men, 561 colon cancer cases	Whole grains	Qu5 vs. Qu1	Colon cancer: 0.75(0.67–1.00) NS	(↓)
(Larsson et al., 2005a)	SE	The Swedish Mammography Cohort	15 years	61 433 women, 805 CRC cases	Whole grain products	>4.5 servings/day vs. <1.5 servings/day	CRC: 0.80 (0.60–1.06) Colon cancer: 0.67 (0.47–0.96) Rectal cancer: 1.11 (0.67–1.83)	→ ↓ →
(McCarl et al., 2006)	US	Iowa Women's Health Study	15 years	35 197 women, 954 CRC cases	Whole grain products	≥19 servings/week vs. ≤3.5 servings/week	CRC:0.81 (0.66–0.99)	↓
(Schatzkin et al., 2007)	US	NIH-AARP Diet and Health Study	5 years	489 611 men and women, 2974 CRC cases	Whole grain (absolute amounts, g/day)	Qu5 (1.3 g/day per 1000 kcal) vs. Qu1 (0.2 g/day per 1000 kcal)	CRC:0.79 (0.70–0.89)	↓

(continued)

Table 11.2 Cohort studies on whole grains and colorectal cancer (in chronological order). (*continued*)

Reference	Country	Population	Follow-up	Participants, cases	Whole grain assessment	Comparison, intake	RR (96% CI)	Effect on risk
(Egeberg et al., 2010) †	DK	The Diet, Cancer and Health Cohort Study	11 years	55 819 men and women, 744 CRC cases	Whole grain products	>160 g/day vs. ≤75 g/day	Colon cancer: ♂: 0.61 (0.43–0.86) ♀: 0.92 (0.63–1.35) Rectal cancer: NS	 ↓ ➔ ➔
(Fung et al., 2010)	US	♂: Health Professional Follow-Up Study & ♀: Nurses' Health Study &	26 years & 20 years	♂:: 45 490 participants, 1032 CRC cases & ♀:: 87 256 participants, 1432 CRC cases	Whole grains	Per serving increase	CRC: ♂: 0.94 (0.88–0.99) ♀: 0.95 (0.89–1.02)	 ↓ ➔
(Kyro et al., 2013)†	SE/NO/ DK	The HELGA cohort	11 years	108 000 men and women, 1123 CRC cases	Whole grain products	Q5 vs. Q1	CRC: 0.77 (0.63-0.93)	↓
(Bakken et al., 2016) †	NO	The Norwegian Women and Cancer Study	9 years	90 592 women, 795 CRC cases	Whole grain bread	High vs. low	Colon cancer: 0.88 (0.66-1.09) Rectal cancer: 0.78 (0.47-1.27)	➔ ➔

*Results published twice; †Study populations overlapping. Abbreviations: RR, relative risk; Q, quartile; Qu, quintile; CRC, colorectal cancer; NS, non-significant; UK, the United Kingdom; FI, Finland; US, the United States; SE, Sweden; DK, Denmark; NO, Norway; ➔, no association; ↓, inverse association; (↓), borderline statistically significant inverse association.

being a rich source of dietary fibre. Recently, dietary fibre was concluded as being convincingly related to a decreased incidence of colorectal cancer, with a 10% lower risk of colorectal cancer (relative risk [RR], 0.90, 95% CI, 0.86–0.94) for each 10 gram of fibre eaten per day (Aune et al., 2011). The same meta-analysis further indicate that dietary fibre originating from cereals show stronger associations towards lower incidence of colorectal cancer than dietary fibre originating from fruits, vegetables or legumes. In the recent WCRF/AICR Continuous Update Project (World Cancer Research Fund/American Institute for Cancer Research [WCRF/AICR], 2017) whole grains as a food group was categorized as probably related to lower risk of colorectal cancer, alongside the more general classification of "Foods containing dietary fibre."

In summary, evidence strongly point towards that whole grain intake entail protection of colorectal cancer. The number of published studies is still relatively low and methodological problems related to confounding by other aspects associated with healthy lifestyle cannot be ruled out. However, the combination of strong mechanistic support and a picture of observational studies pointing almost unequivocally in the direction that whole grains may play a role in the prevention of colorectal cancer. In addition, some evidence points towards that the association seen with whole grains is more consistent than the associations seen with other foods containing dietary fibre.

11.10 Epidemiological evidence – breast cancer

Recently, the literature associating intake of whole grains and incidence of breast cancer was summarized in a meta-analysis, reporting a statistically significant lower incidence of breast cancer related to high intake of whole grains (Xiao et al., 2018). Subgroup analysis by study design, however, found the decreased risk to be evident only in case-control studies (summery RR 0.69 [95% CI: 0.56–0.97]) and not in cohort studies (summary RR 0.96 [95% CI, 0.82–1.14]). Overall, the evidence for a breast cancer protective effect of whole grains must be considered limited. As previously mentioned, a potential role of the phytoestrogen enterolactone has been hypothesized to prevent breast cancer. Enterolactone is derived from plant lignans, especially in whole grain rye, which is an important source. The literature was summarized in 2010, concluding that a high intake of lignans and/or high concentrations of enterolactone in blood or urine may be associated with a reduced breast cancer risk in postmenopausal women, but that further research was needed (Buck et al., 2010).

11.11 Epidemiological evidence – prostate cancer

The association between whole grain intake and incidence of prostate cancer has been evaluated in three prospective studies, one showing no signs of an association (Egeberg et al., 2011), and the second indicating higher incidence of prostate cancer related to higher whole grain intake (Nimptsch et al., 2011). The third study attempted to estimate intake of whole grain rye bread in early life (14–19 years of age) and found a markedly lower risk of being diagnosed with prostate cancer in an clinically advanced stage many years later (mean age of diagnosis 75 years) among those with high intakes (Torfadottir et al., 2012). Recently, a study associating the biomarkers of whole grain intake, plasma alkylresorcinols with prostate cancer incidence found a higher incidence with higher levels (Drake et al., 2013).

The literature on whole grain intake and incidence of prostate cancer must be regarded as inconclusive and further research is needed.

11.12 Epidemiological evidence – endometrial cancer

The association between intake of whole grains and endometrial cancer has been investigated in two cohort studies. In a cohort of American women, a tendency towards lower incidence with higher intakes was seen among women not using hormone replacement therapy (Kasum et al., 2001), whereas no association was seen in a cohort of Danish women (Aarestrup et al., 2012).

11.13 Epidemiological evidence – stomach cancer

A recent meta-analysis concluded that there seem to be a consistent protective effect of dietary fibre on stomach cancer (Zhang et al., 2013), interesting the association seem to be stronger for intake of cereal fibre than for fruit or vegetable fibre, indicating that whole grains may have a potential in stomach cancer prevention. No studies reporting on the direct association between whole grain intake and stomach cancer have been identified, thus more research is from well-conducted cohort studies is needed.

11.14 Epidemiological evidence – whole grains and cancer prognosis

As previously mentioned, intake of whole grains has also been hypothesized to influence prognosis among patients diagnosed with especially prostate or breast cancer.

For prostate cancer, a potential influence of whole grain intake on prognosis has not been studied in observational studies. Two short-term studies have intervened prostate cancer patients with very high amounts of whole grain rye, both indicating very interesting results (Bylund et al., 2003; Landberg et al., 2010). These studies do, however, both rely on intermediate markers of disease progression and further studies are needed. For breast cancer, the primary interest has considered the phytoestrogen enterolactone. Seven studies have associated estimated intake of lignans or blood concentrations of enterolactone to mortality after breast cancer diagnosis (Fink et al., 2007; McCann et al., 2010; Buck et al., 2011; Buck et al., 2011; Olsen et al., 2011; Guglielmini et al., 2012; Seibold et al., 2014), all but one (Fink et al., 2007) showing statistically significantly lower all cause and/or breast cancer specific mortality among postmenopausal breast cancer patients with high intakes/blood concentrations. Summarized in a meta-analysis comparing highest to lowest, a more than 40% lower mortality is reported (Seibold et al., 2014). In some geographical areas, especially in the Nordic countries, whole grains are a very important source of plant lignans. One study has associated prediagnostic whole grain intake to mortality among colorectal cancer patients, indicating no association (Skeie et al., 2014). Another study obtained information about whole grain intake from 1575 patients diagnosed with colorectal cancer in stage I, II or III. During a median of 8 years of followup, they reported a statistically significant 28% lower colorectal cancer specific mortality for per 20 gram higher daily intake of whole grain (HR per 20 g/d increment, 0.72 [95% CI: 0.59–0.88]) (Song et al., 2018). Though further research is highly needed, this finding points towards a potential role in secondary prevention of colorectal cancer.

11.15 Conclusion

To summarize, there is a growing body of evidence, mechanistic as well as epidemiologic, supporting an important role of whole grains in prevention of especially colorectal cancer. For this cancer site, which is among the most frequently occurring cancers in the Western world, the evidence is increasing rapidly and whole grain intake may turn out be the most important preventive dietary factor. The evidence regarding other cancer sites is less clear. With regard to prognosis in cancer patients, interesting prospects are indicated especially for colorectal cancer, but also for prostate and breast cancer, though further research is needed before conclusions can be made.

11.16 Acknowledgments

This work was supported by grants from The Danish Council for Strategic Research (project "ELIN - the effects of enterolignans in chronic disease"), Wereld Kanker Onderzoek Fonds (WCRF NL; grant 2011/436), as part of the WCRF International grant program, NordForsk (Centre of Excellence programme HELGA; 070015), and Danish Cancer Society.

11.17 References

Aarestrup J, Kyro C, Christensen J, Kristensen M, Wurtz AM, Johnsen NF, Overvad K, Tjonneland A, Olsen A (2012) Whole grain, dietary fiber, and incidence of endometrial cancer in a Danish cohort study. *Nutr Cancer* 64:1160–1168.

Adlercreutz H (1995) Phytoestrogens: Epidemiology and a possible role in cancer protection. *Environ Health Perspect* 103 Suppl 7:103–112.

Adlercreutz H (2002) Phyto-oestrogens and cancer. *Lancet Oncol* 3:364–373.

Ahn J, Sinha R, Pei Z, Dominianni C, Wu J, Shi J, Goedert JJ, Hayes RB, Yang L (2013) Human gut microbiome and risk for colorectal cancer. *J Natl Cancer Inst* 105:1907–1911.

Arts CJ, de Bie AT, van den Berg H, van ', V, Bunnik GS, Thijssen JH (1991) Influence of wheat bran on NMU-induced mammary tumor development, plasma estrogen levels and estrogen excretion in female rats. *J Steroid Biochem Mol Biol* 39:193–202.

Aune D, Chan DS, Lau R, Vieira R, Greenwood DC, Kampman E, Norat T (2011) Dietary fibre, whole grains, and risk of colorectal cancer: Systematic review and dose-response meta-analysis of prospective studies. *BMJ* 343:d6617.

Bakken T, Braaten T, Olsen A, Kyrø C, Lund E, Skeie G (2016) Consumption of whole-grain bread and risk of colorectal cancer among Norwegian women (the NOWAC study). *Nutrients* 40.

Barbini L, Lopez P, Ruffa J, Martino V, Ferraro G, Campos R, Cavallaro L (2006) Induction of apoptosis on human hepatocarcinoma cell lines by an alkyl resorcinol isolated from Lithraea molleoides. *World J Gastroenterol* 12:5959–5963.

Bartlomiej S, Justyna RK, Ewa N (2012) Bioactive compounds in cereal grains – Occurrence, structure, technological significance and nutritional benefits – A review. *Food Sci Technol Int* 18:559–568.

Bingham SA (1990) Mechanisms and experimental and epidemiological evidence relating dietary fibre (non-starch polysaccharides) and starch to protection against large bowel cancer. *Proc Nutr Soc* 49:153–171.

Brooks JD, Thompson LU (2005) Mammalian lignans and genistein decrease the activities of aromatase and 17 beta-hydroxysteroid dehydrogenase in MCF-7 cells. *J Steroid Biochem Mol Biol* 94:461–467.

Buck K, Vrieling A, Zaineddin AK, Becker S, Husing A, Kaaks R, Linseisen J, Flesch-Janys D, Chang-Claude J (2011) Serum enterolactone and prognosis of postmenopausal breast cancer. *J Clin Oncol* 29:3730–3738.

Buck K, Zaineddin AK, Vrieling A, Linseisen J, Chang-Claude J (2010) Meta-analyses of lignans and enterolignans in relation to breast cancer risk. *Am J Clin Nutr* 92:141–153.

Burkitt DP (1978) Colonic-rectal cancer: Fiber and other dietary factors. *Am J Clin Nutr* 31:S58–S64.

Bylund A, Lundin E, Zhang JX, Nordin A, Kaaks R, Stenman UH, Aman P, Adlercreutz H, Nilsson TK, Hallmans G, Bergh A, Stattin P (2003) Randomised controlled short-term intervention pilot study on rye bran bread in prostate cancer. *Eur J Cancer Prev* 12:407–415.

Bylund A, Zhang JX, Bergh A, Damber JE, Widmark A, Johansson A, Adlercreutz H, Aman P, Shepherd MJ, Hallmans G (2000) Rye bran and soy protein delay growth and increase apoptosis of human LNCaP prostate adenocarcinoma in nude mice. *Prostate* 42:304–314.

Chen J, Wang L, Thompson LU (2006) Flaxseed and its components reduce metastasis after surgical excision of solid human breast tumor in nude mice. *Cancer Lett* 234:168–175.

Christensen MJ (2014) Selenium and prostate cancer prevention: What next-if anything? *Cancer Prev Res (Phila)* 7:781–785.

Colditz GA (1998) Relationship between estrogen levels, use of hormone replacement therapy, and breast cancer. *J Natl Cancer Inst* 90:814–823.

Drake I, Sonestedt E, Gullberg B, Bjartell A, Olsson H, Adlercreutz H, Tikkanen MJ, Wirfalt E, Wallstrom P (2013) Plasma alkylresorcinol metabolites as biomarkers for whole-grain intake and rheir association with prostate cancer: A Swedish nested case-control study. *Cancer Epidemiol Biomarkers Prev* 23(1):73-83.

Egeberg R, Olsen A, Christensen J, Johnsen NF, Loft S, Overvad K, Tjonneland A (2011) Intake of whole-grain products and risk of prostate cancer among men in the Danish Diet, Cancer and Health cohort study. *Cancer Causes Control*22(8):1133-9.

Egeberg R, Olsen A, Loft S, Christensen J, Johnsen NF, Overvad K, Tjonneland A (2009) Intake of whole grain products and risk of breast cancer by hormone receptor status and histology among postmenopausal women. *Int J Cancer* 124:745–750.

Egeberg R, Olsen A, Loft S, Christensen J, Johnsen NF, Overvad K, Tjonneland A (2010) Intake of wholegrain products and risk of colorectal cancers in the Diet, Cancer and Health cohort study. *Br J Cancer* 103:730–734.

Fardet A (2010) New hypotheses for the health-protective mechanisms of whole-grain cereals: What is beyond fibre? *Nutr Res Rev* 23:65–134.

Ferlay, Soerjomataram I, Ervik M, Dikshit R, Eser S, Mathers C, Rebelo M, Parkin DM, Forman D, Bray F (2013) GLOBOCAN 2012 v1.0, Cancer Incidence and Mortality Worldwide: IARC CancerBase No. 11 [Internet], Lyon, France: International Agency for Research on Cancer; 2013.Available from: http://globocan.iarc.fr,

Fink BN, Steck SE, Wolff MS, Britton JA, Kabat GC, Gaudet MM, Abrahamson PE, Bell P, Schroeder JC, Teitelbaum SL, Neugut AI, Gammon MD (2007) Dietary flavonoid intake and breast cancer survival among women on Long Island. *Cancer Epidemiol Biomarkers Prev* 16:2285–2292.

Fung KY, Cosgrove L, Lockett T, Head R, Topping DL (2012) A review of the potential mechanisms for the lowering of colorectal oncogenesis by butyrate. *Br J Nutr* 108:820–831.

Fung TT, Hu FB, Wu K, Chiuve SE, Fuchs CS, Giovannucci E (2010) The Mediterranean and Dietary Approaches to Stop Hypertension (DASH) diets and colorectal cancer. *Am J Clin Nutr* 92:1429–1435

Gerber M (1998) Fibre and breast cancer. *Eur J Cancer Prev* 7 Suppl 2:S63–S67.

Giacco R, Della PG, Luongo D, Riccardi G (2011) Whole grain intake in relation to body weight: From epidemiological evidence to clinical trials. *Nutr Metab Cardiovasc Dis* 21:901–908.

Guglielmini P, Rubagotti A, Boccardo F (2012) Serum enterolactone levels and mortality outcome in women with early breast cancer: A retrospective cohort study. *Breast Cancer Res Treat* 132:661–668.

Kamal-Eldin A, Pouru A, Eliasson C, Aman P (2000) Alkylresorcinols as antioxidants: hydrogen donation and peroxyl radical-scavenging effects. *Journal of the Science of Food and Agriculture* 81:353–356.

Kasum CM, Nicodemus K, Harnack LJ, Jacobs DR, Jr., Folsom AR (2001) Whole grain intake and incident endometrial cancer: The Iowa Women's Health Study. *Nutr Cancer* 39:180–186.

Kennedy DA, Stern SJ, Matok I, Sarkar M, Nickel C, Koren G (2011) Folate intake and the risk of colorectal cancer: A systematic review and meta-analysis. *Cancer Epidemiol* 35:2–10.

Kozubek A, Nienartowicz B (1995) Cereal grain resorcinolic lipids inhibit H2O2-induced peroxidation of biological membranes. *Acta Biochimica Polonica* 42:309-316

Kozubek A, Tyman JH (1999) Resorcinolic Lipids, the Natural Non-isoprenoid Phenolic Amphiphiles and Their Biological Activity. *Chem Rev* 99:1–26.

Kyro C, Olsen A, Landberg R, Skeie G, Loft S, Aman P, Leenders M, Dik VK, Siersema PD, Pischon T, Christensen J, Overvad K, Boutron-Ruault MC, Fagherazzi G, Cottet V, Kuhn T, Chang-Claude J, Boeing H, Trichopoulou A, Bamia C, Trichopoulos D, Palli D, Krogh V, Tumino R, Vineis P, Panico S, Peeters PH, Weiderpass E, Bakken T, Asli LA, Arguelles M, Jakszyn P, Sanchez MJ, Amiano P, Huerta JM, Barricarte A, Ljuslinder I, Palmqvist R, Khaw KT, Wareham N, Key TJ, Travis RC, Ferrari P, Freisling H, Jenab M, Gunter MJ, Murphy N, Riboli E, Tjonneland A, Bueno-de-Mesquita HB (2014) Plasma alkylresorcinols, biomarkers of whole-grain wheat and rye intake, and incidence of colorectal cancer. J Natl Cancer Inst 106:djt352.

Kyro, C., and A. Tjonneland. 2016. Whole grains and public health. *BMJ*, 353: i3046.

Kyro C, Skeie G, Loft S, Landberg R, Christensen J, Lund E, Nilsson LM, Palmqvist R, Tjonneland A, Olsen A (2013) Intake of whole grains from different cereal and food sources and incidence of colorectal cancer in the Scandinavian HELGA cohort. *Cancer Causes Control* 24:1363–1374.

Landberg R, Andersson SO, Zhang JX, Johansson JE, Stenman UH, Adlercreutz H, Kamal-Eldin A, Aman P, Hallmans G (2010) Rye whole grain and bran intake compared with refined wheat decreases urinary C-peptide, plasma insulin, and prostate specific antigen in men with prostate cancer. *J Nutr* 140(12):2180–6.

Landstrom M, Zhang JX, Hallmans G, Aman P, Bergh A, Damber JE, Mazur W, Wahala K, Adlercreutz H (1998) Inhibitory effects of soy and rye diets on the development of Dunning R3327 prostate adenocarcinoma in rats. *Prostate* 36:151–161.

Larsson SC, Giovannucci E, Bergkvist L, Wolk A (2005a) Whole grain consumption and risk of colorectal cancer: A population-based cohort of 60,000 women. *Br J Cancer* 92:1803–1807.

Larsson SC, Orsini N, Wolk A (2005b) Diabetes mellitus and risk of colorectal cancer: A meta-analysis. *J Natl Cancer Inst* 97:1679–1687.

Leufkens AM, van Duijnhoven FJ, Woudt SH, Siersema PD, Jenab M, Jansen EH, Pischon T, Tjonneland A, Olsen A, Overvad K, Boutron-Ruault MC, Clavel-Chapelon F, Morois S, Palli D, Pala V, Tumino R, Vineis P, Panico S, Kaaks R, Lukanova A, Boeing H, Aleksandrova K, Trichopoulou A, Trichopoulos D, Dilis V, Peeters PH, Skeie G, Gonzalez CA, Arguelles M, Sanchez MJ, Dorronsoro M, Huerta JM, Ardanaz E, Hallmans G, Palmqvist R, Khaw KT, Wareham N, Allen NE, Crowe FL, Fedirko V, Norat T, Riboli E, Bueno-de-Mesquita HB (2012) Biomarkers of oxidative stress and risk of developing colorectal cancer: A cohort-nested case-control study in the European Prospective Investigation into Cancer and Nutrition. *Am J Epidemiol* 175:653–663.

Linko AM, Adlercreutz H (2005) Whole-grain rye and wheat alkylresorcinols are incorporated into human erythrocyte membranes. *Br J Nutr* 93:11–13.

Lippman SM, Klein EA, Goodman PJ, Lucia MS, Thompson IM, Ford LG, Parnes HL, Minasian LM, Gaziano JM, Hartline JA, Parsons JK, Bearden JD, III, Crawford ED, Goodman GE, Claudio J, Winquist E, Cook ED, Karp DD, Walther P, Lieber MM, Kristal AR, Darke AK, Arnold KB, Ganz PA, Santella RM, Albanes D, Taylor PR, Probstfield JL, Jagpal TJ, Crowley JJ, Meyskens FL, Jr., Baker LH, Coltman CA, Jr. (2009) Effect of selenium and vitamin E on risk of prostate cancer and other cancers: The Selenium and Vitamin E Cancer Prevention Trial (SELECT). *JAMA* 301:39–51.

Liu Y, Chang CC, Marsh GM, Wu F (2012) Population attributable risk of aflatoxin-related liver cancer: Systematic review and meta-analysis. *Eur J Cancer* 48:2125–2136.

Ma Y, Yang Y, Wang F, Zhang P, Shi C, Zou Y, Qin H (2013) Obesity and risk of colorectal cancer: A systematic review of prospective studies. *PLoS One* 8:e53916.

McCann SE, Thompson LU, Nie J, Dorn J, Trevisan M, Shields PG, Ambrosone CB, Edge SB, Li HF, Kasprzak C, Freudenheim JL (2010) Dietary lignan intakes in relation to survival among women with breast cancer: The Western New York; Exposures and Breast Cancer (WEB) Study. *Breast Cancer Res Treat* 122:229–235.

McCarl M, Harnack L, Limburg PJ, Anderson KE, Folsom AR (2006) Incidence of colorectal cancer in relation to glycemic index and load in a cohort of women. *Cancer Epidemiol Biomarkers Prev* 15:892–896.

McCullough ML, Robertson AS, Chao A, Jacobs EJ, Stampfer MJ, Jacobs DR, Diver WR, Calle EE, Thun MJ (2003) A prospective study of whole grains, fruits, vegetables and colon cancer risk. *Cancer Causes Control* 14:959–970.

McKeown NM, Meigs JB, Liu S, Wilson PW, Jacques PF (2002) Whole-grain intake is favorably associated with metabolic risk factors for type 2 diabetes and cardiovascular disease in the Framingham Offspring Study. *Am J Clin Nutr* 76:390–398.

Montonen J, Boeing H, Fritsche A, Schleicher E, Joost HG, Schulze MB, Steffen A, Pischon T (2012) Consumption of red meat and whole-grain bread in relation to biomarkers of obesity, inflammation, glucose metabolism and oxidative stress. *Eur J Nutr* 52(1):337–45.

Nicodemus KK, Jacobs DR, Jr., Folsom AR (2001) Whole and refined grain intake and risk of incident postmenopausal breast cancer (United States). *Cancer Causes Control* 12:917–925.

Nimptsch K, Kenfield S, Jensen MK, Stampfer MJ, Franz M, Sampson L, Brand-Miller JC, Willett WC, Giovannucci E (2011) Dietary glycemic index, glycemic load, insulin index, fiber and whole-grain intake in relation to risk of prostate cancer. *Cancer Causes Control* 22:51–61.

Olsen A, Christensen J, Knudsen KE, Johnsen NF, Overvad K, Tjonneland A (2011) Prediagnostic plasma enterolactone levels and mortality among women with breast cancer. *Breast Cancer Res Treat* 128:883–889.

Papas MA, Giovannucci E, Platz EA (2004) Fiber from fruit and colorectal neoplasia. *Cancer Epidemiol Biomarkers Prev* 13:1267–1270.

Parkin DM (2011) 1. The fraction of cancer attributable to lifestyle and environmental factors in the UK in 2010. *Br J Cancer* 105 Suppl 2:S2–S5.

Pietinen P, Malila N, Virtanen M, Hartman TJ, Tangrea JA, Albanes D, Virtamo J (1999) Diet and risk of colorectal cancer in a cohort of Finnish men. *Cancer Causes Control* 10:387–396.

Prasad K (2000) Antioxidant activity of secoisolariciresinol diglucoside-derived metabolites, secoisolariciresinol, enterodiol, and enterolactone. *Int J Angiol* 9:220–225.

Rejman J, Kozubek A (1997) Long-chain orcinol homologues from cereal bran are effective inhibitors of glycerophosphate dehydrogenase. *Cellular & Molecular Biology Letters* 2:411–419.

Rejman J, Kozubek A (2004) Inhibitory effect of natural phenolic lipids upon NAD-dependent dehydrogenases and on triglyceride accumulation in 3T3-L1 cells in culture. *J Agric Food Chem* 52:246–250.

Roberfroid M, Gibson GR, Hoyles L, McCartney AL, Rastall R, Rowland I, Wolvers D, Watzl B, Szajewska H, Stahl B, Guarner F, Respondek F, Whelan K, Coxam V, Davicco MJ, Leotoing L, Wittrant Y, Delzenne NM, Cani PD, Neyrinck AM, Meheust A (2010) Prebiotic effects: Metabolic and health benefits. *Br J Nutr* 104:S1–S63.

Roediger WE (1980) Role of anaerobic bacteria in the metabolic welfare of the colonic mucosa in man. *Gut* 21:793–798.

Ross AB (2012) Present status and perspectives on the use of alkylresorcinols as biomarkers of wholegrain wheat and rye intake. *J Nutr Metab* 2012:462967.

Ross AB, Kamal-Eldin A, Aman P (2004) Dietary alkylresorcinols: absorption, bioactivities, and possible use as biomarkers of whole-grain wheat- and rye-rich foods. *Nutr Rev* 62:81–95.

Ross AB, Kamal-Eldin A, Lundin EA, Zhang JX, Hallmans G, Aman P (2003) Cereal alkylresorcinols are absorbed by humans. *J Nutr* 133:2222–2224.

Sandle GI (1998) Salt and water absorption in the human colon: A modern appraisal. *Gut* 43:294–299.

Schatzkin A, Mouw T, Park Y, Subar AF, Kipnis V, Hollenbeck A, Leitzmann MF, Thompson FE (2007) Dietary fiber and whole-grain consumption in relation to colorectal cancer in the NIH-AARP Diet and Health Study. *Am J Clin Nutr* 85:1353–1360.

Seibold P, Vrieling A, Johnson TS, Buck K, Behrens S, Kaaks R, Linseisen J, Obi N, Heinz J, Flesch-Janys D, Chang-Claude J (2014) Enterolactone concentrations and prognosis after postmenopausal breast cancer: Assessment of effect modification and meta-analysis. *Int J Cancer* 135:923–933.

Skeie G, Braaten T, Olsen A, Kyro C, Tjonneland A, Nilsson LM, Landberg R, Lund E (2014) Whole grain intake and survival among Scandinavian colorectal cancer patients. *Nutr Cancer* 66:6–13.

Slavin J (2003) Why whole grains are protective: Biological mechanisms. *Proc Nutr Soc* 62:129–134.

Slavin J (2004) Whole grains and human health. *Nutr Res Rev* 17:99–110.

Slavin JL (2000) Mechanisms for the impact of whole grain foods on cancer risk. *J Am Coll Nutr* 19:300S–307S.

Sonestedt E, Borgquist S, Ericson U, Gullberg B, Landberg G, Olsson H, Wirfalt E (2008) Plant foods and oestrogen receptor alpha- and beta-defined breast cancer: Observations from the Malmo Diet and Cancer cohort. *Carcinogenesis* 29:2203–2209.

Song M, Wu K, Meyerhardt J, Ogino S, Wang M, Fuchs C, Giovannucci E, Chan A (2018) Fiber intake and survival after colorectal cancer diagnosis. *JAMA Oncology* 4:71–79 .

Sung MK, Lautens M, Thompson LU (1998) Mammalian lignans inhibit the growth of estrogen-independent human colon tumor cells. *Anticancer Res* 18:1405–1408.

Tetens I, Turrini A, Tapanainen H, Christensen T, Lampe JW, Fagt S, Hakansson N, Lundquist A, Hallund J, Valsta LM (2013) Dietary intake and main sources of plant lignans in five European countries. *Food Nutr Res* 57: doi: 10.3402/fnr.v57i0.19805

Topping DL, Clifton PM (2001) Short-chain fatty acids and human colonic function: Roles of resistant starch and nonstarch polysaccharides. *Physiol Rev* 81:1031–1064.

Torfadottir JE, Valdimarsdottir UA, Mucci L, Stampfer M, Kasperzyk JL, Fall K, Tryggvadottir L, Aspelund T, Olafsson O, Harris TB, Jonsson E, Tulinius H, Adami HO, Gudnason V, Steingrimsdottir L (2012) Rye bread consumption in early life and reduced risk of advanced prostate cancer. *Cancer Causes Control* 23:941–950.

US Food and Drug Administration (1996) Food additives permitted for direct addition to food for human consumption: Folic acid, 21 CFR Part 172, Federal Register., 21 CFR Part 172, Federal Register edn.

Waterhouse J, Muir CS, Correa P, Powell, J, eds. (1976) Cancer Incidence in Five Continents, Vol. *III*. IARC Scientific Publications, No. 15, Lyon, IARC.

Wang L, Chen J, Thompson LU (2005) The inhibitory effect of flaxseed on the growth and metastasis of estrogen receptor negative human breast cancer xenograftsis attributed to both its lignan and oil components. *Int J Cancer* 116:793–798.

Wong JM, de SR, Kendall CW, Emam A, Jenkins DJ (2006) Colonic health: Fermentation and short chain fatty acids. *J Clin Gastroenterol* 40:235–243.

World Cancer Research Fund/American Institute for Cancer Research (2018) Food, Nutrition, Physical Activity, and the Prevention of Cancer: A Global Perspective. AICR, Washington DC, https://www.wcrf.org/dietandcancer/cancers ().

World Cancer Research Fund/American Institute for Cancer Research (2009) Policy and Action for Cancer Prevention. Food, Nutrition, and Physical Activity: A Global Perspective. AICR, Washington DC.

World Cancer Research Fund/American Institute for Cancer Research (2017) Continuous Update Project Interim Report Summary. *Food, Nutrition, Physical Activity, and the Prevention of Colorectal Cancer*, available at: https://www.wcrf.org/sites/default/files/Colorectal-cancer-report.pdf. ().

Wu K, Hu FB, Fuchs C, Rimm EB, Willett WC, Giovannucci E (2004) Dietary patterns and risk of colon cancer and adenoma in a cohort of men (United States). *Cancer Causes Control* 15:853–862.

Xiao Y, Ke Y, Wu S, Huang S, Li S, Lv Z, Yeoh EK, Lao X, Wong S, Kim JH, Colditz GA, Tamimi RM, Su X. (2018) Association between whole grain intake and breast cancer risk: A systematic review and meta-analysis of observational studies. *Nutr J*, 17: 87.

Zhang Z, Xu G, Ma M, Yang J, Liu X (2013) Dietary fiber intake reduces risk for gastric cancer: A meta-analysis. *Gastroenterology* 145:113–120.

Zhu Y, Conklin DR, Chen H, Wang L, Sang S (2011) 5-alk(en)ylresorcinols as the major active components in wheat bran inhibit human colon cancer cell growth. *Bioorg Med Chem* 19:3973–3982.

Zur Hausen H (2000) Papillomaviruses causing cancer: Evasion from host-cell control in early events in carcinogenesis. *J Natl Cancer Inst* 92:690–698.

12 Whole Grain Intake and Mortality

Guri Skeie[1*] and David R. Jacobs Jr.[2]

[1]Department of Community Medicine, University of Tromsø – The Arctic University of Norway, Tromsø, Norway
[2]University of Minnesota, School of Public Health, Division of Epidemiology & Community Health, Minneapolis, Minnesota, USA

12.1 Introduction

Is the benefit of whole grain larger than the sum of its fibre? While several studies have associated higher intake of dietary fibre in general, or cereal fibre in particular, with lower risk of death (e.g., Kim and Je, 2014; Liu et al., 2015; Wu et al., 2015b), less attention has been directed to associations between whole grain intake and disease and death. Still, in recent years, cereal consumption has been the subject of much debate, (e.g., Brouns et al., 2013). At the same time as cereal consumption has been advised against in popular diets, review papers have suggested that whole grains could be key ingredients in healthy ageing (Kiefte-de Jong et al., 2014; Ford et al., 2013). Nine (!) recent reviews and/or meta-analyses all conclude that higher whole grain consumption is associated with lower all cause and cause-specific mortality (Aune et al., 2016; Schwingshackl et al., 2017; Zhang et al., 2017; Benisi-Kohansal et al., 2016; Ma et al., 2016; Li et al., 2016; Wei et al., 2016; Chen et al., 2016; Zong et al., 2016). Currently, 49 out of 127 organizations screened give recommendations for whole grain intake (Seal et al., 2016). Some have tried to quantify how much of the cereal consumption could be in the form of refined grains, and concluded that consuming up to 50% of the cereals as refined grains (without significant added fat, sugar or sodium) did not confer any increased risk of disease or death (Williams, 2012). The author did recognize the beneficial effects of whole grains, and that most consumers would need to decrease their refined grain consumption in order to fulfill whole grain recommendations.

In this chapter, we review the evidence for an association between intake of whole grains and both total and cause-specific mortality. The results stem from a PubMed search combining *whole grain* or *whole grains* and *mortality* or *death* or *survival*. We include prospective studies. Issues pertaining to dietary patterns and human intervention studies are briefly mentioned. We have adopted the definitions of *whole grains* used by the various paper authors. In general, they are based on the AACC International definition, where the bran, germ and endosperm should be present in their natural proportions (AACC International, 1999). Most studies have been done in countries where wheat consumption dominates, but some rye could be included in the whole grain breads. In breakfast cereals, oat is a major whole grain component. For whole grain products, some of the studies have

Whole Grains and Health, Second Edition. Edited by Rikard Landberg and Nathalie Scheers.

Additional materials available for download online at https://www.wiley.com/en-gb/Whole+Grains+and+Health-p-9781118939437

a definition where only cold breakfast cereals, including a minimum of 25% whole grains or bran by weight, were included as whole grain products (Jacobs et al., 1998), while others have no restrictions on whole grain content in the foods. Foods like "dark bread" or "wholemeal bread" might differ in whole grain content, and one of the studies pointed to their validation study, which showed that people tended to overestimate the whole grain content of their bread (Jacobs et al., 2001). We have not included results for bran products. Some authors have calculated the intake of whole grain per se, (e.g., Johnsen et al., 2015), while others have used servings of whole grains (e.g., Huang et al., 2015). In other cases, it is not quite clear whether *whole grains* refers to the amount of the grain or the product (e.g., Buil-Cosiales et al., 2014). It is well known that reporting varies a lot in studies of whole grains and health (Ross et al., 2015), so we choose to include and combine results for both total whole grains, total whole grain products and specific whole grain products, regardless of how it was reported.

The focus of this chapter is total mortality, but we have also included cardiovascular mortality and cancer mortality in the figure. In Table 12.1, we include estimates for main causes of mortality when it was reported, except when there were few cases. Some papers reported rates for specific diseases such as stroke or breast cancer, but these have not been tabulated and discussed in detail.

12.2 Epidemiological evidence

12.2.1 Whole grains and mortality

Table 12.1 summarizes the 18 papers from 15 studies on whole grains and whole grain products and mortality (Wang et al., 2016; Zong et al., 2016; Huang et al., 2015; Johnsen et al., 2015; Wu et al., 2015a; Buil-Cosiales et al., 2014; Rebello et al., 2014; Jacobs et al., 2007; Sahyoun et al., 2006; Liu et al., 2003; Steffen et al., 2003; Appleby et al., 2002; Jacobs et al., 2001; Jacobs et al., 1999; Jacobs et al., 1998; Pietinen et al., 1996; Key et al., 1996; Fraser et al., 1992). Most studies have been performed in adult populations in the United States, but there are also some papers on elderly persons, six European studies, and two from Asia. Two of the studies included mainly vegetarians. A general observation is that persons with the highest consumption of whole grains also score high on other health behaviors that are perceived to be positive. Therefore, in an attempt to present the independent effect of the whole grain itself, the results presented are from the fully adjusted models, even though adjustments vary between studies, both in terms of what was relevant, and which variables were available for adjustment. To increase comparability, when multivariable adjustments including and excluding cereal fibre were available, we chose models without this adjustment.

12.2.2 Total mortality

Ten out of 13 papers reported lower mortality with higher consumption of total whole grains, or total or specific whole grain products (Table 12.1). From the Health Professionals Study, the Iowa Women's Study and the Health Food Shoppers Study, there were several reports, either on different exposures or endpoints or with longer followup. In Figure 12.1, the mortality in the highest category of total whole grains or total or specific whole grain products intake is compared with the lowest intake category. In general, effect estimates

Table 12.1 Papers on intake of whole grains and mortality. Results are for comparison of highest and lowest category unless otherwise stated.

Authors	Setting	Exposure	Outcome	Results	Comments
Wang JB, Sci Rep, 2016 (Wang et al., 2016)	2445 participants in the Linxian Nutrition Intervention Trials cohort, aged 40–69 y, up to 26 y of followup, 1501 total deaths, 355 heart disease, 452 stroke deaths China	All grains, non-whole grains, whole grains (daily vs. less often)	Total deaths, esophageal cancer deaths, gastric cancer deaths, heart disease deaths, stroke deaths	*Whole grains:* Total deaths: 0.98 (0.93–1.05) Heart disease: 0.94 (0.83–1.07) Stroke deaths: 0.93 (0.83–1.04)	Non-whole grains products mainly wheat, rice and millet, whole grain products mainly corn (and sorghum).
Zong G, Circulation, 2016 (Zong et al., 2016)	11 666 adults participating in NHANES III – 2545 deaths, and 9954 adults participating in NHANES 1999–2004 – 972 deaths Adults >20 y USA	Whole grain servings based on a single 24HDR	Total deaths, CVD deaths, cancer deaths	*NHANES III* Total deaths: 0.88 (0.77–1.02) CVD deaths: 0.99 (0.71–1.39) Cancer deaths: 0.84 (0.66–1.07) *NHANES 1999-–2004* Total deaths: 0.83 (0.65–1.07) CVD deaths: 0.74 (0.41–1.32) Cancer deaths: 0.63 (0.37-1.09)	Unpublished results from the NHANES included in this review paper.
Huang T, BMC Medicine, 2015 (Huang et al., 2015)	367 442 participants in the NIH-AARP study, aged 50–71 at baseline Average 14 y of followup, 46,067 deaths USA	Whole grains, ounce equivalents/day (and cereal fibre)	Total deaths, cancer deaths, CVD deaths, diabetes deaths, respiratory disease deaths, infectious disease deaths, other causes of death	Total mortality: 0.83 (0.81–0.86) CVD mortality: 0.83 (0.78–0.88) Cancer mortality: 0.85 (0.81–0.89) Diabetes mortality: 0.52 (0.37–0.75) Respiratory disease mortality: 0.89 (0.80–0.98) Infectious diseases mortality: 0.77 (0.62–0.95) Other/unknown causes of death: 0.86 (0.78–0.94)	Excluded participants with one of several prevalent major causes of death. These results are not adjusted for cereal fibre. That adjustment attenuated the associations, suggesting that cereal fibre is responsible for much of the association seen.

(continued)

Table 12.1 Papers on intake of whole grains and mortality. Results are for comparison of highest and lowest category unless otherwise stated. (*continued*)

Authors	Setting	Exposure	Outcome	Results	Comments
Johnsen N, BJN, 2015 (Johnsen et al., 2015)	120 010 members of the HELGA cohort, aged 30–64 at recruitment, 11–14 y of followup in different subcohorts 3658 women and 4181 men died Norway, Sweden and Denmark	Oat Rye Wheat Other Total whole grain Breakfast cereals, non-white bread Crisp bread Total whole grain products	All-cause mortality Cancer mortality CHD mortality Stroke mortality Respiratory disease mortality Diabetes mortality (omitted here due to few cases) Other causes of mortality	*Total whole grains (F/M)* Total mortality: 0.68 (0.62–0.75)/0.75 (0.68–0.81) Cancer mortality: 0.86 (0.74–0.99)/0.70 (0.60–0.81) CHD mortality: 0.56 (0.40–0.78)/0.85 (0.70–1.04) Stroke mortality: 0.85 (0.53–1.37)/0.86 (0.54–1.37) Respiratory disease mortality: 0.82 (0.49–1.37)/0.60 (0.33–1.07) Other causes of mortality: 0.57 (0.47–0.68)/0.70 (0.61–0.80)	The authors also give results for specific types of grain (oat, rye, wheat, other) and whole grain products (bread, breakfast cereals, crispbread) in the paper In general, intake of non-white bread, breakfast cereals, and whole grain oats, rye and wheat were associated with reduced mortality. The results were found in women and men, and for most specific causes of death.
Wu, JAMA Intern Med, 2015 (Wu et al., 2015a)	74 341 women from the Nurses' Health Study and 43 744 men from the Health Professionals Follow-up Study, 26 920 deaths during 2 727 006 person-years of followup USA	Updated every 2–4 years Whole grains Bran Germ	Total mortality, CVD mortality, cancer mortality	Highest/lowest quintile Total mortality: 0.91 (0.88–0.95) CVD mortality: 0.85 (0.78–0.92) Cancer mortality: 0.97 (0.91–1.04)	Free of cancer and CVD at baseline. Presents pooled estimates here, but sex-specific estimates are available in the paper.
Buil-Cosiales, Am J Clin Nutr, 2014 (Buil-Cosiales et al., 2014)	7216 men and women 55–75 y, high CVD risk, but free of CVD – participants of the PREDIMED study Mean followup 5.9 y 425 deaths Spain	Whole grains (quintiles/ quartiles)	Total deaths CVD deaths Cancer deaths Other causes of death	Highest vs. lowest:Total deaths: 0.92 (0.64-1.33), similar results for cumulative diet information CVD deaths: 0.73 (0.34–1.58) Cancer deaths: 0.75 (0.40–1.41) Other causes of death: 0.76 (0.38–1.53)	Participants were originally part of a dietary intervention study.

Rebello SA, Am J Clin Nutr 2014 (Rebello et al., 2014)	53 469 persons 45–74 y 1 660 deaths Singapore Chinese Health Study Average followup 15 y Singapore	Various carbohydrates and carbohydrate-rich foods, including rice, noodles, bread and whole-wheat bread	Ischemic heart disease mortality	Whole-wheat bread decreased risk for women (HR 0.51, 96% CI 0.30–0.89), but not for men (HR 0.94, 95% CI 0.60–1.04), comparing highest and lowest tertile. Increased risk for noodles, no association for rice. Decreased risk with dietary fibre, both for men and women.	Low intake, sex differences for whole grain, but not for dietary fibre.
Jacobs DR Jr., Am J Clin Nutr 2007 (Jacobs et al., 2007)	27 312 US women aged 55–69 y 5552 deaths Iowa Women's study Followed for 17 y USA	Whole grain food, dark bread, WHG breakfast cereal, other WHG food, refined grain food (quintiles)	All-cause mortality, death due to: CVD, CHD, stroke (subtypes), cancer, non-cardiovascular, non-cancer, inflammatory diseases, non-cardiovascular, non-cancer, non-inflammatory diseases	Inflammation-related death was inversely associated with whole grain intake, HR 0.69 (95% CI: 0.57, 0.83) for 4–7 servings/wk, 0.79 (0.66, 0.95) for 7.5–10.5 servings/wk, 0.64 (0.53, 0.79) for 11–18.5 servings/wk, and 0.66 (0.54, 0.81) for ≥19 servings/wk. Corresponding patterns for dark bread, whole grain breakfast cereal, and other whole grain foods. Inverse associations of whole grain intake with total and CHD mortality persisted. Tendencies to increased risk of non-cardiovascular, non-cancer, inflammatory deaths with higher intake of refined grains (HR highest vs. lowest quintile 1.21, 95%CI 0.96–1.53, p trend 0.04).	Among the non-cardiovascular, non-cancer, inflammatory deaths, respiratory deaths, particularly non-infectious showed the most robust associations.

(*continued*)

Table 12.1 Papers on intake of whole grains and mortality. Results are for comparison of highest and lowest category unless otherwise stated. (*continued*)

Authors	Setting	Exposure	Outcome	Results	Comments
Sahyoun NR, Am J Clin Nutr, 2006 (Sahyoun et al., 2006)	535 healthy community-living persons aged 60–98 y 42% died (89 CVD deaths) Boston 12–15 y followup USA	Whole grain, refined grain (quartiles)	CVD mortality	Significant inverse trend between whole grain intake and mortality from cardiovascular disease RR highest vs. lowest quartile: 0.48 (95%CI 0.25–0.96), *P* for trend =0.04. No association with total mortality. No associations with refined grains	Elderly persons. Diet records. Lower prevalence of metabolic syndrome at baseline in high whole grain consumers.
Liu S, Am J Clin Nutr, 2003 (Liu et al., 2003)	86 190 US male physicians aged 40–84 y 3114 deaths (1381 CVD) 5.5 y of followup USA	Breakfast cereals (total, whole grains and refined grains) Continuous and categorical (not quintile)	Total and CVD-specific mortality	RR total and CVD-specific mortality (95% CI) comparing highest and lowest category: 0.83 (0.73–0.94), p-trend <0.01 and 0.80 (0.66–0.97), p-trend <0.001. No associations for total and refined grain breakfast cereals	Results persisted in analyses stratified by disease history. Stronger results for MI mortality.
Steffen LM, Am J Clin Nutr, 2003 (Steffen et al., 2003)	11 940 persons aged 45–64 at baseline 867 deaths 11-y follow-up period USA	Quintiles of whole grain intake (refined grain)	Total mortality	Whole grain intake was inversely associated with total mortality, HRR upper quintile 0.78 (95%CI 0.61–1.01), p trend 0.02. No clear associations with refined grains in adjusted models	One of the first studies to also include African-Americans. No interactions with race and sex. FFQ applied twice, 6 years apart.
Appleby PM, IARC Sci Publ, 2002 (Appleby et al., 2002)	10 771 participants in the Health Food Shoppers study, aged 16–89 at recruitment 2529 deaths before age 90, >213 000 person-years of followup, UK	Wholemeal bread Daily consumers vs. not	Total deaths, cancer deaths, CVD deaths, respiratory disease death, other causes of death	Total deaths: 0.89 (0.82–0.98) Cancer deaths: 1.01 (0.85–1.20) CVD deaths: 0.86 (0.76–0.98) Respiratory disease deaths: 0.88 (0.67–1.14) Other causes of death: 0.79 (0.63–1.00)	Analyzed mortality up to age 90. Participants free from cancer. Paper also gives estimates for some specific sub-groups of cancer and CVD mortality.

Jacobs DR Jr, Eur J Clin Nutr, 2001 (Jacobs et al., 2001)	16 933 men and 16 915 women aged 35–56 y 1342 (M) and 649 (F) deaths Norway	Whole grain bread score based on density and amount of bread, 6 categories	Total mortality, coronary heart disease mortality, total cardiovascular disease mortality, total cancer mortality, deaths from other causes	HRR for total mortality were inverse and graded across whole grain bread score categories (category 5 vs. category 1 HRR: 0.75, 95% CI 0.63–0.89 in men and 0.66, 0.44–0.98 in women). Tendencies of protective effects for all causes of death, significant trends for CVD and CHD deaths	Baseline was population-based screening. Whole grain consumption circa four times that of in the United States. Clearer trends in men than in women.
Jacobs DR Jr, Am J Public Health, 1999 (Jacobs et al., 1999)	38 740 women aged 55–69 years 3320 deaths Iowa Women's study 9 years of followup USA	Whole grain servings per week Refined grain Quintiles	Total mortality, cancer mortality, CVD mortality and other mortality	HRR (95%CI) highest vs. lowest quintile: Total mortality – 0.86 (0.76-0.97), all CVD 0.82 (0.66–1.01), CHD 0.82 (0.63–1.06), all p-values <0.05. No significant associations for other causes of death in adjusted analyses. Rates of total, but not CVD mortality, were higher among frequent consumers of refined grain.	Similar associations when those with baseline diseases were excluded and not. Similar HRRs in the three upper quintiles. The association of whole grain intake with mortality was independent of intake of refined grains.
Jacobs DR Jr, Am J Clin Nutr, 1998 (Jacobs et al., 1998)	34 492 postmenopausal women aged 55–69 y 438 IHD deaths Iowa women's Study Average 9 years follow-up	Quintiles of total whole grain intake, quartiles of dark bread, whole grain breakfast cereal, other whole grains	IHD death	Adjusted relative hazards were 1.0, 0.96, 0.71, 0.64 and 0.70 in ascending quintiles (P for trend = 0.02). Protective effects seen for dark bread, RR=0.67 in upper quartile, P for trend=0.02. No effects for breakfast cereals and other grains in adjusted models.	Intake of fibre or several other constituents of whole grains did not explain the lower risk with higher whole grain intake. Inconsistent associations with refined grains.

(*continued*)

Table 12.1 Papers on intake of whole grains and mortality. Results are for comparison of highest and lowest category unless otherwise stated. (*continued*)

Authors	Setting	Exposure	Outcome	Results	Comments
Pietinen P, Circulation 1996 (Pietinen et al., 1996)	21 930 smoking men aged 50–69 y 635 deaths Followup of the ATBC-study 6.1 y followup Finland	Rye products (plus various dietary fibre variables and food variables)	Coronary death (and major coronary events - combination of incident disease and fatal disease)	Multivariate RR highest vs. lowest quintile: 0.75 (0.58–0.98). P-trend 0.02.	Stronger associations for death than major events (dietary fibre), no association for major events for rye products.
Key TJ, BMJ 1996 (Key et al., 1996)	10 771 participants in the Health Food Shoppers study 1,343 deaths Followed up for an average of 17 years UK	Wholemeal bread, bran cereals, daily vs. not	Total mortality, IHD mortality, cerebrovascular mortality, cancer mortality	Adjusted for age, sex and smoking: Total mortality MR=0.88 95% 0.78–0.98, ischemic heart disease mortality MR=0.85 95% 0.68–1.06. No association for cerebrovascular and cancer mortality.	When adjusted for fruit intake, the association with total mortality lost significance.
Fraser G, Arch Int Med 1992 (Fraser et al., 1992)	26,473 non-Hispanic white California Seventh Day Adventists 463 deaths Followed up for six years USA	Whole-wheat bread White bread	Definite fatal CHD, coronary deaths	RR=0.89 (95% CI 0.60–1.33) for definite fatal CHD compared to those who usually ate white bread, overall p<0.005 in chi-squared test. Determined by death certificate only: RR=0.74 (95% CI 0.56–0.99), p <0.0001	This population is almost non-smoking, and does not drink much alcohol. Many lacto-ovo-vegetarians.

Abbreviations: CAD=coronary artery disease, CHD=coronary heart disease, CI= 95% confidence interval, CVD=cardiovascular disease, F=female FFQ=food frequency questionnaire, HR= Hazard rate, HRR= Hazard rate ratio, IHD=ischemic heart disease, M=male, RR=relative risk.
The results extracted are those for the multivariable adjusted models.

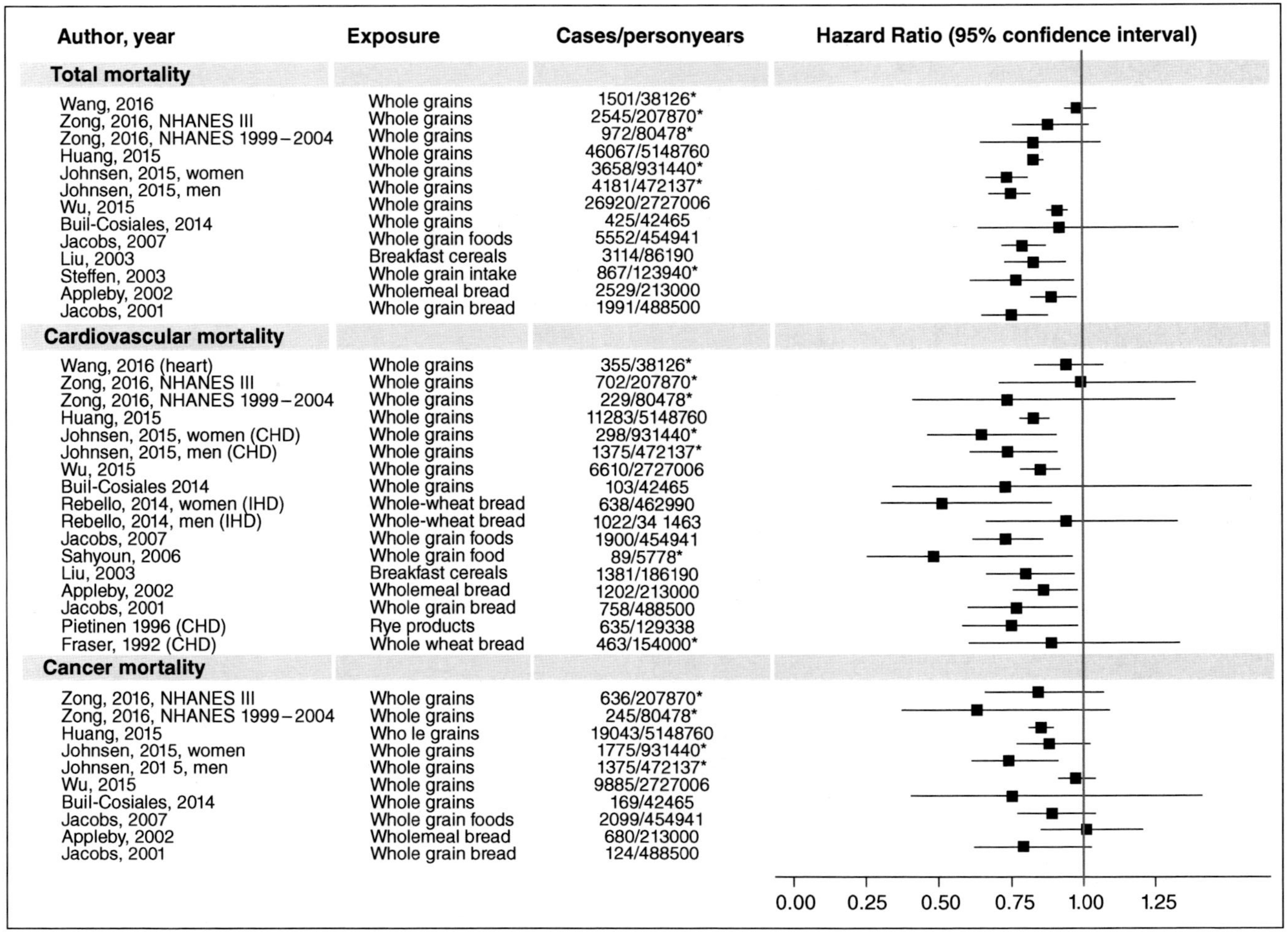

Figure 12.1 Whole grain consumption and total mortality and cardiovascular mortality and cancer. Highest versus lowest category of intake, results from fully adjusted models.* Estimated person-years

between 0.8–0.9 were found, with stronger associations in Scandinavian populations (a mortality rate ratio of 0.68 (0.62–0.75) among women and 0.75 (0.68–0.81) among men in the Helga study, and similar in the Norwegian County study) (Johnsen et al., 2015; Jacobs et al., 2001).

As the studies are heterogeneous, both with respect to which foods or combination of foods or definition of *whole grain*, have been studied, the categorization of the intake groups, and the level of whole grain consumption, no overall estimate has been calculated. Still, a reduction in mortality risk of 13–20% in those who consumed most whole grains seems to be the result across diverse studies. This is supported by other recent reviews (Aune et al., 2016; Ma et al., 2016; Benisi-Kohansal et al., 2016; Zhang et al., 2017; Chen et al., 2016; Wei et al., 2016; Zong et al., 2016), while others report mortality reductions of about 8% per serving (Li et al., 2016; Schwingshackl et al., 2017). In some studies, daily consumers were considered high consumers (Appleby et al., 2002; Wang et al., 2016), while in other studies, several servings a day were necessary in order to be categorized as a high consumer (Johnsen et al., 2015; Jacobs et al., 2001). Aune et al. (2016) reported that even though the benefits seemed largest at lower consumption, benefits of increased whole grain consumption were seen up to as many as 7.5 servings/day.

12.2.3 Cardiovascular mortality

Eleven out of 17 studies reported lower cardiovascular mortality, ischemic heart disease mortality or coronary deaths for high consumers compared to low consumers (Table 12.1). In addition, one study reported lower mortality for women, but not for men (Rebello et al., 2014). The other studies reporting sex-specific estimates did not find different effects (Johnsen et al., 2015; Wu et al., 2015a). Again, there were several papers from some of the studies. The reduction in mortality risk ranged from 1% (non-significant) in NHANES III (Zong et al., 2016) to 52% in an elderly population (Sahyoun et al., 2006). Non-significant results were reported in the first papers from both the vegetarian cohorts (Fraser et al., 1992; Key et al., 1996), but updated papers showed significant associations in both cohorts (the result from the Adventist Health Study is not included due to missing confidence limits) (Fraser, 1999; Appleby et al., 2002). In Chinese women and an elderly US population, the mortality risk was almost halved in the highest consumption category (Rebello et al., 2014; Sahyoun et al., 2006). The other studies showed a risk reduction of around 20%. A clear reduction in fatal coronary heart disease with higher consumption of whole grains has also been reported from the Nurses' Health Study (RR=0.51, 95% CI 0.33–0.80), but no multivariable adjusted results were reported specifically for fatal cases, so this study has not been included in the table and figure (Liu et al., 1999). The results of the studies of cardiovascular mortality or ischemic heart disease mortality display some more variability than for total mortality, but the results are based on fewer cases of death per study (Figure 12.1). The recent reviews have summarized that the mortality reduction is between 12% and 30% (Aune et al., 2016; Chen et al., 2016; Wei et al., 2016; Zong et al., 2016; Benisi-Kohansal et al., 2016; Zhang et al., 2017).

12.2.4 Total cancer mortality

Fewer studies provided estimates for total cancer mortality, and eight out of ten studies had non-significant effects, still, the tendency of a protective association was clear (Table 12.1, Figure 12.1). The two studies that found significant protective associations were both large cohort studies (>100 000 participants) (Johnsen et al., 2015; Huang et al., 2015). Recent reviews have found a mortality risk reduction between 6% and 18% (Aune et al., 2016; Chen et al., 2016; Wei et al., 2016; Zong et al., 2016; Benisi-Kohansal et al., 2016; Zhang et al., 2017). In the latter review, the association was not significant, but the estimate was based on a mixture of studies reporting incidence, or mortality, for one cancer type or for total cancer, and hence likely to be less precise than more stringently performed reviews (Zhang et al., 2017).

12.2.5 Other causes of death

Four papers reported on respiratory disease mortality (Table 12.1). All showed tendencies of protective effects, but only two of them were significant (Appleby et al., 2002; Huang et al., 2015; Jacobs et al., 2007; Johnsen et al., 2015). Aune et al.'s (2016) review summarized the relative mortality risks as 0.78 (0.70– 0.87). Two studies reported on deaths due to infectious diseases, one found reduced mortality and one a more inconsistent association (Johnsen et al., 2015; Jacobs et al., 2007). Two studies presented data for diabetes death, but only the larger one showed consistent protective effects (Huang et al., 2015; Johnsen et al., 2015). Jacobs et al. (2007) found a reduction in deaths due to inflammatory causes by 34%, while there were no effects for the non-cancer, non-cardiovascular, non-inflammatory deaths (many of which are due to injury or other acute causes). Several studies report "other causes of death," unknown causes of death, or, for example, "non-cancer, non-cardiovascular deaths" (e.g., Appleby et al., 2002; Buil-Cosiales et al., 2014; Huang et al., 2015; Jacobs et al., 2001; Jacobs et al., 1999; Johnsen et al., 2015), but what this includes is study-specific. Still, in the largest studies, higher whole grain consumption seems to be associated with lower risk of death also for these causes of death (Huang et al., 2015; Johnsen et al., 2015).

12.2.6 Summary

The prospective cohort studies report a fairly consistent decrease in total mortality, regardless of whether they studied single whole grain products or total whole grains, and at different levels of intake. The observed mortality reduction was around 13–20% for total mortality and cardiovascular mortality, slightly smaller for cancer, and possibly as large as 35% for non-cancer, non-cardiovascular, inflammatory deaths. There are fewer and more inconsistent studies for other causes of death, but also in most of these, high whole grain consumption seems to be associated with lower mortality.

12.3 Types of whole grain products and varieties of grain

The preceding paragraphs, Table 12.1 and Figure 12.1 contain data both on total servings and on grams of whole grains, total whole grain products, and specific whole grain products. Several studies list bread and breakfast cereals as the most consumed whole grain products (Sahyoun et al., 2006; Jacobs et al., 1998; Aune et al., 2016). In other countries, rye bread, oatmeal or brown rice could be the major whole grain sources, and in the paper from China, it was reported that products based on corn were the most frequently consumed whole grain product (Wang et al., 2016). The paper from Finland was based on intake of rye products (Pietinen et al., 1996). There is a lack of studies on whole grains other than wheat, and products besides bread and breakfast cereals (Frolich et al., 2013). The paper based on corn found no associations, but the whole grain intake was low (Wang et al., 2016). Johnsen et al. (2015) reported specific estimates both for whole grain wheat, whole grain rye, whole grain oat and other whole grains, and generally found the same for specific grains as for total grains. A study of a healthy Nordic food index found lower mortality with higher consumption of whole grain rye bread in men, but no difference in women (HR 0.84, 95%CI 0.75–0.94) (Olsen et al., 2011). The Singapore Chinese study estimated that 20% of the ischemic heart disease deaths could have been avoided if a serving of rice was substituted by a serving of whole-wheat bread (Rebello et al., 2014). Aune et al.'s (2016) review concluded that both whole grain bread and whole grain breakfast cereals were associated with reduced risk of all-cause mortality, while this was not the case with refined grains or total grains.

12.4 Dietary patterns with whole grains and mortality

Results from both a priori (hypothesis driven) and a posteriori (data driven) studies of dietary patterns have suggested that whole grains play a role as a part of a healthful dietary pattern (Ford et al., 2013). Among a priori dietary patterns, three groups can be distinguished 1) dietary scores based on national or international dietary guidelines, 2) scores derived from assessment of concordance with nutrients or foods associated with the specific health outcomes and 3) scores based on characteristics of regional diets (Kiefte-de Jong et al., 2014). Whole grains are included as parts of all these types of patterns, if not originally, then in more recent versions (George et al., 2014). As most papers on dietary patterns and mortality focus on the overall pattern, not the specific elements of the patterns that might be more beneficial, we have not tabulated papers on dietary patterns emphasizing whole grains. Given the way in which we conducted our literature search, such tabulation might lead to bias, listing only papers where whole grains have been mentioned, presumably due to a beneficial impact on mortality, and not those with no whole grain mention or no effect. For instance, papers utilizing the Healthy Nordic Food Index found that the whole grain bread component of the index was associated with lower mortality (Olsen et al., 2011; Roswall et al., 2015). A study looking at Mediterranean Diet in elderly Swedes found similar results (Tognon et al., 2011), while a Dutch study on the Mediterranean Diet found no association (van den Brandt, 2011). In a study of African-American women, a high intake of whole grains was the component of the DASH Index most strongly associated with lower mortality (Boggs et al., 2015). Another study of mainly African-Americans and people of low socioeconomic status showed that whole grains were one of the components of the Healthy Eating Index that contributed to lower mortality risks among high adherers (Yu et al., 2015). As previously mentioned, recent reviews of dietary pattern analyses have pointed to whole grains as part of a pattern that predicts longevity (Kiefte-de Jong et al., 2014; Ford et al., 2013). Furthermore, we note that the greater reduction in mortality in less adjusted models than in the full adjusted model presented here correspond, in a sense, to effects of a healthy diet pattern (including whole grain foods) and lifestyle because they include part of the independent effects of these other dietary and behavioral variables.

Many indices are concerned with specific foods or food groups that are considered beneficial or harmful, and give points for, for example, above-median consumption. Some indices, such as the Recommended Food Score, are concerned only with the recommended foods, and regular consumption of any of those contributes to the score, giving also food variety a part in the index (Kant et al., 2004). A study looking at both the Recommended Food Score and Non-Recommended Food Score showed that the recommended foods strongly predicted death, whereas the Non-Recommended food score did not, with the exception of cancer mortality (Michels and Wolk, 2002). The authors suggested that it might be more important to increase the variety of healthy foods rather than decrease the number of unhealthy foods. Coupled with the preceding reviews, whole grain foods would appear to have a place in patterns such as these.

12.5 Human intervention studies

No human intervention study has compared whole grains or a diet high in whole grains with a control diet in order to assess effects on total mortality in healthy adults (Kelly et al., 2017). The Diet and Reinfarction Trial (DART) was an intervention among British men with a history of recent myocardial infarction. The intervention participants were given advice to increase their consumption of fish, particularly fatty fish, or dietary fibre (comparable to six slices of wholemeal bread per day), or to reduce the total fat intake and increase the ratio of polyunsaturated fat to saturated fat, or a combination of these advices (Burr et al., 1989). The intervention managed to change the relevant dietary factors, and after two years, the death rates were lower in the fish group, whereas there was a non-significant increased risk of death in the dietary fibre group. In the long term, there was no clear effect of the fat or fibre advice on coronary or all-cause mortality, and the early reduction of mortality in the fish group was followed by an increase in all-cause mortality in the next three years (Ness et al., 2002). Hence, the authors concluded that the intervention had had no substantial long-term survival benefits. We note that the group that was randomized to follow all three of the fish, fat, and fibre recommendations had reduced outcomes, although fibre in other combinations of the randomized study arms did not do better (Burr et al., 1989). The PREDIMED study was an intervention on Mediterranean Diet among Spanish adults with increased risk for cardiovascular diseases. Their dietary advice included increased cereal consumption, but the paper on fibre and whole grain consumption is a follow-up of the cohort, and does not report results according to intervention groups (Buil-Cosiales et al., 2014). However, results from baseline analyses and from analyses using the average of the yearly food frequency questionnaires, which to some extent should reflect the dietary changes obtained in the intervention, did not differ.

12.6 Cell and animal studies

Other chapters in this book have reviewed the mechanistic evidence for an association between whole grain consumption and various chronic diseases. It is likely that reduced morbidity is the greatest component of the reduced mortality reviewed here, and that the same mechanisms are relevant for the association between whole grain consumption and mortality as for whole grain consumption and morbidity. We therefore refer to the relevant chapters for more details on cell and animal studies. Regarding non-cancer, non-cardiovascular inflammatory deaths, some of the same mechanisms as for cardiovascular death might be relevant (Jacobs et al., 2007). Antioxidants, dietary fibre and many phytochemicals in the whole grain contribute to its anti-inflammatory properties (Okarter and Liu, 2010).

12.7 Conclusion

The studies reviewed suggested a beneficial effect of whole grain intake on mortality, particularly cardiovascular mortality and non-cancer, non-cardiovascular inflammatory mortality. The reduction seems to be around 13–20% for total and cardiovascular mortality, and possibly up to 35% for non-cancer, non-cardiovascular, inflammatory deaths. For cancer mortality, the reduction seems to be in the 6–15% range, while also for the heterogeneous "other causes of death" some protection seems evident. This compares well with recent reviews and meta-analyses (Aune et al., 2016; Chen et al., 2016; Wei et al., 2016; Zong et al., 2016; Schwingshackl et al., 2017; Zhang et al., 2017; Benisi-Kohansal et al., 2016; Ma et al., 2016; Li et al., 2016). In a study by Jacobs et al. (2000), women who consumed their cereal fibre predominantly from whole grain foods rather than from refined-grain foods had a 17% lower risk of death. Huang et al. (2015) adjusted the whole grain intake for cereal fibre, and this attenuated the effect estimates, so that for several, but not all, causes of death the associations were no longer significant. In a paper from the Nurses' Health Study, the authors presented several multivariable adjusted models for the association between whole grains and coronary heart disease (fatal and non-fatal combined), and for smokers, the trend test lost significance when dietary fibre, folate, vitamin B-6 and vitamin E were included in the model (RR=0.79, 95% CI 0.62–1.01, p=0.07). However, in non-smokers, the estimates and p-values were still significant in the fully adjusted model (RR=0.47, 95% CI 0.27–0.79, p=0.006) (Liu et al., 1999). In another interesting paper from the same cohort, the authors looked at a combination of risk factors and their associations with several causes of death in a competing risk model, allowing for different associations between a risk factor and specific causes of death (Baer et al., 2011). Although this analysis looked at cereal fibre, not whole grains, it found that the association was uniform, and beneficial across CVD-deaths, smoking-related cancer deaths, other cancer deaths and deaths from other causes. The risk of mortality was 16% lower per 4 g extra of cereal fibre. Taken together, these results suggest that whole grains help delay death, and that the effect is not solely due to dietary fibre.

Whole grains contain a range of phytochemicals, many of which are not yet well characterized. Okarter and Liu (2010) reviewed beneficial health effects of several whole grain phytochemicals: phenolics (phenolic acids, alkyl(en)resorcinols, flavonoids), carotenoids, vitamin E, γ-oryzanol, and dietary fibre. The content of beneficial substances differs between grains with growing conditions, and varies between varieties of specific grains. As most whole grain products are reconstituted, milling and processing also affect the content of beneficial substances (Okarter and Liu, 2010). New genomic techniques have provided new tools both for characterizing grains and their varieties (Brouns et al., 2013; Scalbert et al., 2014), and for understanding how foods such as whole grains act in physiological pathways or influence our metabolic or genetic profile (Suhre et al., 2011; Stempler et al., 2014). This will give a more detailed characterization of grains and their varieties, and a holistic picture of how whole grain consumption affects us. However, it might also lead to a chase for the best variety, or the single substance in the grain that confers *the* benefit (Topping, 2007). People eat foods, not "bioactive non-nutrient plant compounds," and foods are not only a sum of compounds, but also the synergy of the components (Jacobs and Orlich, 2014). Several studies have shown that isolating one component and giving it separately, particularly in pharmaceutical not nutritional doses, has adverse effects (e.g., Tanvetyanon and Bepler, 2008).

Dietary advice with regards to whole grains is not uncommon, but although 49 out of 127 organizations screened gave advice on whole grains, the format of the advice varied (Seal et al., 2016). Some gave advice on whole grains directly, others more indirectly, in order to fulfill dietary fibre recommendations. Some gave quantitative advice (e.g., servings per day), other "semi-quantitative" advice – choose whole grains over refined grains and some more general qualitative advice like choose whole grains whenever possible. As whole grains appear in most indices of higher diet quality, they tend to replace less healthy foods, and to the extent specific advice is given, it is often to replace refined grains with whole grains. As more sustainable diets are recommended, a substitution also for animal foods could be envisioned. Too much grain could theoretically reduce diet diversity, but the recent review from Aune et al. (2016) stated benefits up to at least 7.5 servings per day, suggesting that for the vast majority additional increases in whole grain consumption would confer beneficial effects. A paper from the United States attempted to quantify the association between dietary factors and mortality from heart disease, stroke and type 2 diabetes, combining published estimates on, for example, whole grain intake with national disease specific mortality data and estimates of the strength of the association (Micha et al., 2017). The researchers estimated that 5.9% of the cardiometabolic deaths in the United States could be attributed to suboptimal whole grain intakes.

In this chapter, we have concentrated on papers in which whole grain consumption was assessed in healthy persons. There are some papers on, for example, diabetics (whole grains) (He et al., 2010), persons with myocardial infarction (dietary fibre, specifically cereal fibre) (Li et al., 2014), women with heart failure (whole grain as part of Mediterranean Diet and DASH Score) (Levitan et al., 2013), and colorectal cancer (Vrieling and Kampman, 2010; van Meer et al., 2013) and their survival. The reviews on colorectal cancer noted a paucity of data on diet and survival, particularly using post-diagnosis diet, and few solid conclusions could be drawn. For myocardial infarction, heart failure and diabetes, the results suggested a benefit for whole grain consumers, also in secondary prevention, but these are single studies. They also point to the lack of evidence for dietary guidelines for survivors (Li et al., 2014).

Grains, and in particular refined wheat, have been the focus of debate lately, partly due to their high glycemic index (Brouns et al., 2013; Brand-Miller et al., 2008). However, different carbohydrates have different glycemic indices, and generally, whole grains have lower glycemic index than refined grains. For rice, the glycemic index varies a lot, due to botanical differences, particularly differences in amylose (Foster-Powell et al., 2002). For wheat and maize, but not for oats, the glycemic index is highly dependent on particle size, so whole grains, even flour, would have a lower glycemic index than the corresponding food in refined format (Heaton et al., 1988). Low-carbohydrate diets have gained a lot of popularity, but their health effects have not been thoroughly studied. A simple cross-classification of high/low whole grain and high/low glycemic index would be illustrative. If such a grouping also was related to, for example, prospective weight loss or mortality, further insight would have been gained. McMillan Price et al. (2006) compared four diets with varying glycemic load on weight loss and cardiovascular risk factors. The results were similar regarding weight loss for a high-carbohydrate low-glycemic index diet (intermediate glycemic load) and a high-protein diet with similar glycemic load, but the latter had adverse effects on the cardiovascular risk factors. More research is needed in this field, but it is important to bear in mind that not all carbohydrates are equal. If current trends towards sustainable diets should be fulfilled, high-protein diets are hardly the way to go (NNR, 2014).

We can never rule out biases, residual confounding and reverse causation as explanations for the results. However, lately, larger cohort studies have published their results where a wide range of confounding factors have been adjusted for. Selection bias is less of a problem in cohort studies, and national identifiers in combination with registries, or detailed systems for staying in touch with participants avoid loss to followup. Most large studies also routinely exclude early cases in order to avoid reverse causality. In addition, many of the studies did not include people with certain diagnoses at baseline in case diagnoses have led to dietary change. For the causes of death we have reviewed in this paper, others have studied the possibilities for small study bias and publication bias, and found no strong indications (Aune et al., 2016).

As this review has shown, most of the research has been performed in wheat-eating populations in the United States. Future research should include studies from other populations with preferences for other grains such as rye. Few studies have been able to estimate associations between specific causes of death other than cancer and cardiovascular disease. Confirmation of such an association in other populations is needed. Furthermore, more studies of persons with higher levels of intake might inform us of any threshold after which increased consumption does not confer any extra benefit. In observational studies, one cannot totally rule out residual confounding, so an intervention study on whole grain foods and total mortality would be needed to demonstrate causality. Although death clearly cannot be prevented, this chapter suggests it may be postponed.

12.8 References

AACC International. (1999) Definition of whole grain [Online]. American Association of Cereal Chemists. Available: http://www.aaccnet.org/initiatives/definitions/Pages/WholeGrain.aspx [Accessed 29.10.2013.

Appleby, P. N., Key, T. J., Burr, M. L. & Thorogood, M. (2002) Mortality and fresh fruit consumption. *IARC Sci Publ* 156, 131–3.

Aune, D., Keum, N., Giovannucci, E. et al. (2016) Whole grain consumption and risk of cardiovascular disease, cancer, and all cause and cause specific mortality: Systematic review and dose-response meta-analysis of prospective studies. *BMJ* 353, i2716.

Baer, H. J., Glynn, R. J., Hu, F. B. et al. (2011) Risk factors for mortality in the Nurses' Health Study: A competing risks analysis. *American Journal of Epidemiology* 173, 319–29.

Benisi-Kohansal, S., Saneei, P., Salehi-Marzijarani, M., Larijani, B. & Esmaillzadeh, A. (2016) Whole-Grain Intake and Mortality from All Causes, Cardiovascular Disease, and Cancer: A systematic review and dose-response meta-analysis of prospective cohort tudies. *Adv Nutr* 7, 1052-65.

Boggs, D. A., Ban, Y., Palmer, J. R. & Rosenberg, L. (2015) Higher diet quality is inversely associated with mortality in African-American women. *The Journal of Nutrition* 145, 547–54.

Brand-Miller, J., Mcmillan-Price, J., Steinbeck, K. & Caterson, I. (2008) Carbohydrates – The good, the bad and the whole grain. *Asia Pacific journal of clinical nutrition* 17 Suppl 1, 16–9.

Brouns, F. J. P. H., Van Buul, V. J. & Shewry, P. R. (2013) Does wheat make us fat and sick? *Journal of Cereal Science* 58, 209–15.

Buil-Cosiales, P., Zazpe, I., Toledo, E. et al. (2014) Fiber intake and all-cause mortality in the Prevencion con Dieta Mediterranea (PREDIMED) study. *American Journal of Clinical Nutrition* 100, 1498–507.

Burr, M. L., Fehily, A. M., Gilbert, J. F. et al. (1989) Effects of changes in fat, fish, and fibre intakes on death and myocardial reinfarction: Diet and reinfarction trial (DART). *Lancet* 2, 757–61.

Chen, G. C., Tong, X., Xu, J. Y. et al. (2016) Whole-grain intake and total, cardiovascular, and cancer mortality: A systematic review and meta-analysis of prospective studies. *American Journal of Clinical Nutrition* 104, 164–72.

Ford, D. W., Jensen, G. L., Hartman, T. J., Wray, L. & Smiciklas-Wright, H. (2013) Association between dietary quality and mortality in older adults: A review of the epidemiological evidence. *Journal of Nutrition in Gerontology and Geriatrics* 32, 85–105.

Foster-Powell, K., Holt, S. H. & Brand-Miller, J. C. (2002) International table of glycemic index and glycemic load values: 2002. *The American Journal of Clinical Nutrition* 76, 5–56.

Fraser, G. E. (1999) Associations between diet and cancer, ischemic heart disease, and all-cause mortality in non-Hispanic white California Seventh-day Adventists. *American Journal of Clinical Nutrition* 70, 532S–38S.

Fraser, G. E., Sabate, J., Beeson, W. L. & Strahan, T. M. (1992) A possible protective effect of nut consumption on risk of coronary heart disease. *The Adventist Health Study. Archives of Internal Medicine* 152, 1416–24.

Frolich, W., Aman, P. & Tetens, I. (2013) Whole grain foods and health – a Scandinavian perspective. *Food & Nutrition Research* 57, 1–10.

George, S. M., Ballard-Barbash, R., Manson, J. E. et al. (2014) Comparing indices of diet quality with chronic disease mortality risk in postmenopausal women in the Women's Health Initiative Observational Study: Evidence to inform national dietary guidance. *American Journal of Epidemiology* 180, 616–25.

He, M., Van Dam, R. M., Rimm, E., Hu, F. B. & Qi, L. (2010) Whole-grain, cereal fiber, bran, and germ intake and the risks of all-cause and cardiovascular disease-specific mortality among women with type 2 diabetes mellitus. *Circulation* 121, 2162–8.

Heaton, K. W., Marcus, S. N., Emmett, P. M. & Bolton, C. H. (1988) Particle size of wheat, maize, and oat test meals: Effects on plasma glucose and insulin responses and on the rate of starch digestion in vitro. *The American Journal of Clinical Nutrition* 47, 675–82.

Huang, T., Xu, M., Lee, A., Cho, S. & Qi, L. (2015) Consumption of whole grains and cereal fiber and total and cause-specific mortality: prospective analysis of 367,442 individuals. *BMC Med* 13, 59.

Jacobs, D. R., Jr., Andersen, L. F. & Blomhoff, R. (2007) Whole-grain consumption is associated with a reduced risk of noncardiovascular, noncancer death attributed to inflammatory diseases in the Iowa Women's Health Study. *American Journal of Clinical Nutrition* 85, 1606–14.

Jacobs, D. R., Jr., Meyer, H. E. & Solvoll, K. (2001) Reduced mortality among whole grain bread eaters in men and women in the Norwegian County Study. *European Journal of Clinical Nutrition* 55, 137–43.

Jacobs, D. R., Jr., Meyer, K. A., Kushi, L. H. & Folsom, A. R. (1998) Whole-grain intake may reduce the risk of ischemic heart disease death in postmenopausal women: the Iowa Women's Health Study. *American Journal of Clinical Nutrition* 68, 248–57.

Jacobs, D. R., Jr., Meyer, K. A., Kushi, L. H. & Folsom, A. R. (1999) Is whole grain intake associated with reduced total and cause-specific death rates in older women? The Iowa Women's Health Study. *American Journal of Public Health* 89, 322–9.

Jacobs, D. R., Jr. & Orlich, M. J. (2014) Diet pattern and longevity: do simple rules suffice? *A commentary. American Journal of Clinical Nutrition* 100 Suppl 1, 313S–9S.

Jacobs, D. R., Pereira, M. A., Meyer, K. A. & Kushi, L. H. (2000) Fiber from whole grains, but not refined grains, is inversely associated with all-cause mortality in older women: The Iowa women's health study. *Journal of the American College of Nutrition* 19, 326S–30S.

Johnsen, N. F., Frederiksen, K., Christensen, J. et al. (2015) Whole-grain products and whole-grain types are associated with lower all-cause and cause-specific mortality in the Scandinavian HELGA cohort. *The British journal of nutrition* 114, 608–23.

Kant, A. K., Graubard, B. I. & Schatzkin, A. (2004) Dietary patterns predict mortality in a national cohort: The National Health Interview Surveys, 1987 and 1992. *The Journal of Nutrition* 134, 1793–9.

Kelly, S. A. M., Hartley, L., Loveman, E. et al. (2017) Whole grain cereals for the primary or secondary prevention of cardiovascular disease. *Cochrane Database of Systematic Reviews.* 8, 1–100

Key, T. J., Thorogood, M., Appleby, P. N. & Burr, M. L. (1996) Dietary habits and mortality in 11,000 vegetarians and health conscious people: results of a 17 year follow up. *BMJ* 313, 775–9.

Kiefte-De Jong, J. C., Mathers, J. C. & Franco, O. H. (2014) Nutrition and healthy ageing: The key ingredients. *Proceedings of the Nutrition Society* 73, 249–59.

Kim, Y. & Je, Y. (2014) Dietary fiber intake and total mortality: A meta-analysis of prospective cohort studies. *American Journal of Epidemiology* 180, 565–73.

Levitan, E. B., Lewis, C. E., Tinker, L. F. et al. (2013) Mediterranean and DASH Diet scores and mortality in women with heart failure: The Women's Health Initiative. *Circulation: Heart Failure* 6, 1116–23.

Li, B., Zhang, G., Tan, M. et al. (2016) Consumption of whole grains in relation to mortality from all causes, cardiovascular disease, and diabetes: Dose–response meta-analysis of prospective cohort studies. *Medicine* 95, e4229.

Li, S., Flint, A., Pai, J. K. et al. (2014) Dietary fiber intake and mortality among survivors of myocardial infarction: Prospective cohort study. *BMJ* 348, g2659.

Liu, L., Wang, S. & Liu, J. (2015) Fiber consumption and all-cause, cardiovascular, and cancer mortalities: A systematic review and meta-analysis of cohort studies. *Mol Nutr Food Res* 59, 139–46.

Liu, S., Sesso, H. D., Manson, J. E., Willett, W. C. & Buring, J. E. (2003) Is intake of breakfast cereals related to total and cause-specific mortality in men? *American Journal of Clinical Nutrition* 77, 594–9.

Liu, S., Stampfer, M. J., Hu, F. B. et al. (1999) Whole-grain consumption and risk of coronary heart disease: Results from the Nurses' Health Study. *American Journal of Clinical Nutrition* 70, 412–9.

Ma, X., Tang, W.-G., Yang, Y., Zhang, Q.-L., Zheng, J.-L. & Xiang, Y.-B. (2016) Association between whole grain intake and all-cause mortality: A meta-analysis of cohort studies. *Oncotarget* 7, 61996–62005.

McMillan-Price, J., Petocz, P., Atkinson, F., O'Neill, K., Samman, S., Steinbeck, K., Caterson, I., Brand-Miller, J. (2006) Comparison of 4 diets of varying glycemic load on weight loss and cardiovascular risk reduction in overweight and obese young adults: a randomized controlled trial. Arch Intern Med. July 24,166(14), 1466–75. doi: 10.1001/archinte.166.14.1466. PMID: 16864756.

Micha, R., Penalvo, J. L., Cudhea, F., Imamura, F., Rehm, C. D. & Mozaffarian, D. (2017) Association between dietary factors and mortality from heart disease, stroke, and type 2 diabetes in the United States. *JAMA:The journal of the American Medical Association* 317, 912–24.

Michels, K. B. & Wolk, A. (2002) A prospective study of variety of healthy foods and mortality in women. *International Journal of Epidemiology* 31, 847–54.

Ness, A. R., Hughes, J., Elwood, P. C., Whitley, E., Smith, G. D. & Burr, M. L. (2002) The long-term effect of dietary advice in men with coronary disease: Follow-up of the Diet and Reinfarction trial (DART). *European Journal of Clinical Nutrition* 56, 512–8.

NNR 2014. Sustainable food consumption – Environmental issues. In: NORDIC COUNCIL OF MINISTRIES (ed.) *Nordic Nutrition Recommendations 2012: Integrating nutrition and physical activity*. 5 ed. Copenhagen: Nordic Council of Ministers.

Okarter, N. & Liu, R. H. (2010) Health benefits of whole grain phytochemicals. *Crit Rev Food Sci Nutr* 50, 193–208.

Olsen, A., Egeberg, R., Halkjaer, J., Christensen, J., Overvad, K. & Tjonneland, A. (2011) Healthy aspects of the Nordic diet are related to lower total mortality. *The Journal of Nutrition* 141, 639–44.

Pietinen, P., Rimm, E. B., Korhonen, P. et al. (1996) Intake of dietary fiber and risk of coronary heart disease in a cohort of Finnish men: The Alpha-Tocopherol, Beta-Carotene Cancer Prevention Study. *Circulation* 94, 2720–7.

Rebello, S. A., Koh, H., Chen, C. et al. (2014) Amount, type, and sources of carbohydrates in relation to ischemic heart disease mortality in a Chinese population: A prospective cohort study. *American Journal of Clinical Nutrition* 100, 53–64.

Ross, A. B., Kristensen, M., Seal, C. J., Jacques, P. & Mckeown, N. M. (2015) Recommendations for reporting whole-grain intake in observational and intervention studies. *American Journal of Clinical Nutrition* 101, 903–7.

Roswall, N., Sandin, S., Lof, M. et al. (2015) Adherence to the healthy Nordic food index and total and cause-specific mortality among Swedish women. *European Journal of Epidemiology* 30, 509–17.

Sahyoun, N. R., Jacques, P. F., Zhang, X. L. L., Juan, W. Y. & Mckeown, N. M. (2006) Whole-grain intake is inversely associated with the metabolic syndrome and mortality in older adults. *American Journal of Clinical Nutrition* 83, 124–31.

Scalbert, A., Brennan, L., Manach, C. et al. (2014) The food metabolome: a window over dietary exposure. *American Journal of Clinical Nutrition* 99, 1286–308.

Schwingshackl, L., Schwedhelm, C., Hoffmann, G. et al. (2017) Food groups and risk of all-cause mortality: A systematic review and meta-analysis of prospective studies. *The American Journal of Clinical Nutrition* 105, 1462–73.

Seal, C. J., Nugent, A. P., Tee, E.-S. & Thielecke, F. (2016) Whole-grain dietary recommendations: The need for a unified global approach. *British Journal of Nutrition* 115, 2031–38.

Steffen, L. M., Jacobs, D. R., Jr., Stevens, J., Shahar, E., Carithers, T. & Folsom, A. R. (2003) Associations of whole-grain, refined-grain, and fruit and vegetable consumption with risks of all-cause mortality and incident coronary artery disease and ischemic stroke: The Atherosclerosis Risk in Communities (ARIC) Study. *American Journal of Clinical Nutrition* 78, 383–90.

Stempler, S., Yizhak, K. & Ruppin, E. (2014) Integrating transcriptomics with metabolic modeling predicts biomarkers and drug targets for Alzheimer's disease. *PLoS One* 9, e105383.

Suhre, K., Shin, S. Y., Petersen, A. K. et al. (2011) Human metabolic individuality in biomedical and pharmaceutical research. *Nature* 477, 54–60.

Tanvetyanon, T. & Bepler, G. (2008) Beta-carotene in multivitamins and the possible risk of lung cancer among smokers versus former smokers: A meta-analysis and evaluation of national brands. *Cancer* 113, 150–7.

Tognon, G., Rothenberg, E., Eiben, G., Sundh, V., Winkvist, A. & Lissner, L. (2011) Does the Mediterranean diet predict longevity in the elderly? A Swedish perspective. *Age (Dordr)* 33, 439-50.

Topping, D. (2007) Cereal complex carbohydrates and their contribution to human health. *Journal of Cereal Science* 46, 220–9.

Van Den Brandt, P. A. (2011) The impact of a Mediterranean diet and healthy lifestyle on premature mortality in men and women. *American Journal of Clinical Nutrition* 94, 913–20.

Van Meer, S., Leufkens, A. M., Bueno-De-Mesquita, H. B., Van Duijnhoven, F. J., Van Oijen, M. G. & Siersema, P. D. (2013) Role of dietary factors in survival and mortality in colorectal cancer: A systematic review. *Nutrition Reviews* 71, 631–41.

Vrieling, A. & Kampman, E. (2010) The role of body mass index, physical activity, and diet in colorectal cancer recurrence and survival: A review of the literature. *American Journal of Clinical Nutrition* 92, 471–90.

Wang, J. B., Fan, J. H., Dawsey, S. M. et al. (2016) Dietary components and risk of total, cancer and cardiovascular disease mortality in the Linxian Nutrition Intervention Trials cohort in China. *Sci Rep* 6, 22619.

Wei, H., Gao, Z., Liang, R., Li, Z., Hao, H. & Liu, X. (2016) Whole-grain consumption and the risk of all-cause, CVD and cancer mortality: A meta-analysis of prospective cohort studies. *The British journal of nutrition* 116, 514–25.

Williams, P. G. (2012) Evaluation of the evidence between consumption of refined grains and health outcomes. *Nutrition Reviews* 70, 80–99.

Wu, H., Flint, A. J., Qi, Q. et al. (2015a) Association between dietary whole grain intake and risk of mortality: Two large prospective studies in US men and women. *JAMA Intern Med* 175, 373–84.

Wu, Y., Qian, Y., Pan, Y. et al. (2015b) Association between dietary fiber intake and risk of coronary heart disease: A meta-analysis. *Clinical nutrition* 34, 603–11.

Yu, D., Sonderman, J., Buchowski, M. S. et al. (2015) Healthy eating and risks of total and cause-specific death among low-income populations of African-Americans and other adults in the southeastern United States: A prospective cohort study. *Plos Medicine* 12, e1001830.

Zhang, B., Zhao, Q., Guo, W., Bao, W. & Wang, X. (2017) Association of whole grain intake with all-cause, cardiovascular, and cancer mortality: A systematic review and dose–response meta-analysis from prospective cohort studies. *European Journal of Clinical Nutrition* 72, 57.

Zong, G., Gao, A., Hu, F. B. & Sun, Q. (2016) Whole grain intake and mortality from all causes, cardiovascular disease, and cancer: A meta-analysis of prospective cohort studies. *Circulation* 133, 2370–80.

13 Whole Grains and Appetite

Sabine Ibrügger[1], Kia Nøhr Iversen[2], Mette Kristensen[1], and Rikard Landberg[2]

[1]Department of Nutrition, Exercise and Sports, Faculty of Science, University of Copenhagen, Frederiksberg, Denmark
[2]Division of Food and Nutrition Science, Department of Biology and Biological Engineering, Chalmers University of Technology, Gothenburg, Sweden

13.1 Introduction

Consumption of whole grain has been suggested to decrease the risk of obesity, indicated by a decreased weight or weight gain in prospective studies (Koh-Banerjee et al., 2004; Ye et al., 2012). In contrast, this has not been substantiated in intervention studies as shown by a recent meta-analysis, although a small effect on body fat was found (Pol et al., 2013). This may, however, be related to limitations in the study design such as a short study duration or a relatively low consumption amounts of whole grain (Pol et al., 2013). Moreover, many of the included studies were not designed for weight loss. Potential effects of whole grain consumption on body weight may be the consequence of a reduction in appetite sensation, and thus a lower energy intake (Giacco et al., 2011; Jonnalagadda et al., 2011). The term *appetite*, as used in this chapter, refers to the comprehensive field of food intake, the motivation to eat, and the selection and preferences of foods (Blundell et al., 2010). *Satiation* relates to processes that terminate eating and control meal size (intra-meal satiety) and *satiety* to processes after meal termination that inhibit further eating (inter-meal satiety) (Blundell et al., 2010). Appetite is controlled by short- and long-term physiological processes as well as by psychological cues, illustrated in a conceptual framework, the so called "satiety cascade," by Blundell et al. (1987). In this chapter, we solely focus on physiological processes of appetite control, that is, not the hedonic aspects.

Appetite sensation may be affected during or immediately after whole grain consumption, potentially mediated by mechanisms related to stomach distension or a lower glycemic response. Further, whole grain may also impact appetite sensation after a subsequent/second meal, which may be associated with the fermentation of whole grain components in the colon and a consequent increase in the satiety hormones glucagon-like peptide-1 (GLP-1) and peptide YY (PYY). Moreover, it is conceivable that regular whole grain intake may change overall appetite sensation due to continuously ongoing colonic fermentation, with effects being apparent even if the meal does not contain whole grain (Sandberg et al., 2017).

Whole Grains and Health, Second Edition. Edited by Rikard Landberg and Nathalie Scheers.

Additional materials available for download online at https://www.wiley.com/en-gb/Whole+Grains+and+Health-p-9781118939437

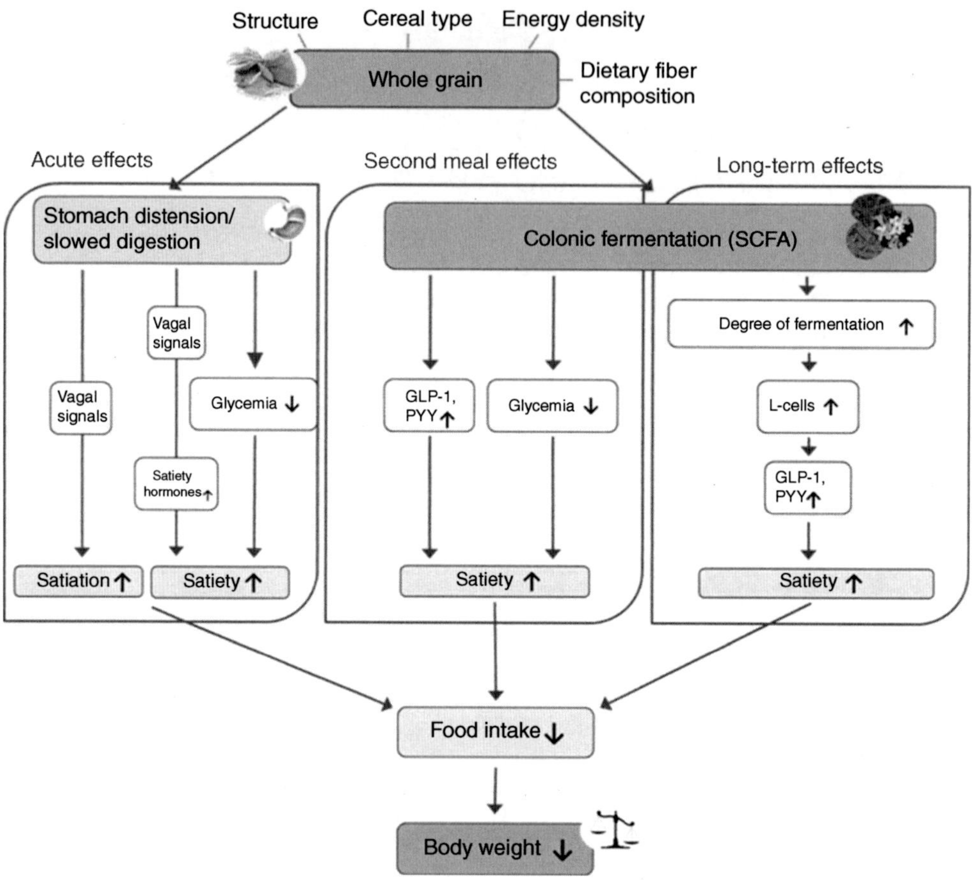

Figure 13.1 Hypothetical mechanistic links between whole grain intake, appetite and long-term body weight.

The hypothetical mechanistic links between whole grain intake, appetite and long-term body weigh are depicted in Figure 13.1.

This chapter describes the current evidence as well as potential underlying mechanisms of acute, second meal and long-term effects of whole grain consumption on appetite sensation.

13.2 Acute effects of whole grain intake on appetite

Various single-meal studies have investigated the effects of different types of whole grain products on subjective appetite sensation and ad libitum energy intake at a subsequent meal in acute settings (Table 13.1). The majority of the studies investigated whole grain rye (13 studies) or wheat products (9 studies). Merely three studies tested the effects of oat and two studies of barley products. Typically, subjects received different types of whole grain breads, porridges, whole kernels or breakfast cereals. The portion sizes varied greatly among studies, from around 50–160 g for breads up to 230–520 g

Table 13.1 Randomized, cross-over studies investigating the effect of whole grain consumption on subjective appetite sensation immediately after consumption as well as on ad libitum energy intake at a subsequent meal.*

Author (Year)	Subjects	Study products	Outcome measures	Main findings (compared to reference product)
Whole grain rye products				
Iversen (2018)	n=23 (8m/15f); age: 32y; BMI: 22.5 kg/m^2; healthy	100 g soft bread served as part of a breakfast meal (+15 g margarine, 20 g cheese, 100 g orange juice) • WWB (ref) (992 kJ, 3.6 g DF, 41.9 g starch) • Rye bread "MS/MR" (42% rye flour, 30% sourdough) (959 kJ, 7.0 g DF, 41.2 g starch) • Rye bread "HS/LR" (35% rye flour, 51% sourdough) (963 kJ, 6.0 g DF, 41.9 g starch) • Rye bread "HS/HR" (48% rye flour, 51% sourdough) (934 kJ, 7.2 g DF, 39.9 g starch) • Rye bread "LS/LR" (35% rye flour, 9% sourdough) (946 kJ, 6.8 g DF, 40.4 g starch) • Rye bread "LS/HR" (48% rye flour, 9% sourdough) (920 kJ, 8.3 g DF, 39.8 g starch)	Subjective appetite (VAS; repeated and AUC 0-240 min) Ad libitum EI	↓Hunger: MS/MR, LS/HR ↑Fullness: MS/MR, HR/HS, LS/HR ↓ Desire: HS/HR, LS/HR EI: no difference
Zamaratskaia (2017)	n=24 (13m/11f); age: 18–70y; BMI: 18.5–30 kg/m^2; healthy	Crispbread served as part of a breakfast meal (incl. cheese, margarine, orange juice) • 52 g yeast fermented refined wheat crisp bread (ref) (1528 kJ, 3.6 g DF, 44.2 g CHO) • 60 g sourdough fermented WG rye crisp bread (1514 kJ, 10.2 g DF, 45.5 g CHO) • 59 g unfermented WG rye crisp bread (1523 kJ, 12.4 g DF, 44.6 g CHO)	Subjective appetite (VAS; repeated and AUC 0–360 min)	Repeated hunger, fullness and desire to eat: no difference Fullness AUC: no difference ↓Hunger, sourdough fermented WG rye compared to ref (unfermented rye: no difference) ↓Desire to eat, sourdough fermented and unfermented WG rye

(continued)

Table 13.1 Randomized, cross-over studies investigating the effect of whole grain consumption on subjective appetite sensation immediately after consumption as well as on ad libitum energy intake at a subsequent meal.* (*continued*)

Author (Year)	Subjects	Study products	Outcome measures	Main findings (compared to reference product)
Whole grain rye products (continued)				
Lee (2017)	n=21 (11m/10f); age: 39y; BMI: 24.9 kg/m^2; healthy	Porridge or WWB bread served as part of an isoenergetic breakfast meal (incl. margarine, jam, milk): • 55 g WWB (ref) (1157 kJ, 3.4 g DF, 39 g CHO) • Porridge from 40 g rye flakes (P40) (1191 kJ, 7.1 g DF, 41.2 g CHO) • Porridge from 55 g rye flakes (P55) (1205 kJ, 9.7 g DF, 50.3 g CHO)	Subjective appetite (VAS; repeated and AUC 0–240 min)	P55: ↓ Hunger ↑Fullness Desire to eat: no difference P40: Hunger, fullness, desire to eat: no difference
Johansson (2015)	n=23 (7m/16f); age: 60y; BMI: 23.8 kg/m^2; healthy	Crispbread served as part of a breakfast meal (+cheese, margarine, orange juice) • 52 g yeast fermented refined wheat crisp bread (ref) (1561 kJ, 3.6 g DF, 43.9 g CHO) • 60 g yeast fermented WG rye crisp bread (1561 kJ, 10.9 g DF, 47.2 g CHO) • 59 g unfermented WG rye crisp bread (1538 kJ, 12.0 g DF, 45.6 g CHO)	Subjective appetite (VAS; repeated and AUC -30–240 min)	↑ Fullness, both WG crisp bread compared to ref (AUC and repeated) ↓ Hunger, both WG crisp bread compared to ref (AUC and repeated) ↓ Desire both WG crisp bread compared to ref (repeated) Desire to eat, AUC: no difference
Forsberg (2014)	Study 1: n=21 (10m/ 11f); age: 39y, BMI: 23 kg/m^2; healthy Study 2: n=20 (6m/ 14f); age: 29y, BMI: 23 kg/m^2; healthy	Study 1: Breakfast meals based on ~1.2MJ per portion (+27 g ham, 25 g cheese, 200 g orange juice: ~1.3MJ) • WWB (ref) (108 g, 3.8 g DF) • WG rye crisp bread (80 g; 13 g DF) • Study 2: Breakfast meals based on ~0.9MJ-1.0MJ per portion (+30 g ham, 100 g orange juice: ~0.6MJ) • WWB (ref) (86 g; 2.6 g DF) • WG rye crisp bread (64 g; 10 g DF)	Study 1 and 2: Subjective appetite (VAS; repeated and AUC 0–240 min)ad libitum EI (240 min after breakfast)	Study 1: ↑ Satiety (repeated) ↓ Hunger (AUC 0-240 min and repeated) ↓ Desire to eat (AUC 0–240 min and repeated) Ad libitum EI: no difference Study 2: ↑Satiety (AUC 0–240 min and repeated) ↓Hunger (AUC 0–240 min and repeated) ↓Desire to eat (AUC 0–240 min and repeated) ↓ Ad libitum EI

Isaksson (2012)	n=24 (5m/ 19f); age: 33y; BMI: 23.4 kg/m^2; healthy	Breakfast meals based on ~0.8MJ per portion (+25 g jam, 10 g 40% fat margarine, 200 g 1.5% fat milk: ~0.1MJ): • WWB (colored with colorit) (ref) (74 g, 3.2g DF) • WG rye flakes porridge (55 g + 300 g water, 10.8 g DF)	Subjective appetite (VAS; repeated 30– 240 min)	↑ Satiety ↓ Hunger ↓ Desire to eat
Whole grain rye products (continued)				
Isaksson (2011)	Bread study: n=24 (2m/ 22f); age: 25y; BMI: 22.7 kg/m^2; healthyPorridge study: n=20 (20f); age: 24y; BMI: 22.2 kg/m^2; healthy	Bread study: Breakfast meals based on ~1.65MJ per portion (+10 g margarine, 24 g cheese, 200 g orange juice:~0.9MJ): • WWB (ref) (144 g, 5.3 g DF) • Milled RK bread (158 g, 13.0 g DF) • Whole RK bread (156 g, 11.0 g DF) Porridge study: Breakfast meals based on ~0.95MJ per portion (+ 10 g 40% fat margarine, 60 g jam, 200 g 1.5% fat milk:~0.9MJ): • WWB (ref) (86 g, 3.4 g DF) • Milled RK porridge (350 g, 11.7 g DF) • Whole RK porridge (137 g, 10.7 g DF)	Subjective appetite (VAS; repeated 30–240 min)	Bread study: ↑ Satiety (milled and whole RK breads) Hunger: no difference ↓ Desire to eat (whole RK bread) Porridge study: ↑ Satiety (milled and whole RK porridges) ↓ Hunger (milled and whole RK porridges) ↓ Desire to eat (milled and whole RK porridges)
Rosén (2011c)	n=14 (7m/ 7f); age: 24y; BMI: 22.0 kg/m^2; healthy	Breakfast meals based on 50 g available starch: • WWB (ref) (123 g, 2.7 g IDF+SDF) • WG rye bread from variety "D.Zlote" (165 g , 12.4 g IDF+SDF) • WG rye bread from variety "H.Loire" (176 g , 15.1 g IDF+SDF) • WG rye bread from variety "Nikita" (169 g , 14.4 g IDF+SDF) • WG rye bread from variety "Rekrut" (171 g , 16.2 g IDF+SDF) • WG rye bread from variety "Amilo" (172 g , 15.6 g IDF+SDF)	Subjective appetite (repeated and AUC 0–180 min)	↓ Hunger (AUC 0–60 min: D. Zlote and Rekrut; AUC 60–120 min: D.Zlote and Rekrut; AUC 120–180 min: D.Zlote) ↑ Fullness (AUC 0–180 min: all WG rye breads; AUC 0–60 min: D.Zlote and Rekrut; AUC 60–120 min: Nikita, D.Zlote and Rekrut; AUC 120–180 min: D.Zlote, Nikita, Rekrut, Amilo) Desire to eat: no differences

(continued)

Table 13.1 Randomized, cross-over studies investigating the effect of whole grain consumption on subjective appetite sensation immediately after consumption as well as on ad libitum energy intake at a subsequent meal.* *(continued)*

Author (Year)	Subjects	Study products	Outcome measures	Main findings (compared to reference product)
Whole grain rye products (continued)				
Rosén (2011b)	n=20 (10m/ 10f); age: 27y; BMI: 22.2 kg/m^2; healthy	Breakfast meals based on 50 g available starch: • WWB (ref) (126 g , 2.8 g IDF+SDF) • WG rye bread from variety "Amilo" (ref) (155 g , 12.6 g IDF+SDF) • WG rye bread from variety "Evolo (153 g , 13.3 g IDF+SDF) • WG rye bread from variety "Kaskelott (154 g , 13.8 g IDF+SDF) • WG rye bread from variety "Picasso (154 g , 13.4 g IDF+SDF) • WG rye bread from variety "Vicello" (149 g , 13.1 g IDF+SDF) • Commercial WG rye bread (158 g , 13.9 g IDF+SDF)	Subjective appetite (VAS; repeated and AUC 0–180 min)	↓Hunger (AUC 0–60 min: commercial bread, Evolo ; AUC 0–180 min: Evolo) ↓Desire to eat (AUC 0–60 min: commercial bread) ↑Fullness (AUC 0–60 min: Amilo, Vicello; AUC 60–120 min: Evolo)
Rosén (2009)	n=12 (9m/ 3f); age 25y, BMI: 23.1 kg/m^2; healthy	Breakfast meals based on 40 g available starch: • WWB (ref) (101 g , 1.8 g DF) • WG rye bread (123 g , 9.6 g DF) • WG rye porridge (warm) (258 g prepared, 10.1 g DF)	Subjective appetite (by bipolar scales from -10 to 10; iAUC 0–180 min)	↑ Satiety (iAUC 0–180 min: WG rye porridge), Hunger: results not reported
Hartvigsen (2014b)	n=15 (8m/ 7f); age: 64y; BMI: 31.3 kg/m^2; MS	Breakfast meals based on 50 g available CHO: • Semolina porridge (ref) (525 g , 5.7 g DF, 1.8 g RS, 1005kJ) • RK porridge (435 g , 12.7 g , 1.4 g RS, 1001kJ)	Subjective appetite (VAS; AUC 0–240 min)	No differences in appetite
Hartvigsen (2014a)	n=15 (7m/ 8f); age: 63y; BMI: 31.1 kg/m^2; MS	Breakfast meals based on 50 g available CHO: • WWB (ref) (107 g ; 2.9 g DF; 1088kJ) • RK bread (147 g ; 12.2 g DF; 1040kJ)	Subjective appetite (VAS; AUC 0–270 min) Ad libitum EI (270 min after breakfast) Cumulative EI (ad libitum EI + breakfast)	↑ Satiety ↓ Hunger ↑ Fullness Ad libitum and cumulative EI: no differences

Whole grain wheat products				
Costabile (2018)	n=14 (7m/7f); age: 30y; BMI: 22 kg/m^2; healthy	Breakfast meal based on 69 g available CHO from pasta: • Refined wheat pasta (ref) (100 g , 3.0 g DF, 1322 kJ) • WG wheat pasta (117 g , 11.0 g DF, 1431 kJ)	Subjective appetite (VAS; repeated and AUC 30–240 min) Self-reported EI over 8 hours (240–720 min).	↓Desire to eat ↓Hunger Satiety: no difference EI: no difference
Cioffi (2016)	n=15 (7m/8f); age: 44y; BMI: 30.1 kg/m^2; healthy	Lunch meal consisting of 100 g pasta and 100 ml tomato sauce: • Refind wheat pasta (ref) (1900 kJ, 3.8 g DF, 75.2 E% CHO) • WG wheat pasta (1900 kJ, 8.g DF, 71.7 E% CHO)	Subjective appetite (VAS; repeated and AUC 0–240 min) Ad libitum EI (240 min after lunch)	↑Satiety ↑Fullness ↑Comfort ↓prospective Hunger: no difference Thirst: no difference EI: no difference
Kristensen (2010)	n=16 (6m/ 10f); age: 24y; BMI: 21.7 kg/m^2; healthy	Breakfast meals based on 50 g available CHO (all 2000kJ): • WWB (ref 1) (119 g + 51 g cheese, 3.6 g DF) • WG wheat bread (146 g + 35 g cheese, 11.7 g DF) • Refined wheat pasta (ref 2) (72 g dry + 69 g cheese, 2.2 g DF) • WG wheat pasta (84 g dry + 60 g cheese, 5.0 g DF)	Subjective appetite (VAS; repeated and AUC 0–180 min)Ad libitum EI	WG wheat bread (compared to ref 1):↑ Satiety (AUC 0–180 min; repeated: trend) ↓ Hunger (AUC 0–180 min) ↑ Fullness (AUC 0–180 min, repeated: trend) ↓ Prospective (AUC 0–180 min; repeated: trend) Ad libitum EI: no difference WG wheat pasta (compared to ref 2): No differences in appetite and ad libitum EI
Freeland (2009)	Study 1: n=17 (17m), age: 25y; BMI: 23.4 kg/m^2, healthyStudy 2: n=16 (16m), age: 25y, BMI: 21.1 kg/m^2, healthy	Study 1 and 2: Preloads based on ~0.77MJ per portion (+125mL 2% fat milk mixed with 125mL water: ~0.27MJ): • Wheatlets (ref) (44 g raw, cooked with 250mL water +2.5 g safflower oil, 2.3 g protein powder, 100 mg sucralose; 1 g DF) • High-DF cereal (FiberOne, General Mills; WG wheat first ingredient) (90g raw + 210mL boiling water, 75 mg sucralose; 41 g DF)	Study 1: Subjective appetite (VAS; iAUC 0-60 min, single time points 15, 30, 45, 60 min); ad libitum EI (60 min after preload)Study 2: Subjective appetite (VAS; iAUC 0–120 min, single time points 15, 30, 45, 60, 90, 120 min) ad libitum EI (120 min after preload)	Study 1: ↑ Fullness (15 min) Hunger: no difference ↓ Ad libitum EI Study 2: No differences in hunger, fullness and ad libitum EI

(*continued*)

Table 13.1 Randomized, cross-over studies investigating the effect of whole grain consumption on subjective appetite sensation immediately after consumption as well as on ad libitum energy intake at a subsequent meal.* (*continued*)

Author (Year)	Subjects	Study products	Outcome measures	Main findings (compared to reference product)
Whole grain wheat products (continued)				
Hlebowicz (2008)	n=13 (6m/ 7f); age: 25y; BMI: 22.8 kg/m^2; healthy	Breakfast meals based on 50 g available CHO (+ 28 g vinegar): • WWB (ref) (106 g , 2.1 g DF) • WG wheat kernel bread (133 g , 7.2 g DF) • WG milled wheat kernel bread (108 g , 7.2 g DF)	Subjective satiety (bipolar scale from -10 to 10; repeated and AUC 0–120 min)	Satiety↑ Satiety (AUC 0–120 min and 15, 30, 45, 60, 90 min: WG wheat kernel bread)
Holm (1992)	n=10 (3m/ 7f); age: 34-44y (m) and 26–49y (f); BMI: 18.5–23.5 kg/m^2(m) and 17.5–23.0 kg/m^2 (f), healthy	Breakfast meals based on 50 g starch (each ~1.7MJ): • WWB (ref) (101 g + 32 g cheese, 7 g margarine; 2.3 g DF) • WG wheat kernel bread (145 g + 26 g cheese, 8 g margarine; 8.1 g DF)	Subjective satiety (bipolar scale from -4 to 4; single time points 15, 95, 180 min)	↑ Satiety (15 min)
Whole grain barley products				
Granfeldt** (1994)	n=10 (5m/ 5f); age: 34y; BMI: 21 kg/m^2; healthy	Breakfast meals based on 50 g available starch (+ cheese and butter; all meals ~1.5MJ): • WWB (ref) (~53 g) • Waxy barley kernels, hull-less (~231 g prepared, 18.6%DM DF) • Ord. barley kernels, covered (~231 g prepared, 14.9%DM DF) • HA barley kernels, covered (~231 g prepared, 17.9%DM DF) • HA barley kernels, hull-less (~231 g prepared,18.4%DM DF) • Ord. barley flour porridge, dehulled (~231 g prepared) • HA barley flour porridge, covered (~231 g prepared, 17.9%DM DF)	Subjective satiety (bipolar scale from -10 to +10; AUC 0-180 min and single time points 15, 45, 95, 120, 180 min)	↑ Satiety (AUC 0-180 min: waxy and HA barley kernels, HA barley flour porridge; 95 min: all barley products)

Whole grain oat products				
Rebello (2013)	n=46 (17m/ 29f); age: 34y; BMI: 26.1 kg/m²; healthy	Breakfast meals based on ~1.0MJ per portion (+ 307 g lactose-free, fat-free milk: ~473 kJ): • RTE cereal (ref) (Honey Nut Cheerios) (64 g , served with 360 g water, 4.5 g DF) • Oatmeal (Old Fashioned, Quaker Old) (67 g raw, heated with 360 g water, 6.7 g DF)	Subjective appetite (VAS; AUC 0–240 min and changes from fasting at single time points 30, 60, 120, 180, 240 min)	↓ Hunger (AUC 0–240 min and 120, 180, 240 min) ↑ Fullness (AUC 0–240 min and 120, 180, 240 min) ↑ Stomach Fullness (AUC 0–240 min; 180, 240 min) ↓ Desire to eat (AUC 0–240mi and; 120, 180, 240 min) ↓ Prospective (AUC 0–40 min and 120, 180, 240 min)
Rebello (2014)	n=43 (20m/ 28f); age: 30y; BMI: 27.1 kg/m²; healthy	Breakfast meals based on ~0.9MJ (+ 184 g lactose-free, fat-free milk: ~282kJ): • RTE cereal (Honey Nut Cheerios) (ref) (38 g , served with 240 g water, 2.7 g DF) • Instant Oatmeal flakes (Quaker) (40 g dry + ca. 250 ml boiling water, 4.0 g DF) • Oatmeal (Old fashioned, Quaker) (40 g dry, cooked with 240 g water, 4.0 g DF)	Subjective appetite (VAS; repeated and AUC 0–240 min)	↓Hunger (60 min: Instant oatmeal flakes) ↑Fullness (AUC 0–240 min and 60 min: Instant oatmeal flakes) ↓Desire to eat (AUC 0–240 min and 60, 120 min: Instant oatmeal flakes) ↓Prospective (AUC 0–240 min and 30, 120 min: Instant oatmeal flakes and Oatmeal; 60 min: Instant oatmeal flakes)
Different whole grain products				
Rosén (2011a)	n=10 (5m/ 5f); age: 26y; BMI: 22.6 kg/m²; healthy	Breakfast meals based on 50 g available starch: • WWB (ref) (124 g , 1.1 g RS, 4.4 g indig. CHO, 1015kJ) • WG rye bread (163 g , 2.5 g RS, 19.8 g indig. CHO, 1078kJ) • Wheat kernel (172 g prepared, 7.5 g RS, 19.8 g indig. CHO, 1170kJ) • RK (227 g prepared, 7.5 g RS, 25.2 g indig. CHO, 1066kJ)	Subjective appetite (VAS; AUC 0–60 min, 120–210 min, 210-270 min, 300–390 min) Ad libitum EI (270 min after breakfast) Cumulative EI (breakfast + ad libitum lunch)	↑ Fullness (AUC 0–60 min: all test products) ↓ Desire to eat (AUC 0–60 min: Wheat kernel, RK; AUC 120–210 min and 210-270 min: RK) ↓ Hunger (AUC 0–60 min: RK, wheat kernel, WG rye bread; AUC 120–210 and 210–270 min: RK) ↓ ad libitum EI: RK ↓ Cumulative EI: RK

(continued)

Table 13.1 Randomized, cross-over studies investigating the effect of whole grain consumption on subjective appetite sensation immediately after consumption as well as on ad libitum energy intake at a subsequent meal.* (*continued*)

Author (Year)	Subjects	Study products	Outcome measures	Main findings (compared to reference product)
Different whole grain products (continued)				
Schroeder (2009)	n=47(12m/ 35f); age: 31y; BMI: 23 kg/m²; healthy	Breakfasts meals based on 56 g -portions (+ 89 ml 2% fat milk) and snack based on 30 g -portions (after 2h): • Refined rice hot cereal (ref) (1 g DF, 879kJ) + snack mix (0 g DF, 502kJ) • WG high-DF barley hot cereal (12 g DF, 921kJ) + snack mix (8 g DF, 502kJ) • WG wheat hot cereal (5 g DF, 837kJ) + snack mix (2 g DF, 460kJ)	Subjective appetite (modified VAS/ SLIM; AUC 0–210 min)ad libitum EI (210 min after breakfast)	No differences in appetite and ad libitum EI
Isaksson (2008)	n=22 (8m/ 14f); age: 41y; BMI: 23.2 kg/m²; healthy	Part 1: Breakfast meals based on ~0.8MJ per portion (+ 45 g apple sauce, 5 g 40% fat margarine, 200 g 1.5% fat milk: ~0.9MJ): • WWB (ref) (71 g , 1.8 g DF) • WG rye flakes porridge (62 g + 250 g water, 8.7 g DF) Part 2: Lunch meals based on ~1.4MJ per portion (+ 210 g tomato sauce, 10 g parmesan: ~0.9MJ) (proceeded by rye flakes porridge breakfast 4h before) • Refined wheat pasta (ref) (94 g dry, 2.8 g DF) • WG wheat pasta (100 g dry, 9.5 g DF)	Subjective appetite (VAS; part 1 and 2: single time points 30 – 240 min) Ad libitum EI (only part 2: 240 min after lunch Self-reported 24h EI (24h from breakfast)	Part 1: ↑ Satiety (all time points) ↓ Hunger (all time points) ↓ Desire to eat (all time points) No differences in self-reported 24h EI Part 2: No differences in appetite and ad libitum and self-reported 24h EI
Hlebowicz (2007)	n=12 (6m/ 6f); age: 28y; BMI: 22kg/m²; healthy	Breakfast meals based on 50 g -portions (+ 300 g sour milk ~565kJ) • Corn flakes (ref) (1.5 g DF, 774kJ) • Cereal WG/ bran wheat flakes (AllBran, Kellogg's) (7.5 g DF, 682kJ) • WG oat flakes (4.0 g DF, 774kJ)	Subjective satiety (bipolar scale from -10 to +10) (iAUC 0–120 min)	No differences in satiety

Jenkins** (1986)	n=16 (9m/ 7f); age: 67y; NIDDM; and n=6 (1m/ 5f); age: 50y; IDDM	Breakfast meals based on 50 g available CHO: • WWG (ref) (67 g) • Milled WG wheat bread (76 g) • WG bulgur (67 g dry) • Wheat kernels (76 g dry) • Pumpernickel bread (110 g) • RK (66 g dry) • Milled WG rye bread (66 g)	Subjective satiety (bipolar scale from -3 to +3; single time points 30, 90, 180 min)	↑ Satiety (30 min: WG bulgur, wheat kernels)

* Only the study products and findings relevant for the acute effects of whole grain intake on appetite sensation were included in the table.

** Not randomized.Abbreviations: ↑, increase; ↓, decrease; %DM, percentage dry matter; AUC, area under the curve; BMI, body mass index; CHO, carbohydrates; DF, dietary fibre; EI, energy intake; E%, percentage of total energy; f, female; HA, high-amylose; iAUC, incremental area under the curve; IDDM, insulin-dependent diabetics; IDF, insoluble dietary fibre; indig., indigestible; m, male; MS, metabolic syndrome; NIDDM, non-insulin dependent diabetics; ord., ordinary; prospective, prospective food intake; ref, reference product; repeated, repeated measures analysis; RK, rye kernels; RS, resistant starch; RTE, ready-to-eat; SDF, soluble dietary fibre; SLIM, Satiety Labeled Intensity Magnitude Scale; VAS, visual analogue scale; WG, whole grain; WWB, white wheat bread.

for porridges and boiled kernels. By far, most of the studies were conducted in young, healthy men and women; only two studies included subjects diagnosed with the metabolic syndrome (Hartvigsen et al., 2014b, 2014a) and one study with diabetic subjects (Jenkins et al., 1986). Some of the studies found whole grain products such as rye-based soft bread or crisp bread (Forsberg et al., 2014; Iversen et al., 2018; Johansson et al., 2015), wheat breads and pasta (Costabile et al., 2018; Hlebowicz et al., 2008; Holm and Björck, 1992; Kristensen et al., 2010), oatmeal (Rebello et al., 2014, 2013), boiled kernels (Jenkins et al., 1986; Rosén et al., 2011a) or rye flakes porridges (Isaksson et al., 2011; Lee et al., 2017; Rosén et al., 2009) to beneficially affect measures of subjective appetite sensation compared with a control product, often refined-wheat bread (WWB). In contrast, in other studies, subjective appetite sensation was not affected after ingestion of different whole grain products, for instance, whole grain wheat pasta (Isaksson et al., 2008; Kristensen et al., 2010), whole grain wheat or rye breads (Hlebowicz et al., 2008; Jenkins et al., 1986) or rye kernel porridge (Hartvigsen et al., 2014b). Fewer studies have investigated the effects of whole grain consumption on ad libitum energy intake at a subsequent meal (Cioffi et al., 2016; Forsberg et al., 2014; Freeland et al., 2009; Hartvigsen et al., 2014a; Isaksson et al., 2008; Kristensen et al., 2010; Rosén et al., 2011a; Schroeder et al., 2009). Results from such studies have been inconsistent, which may be partly due to the low number of participants in the studies resulting in a lack of statistical power to find underlying differences. While the consumption of whole grain rye crisp bread (Forsberg et al., 2014) or boiled rye kernels (Rosén et al., 2011a) was found to reduce ad libitum energy intake at a subsequent meal, no effects on ad libitum energy intake were detected after ingestion of whole grain rye kernel bread (Hartvigsen et al., 2014a), whole grain wheat bread or pasta (Cioffi et al., 2016; Kristensen et al., 2010), or whole grain rye porridge or crisp bread (Forsberg et al., 2014; Isaksson et al., 2008). Remarkably, only one study has investigated the effect of whole grain on satiation (Cioffi et al., 2016). Although, this study found no difference in energy intake at serving ad libitum meals containing refined-wheat pasta or whole grain pasta, more studies are needed to determine whether energy intake is lower during meals containing whole grain compared to meals containing refined grain.

13.3 Potential mechanisms of acute effects of whole grain intake on appetite

13.3.1 Gastric emptying and distension

One suggested mechanism is that whole grain consumption may increase satiety by delaying gastric emptying (Juntunen et al., 2002). A delay in gastric emptying would extend the duration of gastric distension and thus satiety feelings (Delzenne et al., 2010). The presence of dietary fibre and resistant starch as well as the firmer botanical structure of whole grain foods may impair digestion and absorption in the small intestine, which increases the passage of macronutrients to the colon (Chapman et al., 1985; Livesey et al., 1995). This, in turn, will activate the so called "ileal brake," causing a slowing of both gastric emptying and small intestinal transit time (Maljaars et al., 2008). Prolonged exposure of macronutrients in the small intestine may extend the period of secretion of gastrointestinal satiety hormones (Lavin et al., 1998; Lavin and Read, 1995). Nevertheless, relatively few studies have investigated the effects of whole grain consumption on gastric emptying and distension. Marciani et al. (2013) observed a longer gastric half-emptying time after whole meal bread intake compared to rice pudding measured by magnetic resonance imaging. Also Juntunen et al. (2002) found a reduced gastric emptying rate in the later post-prandial period after whole kernel rye bread consumption in comparison to WWB using paracetamol. In contrast, other studies, using paracetamol or ultrasonography, did not find different whole grain products to affect gastric emptying compared to their reference products (Hlebowicz et al., 2009, 2008; Najjar et al., 2009). Thus, more studies are needed to elucidate which features of whole grain foods may lead to slower gastric emptying.

13.3.2 Lower glucose and insulin responses

A prolongation of gastric emptying and small intestinal transit as well as impaired digestion and absorption due to a greater dietary fibre content and a coarser food structure may attenuate glycemic and insulinemic responses after whole grain intake (Juntunen et al., 2003, 2002), which in turn, may contribute to a reduction in appetite (Arumugam et al., 2008; Rosén et al., 2011a). A number of studies have found a lower glycemic response after the consumption of different kinds of whole grain products, which was paralleled by beneficial effects on appetite sensation in several studies (Hartvigsen et al., 2014a; Rosén et al., 2011a, 2009). In contrast, others did not observe a reduced glycemic response after the consumption of different whole grain products (Johansson et al., 2015; Juntunen et al., 2002; Kristensen et al., 2010; Zamaratskaia et al., 2017). This is probably due to differences in food structure of different whole grains (Juntunen et al., 2003, 2002). It has been suggested that the prevention of hypoglycemia in the late-postprandial period may be more important for satiety sensation than the overall glucose response (Arumugam et al., 2008). Indeed, some whole grain studies reported higher late-postprandial glucose concentrations compared to their reference products (Juntunen et al., 2002; Rosén et al., 2011a, 2009), which went along with increased satiety in the two studies also assessing appetite (Rosén et al., 2011a, 2011c). However, the differences in appetite ratings between the different test meals often paralleled during the whole postprandial period; thus, the importance of the late-postprandial glycemic response after whole grain intake needs further investigation.

A number of studies also detected a lower postprandial insulin response following whole grain (rye) consumption (Hartvigsen et al., 2014a; Johansson et al., 2015; Rosén et al., 2011a, 2011c), which was in one study found to be associated with decreased late-postprandial feelings of fullness (Rosén et al., 2011c) and in another with a decreased ad libitum energy intake at lunch (Rosén et al., 2011a). However, a few other studies did not find differences in insulin response in both healthy and diabetic subjects after whole grain consumption compared to the control products (Hagander et al., 1984; Najjar et al., 2009).

13.3.3 Summary of potential mechanisms

A likely mechanism by which whole grain intake may increases satiety is due to a delay in gastric emptying, greater and prolonged stomach distension. Yet, actual evidence from whole grain studies supporting this is sparse. It is also conceivable that an attenuated glucose and insulin response after whole grain intake may affect appetite sensation, but so far this relationship has only been investigated in few studies. Also, not all whole grain products have a lower glycemic or insulinemic index than the corresponding refined-grain products.

13.4 Impact of whole grain characteristics on appetite and suggested mechanisms

Altogether, evidence of the effects of whole grain products on appetite sensation and the potential underlying mechanism is rather inconsistent. Whole grain products are very diverse exhibiting different dietary fibre contents and compositions as well as food structures that suggests that different whole grain products may not necessarily have the same physiological effects (Frølich and Åman, 2010). Factors such as dietary fibre content and composition, particle size and cereal type may determine effects on appetite.

13.4.1 Dietary fibre content

Isolated dietary fibres have often been found to have satiating effects (Wanders et al., 2011), suggesting that the high dietary fibre content of whole grain products may determine the satiating capability of whole grain foods. Dietary fibres are diverse in their structure as well as physico-chemical properties (Kumar et al., 2012), and dietary fibre content and composition vary across cereal types (Frølich et al., 2013). Especially viscous dietary fibres, such as β-glucan, have been found to enhance satiety (Hartvigsen et al., 2014a; Vitaglione et al., 2010). β-Glucans are mainly found in oat and barley (Frølich et al., 2013), and it is conceivable that it may have contributed to the satiating effects found for some whole grain oat and barley products (Granfeldt et al., 1994; Rebello et al., 2013). However in studies investigating other types of whole grain cereals, dietary fibre content did not seem to be a crucial factor for the effectiveness on satiety, indicated by the absence of a dose-response relationship of dietary fibre content of the cereal products and effects on appetite in a study by Kristensen et al. (2010). Further, Hlebowicz et al. (2008) observed that consumption of whole kernel wheat bread enhanced satiety to a greater extent than the consumption of bread with the same dietary fibre content and composition but made from milled kernels. Also, potential underlying mechanisms, such as glucose response and gastric emptying, do not seem to depend on dietary fibre content of whole grain products (Hlebowicz et al., 2008; Kristensen et al., 2010).

13.4.2 Structure and particle size

Food structure and particle size may to a larger extent than the dietary fibre content determine the effects of whole grain products on satiety and underlying mechanisms (Hlebowicz et al., 2008; Juntunen et al., 2002). Indeed, in most studies, ingestion of whole grain products comprising whole or cracked kernels was found to increase satiety (Hartvigsen et al., 2014a; Hlebowicz et al., 2008; Rosén et al., 2011a) with only few exceptions (Hartvigsen et al., 2014b; Jenkins et al., 1986). One may speculate that particle size influences gastric emptying, as particles are first released from the stomach when their size is reduced to a size of 1–2 mm by peristaltic stomach movements. Moreover, harder particles empty slower than softer particles (Kong and Singh, 2008). This is supported by the observation of delayed gastric emptying after whole grain rye kernel bread consumption

(Juntunen et al., 2002) and an unaffected gastric emptying rate after consumption of whole grain wheat bread made of milled flour (Najjar et al., 2009). Also, the glycemic and insulinemic response may decrease with greater particle size (Heaton et al., 1988; Jenkins et al., 1988), which is supported by the lower postprandial glucose and insulin response observed in many studies administering coarse whole grain products (Hlebowicz et al., 2008; Juntunen et al., 2002; Rosén et al., 2011a) and no effects after ingestion of products made from finely milled whole grain flour (Hlebowicz et al., 2007; Kristensen et al., 2010; Najjar et al., 2009). Both, slowing of gastric emptying and an impediment of starch hydrolysis due to the intact botanical structure, may reduce the glycemic response (Juntunen et al., 2002; Snow and O'Dea, 1981). However, since some whole grain products made of milled flour have been reported to increase satiety (Forsberg et al., 2014; Isaksson et al., 2011; Rosén et al., 2011a), further factors may influence the effects of whole grain intake on appetite.

13.4.3 Cereal type

Different types of cereals differ in their biochemical composition, including dietary fibre as well as other bioactive components, making them unique (Frølich et al., 2013; Pascoe and Fulcher, n.d.). Remarkably, the vast majority of studies observed satiety enhancing effects of whole grain rye products regardless of their structure (Forsberg et al., 2014; Hartvigsen et al., 2014a; Isaksson et al., 2011; Johansson et al., 2015; Rosén et al., 2011a; Zamaratskaia et al., 2017). Merely in few cases, whole grain rye products did not affect appetite feelings (Hartvigsen et al., 2014b; Rosén et al., 2009). Whole grain rye has also been associated with a reduced insulinemic response (Hartvigsen et al., 2014a; Rosén et al., 2009), which may be one potential reason for the increased satiety sensation. Interestingly, effects on insulin often occurred without a corresponding effect on the glycemic response (Johansson et al., 2015; Juntunen et al., 2003, 2002; Leinonen et al., 1999). Results on wheat are less consistent, as intake of some whole grain wheat products seemed to increase satiety (Costabile et al., 2018; Hlebowicz et al., 2008; Kristensen et al., 2010), whereas others did not have an effect (Kristensen et al., 2010; Schroeder et al., 2009). As already mentioned, whole grain oat and barley products may have different effects than other whole grains due to their high β-glucan content (Frølich et al., 2013). Relatively few studies have investigated the impact of whole grain oat and barley on appetite, of which the majority observed a reduction in appetite (Granfeldt et al., 1994; Rebello et al., 2014, 2013).

13.5 Second-meal effects of whole grain intake on appetite

Consumption of certain whole grain foods has been reported to influence appetite sensation after the following meal, the so-called "second-meal effect." Studies commonly apply two different designs of second meal studies. In an "evening meal design," it is investigated how whole grain evening meals affect appetite sensation after a standardized breakfast at the subsequent day, while studies with a "breakfast design" examine the effects of whole grain breakfasts on appetite sensation after a standardized lunch.

13.5.1 Evidence from second meal studies

Several studies have investigated the effects of consumption of different whole grain products on appetite sensation after a second meal, in which the majority applied a "breakfast

Table 13.2 Randomized, cross-over studies investigating the effect of whole grain consumption on subjective appetite sensation after a second meal as well as on ad libitum energy intake at a third meal.*

Author	Subjects	Intervention products	Outcome measures	Main findings (compared to reference product)
Breakfast design				
Lee (2017)	n=21 (11m/10f); age: 39y; BMI: 24.9 kg/m^2; healthy	Porridge or WWB bread served as part of an isoenergetic breakfast meal (incl. margarine, jam, milk): • 55 g WWB (ref) (1157 kJ, 3.4 g DF, 39 g CHO) • Porridge with 40 g rye flake (P40) (1191 kJ, 7.1 g DF, 41.2 g CHO) • Porridge from 55 g rye flakes (P55) (1205 kJ, 9.7 g DF, 50.3 g CHO)	Subjective appetite after stand. Lunch served 240 minutes after breakfast (VAS; repeated and AUC 270–480 min after breakfast) Ad libitum EI served 480 min after breakfast	No difference in appetite Ad libitum EI: no difference
Hartvigsen(2014b)	n=15 (8m/ 7f); age: 64y; BMI: 31.3 kg/m^2; MS	Breakfast meals based on 50 g available CHO: • Semolina porridge (ref) (525 g , 5.7 g DF, 1.8 g RS, 1005kJ) • RK porridge (435 g , 12.7 g , 1.4 g RS, 1001kJ)	Subjective appetite after stand. Lunch (VAS; AUC 0–120 min)	No differences in appetite
Isaksson (2012)	n=24 (5m/ 19f); age: 33y; BMI: 23.4 kg/m^2; healthy	Breakfast meals based on ~0.8MJ per portion (+ 25 g jam, 10 g 40% fat margarine, 200 g 1.5% fat milk: ~0.1MJ): • WWB (colored with colorit) (ref) (74 g , 3.2 g DF) • WG rye flakes porridge (55 g + 300 g water, 10.8 g DF)	Subjective appetite after stand. Lunch (VAS; repeated 30–240 min)	No differences in appetite

Isaksson (2011)	<u>Bread study:</u> n=24 (2m/ 22f); age: 25y; BMI: 22.7 kg/m^2; healthy <u>Porridge study:</u> n=20 (20f); age: 24y; BMI: 22.2 kg/m^2; healthy	<u>Bread study:</u> Breakfast meals based on ~1.7MJ per portion (+ 10g margarine, 24g cheese, 200g orange juice: ~0.9MJ): • WWB (ref) (144 g , 5.3 g DF) • Milled RK bread (158 g ; 13.0 g DF) • Whole RK bread (156 g ; 1600 kJ; 11.0 g DF) <u>Porridge study:</u> Breakfast meals based on ~1.0MJ per portion (+10 g 40% fat margarine, 60 g jam, 200 g 1.5% fat milk:~0.9MJ): • WWB (ref) (86 g ; 3.4 g DF) • Milled RK porridge (350g ; 11.7 g DF) • Whole RK porridge (137 g ; 10.7 g DF)	Subjective appetite after stand. Lunch (VAS; repeated 30–240 min)	<u>Bread study:</u> ↑ Satiety (milled and whole RK breads) ↓ Hunger: (whole RK bread) ↓ Desire to eat (milled and whole RK breads) <u>Porridge study:</u> ↑ Satiety (Milled and whole RK porridges) ↓ Hunger (Whole RK porridge) ↓ Desire to eat (Whole RK porridge)
Isaksson (2008)	n=22 (8m/ 14f); age: 41y; BMI: 23.2 kg/m^2; healthy	Breakfast test meals based on ~0.8MJ per portion(+45 g apple sauce, 5 g 40% fat margarine, 200 g 1.5% fat milk: ~0.9MJ) • WWB (ref) (71 g , 1.8 g DF) • WG rye flakes porridge (62 g + 250 g water, 8.7 g DF)	Subjective appetite after stand. Lunch (VAS; single time points 30–240 min) Ad libitum EI (240 min after lunch)	↑ Satiety (all time points) ↓ Hunger (all time points except 60 and 210 min) ↓ Desire to eat (all time points except 60 and 150 min) Ad libitum EI: no difference
Liljeberg (1999)	n=10 (4m/ 6f); age: 22-57y, BMI: 21.6 kg/ m^2; healthy	Breakfast meals based on 50 g available starch (+100 ml 0.5% fat milk; complete meals: ~1.5 MJ): • WWB (ref) (123 g + 27 g cheese, 7 g butter, 2 g DF, 0.1 g RS) • WG HA-barley bread (159 g + 20 g cheese, 7 g butter, 10 g DF, 1.4 g RS) • WG HA barley bread-long (164 g + 19 g cheese, 7 g butter; 11 g DF, 5.1 g RS) • WG HA barley bread with preb. Barley flour-long (212 g + 15 g cheese, 7 g butter; 12 g DF; 6.8 g RS) • WG HA barley bread with HBG barley flakes-long (115 g + 5 g butter; 25 g DF; 11.2 g RS)	Subjective satiety after stand. Lunch (bipolar scale from -10 to +10; single time points 15, 45, 95, 120, 180 min)	↑ Satiety (45 min: WG HA barley bread-long, WG HA barley bread with HBG barley flakes-long; 95 min: WG HA barley bread with preb. Barley flour-long, WG HA barley bread with HBG barley flakes-long)

(*continued*)

Table 13.2 Randomized, cross-over studies investigating the effect of whole grain consumption on subjective appetite sensation after a second meal as well as on ad libitum energy intake at a third meal.* (*continued*)

Author	Subjects	Intervention products	Outcome measures	Main findings (compared to reference product)
Evening design				
Sandberg (2016)	n=19 (9m/10f); age: 26y; BMI: 21.9 kg/m^2; healthy	Evening meals based on 50 g available starch: • WWB (ref) (121.4 g, 3.9 g DF, 1.3 g RS) • RK bread (142.5 g, 15.6 g DF, 3.9 g RS)	Subjective satiety of WWB breakfast (VAS, AUC 0–180 min)	↑Satiety (RK bread, AUC 0–180) ↓Hunger (RK bread, AUC 0–180) ↓Desire to eat (RK bread, AUC 0–180)
Ibrügger (2014)	n=12 (m); age: 26y, BMI: 23.1 kg/m^2; healthy	Evening meals based on 50 g starch: • WWB (ref) (111 g , 3 g DF, 4.0 g RS) • WG rye kernel bread (143 g , 11 g DF, 7.6 g RS) • Rye kernels (147 g prepared, 12 g DF, 11.1 g RS)	Subjective appetite after stand. Breakfast (VAS; repeated 0–180 min) Ad libitum EI (180 min after breakfast)	No differences in appetite ↓ Ad libitum EI at lunch
Johansson** (2013)	n=19 (6f/ 13f); age: 24y, BMI: 22.3 kg/m^2; healthy	Evening meals based on 50 g available starch: • WWB (ref) (119.7 g , 1.2 g DF, 3.0 g RS) • Barley kernel (96.8 g barley kernel +150 ml water)(146.8 g , 12.2 g DF, 10.1 g RS)	Subjective appetite after ad libitum breakfast (VAS; AUC 0–120 min , AUC 210–330 min , AUC 0-300 min) Ad libitum EI (at breakfast and lunch 210 min after breakfast)	Satiety: no difference ↓ Hunger (AUC 0–300 min, AUC 120–210 min) Desire to eat: no difference Ad libitum EI at breakfast: no difference ↓ Ad libitum EI at lunch

Nilsson (2008c)	n=17 (11m/ 6f); age: 26y, BMI: 22.5 kg/m^2; healthy	Evening meals based on 50 g available starch: • WWB (ref) (117 g , 2.6 g DF, 1.3 g RS) • Whole ord. barley kernel bread (161 g , 10.7 g DF, 9.5 g RS) • Cut ord. barley kernel bread (190 g , 10.6 g DF, 8.8 g RS) • HA barley kernel bread (213 g , 16.1 g DF, 22.0 g RS) • HBG barley kernel bread (388 g , 50.1 g DF, 30.9 g RS)	Subjective satiety after stand. Breakfast (bipolar scale from -4 to 4; AUC 0-180 min)	↑ Satiety (iAUC: HBG barley kernel bread)

*Only the study products and findings relevant for the second meal effects of whole grain intake on appetite sensation were included in the table.

**Ad libitum breakfast. Abbreviations: ↑, increase; ↓, decrease; AUC, area under the curve; CHO, carbohydrates; DF, dietary fibre; EI, energy intake; iAUC, incremental area under the curve; HA, high-amylose; HBG, high-β-glucan; long, baked for 20h at 120°C; ord., ordinary; preb., preboiled; ref, reference product; repeated, repeated measures analysis; RK, rye kernels; RS, resistant starch; stand., standardized; VAS, visual analogue scale; WG, whole grain; WWB, white wheat bread.

design" (Table 13.2). All second meal studies administered either whole grain rye (7 studies) or barley products (3 studies); hence, none investigated wheat or oat products. All, but one study (Hartvigsen et al., 2014b) were conducted in healthy young to middle-aged subjects. Increased satiety after a standardized lunch has been reported following breakfasts of milled or whole kernel rye porridges (Isaksson et al., 2011, 2008), breads made from milled or whole rye kernels (Isaksson et al., 2011; Sandberg et al., 2016) or different high-amylose barley breads (Johansson et al., 2013; Nilsson et al., 2008c). In contrast, while a rye kernel porridge breakfast reduced hunger in the afternoon in one study (Isaksson et al., 2008), this was not observed in another study by the same study group (Isaksson et al., 2012), possibly due to a 12% smaller amount of rye flakes in the porridge in the latter study, illustrating the importance of portion size (Isaksson et al., 2012). Also Hartvigsen et al. (2014b) did not find effects on appetite after a standardized lunch following a whole grain rye kernel porridge breakfast.

Relatively few studies have applied an "evening meal design." Nilsson et al. (2008c) observed an increased satiety after a standardized breakfast following an evening meal of whole grain barley bread made from a high-β-glucan variety. In another study by Ibrügger et al. (2014), evening meals containing whole grain rye kernel bread or boiled rye kernels reduced both ad libitum energy intake at lunch, although they did not affect subjective appetite after a standardized breakfast. Sandberg et al (2016) found increased satiety after standardized breakfast, following an evening meal containing rye kernel bread. Johansson et al. (2013) applied a slightly different design in which a barley kernel evening meal was succeeded by an ad libitum breakfast and ad libitum lunch meal. At breakfast ad libitum energy intake was not affected, but postprandial hunger as well as ad libitum energy intake at lunch were reduced following the barley kernel evening meal (Johansson et al., 2013). In contrast, evening meals consisting of breads made from ordinary whole or cut barley kernels as well as high-amylose barley kernels did not have an effect on satiety at the following morning (Nilsson et al., 2008c).

13.5.2 Potential Mechanisms of second-meal effects on appetite

Whole grain foods are rich in fermentable components such as fructans, arabinoxylans and resistant starch (Frølich et al., 2013) that are broken down by the colonic microflora leading to the formation of short-chain fatty acids (SCFA) gasses, for example, hydrogen and methane, and other metabolites (Macfarlane and Macfarlane, 2003). It has been suggested that the effects of whole grain consumption on appetite after a second meal may be mediated by colonic fermentation (Jonnalagadda et al., 2011). This is also indicated by positive correlations between satiety and breath hydrogen concentrations or plasma butyrate (Hartvigsen et al., 2014b; Nilsson et al., 2008c) after the consumption of different whole grain products. However, such correlations are typically confounded by other effects mediated by dietary fibre.

13.5.2.1 GLP-1, PYY and gastric emptying

Effects of colonic fermentation of whole grain components on appetite sensation may be the consequence of increases in the satiety hormones GLP-1 and PYY. The fermentation products SCFA have been found to bind to the G-protein-coupled receptors (GPR) GPR41 and GPR43 (Brown et al., 2003), which are expressed on entero-endocrine L-cells in the colon (Karaki et al., 2008; Tazoe et al., 2009). In vitro results indicate that the binding of SCFA to these receptors stimulates the expression of the genes of the GLP-1 precursor proglucagon and PYY in a dose-dependent manner (Zhou et al., 2008, 2006). In fact, animal studies show that expression of the proglucagon gene and secretion of GLP-1 and PYY were increased after consumption of different fermentable dietary fibres over different time periods (Cani et al., 2005; Parnell and Reimer, 2012; Zhou et al., 2008). Also in humans, it has been reported that ingestion of fermentable dietary fibres for one to twelve weeks increased concentrations of GLP-1 and PYY (Cani et al., 2009; Parnell and Reimer, 2009; Piche et al., 2003), which may explain the enhanced satiety, and the decreased hunger and ad libitum energy intake observed after the 2-week consumption of inulin-like fructans or oligofructose (Cani et al., 2009, 2006). Similarly as the "ileal brake" is activated by macronutrients, SCFA are suggested to activate the so called "colonic brake" leading to a slowing in gastric emptying, which is potentially mediated by GLP-1 (Cani et al., 2009, 2004; Ropert et al., 1996).

However, only few whole grain second meal studies measured the postprandial GLP-1 response, even fewer assessed gastric emptying, and none measured PYY. Johansson et al. (2013) observed raised fasting and postprandial GLP-1 concentrations at the subsequent morning after a barley kernel evening meal, although effects on hunger first became apparent in the later post-prandial period. Similarly, Nilsson et al. (2008c) found increased postprandial GLP-1 concentrations after a barley kernel bread evening meal during the subsequent morning, which, however, was not accompanied by an increase in satiety or a delay in gastric emptying. In contrast, in the same study other types of barley kernel bread evening meals did not affect the GLP-1 response. Interestingly, although no effects on GLP-1 were observed, the ingestion of a high-amylose barley kernel bread evening meal slowed gastric emptying the next day, which was inversely correlated with breath hydrogen excretion and positively with satiety (Nilsson et al., 2008c). Differently, Priebe et al. (2010) did not report changes in gastric emptying after a standardized breakfast following a barley kernel evening meal. Also Hartvigsen et al. (2014b) did not find changes in GLP-1 concentrations in the afternoon after a standardized lunch following consumption of a rye kernel porridge breakfast. The lack of effect on GLP-1 second meal response after ingestion of most whole grain products agrees with the suggestion that fermentable components may need to be ingested over a prolonged period of time in order to considerably stimulate GLP-1 and PYY secretion (Freeland et al., 2010; Zhou et al., 2006). This is also supported by the lack of effect on GLP-1 response and subjective satiety after short-term ingestion of fermentable dietary fibres (Hess et al., 2011; Peters et al., 2009; Tarini and Wolever, 2010).

13.5.2.2 Ghrelin

Animal studies indicate that colonic production of SCFA may also influence concentrations of the orexigenic hormone ghrelin (Cani et al., 2005; Parnell and Reimer, 2012). In humans, Parnell et al. (2009) observed decreased ghrelin concentrations after 12-week oligofructose consumption, and Tarini et al. (2010) found reduced postprandial ghrelin concentrations already 4.5 hours after single ingestion of 24 g inulin. Supposedly, this may be due to a decreased expression of the enzyme ghrelin *O*-acyltransferase that acetylates ghrelin, which is thought to be crucial for the orexigenic actions of ghrelin (Parnell and

Reimer, 2012). Only few studies measured ghrelin response after a second meal following whole grain consumption. Johansson et al. (2013) found, in fact, a tendency for lower fasting ghrelin concentrations in the next morning after a barley kernel evening meal, whereas postprandial concentrations were unaffected. Also Hartvigsen et al. (2014b) did not observe effects on the postprandial ghrelin response after a standardized lunch following a rye kernel porridge breakfast.

13.5.2.3 Glucose and insulin response

Also glucose metabolism, which is thought to affect appetite sensation (Arumugam et al., 2008; Rosén et al., 2011a), has been shown to be affected by colonic fermentation (Kovatcheva-Datchary et al., 2015; Zeevi et al., 2015; Hartvigsen et al., 2014b; Nilsson et al., 2008c). Potentially, SCFA may reduce hepatic glucose production (Anderson and Bridges, 1984; Thorburn et al., 1993), enhance peripheral insulin sensitivity (Priebe et al., 2010) and decrease circulating free-fatty acid concentrations, which in turn, may improve the insulin-stimulated glucose uptake (Homko et al., 2003; Nilsson et al., 2008c). A number of studies reported a lowered glucose response after a second meal following the consumption of different whole grain products as breakfast (Liljeberg et al., 1999; Nilsson et al., 2008b) or evening meals (Granfeldt et al., 2006; Nilsson et al., 2008c), although not all whole grain products affected the glycemic response (Hartvigsen et al., 2014b; Nilsson et al., 2008b). It needs to be noted that an attenuated second meal glucose response in "breakfast design" studies may also have been induced by a lower first meal glycaemia rather than by colonic fermentation (Higgins, 2012), as indicated by positive correlations between first and second meal glucose response (Hartvigsen et al., 2014b; Nilsson et al., 2008b). Only few whole grain studies have examined both second meal glucose response and appetite sensation. Nilsson et al. (2008c) found a decreased second meal glucose response after different kinds of barley kernel bread evening meals. However, only one of these breads, made from a high β-glucan barley variety, also enhanced satiety. In a study by Hartvigsen et al. (2014b) a rye kernel porridge breakfast neither affected glucose response after lunch nor appetite sensation.

13.5.2.4 Summary of potential mechanisms

The underlying mechanisms by which whole grain intake may influence second meal appetite are not clear. Although it often is suggested that second meal appetite may be influenced by increased concentrations of GLP-1 and PYY due to colonic fermentation, there is a need for more evidence from whole grain studies supporting this assumption. In addition, the suggestions of a reduced gastric emptying rate or lower ghrelin concentrations after a second meal need to be examined in future studies. A number of studies have shown that whole grain intake may attenuate second glucose and insulin response; however, a direct association with appetite sensation still needs to be established.

13.6 Influence of whole grain characteristics on appetite and suggested mechanisms

The effects of whole grain consumption on second meal appetite sensation have not been entirely consistent. Possibly, outcomes may depend on certain characteristics of the whole grain products such as dietary fibre content, structure or cereal type. The content of fermentable dietary fibres and resistant starch is thought to be crucial for second meal effects. Both, resistant starch and total dietary fibre content of evening meals, have been found to be correlated with plasma butyrate and acetate concentrations the next morning (Nilsson et al., 2010). In a study by Isaksson et al. (2011), the consumption of a whole-rye kernel porridge for breakfast increased satiety to a greater extent than a rye porridge made of milled rye. The porridges did not differ in dietary fibre content and composition; thus, the greater effects of the whole kernel porridge might be attributed to food structure and consequently resistant starch content that is known to be higher in whole kernels (Granfeldt et al., 2006; Nilsson et al., 2008b). Effects of an intact food structure are further supported by the increased breath hydrogen excretion as an indicator of gut fermentation and decreased second meal glucose response after different kernel breakfasts (Nilsson et al., 2008b), but not whole grain barley flour porridge breakfasts or evening meals (Nilsson et al., 2008a, 2008b). The kernel products were high in resistant starch while the content was low in the milled barley porridges (Nilsson et al., 2008a, 2008b). On the contrary, Hartvigsen et al. (2014b) did not observe second meal effects of rye kernel breakfasts on glucose response and satiety despite greater breath hydrogen excretion.

It needs to be noted that second meal effects on appetite sensation have only been investigated for whole grain rye and barley products. Further, a number of the tested barley products were made of barley breeds being particularly high in β-glucan or amylose, the latter resulting in a high content of resistant starch (Liljeberg et al., 1999; Nilsson et al., 2008c). Therefore, the results of these studies may not necessarily apply for ordinary whole grain barley products or whole grain products made from other cereal types calling for further studies.

13.7 Long-term effects of regular whole grain intake on appetite

Conceivably, the regular consumption of whole grains over a prolonged period of time may cause physiological alterations that beneficially influence overall appetite sensation that might even be apparent after non-whole grain meals. This may potentially be mediated by colonic fermentation of whole grain components.

13.7.1 Evidence from intervention studies

So far, little is known of how regular whole grain consumption influences appetite sensation, as this has not been investigated in observational studies and only in few intervention studies (Table 13.3). Bodinham et al. (2011) investigated the effect of three-week daily consumption of two whole grain wheat bread rolls or two refined wheat bread rolls on appetite sensation after a non-fibre, liquid meal and ad libitum energy intake at a subsequent lunch meal in healthy subjects. They found neither differences in subjective appetite sensation nor in ad libitum energy intake after the two intervention periods (Bodinham et al., 2011). However, these results are of rather low validity, as the study was of short duration, included only few subjects, and served a relatively low daily amount of whole grain. Isaksson et al. (2012) compared the effects on appetite of consumption of a whole grain rye porridge breakfast or a WWB breakfast for three weeks. In contrast to the study by Bodinham et al. (2011) the test meals before and after the two intervention periods comprised the corresponding treatment products (Isaksson et al., 2012). Hence, the study investigated whether the intervention

Table 13.3 Intervention studies investigating the effect of regular whole grain consumption on subjective appetite sensation and ad libitum energy intake.

Author (year)	Subjects	Study design	Intervention	Outcome measures	Main findings
Suhr (2017)	n=70 (32m;38f); age: 51y; BMI: 28 kg/m^2; healthy	Parallel RCT (6 weeks, 3 arms); after 0 weeks and 6 weeks; Test breakfast according to intervention product	Replacement of habitual cereal products, with ad libitum study products: • Refined wheat (control): Soft bread, crisp bread, pasta, spelt kernels, puffed breakfast cereal • WG wheat: Soft bread, crisp bread, pasta, kernels, flaked breakfast cereal • WG rye: Soft bread, crisp bread, pasta, kernels, flaked breakfast cereal	Subjective appetite after test breakfast (VAS, repeated and AUC 0–240 min)	No differences in appetite at week 0 or week 6
Bodinham (2011)	n=14 (5m/ 9f); age: 26 y; BMI: 21.8 kg/m^2; healthy	Cross-over RCT (2 x 3 weeks); after 0 and 3 weeks: Stand. test breakfast	Daily consumption of 2 iso-energetic bread rolls (~2.3 MJ): • Control period: Refined grain rolls (214 g ; 5.8 g DF) • WG period: WG wheat rolls (194 g , 10.5 g DF)	Subjective appetite after test breakfast (VAS; repeated 0–180 min) Ad libitum EI (180 min after stand. test breakfast)	No differences in appetite at 0 and 3 weeks
Isaksson (2012)	n=24 (5m, 19f); age: 33y; BMI: 23.4 kg/m^2; healthy	Cross-over RCT (2 x 3 weeks); after 0 and 3 weeks: Test breakfast incl. accord. intervention product	Daily consumption of iso-energetic breakfast foods (~0.8MJ): • Control period: WWB (colored with colorit) (74 g , 3.2 g DF) • WG period: WG rye flakes porridge (55 g , 10.8 g DF)	Subjective appetite after test breakfast (VAS; repeated 30–240 min)	↑ Satiety, ↓ hunger, ↓ desire to eat at 0 and 3 weeks after WG rye flakes porridge test meal compared to WWB test meal No difference in appetite ratings after WG rye flakes porridge test meal after 0 and 3 weeks WG rye flakes porridge breakfast intervention ↑ Satiety, ↓ hunger, ↓ desire to eat after WWB test meal after 3 weeks WWB intervention compare to 0 weeks

Giacco (2010)	n=15 (12m; 3f); age: 55y; BMI: 27.4 kg/m^2; healthy	Cross-over RCT (2 x 3 weeks + 2-week run-in); after 3 weeks: Test meal incl. accord. intervention product	Daily consumption of fixed, iso-energetic amount of provided cereals: • Control period: WWB, pasta, rusks, crackers • WG period: WG wheat bread, WG pasta, WG rusks, WG crackers	Subjective appetite after test meal (VAS; iAUC 0–240 min)	No differences in appetite

Abbreviations: ↑, increase; ↓, decrease; accord., according; AUC, area under the curve; DF, dietary fibre; EI, energy intake; iAUC, incremental area under the curve; incl., including; RCT, randomized control trial; repeated, repeated measures analysis; stand., standardized; VAS, visual analogue scale; WG, whole grain; WWB, white wheat bread.

modified acute effects of whole grain on satiety rather than effects on overall appetite sensation. However, the acute appetite response after whole grain intake was not different before and after the whole grain period (Isaksson et al., 2012). Also in a study by Giacco et al. (2010), appetite sensation was not affected after a test meal including the corresponding treatment products following the consumption of iso-energetic amounts of whole grain or refined-grain products for three weeks. However, also this study was underpowered due to a small number of subjects. Similarly, Suhr et al. (2017) found no effect of appetite in a six-week ad libitum study, but it can be speculated that the study was underpowered due to the parallel design that is generally considered less optimal than cross-over designs for investigating appetite.

13.7.2 Potential mechanisms of long-term effects on appetite

Hypothetically, colonic fermentation of whole grain components may play a role in affecting overall appetite sensation on regular whole grain consumption. Although direct evidence from whole grain studies does not exist, this hypothesis is supported by studies administering fermentable dietary fibres over a certain span of time. The consumption of 16 g oligofructose over two weeks was found to reduce ad libitum energy intake at both a breakfast and lunch buffet meal. Despite the lower energy intake, satiety after breakfast was greater after oligofructose treatment compared to placebo (Cani et al., 2006). Also, another study found a decrease in hunger after two-week ingestion of 16 g oligofructose (Cani et al., 2009). These studies imply that regular intake of non-digestible, fermentable carbohydrates may lead to an overall enhancement of satiety and a decrease in food intake due to colonic fermentation. Furthermore, a higher substrate availability on regular intake of fermentable components may lead to the growth of certain saccharolytic bacteria in the colon (Hughes et al., 2007; Shen et al., 2012). Thus, regular consumption of whole grain may induce an adaption of the colonic microflora and an increase in the overall fermentation potential, which may potentially cause more pronounced effects on overall appetite sensation over time (Freeland et al., 2010; Le Blay et al., 1999; Zhou et al., 2008).

13.7.2.1 PYY and GLP-1

It has been suggested that steadily increased SCFA, due to continuously occurring colonic fermentation on regular whole grain intake, may lead to a chronic activation of the SCFA receptors GPR41 and GPR43 in the colon, which in turn, may increase the postprandial GLP-1 response (Tolhurst et al., 2012). Furthermore, continuously prevalent colonic fermentation may also increase the number of intestinal L-cells as observed in rats after the feeding of oligofructose for four weeks (Cani et al., 2007). Both, proliferation and continuous stimulation of L-cells may be reasons for the increases in proglucagon and PYY gene expression, and concomitantly greater intestinal and portal concentrations of GLP-1 and PYY found after consumption of fermentable dietary fibre over certain periods of time in animal studies (Cani et al., 2005; Parnell and Reimer, 2012; Zhou et al., 2008). Also, two human studies found increases in plasma GLP-1 and PYY concentrations after prolonged consumption of fermentable dietary fibre (Cani et al., 2009; Parnell and Reimer, 2009). Freeland et al. (2010) first showed increases in GLP-1 after nine months consumption of a high wheat-fibre cereal breakfast, which was accompanied with increases in plasma acetate and butyrate. The latter study supports the notion that the microflora first needs to adapt to greater substrate availability (Freeland et al., 2010). However, no intervention studies have investigated how regular whole grain consumption influences GLP-1 and PYY concentrations.

13.7.2.2 Leptin

The SCFA receptors GPR41 and GPR43 are also expressed on adipocytes in the adipose tissue (Al-Lahham et al., 2010; Xiong et al., 2004). in vitro and animal studies suggest that SCFA may stimulate the production of leptin by adipocytes (Al-Lahham et al., 2010; Xiong et al., 2004). Since leptin acts as a long-term satiety hormone (Strader and Woods, 2005), one may speculate that chronic colonic fermentation on regular whole grain intake increases leptin concentrations, and consequently, enhances the overall satiety response. Contrary to this hypothesis, Parnell et al. (2009) found reduced leptin concentrations after 12-week oligofructose consumption in a human study. There occurred, however, a significant loss in body weight in the oligofructose group compared to the placebo group, which may have counteracted potential leptin-enhancing effects of colonic fermentation (Parnell and Reimer, 2009). Also against the hypothesis, Moazzami et al. (2011) found a tendency for reduced leptin concentrations after six weeks daily consumption of a diet high in whole grain rye and rye-bran products compared to a refined-grain diet in prostate cancer patients. However, so far, no study has investigated the effects of sustained whole grain consumption on leptin concentrations in healthy subjects.

13.7.3 Potential adaption of appetite sensation to whole grain intake

It is still an open question whether short-term effects actually are sustained on regular whole grain consumption, as effects might diminish over time due to an adaption to whole grain in the diet (Blundell et al., 2010). The only studies investigating whether appetite adapts to regular whole grain intake did not find difference in appetite response in breakfast meal tests conducted before and after the interventions period (Isaksson et al., 2012; Suhr et al., 2017). However, the study by Isaksson et al (2012) was of relative short duration, which may not be long enough to draw conclusions on longer term adaptions. The study by Suhr et al (2017) had a longer six weeks intervention period, but might be underpowered due to the parallel design. Thus, adaptions of acute appetite sensation in the long run clearly need further investigation.

13.8 Concluding remarks

Whole grain intake may potentially influence appetite sensation in the short term, that is, immediately after the meal or after a subsequent meal as well as in the long term. The evidence from studies of short-term effects of whole grain intake on appetite is not overall consistent. Although many whole grain products were found to be more satiating compared to their control products in both acute and second meal studies, there are still a considerable number of products not showing effects compared to their reference products. The reason for these inconsistencies may be on the one hand related to the study settings and participant characteristics, for example, age, gender or health status, but on the other hand, also to the different types and characteristics of whole grain products as well as the serving amounts. There are indications that especially particle size, rather than dietary fibre content, is a determining factor for the effectiveness of whole grain on acute and second meal appetite. Further, whole grain rye products appear to be consistently more satiating than refined wheat control products, likely due to the dietary fibre composition of rye as well as other contained bioactive components. Evidence for second meal effects of whole grain wheat and oat is so far lacking.

Despite these apparently relevant factors, the overall effectiveness of whole grain consumption on appetite is most likely the consequence of an interplay of different factors. One important aspect regarding the results from single-meal studies is also the chosen reference product. In general, the choice may either be motivated by a public health perspective or by clarifying the underlying mechanisms. From a public health point of view, the studied whole grain products should ideally be compared to a refined-grain product that is consumed in a similar way, in order to be a likely and desirable substitute in the diet. The majority of the single-meal studies used white wheat bread as a control product. This may be a sensible choice when investigating the satiating effect of whole grain breads. It seems, however, less meaningful when studying the impact of food structure, such as boiled grain kernels versus white-wheat bread. Studies designed to show the effectiveness of whole grain per se on appetite should assure that the reference product shares important characteristics, such as particle size and cereal type, with the studied whole grain products. Also, if investigating the role of certain whole grain characteristics, the control product needs to be chosen deliberately. Thus, results of single-meal whole grain studies strongly depend on the reference product and results might differ greatly when compared with other types of refined-grain products. Besides short-term effects, it is also conceivable that regular whole grain intake may affect appetite in the long term. One hypothesis suggests that sustained whole grain consumption exerts beneficial effects on appetite due to mechanisms related to steadily occurring colonic fermentation. Contrary, it is also conceivable that effects of whole grain observed in acute studies disappear over time on chronic consumption due to an adaption to the diet. Both hypotheses need further investigation as to date evidence from intervention studies is sparse.

Overall, there seems to be an impact of whole grain intake on appetite. However, it may be disputed whether one should refer to satiating effects of whole grain per se, or rather of certain whole grain products. We advocate to be more specific on the type of whole grain, rather than referring solely to *whole grain*. This is supported by the fact the grains are quite different from each other and that the European Food Safety Authority therefore rejected any claims on "whole grain" (EFSA, Parma, 2010). Furthermore, also refined-grain foods are satiating, therefore effects of whole grains on appetite should always be regarded in reference to an appropriate control product. There still is a great need for investigation of short- and long-term effects of whole grains on appetite as well as the underlying mechanisms.

13.9 References

Al-Lahham, S.H., Roelofsen, H., Priebe, M., Weening, D., Dijkstra, M., Hoek, A., Rezaee, F., Venema, K., Vonk, R.J., 2010. Regulation of adipokine production in human adipose tissue by propionic acid. *Eur. J. Clin. Invest.* 40, 401–407. https://doi.org/10.1111/j.1365-2362.2010.02278.x

Anderson, J.W., Bridges, S.R., 1984. Short-chain fatty acid fermentation products of plant fiber affect glucose metabolism of isolated rat hepatocytes. *Proc. Soc. Exp. Biol. Med.* 177, 372–376.

Arumugam, V., Lee, J.-S., Nowak, J.K., Pohle, R.J., Nyrop, J.E., Leddy, J.J., Pelkman, C.L., 2008. A high-glycemic meal pattern elicited increased subjective appetite sensations in overweight and obese women. *Appetite* 50, 215–222. https://doi.org/10.1016/J.APPET.2007.07.003

Blundell, J., de Graaf, C., Hulshof, T., Jebb, S., Livingstone, B., Lluch, A., Mela, D., Salah, S., Schuring, E., van der Knaap, H., Westerterp, M., 2010. Appetite control: Methodological aspects of the evaluation of foods. *Obes. Rev.* 11, 251–270. https://doi.org/10.1111/j.1467-789X.2010.00714.x

Blundell, J., Rogers, P., Hill, A., 1987. Evaluating the satiating power of foods: Implications for acceptance and consumption. *Food Accept. Nutr.* 205–219.

Bodinham, C.L., Hitchen, K.L., Youngman, P.J., Frost, G.S., Robertson, M.D., 2011. Short-term effects of whole-grain wheat on appetite and food intake in healthy adults: A pilot study. *Br. J. Nutr.* 106, 327–330. https://doi.org/10.1017/S0007114511000225

Brown, A.J., Goldsworthy, S.M., Barnes, A.A., Eilert, M.M., Tcheang, L., Daniels, D., Muir, A.I., Wigglesworth, M.J., Kinghorn, I., Fraser, N.J., Pike, N.B., Strum, J.C., Steplewski, K.M., Murdock, P.R., Holder, J.C., Marshall, F.H., Szekeres, P.G., Wilson, S., Ignar, D.M., Foord, S.M., Wise, A., Dowell, S.J., 2003. The orphan G protein-coupled receptors GPR41 and GPR43 are activated by propionate and other short chain carboxylic acids. *J. Biol. Chem.* 278, 11312–11319. https://doi.org/10.1074/jbc.M211609200

Cani, P.D., Dewever, C., Delzenne, N.M., 2004. Inulin-type fructans modulate gastrointestinal peptides involved in appetite regulation (glucagon-like peptide-1 and ghrelin) in rats. *Br. J. Nutr.* 92, 521–526.

Cani, P.D., Hoste, S., Guiot, Y., Delzenne, N.M., 2007. Dietary non-digestible carbohydrates promote L-cell differentiation in the proximal colon of rats. *Br. J. Nutr.* 98, 32. https://doi.org/10.1017/S0007114507691648

Cani, P.D., Joly, E., Horsmans, Y., Delzenne, N.M., 2006. Oligofructose promotes satiety in healthy human: A pilot study. *Eur. J. Clin. Nutr.* 60, 567–572. https://doi.org/10.1038/sj.ejcn.1602350

Cani, P.D., Lecourt, E., Dewulf, E.M., Sohet, F.M., Pachikian, B.D., Naslain, D., De Backer, F., Neyrinck, A.M., Delzenne, N.M., 2009. Gut microbiota fermentation of prebiotics increases satietogenic and incretin gut peptide production with consequences for appetite sensation and glucose response after a meal. *Am. J. Clin. Nutr.* 90, 1236–1243. https://doi.org/10.3945/ajcn.2009.28095

Cani, P.D., Neyrinck, A.M., Maton, N., Delzenne, N.M., 2005. Oligofructose promotes satiety in rats fed a high-fat diet: Involvement of glucagon-like peptide-1. *Obes. Res.* 13, 1000–1007. https://doi.org/10.1038/oby.2005.117

Chapman, R.W., Sillery, J.K., Graham, M.M., Saunders, D.R., 1985. Absorption of starch by healthy ileostomates: Effect of transit time and of carbohydrate load. *Am. J. Clin. Nutr.* 41, 1244–1248. https://doi.org/10.1093/ajcn/41.6.1244

Cioffi, I., Ibrugger, S., Bache, J., Thomassen, M.T., Contaldo, F., Pasanisi, F., Kristensen, M., 2016. Effects on satiation, satiety and food intake of wholegrain and refined grain pasta. *Appetite* 107, 152–158. https://doi.org/10.1016/J.APPET.2016.08.002

Costabile, G., Griffo, E., Cipriano, P., Vetrani, C., Vitale, M., Mamone, G., Rivellese, A.A., Riccardi, G., Giacco, R., 2018. Subjective satiety and plasma PYY concentration after wholemeal pasta. *Appetite* 125, 172–181. https://doi.org/10.1016/J.APPET.2018.02.004

Delzenne, N., Blundell, J., Brouns, F., Cunningham, K., De Graaf, K., Erkner, A., Lluch, A., Mars, M., Peters, H.P.F., Westerterp-Plantenga, M., 2010. Gastrointestinal targets of appetite regulation in humans. *Obes. Rev.* 11, 234–250. https://doi.org/10.1111/j.1467-789X.2009.00707.x

European Food Safety Authority (EFSA), Parma, I., 2010. Scientific Opinion on the substantiation of health claims related to whole grain (ID 831, 832, 833, 1126, 1268, 1269, 1270, 1271, 1431) pursuant to Article 13(1) of Regulation (EC) No 1924/2006. *EFSA J.* 8, 1766. https://doi.org/10.2903/j.efsa.2010.1766

Forsberg, T., Åman, P., Landberg, R., 2014. Effects of whole grain rye crisp bread for breakfast on appetite and energy intake in a subsequent meal: Two randomised controlled trails with different amounts of test foods and breakfast energy content. *Nutr. J.* 13, 26. https://doi.org/10.1186/1475-2891-13-26

Freeland, K.R., Anderson, G.H., Wolever, T.M.S., 2009. Acute effects of dietary fibre and glycaemic carbohydrate on appetite and food intake in healthy males. *Appetite* 52, 58–64. https://doi.org/10.1016/j.appet.2008.08.001

Freeland, K.R., Wilson, C., Wolever, T.M.S., 2010. Adaptation of colonic fermentation and glucagon-like peptide-1 secretion with increased wheat fibre intake for 1 year in hyperinsulinaemic human subjects. *Br. J. Nutr.* 103, 82. https://doi.org/10.1017/S0007114509991462

Frølich, W., Åman, P., 2010. Whole grain for whom and why? *Food Nutr. Res.* 54. https://doi.org/10.3402/fnr.v54i0.5056

Frølich, W., Åman, P., Tetens, I., 2013. Whole grain foods and health – A Scandinavian perspective. *Food Nutr. Res.* 57. https://doi.org/10.3402/fnr.v57i0.18503

Giacco, R., Clemente, G., Cipriano, D., Luongo, D., Viscovo, D., Patti, L., Di Marino, L., Giacco, A., Naviglio, D., Bianchi, M.A., Ciati, R., Brighenti, F., Rivellese, A.A., Riccardi, G., 2010. Effects of the regular consumption of wholemeal wheat foods on cardiovascular risk factors in healthy people. *Nutr. Metab. Cardiovasc. Dis.* 20, 186–194. https://doi.org/10.1016/j.numecd.2009.03.025

Giacco, R., Della Pepa, G., Luongo, D., Riccardi, G., 2011. Whole grain intake in relation to body weight: From epidemiological evidence to clinical trials. *Nutr. Metab. Cardiovasc. Dis.* 21, 901–908. https://doi.org/10.1016/j.numecd.2011.07.003

Granfeldt, Y., Liljeberg, H., Drews, A., Newman, R., Björck, I., 1994. Glucose and insulin responses to barley products: Influence of food structure and amylose-amylopectin ratio. *Am. J. Clin. Nutr.* 59, 1075–1082. https://doi.org/10.1093/ajcn/59.5.1075

Granfeldt, Y., Wu, X., Björck, I., 2006. Determination of glycaemic index; some methodological aspects related to the analysis of carbohydrate load and characteristics of the previous evening meal. *Eur. J. Clin. Nutr.* 60, 104–112. https://doi.org/10.1038/sj.ejcn.1602273

Hagander, B., Scherstén, B., Asp, N.G., Sartor, G., Agardh, C.D., Schrezenmeir, J., Kasper, H., Ahrén, B., Lundquist, I., 1984. Effect of dietary fibre on blood glucose, plasma immunoreactive insulin, C-peptide and GIP responses in non insulin dependent (type 2) diabetics and controls. *Acta Med. Scand.* 215, 205–213.

Hartvigsen, M.L., Gregersen, S., Laerke, H.N., Holst, J.J., Knudsen, K.E.B., Hermansen, K., 2014a. Effects of concentrated arabinoxylan and beta-glucan compared with refined wheat and whole grain rye on glucose and appetite in subjects with the metabolic syndrome: A randomized study. *Eur. J. Clin. Nutr.* 68, 84–90. https://doi.org/10.1038/ejcn.2013.236

Hartvigsen, M.L., Lærke, H.N., Overgaard, A., Holst, J.J., Bach Knudsen, K.E., Hermansen, K., 2014b. Postprandial effects of test meals including concentrated arabinoxylan and whole grain rye in subjects with the metabolic syndrome: A randomised study. *Eur. J. Clin. Nutr.* 68, 567–574. https://doi.org/10.1038/ejcn.2014.25

Heaton, K.W., Marcus, S.N., Emmett, P.M., Bolton, C.H., 1988. Particle size of wheat, maize, and oat test meals: Effects on plasma glucose and insulin responses and on the rate of starch digestion in vitro. *Am. J. Clin. Nutr.* 47, 675–682. https://doi.org/10.1093/ajcn/47.4.675

Hess, J.R., Birkett, A.M., Thomas, W., Slavin, J.L., 2011. Effects of short-chain fructooligosaccharides on satiety responses in healthy men and women. *Appetite* 56, 128–134. https://doi.org/10.1016/j.appet.2010.12.005

Higgins, J.A., 2012. Whole grains, legumes, and the subsequent meal effect: Implications for blood glucose control and the role of fermentation. *J. Nutr. Metab.* 2012, 829238. https://doi.org/10.1155/2012/829238

Hlebowicz, J., Jönsson, J.M., Lindstedt, S., Björgell, O., Darwich, G., Almér, L.-O., 2009. Effect of commercial rye whole-meal bread on postprandial blood glucose and gastric emptying in healthy subjects. *Nutr. J.* 8, 26. https://doi.org/10.1186/1475-2891-8-26

Hlebowicz, J., Lindstedt, S., Björgell, O., Höglund, P., Almér, L.-O., Darwiche, G., 2008. The botanical integrity of wheat products influences the gastric distention and satiety in healthy subjects. *Nutr. J.* 7, 12. https://doi.org/10.1186/1475-2891-7-12

Hlebowicz, J., Wickenberg, J., Fahlström, R., Björgell, O., Almér, L.-O., Darwiche, G., 2007. Effect of commercial breakfast fibre cereals compared with corn flakes on postprandial blood glucose, gastric emptying and satiety in healthy subjects: A randomized blinded crossover trial. *Nutr. J.* 6, 22. https://doi.org/10.1186/1475-2891-6-22

Holm, J., Björck, I., 1992. Bioavailability of starch in various wheat-based bread products: Evaluation of metabolic responses in healthy subjects and rate and extent of in vitro starch digestion. *Am. J. Clin. Nutr.* 55, 420–429. https://doi.org/10.1093/ajcn/55.2.420

Homko, C.J., Cheung, P., Boden, G., 2003. Effects of free fatty acids on glucose uptake and utilization in healthy women. *Diabetes* 52, 487–491.

Hughes, S.A., Shewry, P.R., Li, L., Gibson, G.R., Sanz, M.L., Rastall, R.A., 2007. In vitro fermentation by human fecal microflora of wheat arabinoxylans. *J. Agric. Food Chem.* 55, 4589–4595. https://doi.org/10.1021/jf070293g

Ibrugger, S., Vigsnaes, L.K., Blennow, A., Skuflic, D., Raben, A., Lauritzen, L., Kristensen, M., 2014. Second meal effect on appetite and fermentation of wholegrain rye foods. *Appetite* 80, 248–256. https://doi.org/10.1016/j.appet.2014.05.026

Isaksson, H., Rakha, A., Andersson, R., Fredriksson, H., Olsson, J., Åman, P., 2011. Rye kernel breakfast increases satiety in the afternoon – An effect of food structure. *Nutr. J.* 10, 31. https://doi.org/10.1186/1475-2891-10-31

Isaksson, H., Sundberg, B., Aman, P., Fredriksson, H., Olsson, J., 2008. Whole grain rye porridge breakfast improves satiety compared to refined wheat bread breakfast. *Food Nutr. Res.* 52. https://doi.org/10.3402/fnr.v52i0.1809

Isaksson, H., Tillander, I., Andersson, R., Olsson, J., Fredriksson, H., Webb, D.-L., Åman, P., 2012. Whole grain rye breakfast – Sustained satiety during three weeks of regular consumption. *Physiol. Behav.* 105, 877–884. https://doi.org/10.1016/J.PHYSBEH.2011.10.023

Iversen, K.N., Johansson, D., Brunius, C., Andlid, T., Andersson, R., Langton, M., Landberg, R., 2018. Appetite and subsequent food intake were unaffected by the amount of sourdough and rye in soft bread – A randomized cross-over breakfast study. *Nutrients* 10, 1594. https://doi.org/10.3390/nu10111594

Jenkins, D.J.A., Wesson, V., Wolever, T.M.S., Jenkins, A.L., Kalmusky, J., Guidici, S., Csima, A., Josse, R.G., Wong, G.S., 1988. Wholemeal versus wholegrain breads: proportion of whole or cracked grain and the glycaemic response. *Br. Med. J.* 297, 958–960.

Jenkins, D.J.A., Wolever, T.M.S., Jenkins, A.L., Giordano, C., Giudici, S., Thompson, L.U., Kalmusky, J., Josse, R.G., Wong, G.S., 1986. Low glycemic response to traditionally processed wheat and rye products: bulgur and pumpernickel bread. *Am. J. Clin. Nutr.* 43, 516–520. https://doi.org/10.1093/ajcn/43.4.516

Johansson, D.P., Lee, I., Risérus, U., Langton, M., Landberg, R., 2015. Effects of unfermented and fermented whole grain rye crisp breads served as part of a standardized breakfast, on appetite and postprandial glucose and insulin responses: A randomized cross-over trial. *PLoS One* 10, e0122241. https://doi.org/10.1371/journal.pone.0122241

Johansson, E. V, Nilsson, A.C., Östman, E.M., Björck, I.M.E., 2013. Effects of indigestible carbohydrates in barley on glucose metabolism, appetite and voluntary food intake over 16 h in healthy adults. *Nutr. J.* 12, 46. https://doi.org/10.1186/1475-2891-12-46

Jonnalagadda, S.S., Harnack, L., Liu, R.H., McKeown, N., Seal, C., Liu, S., Fahey, G.C., 2011. Putting the whole grain puzzle together: Health benefits associated with whole grains summary of American Society for Nutrition 2010 Satellite Symposium. *J. Nutr.* 141, 1011S–1022S. https://doi.org/10.3945/jn.110.132944

Juntunen, K.S., Laaksonen, D.E., Autio, K., Niskanen, L.K., Holst, J.J., Savolainen, K.E., Liukkonen, K.-H., Poutanen, K.S., Mykkänen, H.M., 2003. Structural differences between rye and wheat breads but not total fiber content may explain the lower postprandial insulin response to rye bread. *Am. J. Clin. Nutr.* 78, 957–964. https://doi.org/10.1093/ajcn/78.5.957

Juntunen, K.S., Niskanen, L.K., Liukkonen, K.H., Poutanen, K.S., Holst, J.J., Mykkänen, H.M., 2002. Postprandial glucose, insulin, and incretin responses to grain products in healthy subjects. *Am. J. Clin. Nutr.* 75, 254–262. https://doi.org/10.1093/ajcn/75.2.254

Karaki, S., Tazoe, H., Hayashi, H., Kashiwabara, H., Tooyama, K., Suzuki, Y., Kuwahara, A., 2008. Expression of the short-chain fatty acid receptor, GPR43, in the human colon. *J. Mol. Histol.* 39, 135–142. https://doi.org/10.1007/s10735-007-9145-y

Koh-Banerjee, P., Franz, M., Sampson, L., Liu, S., Jacobs, D.R., Spiegelman, D., Willett, W., Rimm, E., 2004. Changes in whole-grain, bran, and cereal fiber consumption in relation to 8-y weight gain among men. *Am. J. Clin. Nutr.* 80, 1237–1245. https://doi.org/10.1093/ajcn/80.5.1237

Kong, F., Singh, R.P., 2008. Disintegration of solid foods in human stomach. *J. Food Sci.* 73, R67–R80. https://doi.org/10.1111/j.1750-3841.2008.00766.x

Kovatcheva-Datchary, P., Nilsson, A., Akrami, R., Lee, Ying, S., De VaddeR, F., Arora, T., Hallen, A., Martens, E., Björck, I. & Bäckhed, F., 2015. Dietary fiber-induced improvement in glucose metabolism is associated with increased abundance of prevotella. *Cell Metabolism*, 22, 971–982.

Kristensen, M., Jensen, M.G., Riboldi, G., Petronio, M., Bügel, S., Toubro, S., Tetens, I., Astrup, A., 2010. Wholegrain vs. refined wheat bread and pasta: Effect on postprandial glycemia, appetite, and subsequent ad libitum energy intake in young healthy adults. *Appetite* 54, 163–169. https://doi.org/10.1016/j.appet.2009.10.003

Kumar, V., Sinha, A.K., Makkar, H.P.S., de Boeck, G., Becker, K., 2012. Dietary roles of non-starch polysaccharides in human nutrition: A review. *Crit. Rev. Food Sci. Nutr.* 52, 899–935. https://doi.org/10.1080/10408398.2010.512671

Lavin, J.H., Read, N.W., 1995. The effect on hunger and satiety of slowing the absorption of glucose: Relationship with gastric emptying and postprandial blood glucose and insulin responses. *Appetite* 25, 89–96. https://doi.org/10.1006/appe.1995.0043

Lavin, J.H., Wittert, G.A., Andrews, J., Yeap, B., Wishart, J.M., Morris, H.A., Morley, J.E., Horowitz, M., Read, N.W., 1998. Interaction of insulin, glucagon-like peptide 1, gastric inhibitory polypeptide, and appetite in response to intraduodenal carbohydrate. *Am. J. Clin. Nutr.* 68, 591–598. https://doi.org/10.1093/ajcn/68.3.591

Le Blay, G., Michel, C., Blottière, H.M., Cherbut, C., 1999. Enhancement of butyrate production in the rat caecocolonic tract by long-term ingestion of resistant potato starch. *Br. J. Nutr.* 82, 419–426.

Lee, I., Shi, L., Webb, D.-L., Hellström, P.M., Risérus, U., Landberg, R., 2017. Effects of whole-grain rye porridge with added inulin and wheat gluten on appetite, gut fermentation and postprandial glucose metabolism: A randomised, cross-over, breakfast study. *Br. J. Nutr.* 116, 2139–2149. https://doi.org/10.1017/S0007114516004153

Leinonen, K., Liukkonen, K., Poutanen, K., Uusitupa, M., Mykkänen, H., 1999. Rye bread decreases postprandial insulin response but does not alter glucose response in healthy Finnish subjects. *Eur. J. Clin. Nutr.* 53, 262–267.

Liljeberg, H.G., Åkerberg, A.K., Björck, I.M., 1999. Effect of the glycemic index and content of indigestible carbohydrates of cereal-based breakfast meals on glucose tolerance at lunch in healthy subjects. *Am. J. Clin. Nutr.* 69, 647–655. https://doi.org/10.1093/ajcn/69.4.647

Livesey, G., Wilkinson, J.A., Roe, M., Faulks, R., Clark, S., Brown, J.C., Kennedy, H., Elia, M., 1995. Influence of the physical form of barley grain on the digestion of its starch in the human small intestine and implications for health. *Am. J. Clin. Nutr.* 61, 75–81. https://doi.org/10.1093/ajcn/61.1.75

Macfarlane, S., Macfarlane, G.T., 2003. Regulation of short-chain fatty acid production. *Proc. Nutr. Soc.* 62, 67–72. https://doi.org/10.1079/PNS2002207

Maljaars, P.W.J., Peters, H.P.F., Mela, D.J., Masclee, A.A.M., 2008. Ileal brake: A sensible food target for appetite control. A review. *Physiol. Behav.* 95, 271–281. https://doi.org/10.1016/J.PHYSBEH.2008.07.018

Marciani, L., Pritchard, S.E., Hellier-Woods, C., Costigan, C., Hoad, C.L., Gowland, P.A., Spiller, R.C., 2013. Delayed gastric emptying and reduced postprandial small bowel water content of equicaloric whole meal bread versus rice meals in healthy subjects: Novel MRI insights. *Eur. J. Clin. Nutr.* 67, 754–758. https://doi.org/10.1038/ejcn.2013.78

Moazzami, A.A., Zhang, J.-X., Kamal-Eldin, A., Åman, P., Hallmans, G., Johansson, J.-E., Andersson, S.-O., 2011. Nuclear magnetic resonancebased metabolomics enable Detection of the Effects of a Whole Grain Rye and Rye Bran Diet on the Metabolic Profile of plasma in prostate cancer patients. *J. Nutr.* 141, 2126–2132. https://doi.org/10.3945/jn.111.148239

Najjar, A.M., Parsons, P.M., Duncan, A.M., Robinson, L.E., Yada, R.Y., Graham, T.E., 2009. The acute impact of ingestion of breads of varying composition on blood glucose, insulin and incretins following first and second meals. *Br. J. Nutr.* 101, 391–308. https://doi.org/10.1017/S0007114508003085

Nilsson, A.C., Östman, E., Preston, T., Björck, I., 2008a. Effects of GI vs content of cereal fibre of the evening meal on glucose tolerance at a subsequent standardized breakfast. *Eur. J. Clin. Nutr.* 62, 712–720. https://doi.org/10.1038/sj.ejcn.1602784

Nilsson, A.C., Östman, E.M., Granfeldt, Y., Björck, I.M.E., 2008b. Effect of cereal test breakfasts differing in glycemic index and content of indigestible carbohydrates on daylong glucose tolerance in healthy subjects. *Am. J. Clin. Nutr.* 87, 645–654. https://doi.org/10.1093/ajcn/87.3.645

Nilsson, A.C., Ostman, E.M., Holst, J.J., Björck, I.M.E., 2008c. Including indigestible carbohydrates in the evening meal of healthy subjects improves glucose tolerance, lowers inflammatory markers, and increases satiety after a subsequent standardized breakfast. *J. Nutr.* 138, 732–739. https://doi.org/10.1093/jn/138.4.732

Nilsson, A.C., Östman, E.M., Knudsen, K.E.B., Holst, J.J., Björck, I.M.E., 2010. A cereal-based evening meal rich in indigestible carbohydrates increases plasma butyrate the next morning. *J. Nutr.* 140, 1932–1936. https://doi.org/10.3945/jn.110.123604

Parnell, J.A., Reimer, R.A., 2012. Prebiotic fibres dose-dependently increase satiety hormones and alter Bacteroidetes and Firmicutes in lean and obese JCR:LA-cp rats. *Br. J. Nutr.* 107, 601–613. https://doi.org/10.1017/S0007114511003163

Parnell, J.A., Reimer, R.A., 2009. Weight loss during oligofructose supplementation is associated with decreased ghrelin and increased peptide YY in overweight and obese adults. *Am. J. Clin. Nutr.* 89, 1751–1759. https://doi.org/10.3945/ajcn.2009.27465

Pascoe, D.A., Fulcher, R.G., n.d. Biochemistry and compartmentalization of cereal grain components and their functional relationship to, ammalian health, in: *Whole Grains and Health*. Blackwell Publishing Professional, Ames, Iowa, USA, pp. 89–114. https://doi.org/10.1002/9780470277607.ch8

Peters, H.P., Boers, H.M., Haddeman, E., Melnikov, S.M., Qvyjt, F., 2009. No effect of added β-glucan or of fructooligosaccharide on appetite or energy intake. *Am. J. Clin. Nutr.* 89, 58–63. https://doi.org/10.3945/ajcn.2008.26701

Piche, T., des Varannes, S.B., Sacher-Huvelin, S., Holst, J.J., Cuber, J.C., Galmiche, J.P., 2003. Colonic fermentation influences lower esophageal sphincter function in gastroesophageal reflux disease. *Gastroenterology* 124, 894–902. https://doi.org/10.1053/gast.2003.50159

Pol, K., Christensen, R., Bartels, E.M., Raben, A., Tetens, I., Kristensen, M., 2013. Whole grain and body weight changes in apparently healthy adults: A systematic review and meta-analysis of randomized controlled studies. *Am. J. Clin. Nutr.* 98, 872–884. https://doi.org/10.3945/ajcn.113.064659

Priebe, M.G., Wang, H., Weening, D., Schepers, M., Preston, T., Vonk, R.J., 2010. Factors related to colonic fermentation of nondigestible carbohydrates of a previous evening meal increase tissue glucose uptake and moderate glucose-associated inflammation. *Am. J. Clin. Nutr.* 91, 90–97. https://doi.org/10.3945/ajcn.2009.28521

Rebello, C.J., Chu, Y.-F., Johnson, W.D., Martin, C.K., Han, H., Bordenave, N., Shi, Y., O'Shea, M., Greenway, F.L., 2014. The role of meal viscosity and oat β-glucan characteristics in human appetite control: A randomized crossover trial. *Nutr. J.* 13, 49. https://doi.org/10.1186/1475-2891-13-49

Rebello, C.J., Johnson, W.D., Martin, C.K., Xie, W., O'Shea, M., Kurilich, A., Bordenave, N., Andler, S., Klinken, B.J.W. van, Chu, Y.-F., Greenway, F.L., 2013. Acute effect of oatmeal on subjective measures of appetite and satiety compared to a ready-to-eat breakfast cereal: A randomized crossover trial. *J. Am. Coll. Nutr.* 32, 272–279. https://doi.org/10.1080/07315724.2013.816614

Ropert, A., Cherbut, C., Rozé, C., Le Quellec, A., Holst, J.J., Fu-Cheng, X., Bruley des Varannes, S., Galmiche, J.P., 1996. Colonic fermentation and proximal gastric tone in humans. *Gastroenterology* 111, 289–296.

Rosén, L.A., Östman, E.M., Björck, I.M., 2011a. Effects of cereal breakfasts on postprandial glucose, appetite regulation and voluntary energy intake at a subsequent standardized lunch; focusing on rye products. *Nutr. J.* 10, 7. https://doi.org/10.1186/1475-2891-10-7

Rosén, L.A., Östman, E.M., Björck, I.M., 2011b. Postprandial glycemia, insulinemia, and satiety responses in healthy subjects after whole grain rye bread made from different rye varieties. 2. *J. Agric. Food Chem.* 59, 12149–12154. https://doi.org/10.1021/jf2019837

Rosén, L.A., Östman, E.M., Shewry, P.R., Ward, J.L., Andersson, A.A.M., Piironen, V., Lampi, A.-M., Rakszegi, M., Bedö, Z., Björck, I.M.E., 2011c. Postprandial glycemia, insulinemia, and satiety responses in healthy subjects after whole grain rye bread made from different rye varieties. 1. *J. Agric. Food Chem.* 59, 12139–12148. https://doi.org/10.1021/jf2019825

Rosén, L.A., Silva, L.O.B., Andersson, U.K., Holm, C., Östman, E.M., Björck, I.M., 2009. Endosperm and whole grain rye breads are characterized by low post-prandial insulin response and a beneficial blood glucose profile. *Nutr. J.* 8, 42. https://doi.org/10.1186/1475-2891-8-42

Sandberg, J.C., Björck, I.M.E., Nilsson, A.C., 2016. Rye-based evening meals favorably affected glucose regulation and appetite variables at the following breakfast: A randomized controlled study in healthy subjects. *PLoS One* 11, e0151985. https://doi.org/10.1371/journal.pone.0151985

Sandberg, J.C., Björck, I.M.E., NilssoN, A.C., 2017. Effects of whole grain rye, with and without resistant starch type 2 supplementation, on glucose tolerance, gut hormones, inflammation and appetite regulation in an 11–-14.5 hour perspective: A randomized controlled study in healthy subjects. Nutrition Journal 16:25. doi.10.1186/s12937-017-0246-5

Schroeder, N., Gallaher, D.D., Arndt, E.A., Marquart, L., 2009. Influence of whole grain barley, whole grain wheat, and refined rice-based foods on short-term satiety and energy intake. *Appetite* 53, 363–369. https://doi.org/10.1016/j.appet.2009.07.019

Shen, Q., Zhao, L., Tuohy, K.M., 2012. High-level dietary fibre up-regulates colonic fermentation and relative abundance of saccharolytic bacteria within the human faecal microbiota in vitro. *Eur. J. Nutr.* 51, 693–705. https://doi.org/10.1007/s00394-011-0248-6

Snow, P., O'Dea, K., 1981. Factors affecting the rate of hydrolysis of starch in food. *Am. J. Clin. Nutr.* 34, 2721–2727. https://doi.org/10.1093/ajcn/34.12.2721

Strader, A.D., Woods, S.C., 2005. Gastrointestinal hormones and food intake. *Gastroenterology* 128, 175–191.

Suhr, J., Vuholm, S., Iversen, K.N., Landberg, R., Kristensen, M., 2017. Wholegrain rye, but not wholegrain wheat, lowers body weight and fat mass compared with refined wheat: A 6-week randomized study. *Eur. J. Clin. Nutr.* 71, 959–967. https://doi.org/10.1038/ejcn.2017.12

Tarini, J., Wolever, T.M.S., 2010. The fermentable fibre inulin increases postprandial serum short-chain fatty acids and reduces free-fatty acids and ghrelin in healthy subjects. *Appl. Physiol. Nutr. Metab.* 35, 9–16. https://doi.org/10.1139/H09-119

Tazoe, H., Otomo, Y., Karaki, S.-I., Kato, I., Fukami, Y., Terasaki, M., Kuwahara, A., 2009. Expression of short-chain fatty acid receptor GPR41 in the human colon. *Biomed. Res.* 30, 149–156.

Thorburn, A., Muir, J., Proietto, J., 1993. Carbohydrate fermentation decreases hepatic glucose output in healthy subjects. *Metabolism.* 42, 780–785.

Tolhurst, G., Heffron, H., Lam, Y.S., Parker, H.E., Habib, A.M., Diakogiannaki, E., Cameron, J., Grosse, J., Reimann, F., Gribble, F.M., 2012. Short-chain fatty acids stimulate glucagon-like peptide-1 secretion via the G-protein-coupled receptor FFAR2. *Diabetes* 61, 364–371. https://doi.org/10.2337/db11-1019

Vitaglione, P., Lumaga, R.B., Montagnese, C., Messia, M.C., Marconi, E., Scalfi, L., 2010. Satiating effect of a barley beta-glucan-enriched snack. *J. Am. Coll. Nutr.* 29, 113–121.

Wanders, A.J., van den Borne, J.J.G.C., de Graaf, C., Hulshof, T., Jonathan, M.C., Kristensen, M., Mars, M., Schols, H.A., Feskens, E.J.M., 2011. Effects of dietary fibre on subjective appetite, energy intake and body weight: A systematic review of randomized controlled trials. *Obes. Rev.* 12. https://doi.org/10.1111/j.1467-789X.2011.00895.x

Xiong, Y., Miyamoto, N., Shibata, K., Valasek, M.A., Motoike, T., Kedzierski, R.M., Yanagisawa, M., 2004. Short-chain fatty acids stimulate leptin production in adipocytes through the G protein-coupled receptor GPR41. *Proc. Natl. Acad. Sci.* 101, 1045–1050. https://doi.org/10.1073/pnas.2637002100

Ye, E.Q., Chacko, S.A., Chou, E.L., Kugizaki, M., Liu, S., 2012. Greater whole-grain intake is associated with lower risk of type 2 diabetes, cardiovascular disease, and weight gain. *J. Nutr.* 142, 1304–1313. https://doi.org/10.3945/jn.111.155325

Zamaratskaia, G., Johansson, D.P., Junqueira, M.A., Deissler, L., Langton, M., Hellström, P.M., Landberg, R., 2017. Impact of sourdough fermentation on appetite and postprandial metabolic responses – A randomised cross-over trial with whole grain rye crispbread. *Br. J. Nutr.* 118, 686–697. https://doi.org/10.1017/S000711451700263X

Zeevi, D., Korem, T., Zmora, N., Israel, I.D., Rothschild, D., Weinberge, R. A., BeN-Yacov, O., LadoR, D., Avnit-Sagi, T., Lotan-Pompan, M., Suez, J., Mahdi, J. A., Mato, T. E., Malka, G., Kosower, N., Rein, M., Zilberman, Schapira, G., Dohnalová, L., Pevsner-FischeR, M., Bikovsky, R., Halpern, Z., Elinav, E., Segal, E. 2015. *Personalized nutrition by prediction of glycemic responses. Cell*, 163, 1079–1094.

Zhou, J., Hegsted, M., McCutcheon, K.L., Keenan, M.J., Xi, X., Raggio, A.M., Martin, R.J., 2006. Peptide YY and proglucagon mRNA expression patterns and regulation in the gut. *Obesity* 14, 683–689. https://doi.org/10.1038/oby.2006.77

Zhou, J., Martin, R.J., Tulley, R.T., Raggio, A.M., McCutcheon, K.L., Shen, L., Danna, S.C., Tripathy, S., Hegsted, M., Keenan, M.J., 2008. Dietary resistant starch upregulates total GLP-1 and PYY in a sustained day-long manner through fermentation in rodents. *Am. J. Physiol. Metab.* 295, E1160–E1166. https://doi.org/10.1152/ajpendo.90637.2008

Kovatcheva-Datchary, P., Nilsson, A., Akrami, R., Lee, Ying S., De VaddeR, F., Arora, T., Hallen, A., Martens, E., Björck, I. & Bäckhed, F. 2015. Dietary Fiber-Induced Improvement in Glucose Metabolism Is Associated with Increased Abundance of Prevotella. *Cell Metabolism*, 22, 971-982.

Sandberg, J. C., Björck, I. M. E. & NilssoN, A. C. 2017. Effects of whole grain rye, with and without resistant starch type 2 supplementation, on glucose tolerance, gut hormones, inflammation and appetite regulation in an 11-14.5 hour perspective; a randomized controlled study in healthy subjects. Nutrition journal, 16, 1-1125-25.

Zeevi, D., Korem, T., Zmora, N., IsraelI, D., Rothschild, D., WeinbergeR, A., BeN-Yacov, O., LadoR, D., Avnit-Sagi, T., Lotan-Pompan, M., Suez, J., Mahdi, J. A., MatoT, E., Malka, G., Kosower, N., Rein, M., ZilbermaN-Schapira, G., Dohnalová, L., PEVSNER-FischeR, M., Bikovsky, R., Halpern, Z., Elinav, E. & Segal, E. 2015. *Personalized Nutrition by Prediction of Glycemic Responses. Cell*, 163, 1079-1094.

14 Modulating Glycaemia with Cereal Products

Marion G. Priebe, Coby Eelderink, and Roel J. Vonk

University Medical Center Groningen, Groningen, The Netherlands

14.1 Introduction

Whole grain products and products with cereal fibre are associated with beneficial health effects (Aune et al. 2011; Jacobs, Jr. and Gallaher 2004; Koh-Banerjee and Rimm 2003; Priebe et al. 2008a). These health effects could be mediated by the content of cereal fibre in the products, by the presence of fibre-associated bioactive components ("co-passengers") and by the reduction of the glycemic response (Fardet 2010; Slavin 2003). Reduced postprandial glycaemia is ascribed to slow or reduced starch digestion in the small intestine. Slow or reduced starch digestion after ingestion of whole grain starchy products can be due to the presence of soluble fibre and/or to the large particle size of grains in case of products made with intact, cracked or coarsely ground grains (Holt and Miller 1994; Wood 2007). In addition to low postprandial glycaemia, reduced glycaemia is also observed after a *subsequent* meal in case of certain whole grain or cereal fibre-rich meals (the so-called second-meal effect). As repeated high glucose concentrations and related high insulin concentrations can impact insulin sensitivity and β-cell function in susceptible persons reduction of postprandial glucose and/or insulin concentrations are considered beneficial (Ludwig 2002; Willett et al. 2002). However, commonly consumed starchy foods like many breads are eliciting a high glucose and high insulin response (Fardet et al. 2006); therefore, efforts to modulate starch digestibility are highly relevant.

14.2 Postprandial glucose fluxes and hormonal responses determining glycaemia

To be able to understand how glycaemia can be modulated, it is necessary to first analyze the underlying mechanisms involved. Postprandial glycaemia after consumption of a starchy meal is determined by three different glucose fluxes (Figure 14.1), which occur at the same time.

First, glucose derived from small intestinal starch digestion is an important factor in the total glucose response. This is dependent on person-related characteristics like small-intestinal transit time, gastric emptying and intestinal α-amylase activity, but is mainly determined by food-related factors. Food-related factors, like the presence of organic acids or fat in the product (Cunningham and Read 1989; Liljeberg and Bjorck 1998) can influence the rate of gastric emptying. Soluble fibre can interfere with glucose absorption in the small

Whole Grains and Health, Second Edition. Edited by Rikard Landberg and Nathalie Scheers.

Additional materials available for download online at https://www.wiley.com/en-gb/Whole+Grains+and+Health-p-9781118939437

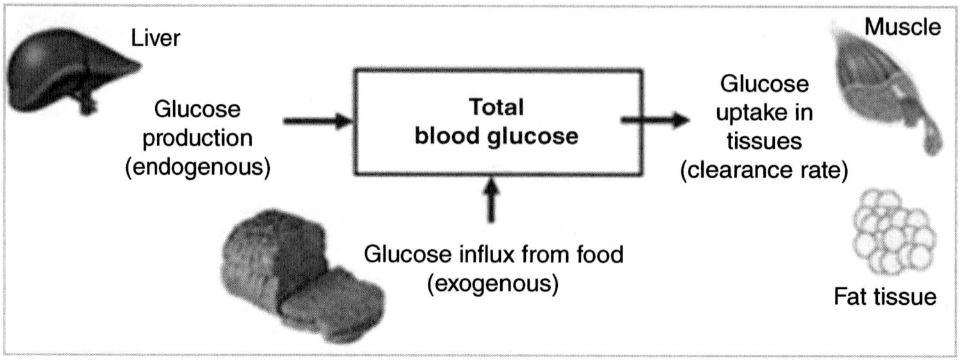

Figure 14.1 Glucose fluxes after a meal determining total blood glucose response.

intestine by increasing viscosity (Wood 2007) and the rate of starch hydrolysis can be reduced by, for example, the preservation of the physical structure of grains, choosing cultivars rich in amylose or applying processing methods that reduce the degree of gelatinization of starch (Bjorck et al. 2000).

Second, glucose produced in the liver (endogenous glucose production, EGP) contributes to postprandial glycaemia. During consumption of starchy meals, insulin is secreted and suppresses EGP. Insulin is the primary determinant of EGP and influences it mainly in a direct, but also in an indirect, manner. Indirect effects are, among others, the inhibition of secretion of glucagon, a hormone that stimulates hepatic glucose secretion, and the inhibition of the release of precursors of gluconeogenesis in the liver (non-esterified fatty acids and glycerol from adipose tissue and amino acids from muscle) (Edgerton et al. 2006). The third flux is glucose uptake into tissues, which can be insulin-independent, but is mainly stimulated by insulin. The most important factors influencing glucose uptake into tissue is the insulin sensitivity state of the individual and the degree of insulin secretion.

As insulin is a crucial driver of postprandial glucose fluxes and subsequent metabolism, it is important to realize that the insulin response is only partly determined by blood glucose. Other important determinants are the incretin hormones glucose-dependent insulinotropic polypeptide (GIP) and glucagon-like peptide (GLP-1), which can account for up to 70% of the rise in postprandial glucose-induced insulin secretion in healthy persons (Deacon and Ahren 2011). GIP is produced by the K-cells located in the proximal intestine and its secretion is stimulated by absorbable carbohydrates, protein and lipids (Holst and Orskov 2001). Schirra et al. (1996) demonstrated that GIP release is proportional to glucose delivery in the duodenum using duodenal glucose perfusion. GLP-1 is synthesized in L-cells that are found in high density in the ileum and colon, but were also reported to be present in the duodenum in comparable amounts as K-cells (Theodorakis et al. 2006). Glucose and other nutrients stimulate GLP-1 secretion and it seems that the presence of nutrients in the intestinal lumen – independent from their absorption – is sufficient to stimulate secretion (Deacon and Ahren 2011). Table 14.1 summarizes location and mode of secretion of the incretin hormones.

Thus, regulation of postprandial glycaemia is a complex process. Exploring food factors that influence this process will help to understand mechanisms that are related to health effects of whole grain/cereal fibre rich products. In addition, to be able to understand the results of attempts to modulate glycaemia, it is useful to monitor this process in detail by

Table 14.1 Overview location and mode of stimulation of GIP and GLP-1 (derived from Deacon and Ahren 2011).

	GIP	GLP-1
Secreting cells	K-cells	L-cells
Location	Throughout whole intestine, highest density in duodenum	Throughout whole intestine, highest density in ileum and colon
Stimulated by	Carbohydrates, protein and fat	Carbohydrates, protein, fat and bile acids
Mode of stimulation by carbohydrates	Rate of absorption	Mere presence

measuring glucose fluxes and hormonal responses. This opens avenues to optimize industrial processing of whole grain or cereal fibre towards health targets.

14.3 Postprandial glucose fluxes – monitoring with the stable isotope technique

Postprandial glucose fluxes can be assessed in humans with the use of stable isotopes.

In a single label study, a tracer amount of deuterated glucose (D-[6,6-$^2H_2$]-glucose) is continuously infused. This makes it possible to measure the impact of the insulin response on glucose uptake into tissue (derived from the kinetics of deuterated glucose). Thus, the rate of appearance and disappearance of total glucose (RaT and RdT, respectively) can be calculated using the one-pool, non–steady state equations of Steele (De Bodo et al. 1963; Steele et al. 1956). RaT and RdT comprise both exogenous and endogenous glucose fluxes. In addition, the glucose clearance rate can be calculated, which reflects the rate of glucose uptake into tissue relative to plasma glucose concentration (Schenk et al. 2003).

Administrating a starchy product labeled with ^{13}C makes it possible to distinguish exogenous glucose from endogenous produced glucose. When combined with the infusion of deuterated glucose (dual isotope technique), the rate of appearance and disappearance of exogenous glucose can be calculated (RaEx and RdEx, respectively) (Tissot et al. 1990). Endogenous glucose production can be derived by subtracting RaEx from RaT (Tissot et al. 1990). Figure 14.2 illustrates the course of ^2H- and ^{13}C-enrichment of glucose as compared to total glucose concentrations – all of which are used for calculating the parameters described above.

14.4 Glycaemia and underlying glucose fluxes – results of isotope studies

14.4.1 Postprandial glycaemia and glucose fluxes

There are several studies that applied stable-isotope techniques to monitor glucose fluxes after consumption of starchy products. Results of some of these studies are summarized in the following.

In a single label study, Schenk et al. (2003) explored the glucose fluxes of two breakfast cereals with different glycemic index (GI) and wheat fibre content: corn flakes (GI 131.5 ± 33.0, 1.6 g total fibre/portion) and bran flakes (GI: 54.5 ± 7.2, 38.5 g total fibre/portion) in

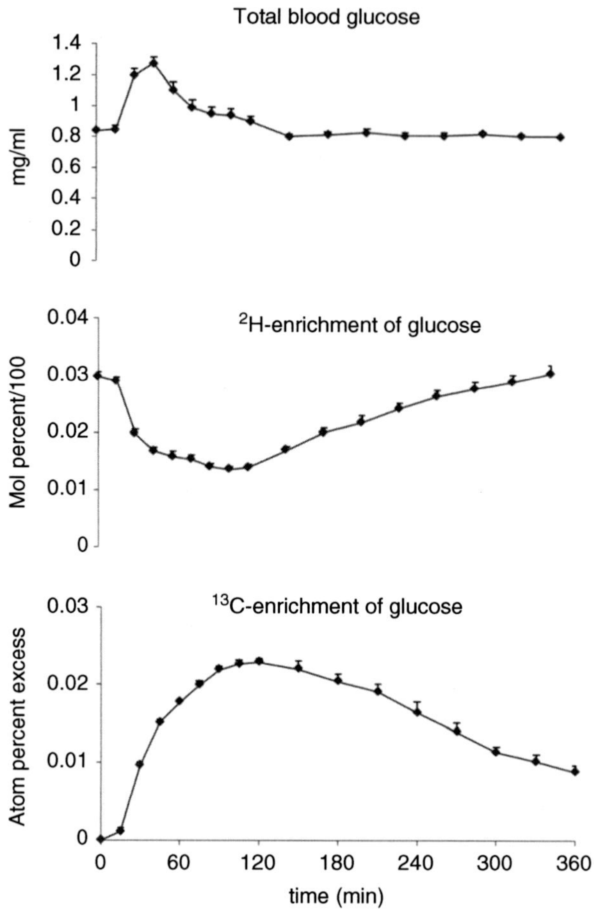

Figure 14.2 Total glucose, ^{2}H- and ^{13}C-enrichment of glucose after ingestion of 138 g of fibre-rich bread (n = 9, mean ± SD).

a cross-over manner in six healthy males. Unexpectedly, they did not find a difference in the rate of appearance of total glucose, but an early increase of the rate of disappearance of total glucose after bran flakes, explaining the difference in total blood glucose response. The 180-min areas under the curves of insulin were not different but an early (t = 0 – 20 min) and marked insulin response after the bran flakes was observed, which strongly correlated with this early increase in glucose clearance. This effect was hypothesized to be due to the higher wheat protein content of bran flakes (15.4 vs. 4.3 g).

Nazare et al. (2010) conducted a dual isotope study in 2 groups of 19 healthy overweight persons in a parallel manner and compared glucose kinetics after ^{13}C-labeled low GI breakfast biscuits (GI 47) with that after "high" GI breakfast flakes (GI 66). Biscuits and flakes were consumed with half-skimmed milk, and the breakfasts did not differ in dietary fibre or macronutrient composition. In this study, glycaemia was lower after the biscuits. This could be explained by a markedly lower rate of appearance of exogenous glucose, despite the fact that endogenous glucose production was less suppressed and the rate of disappearance of total glucose slower after the biscuits. Similar results were obtained in a cross-over study in 16 healthy young women comparing the postprandial glucose kinetics after consumption of ^{13}C-labeled extruded cereals with a low content of slowly digestible starch (SDS, 0,3 %) with that of biscuits with a high content of slowly digestible starch (39–45 % SDS) (Peronnet et al. 2015). The only difference was that, in this population, the endogenous glucose production was more suppressed after the biscuits.

The dual isotope technique was applied to monitor the rate of glucose appearance after the ingestion of ^{13}C- labeled whole meal wheat bread in comparison to that of ^{13}C- labeled glucose (Priebe et al. 2008b) in four healthy males in a cross-over manner. Total glycaemia was lower after bread than after glucose, but did not reach statistically significance – probably because of the few subjects and the known high variability in postprandial glucose responses. The rate of appearance of total glucose, however, was statistically significant lower after bread, whereas the rate of appearance of exogenous glucose was the same after both test products in the early postprandial phase (0–2 h). Endogenous glucose production, which was more suppressed after bread, could explain the lower rate of appearance of total glucose. In addition, it was found that the influx of exogenous glucose was higher after wheat bread in the late postprandial phase (2–4 h) and comparable to that of uncooked corn starch measured in a previous study (Wachters-Hagedoorn et al. 2006). This indicated that the starch in the wholemeal wheat bread was partly rapidly and partly slowly digestible, which could not be derived from in vitro determination of starch digestibility.

In another dual isotope study, glucose kinetics after ingestion of ^{13}C- labeled fibre-rich pasta and wheat bread (Eelderink et al. 2012a; Eelderink et al. 2012b) was explored. The cross-over study in 10 healthy males showed that total blood glucose after both products was the same, despite the fact that the rate of appearance of exogenous glucose was lower after pasta than after bread. The endogenous glucose production was slightly more suppressed after pasta than after bread and could therefore not explain the difference in glycaemia. However, after pasta, the uptake of glucose into tissue (glucose clearance) was much slower than after wheat bread and by that it "counterbalanced" the slow rate of appearance of exogenous glucose. The result was a similar glycemic response after both products. To investigate the impact of a more compact food structure on postprandial glucose kinetics a flat bread was tested and compared with the results of wheat bread (low density) and pasta (high density) (Eelderink et al. 2015). The glucose and insulin response after the flat bread resembled that of pasta whereas the rate of appearance of exogenous glucose was lower only in the first hour. The uptake of glucose into tissue was similar to that after wheat bread and unexpectedly high given the low insulin response, indicating either increased peripheral insulin sensitivity or increased insulin-independent glucose absorption.

Boers et al. (2017) conducted a dual isotope study to investigate the effect of fibre additions to flatbread flour mixes on glucose kinetics in a cross-over study in 12 healthy men. ^{13}C-labeled control flat breads were compared to flat breads in which 15% chickpea flour and 2% (GG2) or 4% (GG4) guar gum was incorporated. GG4-breads significantly reduced the rate of all the kinetic parameters as well as postprandial glucose response compared to the control breads, whereas the GG2-breads had minor effects.

These studies demonstrate that:

- a low glycemic response is *not necessarily* caused by a slow digestion rate of starch;
- a difference in either endogenous glucose production or rate of glucose uptake into tissues can explain a difference in total blood glucose response; and
- slow digestion of starch does not necessarily result in lower glycaemia because a slower uptake of glucose into tissue can counterbalance the slow digestion.

14.4.2 Second-meal glycaemia and glucose fluxes

Several studies demonstrated that certain starchy foods are able to lower the glycemic response after a subsequent meal. Dependent on the timing of the subsequent meal, these studies can be divided in the "early second-meal studies" and "the overnight second-meal studies."

Early second-meal studies investigate the effect of a breakfast on glycaemia of a standardized lunch (Brighenti et al. 2006; Liljeberg and Bjorck 2000; Liljeberg et al. 1999; Nilsson et al. 2008a; Tissot et al. 1990; Wolever et al. 1995). Based on the results of these studies, it seems that glycaemia at lunch can be modulated with breakfasts with a low GI. Breakfasts with a GI lower than 69 resulted in lower glycaemia at lunch independent of the amount of resistant starch and dietary fibre in the breakfast products. It is proposed that insulin sensitivity at lunch could be increased due to lower plasma concentrations of non-esterified fatty acids (NEFA) before lunch as observed by Wolever et al. (1995). After a low GI meal, the short decrease of glucose concentrations below baseline, which is normally occurring after a high GI meal, is prevented. The subsequent release of counter-regulatory hormones, which stimulates the release of NEFA from adipose tissue, is therefore also blunted and can explain the lower concentrations of NEFA (Wolever et al. 1995). This is a plausible explanation, however, none of these studies was conducted with a stable-isotope technique, therefore the effects on the glucose kinetics at lunch are not known and improved insulin sensitivity could not yet be demonstrated.

A large number of overnight second-meal studies investigated the effect of an evening meal on glycaemia at a following standardized breakfast (Nilsson et al. 2006; Nilsson et al. 2007; Nilsson et al. 2008a; Nilsson et al. 2008b; Robertson et al. 2003; Stevenson et al. 2005; Stevenson et al. 2007; Weickert et al. 2005; Wolever et al. 1995). Contrary to the early second-meal studies, glycaemia after the standard breakfasts was not related to the GI of the evening meal and the presence of a high amount of resistant starch and cereal fibre (13.4–81 g) seemed to be more important. To clarify the underlying mechanism of the reduced glycaemia at breakfast a dual isotope study was conducted in 10 healthy male with ^{13}C-labeled glucose (50 g) as standard breakfast and barley kernels or white wheat bread as evening meal (Priebe et al. 2010). The plasma glucose response after the glucose load in the morning was 29% lower after the barley evening meal. The endogenous glucose production and the insulin response was the same, whereas the uptake of glucose into the tissue was 30% higher after the barley evening meal, indicating higher peripheral insulin sensitivity. Fasting NEFA concentrations were not different, which was consistent with the results of three other overnight second-meal studies (Nilsson et al. 2007; Robertson et al. 2003; Weickert et al. 2005), but inconsistent with those of three other similar studies (Nilsson et al. 2006; Stevenson et al. 2007; Thorburn et al. 1993). Hydrogen excretion in the breath, an indicator of colonic carbohydrate fermentation, as well as plasma butyrate concentrations were higher in the morning after the barley evening meal supporting the hypothesis that colonic fermentation might be involved in the overnight second-meal effect.

Thus, in summary, decreasing glycaemia after an early subsequent meal can be achieved by starchy food with a low GI and it is thought that improved insulin sensitivity causes this effect. Starchy foods rich in resistant starch and cereal fibre have been shown to decrease glycaemia in an overnight perspective. Increased glucose uptake into tissue has been demonstrated to cause this effect, indicating increased insulin sensitivity, which could be caused by products of colonic fermentation.

14.4.3 Postprandial glycaemia and hormonal response

Approaches to lower postprandial glycaemia are expected to also lower postprandial insulinemia. Indeed, in general it is observed that kinetics of the insulin response follow that of the glucose response after ingestion of starchy products (without addition of milk products) (Bjorck et al. 2000). Products with a low GI generally also have a low insulinemic index (Bjorck et al. 2000). However, there are several studies reporting no difference in glycaemia but an unexpected lower postprandial insulinemia after certain starchy products as compared to the control. A reduced postprandial insulin response, despite a high glucose response, could be also considered as being beneficial as it would be less demanding for the pancreatic β-cells (Willett et al. 2002). Furthermore, a reduced postprandial insulin response would prevent postprandial hypoglycaemia leading to increased food intake (Ludwig 2002) and could play a role in preventing insulin resistance (Zammit et al. 2001). In addition, diets with a low-insulin demand were reported to beneficially affect plasma lipids especially in obese (Nimptsch et al. 2011), prevent an increase in body fat during puberty (Joslowski et al. 2012) and assist weight loss in obese, insulin-resistant adolescents (Joslowski et al. 2015).

The consumption of differently processed wheat breads resulted in a similar glucose response, but lower insulin response in comparison with conventional breads (Rizkalla et al. 2007). In addition, whole-wheat pasta and several rye breads elicited glycemic responses comparable to that of white wheat bread, whereas the insulin responses were significantly lower (Juntunen et al. 2002; Juntunen et al. 2003; Leinonen et al. 1999). Furthermore, consumption of fresh fibre-rich pasta resulted in the same blood glucose response, but lower insulin response than that after fibre-rich wheat bread (Eelderink et al. 2012b). The lower insulin response could be due to a lower response in incretin hormones. Indeed, lower GIP concentrations were observed after the rye breads and the two types of pasta as compared to the control breads concentrations (Eelderink et al. 2012b; Juntunen et al. 2002; Juntunen et al. 2003). The question then arises: What are the characteristics of the starchy products that result in a lower GIP and consequently in a lower insulin response?

14.5 Food factors influencing GIP release

Duodenal infusion studies with glucose showed that GIP secretion is dependent on the glucose load (Pilichiewicz et al. 2007; Trahair et al. 2012). In accordance with that, GIP concentrations were positively correlated with the rate of appearance of exogenous glucose in the study with fibre-rich pasta (Eelderink et al. 2012b; Eelderink et al. 2015) and high-SDS biscuits (Peronnet et al. 2015). Glucose fluxes were not assessed in the studies with rye breads, whole-wheat pasta and wheat breads, but slower gastric emptying or starch digestion were assumed to be due to specific characteristics of these products. The lower insulin response after consumption of the breads with added rye kernels (60 %), added β-glucan (20%) and whole-wheat pasta as compared to white wheat bread was explained by "structural and compositional properties of fibre" and not the amount of fibre (Juntunen et al. 2002). These results were confirmed in a second study (Juntunen et al. 2003) in which endosperm rye bread, traditional rye bread and high-fibre rye bread was compared to white wheat bread. In both studies, the in vitro hydrolysis index of starch from the different products was determined and found to be lower compared to control for all but one product (rye bread with β-glucan) – indicating slower starch digestion. Rizkalla et al. (2007) explained the lower insulin response after a traditional French bread compared to that of a conventional French bread to the modified texture. The crumb of the traditional French bread was more rigid, tense and with irregular alveoli due to the artisanal processing procedure, which might have decreased the rate of starch digestion. The reason for the lower insulin response after the French bread fermented with sourdough was assumed to be due to a slower gastric emptying rate as consequence of the presence of organic acids in the bread. Thus, it can be concluded that as a consequence of a slower delivery of starch to the small intestine, a slower digestion of starch or a slower absorption of starch-derived glucose less GIP is secreted, which results in a lower insulin response. As a consequence of that glucose uptake into tissue is also reduced – as assessed in the study with fibre-rich pasta – and can explain the discrepancy with the total blood glucose response (Eelderink et al. 2012b).

14.6 Food factors influencing GLP-1 release

Next to lower concentrations of GIP, lower concentrations of GLP-1 could also have contributed to the lower insulin response. However, GLP-1 concentrations were only monitored in the studies with rye-bread and whole-wheat pasta (Juntunen et al. 2002; Juntunen et al. 2003) and showed inconsistent effects. In agreement with lower GIP values, peak concentrations of GLP-1 were lower after the whole-wheat pasta and high-fibre rye bread compared to control. However, after the β-glucan bread the GLP-1 response – in contrary to the GIP response – was not different compared to the control (Juntunen et al. 2002). No differences in GLP-1 concentrations were found after different rye breads as compared to the control bread except of higher concentrations at t = 150 and 180 min after the high fibre bread, whereas GIP concentrations were lower after the rye breads (Juntunen et al. 2003). These observations are in agreement with that of Bakhoj et al. (2003) who also found differential effects of GIP and GLP-1 after different breads (Einkorn and wheat). Thus, the exact role of GLP-1 contributing to the insulin response in these studies is not clear. Differential effects of the GIP and GLP-1 response can be expected based on the mode of stimulation of their secretion and the location of the incretin releasing cells. It has been shown that GLP-1 is only secreted when the carbohydrate load reaching the small intestine is high (2,5 kcal/min) (Schirra et al. 1996) and when a long segment (>60 cm) of the small intestine is exposed to carbohydrates in contrary to GIP when a load of 1 kcal/min and an exposure of <60 cm is enough (Little et al. 2006). Thus, presence of carbohydrates in the more distal small intestine should stimulate GLP-1 release. In agreement with that, a late and prolonged increase of GLP-1 was seen, for example, when digestion of sucrose was delayed by the α-glucosidase inhibitor acarbose (Qualmann et al. 1995; Seifarth et al. 1998) and after consumption of slowly digestible uncooked corn starch (Wachters-Hagedoorn et al. 2006). However, when sugars or starch are ingested in a complex food matrix the GLP-1 stimulating effects seem to be less clear. Starchy foods often contain different types of fibre which can or cannot influence viscosity of the small intestinal contents. In case of products rich in soluble fibre, viscosity was shown to influence GLP-1 secretion as a 300 ml high viscosity drink (30 g oat β-glucan) with the same macronutrient composition and energy density (300 kcal) as a low viscosity drink (30 g oat β-glucan treated with 0.2 g of β-glucanase enzyme [endo-(1,4)- ß-glucanase) resulted in a lower GLP-1 response (Zijlstra et al. 2008). In contrast, studies investigating the effect of soluble fibres in solid meals do not show consistent effects (Frost et al. 2003; Karhunen et al. 2010; Klosterbuer et al. 2012; Lafond et al. 2015; Raben et al. 1994), also perhaps because they are quite diverse as to the amount and type of soluble fibre used. Furthermore, the particle size of fibre or grains may play a role. Substitution of 85% fibre-enriched wheat flour by broken kernels in bread has been shown to result in a lower GLP-1 responses, whereas no differences in postprandial glucose, insulin, GIP and glucose kinetics were observed (Eelderink et al. 2017). In addition to the presence of nutrients, GLP-1 release in the small intestine can also be stimulated by bile acids. Bile acids are secreted after ingestion of a meal and it was shown that activation of the bile acid receptor TGR5 can potentiate GLP-1 release (Rafferty et al. 2011; Thomas et al. 2009). As fibre was shown to have bile acid–binding capacity (Story and Kritchevsky 1976), it is hypothesized that by means of preventing bile acid reabsorption prolonged exposure to bile acids could contribute to increased GLP-1 release. However, differential effects of various types of fibre, as well of different particle sizes (Kahlon et al. 2006) can be expected. To date, there is little information about the relationship between postprandial plasma concentrations of bile acid and GLP-1 after fibre-rich products in humans. Eelderink et al. (2017) found a moderate correlation between bile acids and GLP-1 after a fibre-rich wheat bread that was lower after a bread in which 85% of the wheat flour was substituted by broken kernels. The concentrations of bile acids tended to be lower after the kernel bread and large inter-individual differences were shown.

To summarize, certain product characteristics lower postprandial insulinemia without having an effect on glycaemia. This effect is influenced by a modulated release of incretin hormones. GIP secretion is related especially to the rate of appearance of starch-derived glucose, whereas the mode of stimulation of GLP-1 after starchy foods is apparently very complex. Presence of dietary fibre in food products could modulate the response and this makes it impossible to predict the GLP-1 response based on studies with carbohydrates that were administered without a food matrix.

14.7 Conclusion

Based on the underlying physical processes regulating postprandial glycaemia, glycaemia can be modulated by targeting exogenous glucose appearance, endogenous glucose production and uptake of glucose into tissue as well as the insulin and incretin response. Studies examining glucose fluxes after starchy products with stable isotopes are limited and the incretin response is not always assessed. So far, results indicate that the decrease of glycaemia after consumption of starchy products can be due to slow starch digestion (Nazare et al. 2010; Peronnet et al. 2015), as expected. However, decreased glycaemia can also be caused by increased glucose uptake into tissue, either through increased insulin sensitivity (overnight second-meal studies) (Priebe et al. 2010) or increased initial insulin response (Schenk et al. 2003), which is related to the presence of resistant starch/cereal fibre or protein in the food products, respectively. Furthermore, the effect of slow starch digestion on glycaemia can apparently be "counterbalanced" by a slow tissue uptake of glucose caused by a low GIP-related insulin response. As result, glycaemia is not altered and comparable to that of a product with rapidly digestible starch (Eelderink et al. 2012b). Apparently, to achieve low glycaemia, starch digestibility needs to be even lower than in this study or the glucose uptake rate less reduced.

14.8 General implications

An important fact seems to be that slow starch digestion is not per se reflected by total blood glucose concentrations. Results of studies using this parameter to assess the effect of, for example, different types of fibre or certain processing methods on intestinal glucose absorption or the rate and extent of starch digestion need to be interpreted with caution. Thus, monitoring glucose fluxes seems to be necessary in experimental studies examining underlying mechanisms.

Another implication of this fact is that not only the glycemic response should be considered when assessing health-related effects of starchy foods. Products exerting the same relatively high postprandial glucose concentration can have differential effects on other metabolic parameters due to differences in underlying glucose kinetics. Examples of this are products eliciting the same postprandial glucose concentration but differing in starch digestibility. The resulting differential GIP and insulin responses affect metabolism in different ways. This was already addressed by the formulation of an insulinemic index (Indar-Brown et al. 1992). In addition to beneficial effects of lower insulin concentrations, beneficial effects of lower GIP concentration could be expected. Besides its role as incretin hormone, elevated GIP concentrations are implicated with a number of deleterious effects, for example, promotion of fatty liver, increased fat storage in adipose tissue, increased insulin resistance and postprandial inflammation (Asmar et al. 2010; Asmar et al. 2017; Deacon and Ahren 2011; Gogebakan et al. 2015; Musso et al. 2009; Pfeiffer and Keyhani-Nejad 2018).

Whereas GIP secretion can be linked to the rate of glucose absorption also in intervention studies with starchy foods, it is until now not clear how characteristics of starchy foods influence GLP-1 release. In addition, it is difficult to define in which direction modulation of GLP-1 secretion should be seen as beneficial. In view of advantageous low insulin concentrations, a lower GLP-1 response could be regarded as advantageous. But increased GLP-1 concentrations also have positive effects because GLP-1 is implicated with, for example, decreased gastric emptying, decreased food intake and beneficial cardiovascular actions (Deacon and Ahren 2011).

Thus, processing methods that reduce starch digestibility have the potency to influence health-related processes not only by modulating glycaemia, but also by modulating the insulin and incretin response.

14.9 References

Asmar, M., Asmar, A., Simonsen, L., Gasbjerg, L.S., Sparre-Ulrich, A.H., Rosenkilde, M.M., Hartmann, B., Dela, F., Holst, J.J., & Bulow, J. 2017. The gluco- and liporegulatory and vasodilatory effects of glucose-dependent insulinotropic polypeptide (GIP) are abolished by an antagonist of the human GIP receptor. *Diabetes*, 66, (9) 2363–2371 available from: PM:28667118.

Asmar, M., Simonsen, L., Madsbad, S., Stallknecht, B., Holst, J.J., & Bulow, J. 2010. Glucose-dependent insulinotropic polypeptide may enhance fatty acid re-esterification in subcutaneous abdominal adipose tissue in lean humans. *Diabetes*, 59, (9) 2160–2163 available from: PM:20547981.

Aune, D., Chan, D.S., Lau, R., Vieira, R., Greenwood, D.C., Kampman, E., & Norat, T. 2011. Dietary fibre, whole grains, and risk of colorectal cancer: Systematic review and dose-response meta-analysis of prospective studies. *BMJ*, 343, d6617 available from: PM:22074852.

Bakhoj, S., Flint, A., Holst, J.J., & Tetens, I. 2003. Lower glucose-dependent insulinotropic polypeptide (GIP) response but similar glucagon-like peptide 1 (GLP-1), glycaemic, and insulinaemic response to ancient wheat compared to modern wheat depends on processing. *Eur J Clin Nutr*, 57, (10) 1254–1261 available from: PM:14506486.

Bjorck, I., Liljeberg, H., & Ostman, E. 2000. Low glycaemic-index foods. *Br.J.Nutr.*, 83 Suppl 1, S149–S155 available from: PM:10889806.

Boers, H.M., van Dijk, T.H., Hiemstra, H., Hoogenraad, A.R., Mela, D.J., Peters, H.P.F., Vonk, R.J., & Priebe, M.G. 2017. Effect of fibre additions to flatbread flour mixes on glucose kinetics: A randomised controlled trial. *Br.J.Nutr.*, 118, (10) 777–787 available from: PM:29110741.

Brighenti, F., Benini, L., Del Rio, D., Casiraghi, C., Pellegrini, N., Scazzina, F., Jenkins, D.J., & Vantini, I. 2006. Colonic fermentation of indigestible carbohydrates contributes to the second-meal effect. Am.J Clin.Nutr., 83, (4) 817–822 available from: PM:16600933.

Cunningham, K.M. & Read, N.W. 1989. The effect of incorporating fat into different components of a meal on gastric emptying and postprandial blood glucose and insulin responses. *Br J Nutr*, 61, (2) 285–290 available from: PM:2650735.

De Bodo, R.C., Steele, R., Altszuler, N., Dunn, A., & Bishop, J.S. 1963. On the hormonal regulation of carbohydrate metabolism: Studies with C14 gluocse. *Recent.Prog.Horm.Res.*, 19, 445–448.

Deacon, C.F. & Ahren, B. 2011. Physiology of incretins in health and disease. *Rev Diabet.Stud*, 8, (3) 293–306 available from: PM:22262068.

Edgerton, D.S., Lautz, M., Scott, M., Everett, C.A., Stettler, K.M., Neal, D.W., Chu, C.A., & Cherrington, A.D. 2006. Insulin's direct effects on the liver dominate the control of hepatic glucose production. *J Clin Invest*, 116, (2) 521–527 available from: PM:16453026.

Eelderink, C., Moerdijk-Poortvliet, T.C., Wang, H., Schepers, M., Preston, T., Boer, T., Vonk, R.J., Schierbeek, H., & Priebe, M.G. 2012a. The glycemic response does not reflect the in vivo starch digestibility of fiber-rich wheat products in healthy men. *J Nutr*, 142, (2) 258–263 available from: PM:22223569.

Eelderink, C., Noort, M.W., Sozer, N., Koehorst, M., Holst, J.J., Deacon, C.F., Rehfeld, J.F., Poutanen, K., Vonk, R.J., Oudhuis, L., & Priebe, M.G. 2015. The structure of wheat bread influences the postprandial metabolic response in healthy men. *Food Funct.*, 6, (10) 3236–3248 available from: PM:26288992.

Eelderink, C., Noort, M.W., Sozer, N., Koehorst, M., Holst, J.J., Deacon, C.F., Rehfeld, J.F., Poutanen, K., Vonk, R.J., Oudhuis, L., & Priebe, M.G. 2017. Difference in postprandial GLP-1 response despite similar glucose kinetics after consumption of wheat breads with different particle size in healthy men. *Eur.J.Nutr.*, 56, (3) 1063–1076 available from: PM:26857762.

Eelderink, C., Schepers, M., Preston, T., Vonk, R.J., Oudhuis, L., & Priebe, M.G. 2012b. Slowly and rapidly digestible starchy foods can elicit a similar glycemic response because of differential tissue glucose uptake in healthy men. *Am J Clin Nutr*, 96, (5) 1017–1024 available from: PM:22990033.

Fardet, A. 2010. New hypotheses for the health-protective mechanisms of whole-grain cereals: What is beyond fibre? *Nutr Res Rev*, 23, (1) 65–134 available from: PM:20565994.

Fardet, A., Leenhardt, F., Lioger, D., Scalbert, A., & Remesy, C. 2006. Parameters controlling the glycaemic response to breads. *Nutr Res Rev*, 19, (1) 18–25 available from: PM:19079873.

Frost, G.S., Brynes, A.E., Dhillo, W.S., Bloom, S.R., & McBurney, M.I. 2003. The effects of fiber enrichment of pasta and fat content on gastric emptying, GLP-1, glucose, and insulin responses to a meal. *Eur J Clin Nutr*, 57, (2) 293–298 available from: PM:12571662.

Gogebakan, O., Osterhoff, M.A., Schuler, R., Pivovarova, O., Kruse, M., Seltmann, A.C., Mosig, A.S., Rudovich, N., Nauck, M., & Pfeiffer, A.F. 2015. GIP increases adipose tissue expression and blood levels of MCP-1 in humans and links high energy diets to inflammation: A randomised trial. *Diabetologia*, 58, (8) 1759–1768 available from: PM:25994074.

Holst, J.J. & Orskov, C. 2001. Incretin hormones – An update. *Scand J Clin Lab Invest Suppl*, 234, 75–85 available from: PM:11713984 .

Holt, S.H. & Miller, J.B. 1994. Particle size, satiety and the glycaemic response. *Eur J Clin Nutr*, 48, (7) 496–502 available from: PM:7956991.

Indar-Brown, K., Noreberg, C., & Madar, Z. 1992. Glycemic and insulinemic responses after ingestion of ethnic foods by NIDDM and healthy subjects. *Am J Clin Nutr*, 55, (1) 89–95 available from: PM:1728824.

Jacobs, D.R., Jr. & Gallaher, D.D. 2004. Whole grain intake and cardiovascular disease: A review. *Curr. Atheroscler.Rep.*, 6, (6) 415–423 available from: PM:15485586.

Joslowski, G., Goletzke, J., Cheng, G., Gunther, A.L., Bao, J., Brand-Miller, J.C., & Buyken, A.E. 2012. Prospective associations of dietary insulin demand, glycemic index, and glycemic load during puberty with body composition in young adulthood. Int J Obes.(Lond), 36, (11) 1463–1471 available from: PM:22249223.

Joslowski, G., Halim, J., Goletzke, J., Gow, M., Ho, M., Louie, J.C., Buyken, A.E., Cowell, C.T., & Garnett, S.P. 2015. Dietary glycemic load, insulin load, and weight loss in obese, insulin resistant adolescents: RESIST study. *Clin.Nutr.*, 34(1), 89–94.

Juntunen, K.S., Laaksonen, D.E., Autio, K., Niskanen, L.K., Holst, J.J., Savolainen, K.E., Liukkonen, K.H., Poutanen, K.S., & Mykkanen, H.M. 2003. Structural differences between rye and wheat breads but not total fiber content may explain the lower postprandial insulin response to rye bread. *Am.J.Clin.Nutr.*, 78, (5) 957–-964 available from: PM:14594782.

Juntunen, K.S., Niskanen, L.K., Liukkonen, K.H., Poutanen, K.S., Holst, J.J., & Mykkanen, H.M. 2002. Postprandial glucose, insulin, and incretin responses to grain products in healthy subjects. *Am.J.Clin.Nutr.*, 75, (2) 254–262 available from: PM:11815315.

Kahlon, T., de Berrios, J., Smith, G., & Pan, J. 2006. In vitro bile acid binding capacity of milled wheat bran and milled extruded wheat bran at five specific mechanical energy levels. *Cereal Chem*, 83, 434–438.

Karhunen, L.J., Juvonen, K.R., Flander, S.M., Liukkonen, K.H., Lahteenmaki, L., Siloaho, M., Laaksonen, D.E., Herzig, K.H., Uusitupa, M.I., & Poutanen, K.S. 2010. A psyllium fiber-enriched meal strongly attenuates postprandial gastrointestinal peptide release in healthy young adults. *J Nutr*, 140, (4) 737–744 available from: PM:20147463.

Klosterbuer, A.S., Thomas, W., & Slavin, J.L. 2012. Resistant starch and pullulan reduce postprandial glucose, insulin, and GLP-1, but have no effect on satiety in healthy humans. *J Agric.Food Chem*, 60, (48) 11928–11934 available from: PM:23136915.

Koh-Banerjee, P. & Rimm, E.B. 2003. Whole grain consumption and weight gain: A review of the epidemiological evidence, potential mechanisms and opportunities for future research. *Proc Nutr.Soc*, 62, (1) 25–29 available from: PM:12740053.

Lafond, D.W., Greaves, K.A., Maki, K.C., Leidy, H.J., & Romsos, D.R. 2015. Effects of two dietary fibers as part of ready-to-eat cereal (RTEC) breakfasts on perceived appetite and gut hormones in overweight women. *Nutrients.*, 7, (2) 1245–1266 available from: PM:25689743.

Leinonen, K., Liukkonen, K., Poutanen, K., Uusitupa, M., & Mykkanen, H. 1999. Rye bread decreases postprandial insulin response but does not alter glucose response in healthy Finnish subjects. *Eur J Clin Nutr*, 53, (4) 262–267 available from: PM:10334650.

Liljeberg, H. & Bjorck, I. 1998. Delayed gastric emptying rate may explain improved glycaemia in healthy subjects to a starchy meal with added vinegar. *Eur J Clin Nutr*, 52, (5) 368–371 available from: PM:9630389.

Liljeberg, H. & Bjorck, I. 2000. Effects of a low-glycaemic index spaghetti meal on glucose tolerance and lipaemia at a subsequent meal in healthy subjects. *Eur.J Clin.Nutr.*, 54, (1) 24–28 available from: PM:10694768.

Liljeberg, H.G., Akerberg, A.K., & Bjorck, I.M. 1999. Effect of the glycemic index and content of indigestible carbohydrates of cereal-based breakfast meals on glucose tolerance at lunch in healthy subjects. *Am.J Clin. Nutr.*, 69, (4) 647-655 available from: PM:10197565.

Little, T.J., Doran, S., Meyer, J.H., Smout, A.J., O'Donovan, D.G., Wu, K.L., Jones, K.L., Wishart, J., Rayner, C.K., Horowitz, M., & Feinle-Bisset, C. 2006. The release of GLP-1 and ghrelin, but not GIP and CCK, by glucose is dependent upon the length of small intestine exposed. *Am J Physiol Endocrinol.Metab*, 291, (3) E647–E655 available from: PM:16684852.

Ludwig, D.S. 2002. The glycemic index: Physiological mechanisms relating to obesity, diabetes, and cardiovascular disease. *JAMA*, 287, (18) 2414–2423 available from: PM:11988062.

Musso, G., Gambino, R., Pacini, G., De, M.F., & Cassader, M. 2009. Prolonged saturated fat-induced, glucose-dependent insulinotropic polypeptide elevation is associated with adipokine imbalance and liver injury in nonalcoholic steatohepatitis: Dysregulated enteroadipocyte axis as a novel feature of fatty liver. *Am.J.Clin.Nutr.*, 89, (2) 558–567 available from: PM:19141695.

Nazare, J.A., de, R.A., Normand, S., Sauvinet, V., Sothier, M., Vinoy, S., Desage, M., & Laville, M. 2010. Effect of postprandial modulation of glucose availability: Short- and long-term analysis. *Br J Nutr*, 103, (10) 1461–1470 available from: PM:20030904.

Nilsson, A., Granfeldt, Y., Ostman, E., Preston, T., & Bjorck, I. 2006. Effects of GI and content of indigestible carbohydrates of cereal-based evening meals on glucose tolerance at a subsequent standardised breakfast. *Eur.J Clin.Nutr.*, 60, (9) 1092–1099 available from: PM:16523203.

Nilsson, A., Ostman, E., Preston, T., & Bjorck, I. 2007. Effects of GI vs content of cereal fibre of the evening meal on glucose tolerance at a subsequent standardized breakfast. *Eur.J Clin.Nutr.* available from: PM:17522615.

Nilsson, A.C., Ostman, E.M., Granfeldt, Y., & Bjorck, I.M. 2008a. Effect of cereal test breakfasts differing in glycemic index and content of indigestible carbohydrates on daylong glucose tolerance in healthy subjects. *Am.J Clin.Nutr.*, 87, (3) 645–654 available from: PM:18326603.

Nilsson, A.C., Ostman, E.M., Holst, J.J., & Bjorck, I.M. 2008b. Including indigestible carbohydrates in the evening meal of healthy subjects improves glucose tolerance, lowers inflammatory markers, and increases satiety after a subsequent standardized breakfast. *J Nutr.*, 138, (4) 732–739 available from: PM:18356328.

Nimptsch, K., Brand-Miller, J.C., Franz, M., Sampson, L., Willett, W.C., & Giovannucci, E. 2011. Dietary insulin index and insulin load in relation to biomarkers of glycemic control, plasma lipids, and inflammation markers. *Am J Clin Nutr*, 94, (1) 182–190 available from: PM:21543531.

Peronnet, F., Meynier, A., Sauvinet, V., Normand, S., Bourdon, E., Mignault, D., St-Pierre, D.H., Laville, M., Rabasa-Lhoret, R., & Vinoy, S. 2015. Plasma glucose kinetics and response of insulin and GIP following a cereal breakfast in female subjects: Effect of starch digestibility. *Eur.J.Clin.Nutr.*, 69, (6) 740–745 available from: PM:25852025.

Pfeiffer, A.F.H. & Keyhani-Nejad, F. 2018. High glycemic index metabolic damage – A pivotal role of GIP and GLP-1. *Trends Endocrinol.Metab*, 29, (5) 289–299 available from: PM:29602522.

Pilichiewicz, A.N., Chaikomin, R., Brennan, I.M., Wishart, J.M., Rayner, C.K., Jones, K.L., Smout, A.J., Horowitz, M., & Feinle-Bisset, C. 2007. Load-dependent effects of duodenal glucose on glycemia, gastrointestinal hormones, antropyloroduodenal motility, and energy intake in healthy men. *Am.J Physiol Endocrinol. Metab*, 293, (3) E743–E753 available from: PM:17609258.

Priebe, M.G., van Binsbergen, J.J., de, V.R., & Vonk, R.J. 2008a. Whole grain foods for the prevention of type 2 diabetes mellitus. *Cochrane.Database.Syst.Rev* (1) CD006061 available from: PM:18254091.

Priebe, M.G., Wachters-Hagedoorn, R.E., Heimweg, J.A., Small, A., Preston, T., Elzinga, H., Stellaard, F., & Vonk, R.J. 2008b. An explorative study of in vivo digestive starch characteristics and postprandial glucose kinetics of wholemeal wheat bread. *Eur J Nutr*, 47, (8) 417–423 available from: PM:18853232.

Priebe, M.G., Wang, H., Weening, D., Schepers, M., Preston, T., & Vonk, R.J. 2010. Factors related to colonic fermentation of nondigestible carbohydrates of a previous evening meal increase tissue glucose uptake and moderate glucose-associated inflammation. *Am J Clin Nutr*, 91, (1) 90–97 available from: PM:19889821.

Qualmann, C., Nauck, M.A., Holst, J.J., Orskov, C., & Creutzfeldt, W. 1995. Glucagon-like peptide 1 (7-36 amide) secretion in response to luminal sucrose from the upper and lower gut: A study using alpha-glucosidase inhibition (acarbose). *Scand J Gastroenterol*, 30, (9) 892–896 available from: PM:8578189 .

Raben, A., Christensen, N.J., Madsen, J., Holst, J.J., & Astrup, A. 1994. Decreased postprandial thermogenesis and fat oxidation but increased fullness after a high-fiber meal compared with a low-fiber meal. *Am J Clin Nutr*, 59, (6) 1386–1394 available from: PM:8198065.

Rafferty, E.P., Wylie, A.R., Hand, K.H., Elliott, C.E., Grieve, D.J., & Green, B.D. 2011. Investigating the effects of physiological bile acids on GLP-1 secretion and glucose tolerance in normal and GLP-1R(-/-) mice. *Biol. Chem*, 392, (6) 539–546 available from: PM:21521075.

Rizkalla, S.W., Laromiguiere, M., Champ, M., Bruzzo, F., Boillot, J., & Slama, G. 2007. Effect of baking process on postprandial metabolic consequences: Randomized trials in normal and type 2 diabetic subjects. *Eur.J Clin. Nutr.*, 61, (2) 175–183 available from: PM:16943848.

Robertson, M.D., Currie, J.M., Morgan, L.M., Jewell, D.P., & Frayn, K.N. 2003. Prior short-term consumption of resistant starch enhances postprandial insulin sensitivity in healthy subjects. *Diabetologia*, 46, (5) 659-665 available from: PM:12712245.

Schenk, S., Davidson, C.J., Zderic, T.W., Byerley, L.O., & Coyle, E.F. 2003. Different glycemic indexes of breakfast cereals are not due to glucose entry into blood but to glucose removal by tissue. *Am.J Clin.Nutr.*, 78, (4) 742–748 available from: PM:14522732.

Schirra, J., Katschinski, M., Weidmann, C., Schafer, T., Wank, U., Arnold, R., & Goke, B. 1996. Gastric emptying and release of incretin hormones after glucose ingestion in humans. *J Clin Invest*, 97, (1) 92–103 available from: PM:8550855.

Seifarth, C., Bergmann, J., Holst, J.J., Ritzel, R., Schmiegel, W., & Nauck, M.A. 1998. Prolonged and enhanced secretion of glucagon-like peptide 1 (7-36 amide) after oral sucrose due to alpha-glucosidase inhibition (acarbose) in Type 2 diabetic patients. *Diabet.Med*, 15, (6) 485–491 available from: PM:9632123.

Slavin, J. 2003. Why whole grains are protective: biological mechanisms. *Proc Nutr.Soc*, 62, (1) 129–134 available from: PM:12740067.

Steele, R., Wall, J.S., De Bodo, R.C., & Altszuler, N. 1956. Measurement of size and turnover rate of body glucose pool by the isotope dilution method. *Am.J.Physiol.*, 187, 15–24.

Stevenson, E., Williams, C., & Nute, M. 2005. The influence of the glycaemic index of breakfast and lunch on substrate utilisation during the postprandial periods and subsequent exercise. *Br.J Nutr.*, 93, (6) 885–893 available from: PM:16022758.

Stevenson, E., Williams, C., Nute, M., Humphrey, L., & Witard, O. 2007. Influence of the glycaemic index of an evening meal on substrate oxidation following breakfast and during exercise the next day in healthy women. *Eur.J Clin.Nutr*. available from: PM:17440522.

Story, J.A. & Kritchevsky, D. 1976. Comparison of the binding of various bile acids and bile salts in vitro by several types of fiber. *J Nutr*, 106, (9) 1292–1294 available from: PM:956912.

Theodorakis, M.J., Carlson, O., Michopoulos, S., Doyle, M.E., Juhaszova, M., Petraki, K., & Egan, J.M. 2006. Human duodenal enteroendocrine cells: source of both incretin peptides, GLP-1 and GIP. *Am J Physiol Endocrinol.Metab*, 290, (3) E550–E559 available from: PM:16219666.

Thomas, C., Gioiello, A., Noriega, L., Strehle, A., Oury, J., Rizzo, G., Macchiarulo, A., Yamamoto, H., Mataki, C., Pruzanski, M., Pellicciari, R., Auwerx, J., & Schoonjans, K. 2009. TGR5-mediated bile acid sensing controls glucose homeostasis. *Cell Metab*, 10, (3) 167–177 available from: PM:19723493.

Thorburn, A., Muir, J., & Proietto, J. 1993. Carbohydrate fermentation decreases hepatic glucose output in healthy subjects. *Metabolism*, 42, (6) 780–785 available from: PM:8510524.

Tissot, S., Normand, S., Guilluy, R., Pachiaudi, C., Beylot, M., Laville, M., Cohen, R., Mornex, R., & Riou, J.P. 1990. Use of a new gas chromatograph isotope ratio mass spectrometer to trace exogenous 13C labelled glucose at a very low level of enrichment in man [published erratum appears in Diabetologia 1991 May;34(5):372]. *Diabetologia*, 33, (8) 449–456.

Trahair, L.G., Horowitz, M., Rayner, C.K., Gentilcore, D., Lange, K., Wishart, J.M., & Jones, K.L. 2012. Comparative effects of variations in duodenal glucose load on glycemic, insulinemic, and incretin responses in healthy young and older subjects. *J Clin Endocrinol.Metab*, 97, (3) 844–851 available from: PM:22238398.

Wachters-Hagedoorn, R.E., Priebe, M.G., Heimweg, J.A., Heiner, A.M., Englyst, K.N., Holst, J.J., Stellaard, F., & Vonk, R.J. 2006. The rate of intestinal glucose absorption is correlated with plasma glucose-dependent insulinotropic polypeptide concentrations in healthy men. *J.Nutr.*, 136, (6) 1511–1516 available from: PM:16702313.

Weickert, M.O., Mohlig, M., Koebnick, C., Holst, J.J., Namsolleck, P., Ristow, M., Osterhoff, M., Rochlitz, H., Rudovich, N., Spranger, J., & Pfeiffer, A.F. 2005. Impact of cereal fibre on glucose-regulating factors. *Diabetologia*, 48, (11) 2343–2353 available from: PM:16172868.

Willett, W., Manson, J., & Liu, S. 2002. Glycemic index, glycemic load, and risk of type 2 diabetes. *Am.J Clin. Nutr.*, 76, (1) 274S–280S available from: PM:12081851.

Wolever, T.M., Bentum-Williams, A., & Jenkins, D.J. 1995. Physiological modulation of plasma free fatty acid concentrations by diet: Metabolic implications in nondiabetic subjects. *Diabetes Care*, 18, (7) 962–970 available from: PM:7555557.

Wood, P.J. 2007. Cereal β-glucans in diet and health. *J Cereal Sci* 46, 230–238.

Zammit, V.A., Waterman, I.J., Topping, D., & McKay, G. 2001. Insulin stimulation of hepatic triacylglycerol secretion and the etiology of insulin resistance. *J Nutr*, 131, (8) 2074–2077 available from: PM:11481396.

Zijlstra, N., Mars, M., de Wijk, R.A., Westerterp-Plantenga, M.S., & de, G.C. 2008. The effect of viscosity on ad libitum food intake. *Int J Obes.(Lond)*, 32, (4) 676–683 available from: PM:18071342.

15 Whole Grains, Cereal Fibre and the Gut Function

Johan Dicksved and Emma Ivarsson

Department of Animal Nutrition and Management, Swedish University of Agricultural Sciences, Uppsala, Sweden

15.1 Introduction

Consumption of whole grain cereals has repeatedly been associated with a reduced risk of developing metabolic disorders and improvement of the metabolic parameters associated with these disorders (Jacobs et al., 2007; Slavin, 2004). For example, intake of soluble fibres has been associated with decreased serum cholesterol levels (Othman et al., 2011), lower postprandial glucose and insulin responses and improved gut health (Gemen et al., 2011). The mechanism behind this protective effect is not completely understood, but it is most probably dependent on a combination of factors. One mechanism of importance is likely attributed to the physicochemical properties. Whole grains have a high content of dietary fibre that increases the viscosity of the digesta, which subsequently contributes to a delayed gastric emptying and decreased sugar and lipid absorption from the small bowel (Smith and Tucker, 2011). Phytochemicals and other bioactive compounds have also been indicated as important contributors (Neacsu et al., 2013). In addition, dietary fibre can also increase satiety, which will likely contribute to a decreased food intake (Isaksson et al., 2009). In the past decade, an increased focus has also been directed towards the role of the intestinal microbiome for health and disease. Throughout evolution, mammals and microbes have co-existed and evolved together. This common deep ancestry has contributed to the symbiotic relationship that exists between mammals and their gut bacteria. Microbes support their host by extracting energy and nutrients from the diet and contribute both to their hosts' physiological and immunological development (Sommer and Bäckhed, 2013). The microbiota has also been linked with various metabolic disorders and dysfunctions (Tremaroli and Bäckhed, 2012). The intersection between the gut microbiota and host metabolism and the ability of whole grains to influence both may therefore be one of the important mechanisms explaining beneficial effects of whole grains (Figure 15.1). In this chapter, we review the current knowledge how whole grain cereals and dietary fibre influence gut function and interactions with the gut microbiome.

Whole Grains and Health, Second Edition. Edited by Rikard Landberg and Nathalie Scheers.

Additional materials available for download online at https://www.wiley.com/en-gb/Whole+Grains+and+Health-p-9781118939437

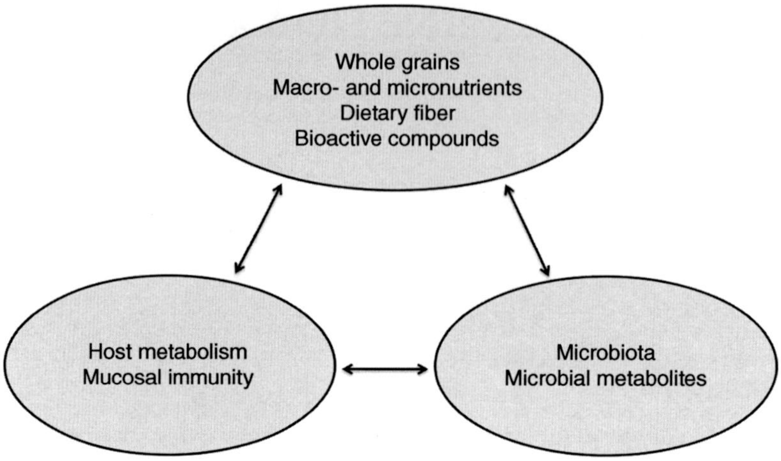

Figure 15.1 Interactions among diet, microbiota and host immunity, where a state of equilibrium and lack of disease commonly is referred to as gut health.

15.2 Whole grains and influence on gut physiology

15.2.1 Importance of molecular structure and solubility

Whole grain cereals have a very complex composition of dietary fibre, which is commonly defined as polysaccharides and lignin resistant to digestion by endogenous secretions of the human digestive tract (Trowell et al., 1976). Dietary fibre is one of the most diverse and heterogenous group of linked molecules found in nature and has a composition consisting of oligosaccharides, resistant starch, lignin and non-starch polysaccharides (NSPs), where the most important NSPs are arabinoxylans, β-glucan and cellulose. Insoluble NSP and lignin is primarily found in the outer cell layer of the grain and the refined flour thus contains a low proportion of insoluble dietary fibre components. Monomeric composition, chain length, type of binding, branching, side chains, anomeric composition and association with other compounds are all factors that introduce a large amount of possible variations in chemical structures (Gemen et al., 2011; Hamaker and Tuncil, 2014). Consequently, the chemical structure affects the physiochemical properties like cation exchange capacity, hydration properties, viscosity, organic compound adsorptive properties, utilization by the gut microbiota and its fermentation end-products (Awati et al., 2005; Bach Knudsen, 2001; Hamaker and Tuncil, 2014). Many studies concerning effects of dietary fibres focusing on a specific fibre type and its effect on gut microbiota, short chain fatty acid (SCFA) profiles and other metabolic effects. However, in many of these studies, the molecular structure is poorly described and it is therefore difficult to link a specific structure to a certain health effect (Gemen et al., 2011), which exemplifies the gap among carbohydrate science, microbiota research and health science.

To be able to manipulate the microbiota in a controlled way, a better understanding about the link between specific structures and the microbial composition is needed. For this reason, Hamaker and Tuncil (2014) introduced the concept of *discrete structure* and defined it as a unique chemical structure, often within a fibre molecule, which aligns with encoded gene clusters in bacterial genomes.

15.2.2 Gastrointestinal transit time

The gastrointestinal (GI) transit time can be described as the passage time from one segment to another; whereas the retention time is the time the digesta stays in the same segment. The mean retention time (MRT) or the mean transit time (MTT) differs substantially between different gut segments, between the liquid and the solid phase of the digesta, and can also be affected by dietary factors (Bach Knudsen, 2001). A summary of reported MRT and MTT in both pig and human studies is shown in Table 15.1. In general, the reported MRT in stomach is about 1 h, the corresponding value in the small intestine is about 4 h, and about 25 h for the large intestine (Glitso et al., 199; Le Gall et al., 2009; Lupton et al., 1993; Spiller et al., 1986; Wilfart et al., 2007). The solubility of the fibre has major impact on the transit time in different parts of the GI-tract. Generally, insoluble fibre decreases the MRT in both small and large intestine (Bach Knudsen, 2001; McIntyre et al., 1997), whereas soluble fibre results in increased MRT in the small intestine (Tosh, 2013), while the effects of soluble fibre on MRT in large intestine is insignificant (Bach Knudsen, 2001). Moreover, the physiochemical properties of fibre have a high influence on the MRT, with a shorter MRT in the small intestine of low viscose fibre compared to high viscose fibre (Metzler-Zebeli et al., 2010). A similar result has been reported for the stomach where soluble fibre that increases the viscosity increase MRT and delay gastric emptying (Tosh, 2013). However, Bach Knudsen (2001) reported that only a small portion of the soluble fibre occurring in natural feeds solubilizes in the stomach, and the same author concluded that the major effect on viscosity in delaying gastric emptying is related to the liquid phase of the digesta. This is in agreement with another study reporting that addition of dietary fibre to a liquid diet delays gastric emptying (Benini et al., 1995). However, the effect on solid digesta is more uncertain, which is shown by divergent results in different studies and several authors have reported delayed gastric emptying with increasing amount of whole grain and natural-occurring fibre (Benini et al., 1995; Hlebowicz et al., 2007; McIntyre et al., 1997). On the other hand, other authors reported no effect of whole grain fibre on MRT (Hlebowicz et al., 2007; Wilfart et al., 2007). Differences in study designs as well as physiochemical properties of the fibres used in the different studies may explain the contrasting results. Apart from the physiochemical properties of fibre, the particle size is also an important factor determining the MRT. McIntyre et al. (1997) used plastic particles to show that the actual particles can stimulate enteric nerves and increase the passage rate in the whole GI-tract (McIntyre et al., 1997).

15.2.3 Nutrient absorption

There is a close association between delayed gastric emptying and delayed nutrient absorption, which is closely linked to lowered post-prandial peripheral glucose and insulin response (Bach Knudsen, 2001). Soluble cereal fibre, especially β-glucans and arabinoxylans, increase the digesta viscosity that physically delays mixing the food with enzymes and delays gastric emptying. Moreover, the proportion of fat and protein in the diet as well as the food microstructure affects the glucose absorption (Tosh, 2013). Furthermore, the presence of intact kernels may physically slow the rate of starch hydrolysis in the gut (Hartvigsen et al., 2014) and it has been shown that the change in glycemic response was greater for intact grains than processed products (Tosh, 2013). In intact kernels, the changed glycemic response was linked to the total dietary fibre content and slowly digestible starch,

Table 15.1 Reported mean retention time (MRT) or mean transit time (MTT) h in different segments of the gastrointestinal tract.

	MRT	MTT	MTT	MTT	MTT	MTT
Species	Pig	Pig	Pig	Human	Human	Human
Stomach						
Solid phase	1.0–1.3					
Liquid phase	0.8–0.9					
Small Intestine						
Solid phase	3.7–4.3					
Liquid phase	3.9–4.4					
Total*				6.10–7.11		
Large intestine						
Solid phase	40.5–49.7					
Liquid phase	24.9–41.3					
Total*		25.1–60.2	21.1–32.8			
Total tract					38.8–47.2	24.6–38.16
Fiber source	Wheat bran 0–400 g/kg	Wheat flour, wheat whole grain, wheat and rye aleurone flour.	Rye products (Whole rye, pericarp/testa, aleurone, endosperm)	Oats, cornflakes, white bread.	Barley bran and cellulose	Hard wheat fiber
Reference	Wilfart et al. (2007)	Le Gall et al. (2009)	Glitsø et al. (1998)	Englyst and Cummings (1985)	Lupton et al. (1993)	Spiller et al. (1986)

*Liquid and solid phase was not separated.

rather than the β-glucan content as in processed products. In the intact grains, the intact cell wall may act as a physical barrier to starch degrading enzymes.

In addition, the digestibility of macronutrients is influenced both by the botanical source of arabinoxylan and by origin tissues of arabinoxylan (whole grain vs. aleurone layer); the firm nature of aleurone cell walls captures nutrients to a higher extent than diets with whole grains, resulting in lower digestibility of protein and fat in diets with aleurone layer. (Le Gall et al., 2009). A study comparing the gastrointestinal and physiological effects of rye- and wheat-based diets showed a lower digestibility of protein and fat in small intestine on rye bread diets which could be subjected to an increased digesta viscosity (Bach Knudsen et al., 2005). Moreover, the part digested in the small intestine differed for different NSP origins; the NSP disappearance in small intestine was 25% in pigs fed on whole grain wheat, whereas neither wheat or rye aleurone bread was degraded at all in small intestine. The rye aleurone bread was easily degraded in ceacum, whereas the wheat aleurone bread was degraded slower and to a higher extent in colon.

15.3 The intestinal gut microbiome

The mammalian GI tract is one of the most densely populated microbial ecosystems that exists. This "meta-genome" develops from birth and onwards to finally encompass trillions of microorganisms that harbor a repertoire of protein-encoding genes that by far exceeds the gene pool of the mammalian genome. Of the dozens of microbial phyla that can be found in the environment, less than ten colonize the mammalian gut of which *Firmicutes* and *Bacteroidetes* are the most dominating. The microbiome provides many important functions for the host (Figure 15.2). For example, gut microbes contribute to the host metabolism by extracting energy, increasing nutrient accessibility from the diet and by

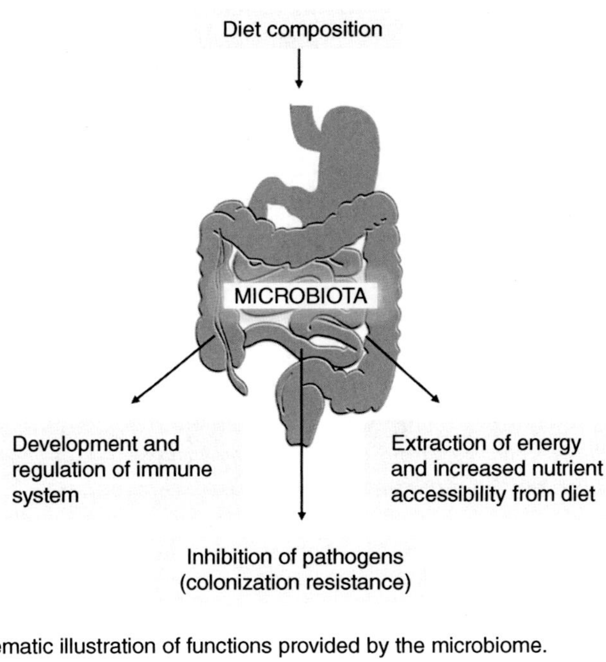

Figure 15.2 Schematic illustration of functions provided by the microbiome.

producing essential vitamins and other bioactive compounds (Sommer and Bäckhed, 2013). Besides the metabolic effects, the gut microbiota also helps to protect against infections from enteric pathogens; it influences gut motility and permeability, and furthermore the gut microbiota have an important role for shaping the structure and dynamic operation of the innate and adaptive immune system (Ivanov and Honda, 2012; Sekirov et al., 2010). A disrupted composition of the microbiota has been associated with a range of disturbances such as, inflammatory bowel disease, cardiovascular diseases, diabetes, obesity, autoimmune diseases and cancers (Sekirov et al., 2010). Diet contributes to the composition and function of the intestinal microbiome. It is therefore important to better understand diet-microbe interactions and the underlying mechanisms of importance, which could contribute to prevent development of metabolic disorders.

15.3.1 Whole grain cereals and the intestinal microbiome

Dietary fibre, such as resistant starch and plant polysaccharides, escapes digestion by indigenous enzymes, but is instead metabolized by the intestinal microbiota. Sequence analyses of various microbial genomes has revealed that our microbial symbionts are equipped with a tremendous arsenal of polysaccharide degrading enzymes (Lombard et al., 2014). As whole grain cereal is rich in dietary fibre, it serves as an important link between diet and the microbiota. Yet, until recently, the microbiota has been neglected in most nutritional studies. Recent research have however highlighted that essentially all diseases negatively correlated with whole grain consumption are also associated with the microbiota and highlights the importance of including the microbiota as a factor in nutritional studies (Walter et al., 2013). The composition of the intestinal microbiota is linked with fibre intake; this is best exemplified from studies comparing populations that have a high natural intake of fibres (Rural Africa, Rural Papua New Guinea) with those having a low intake of fibres (USA). The most striking difference between these populations was associated with differences in microbial diversity (lower in the US population) and the abundance of specific bacterial groups of importance for fibre utilization (lower in the US population) (De Filippo et al., 2010; Martinez et al., 2015). Differences have also been found in intervention studies performed within the same population. Martinez and coworkers (2013) performed a human intervention study on whole grain barley and brown rice to study the impact on the fecal microbiota and further associations between the gut microbiota, inflammatory and metabolic markers in blood. They showed that the microbial diversity increased after consumption of diets, including either whole grain barley, whole grain brown rice or a combination of both. Intake of the WG products was associated with an increased abundance of *Firmicutes* and reduced abundance of *Bacteroidetes*. Interestingly, consumption of whole grain barley and brown rice in combination was associated with reduced levels of the pro-inflammatory cytokine IL-6 in plasma and this feature coincided with compositional alterations of the gut microbiota (Martinez et al., 2013). A placebo-controlled randomized trial comparing the influence of whole grain wheat and wheat bran showed that whole grain wheat consumption increased the amount of bifidobacteria and lactobacilli in the gut (Costabile et al., 2008). By contrast, several studies have failed to show effects of WG cereals on the microbiota (Ampatzoglou et al., 2015; Lappi et al., 2013). Lappi et al. (2013) performed an intervention study for 12 weeks comparing fibre-rich rye bread with refined wheat bread did not illustrate any apparent effects on the microbiota (Lappi et al., 2013). The discrepancies in results between studies can have several explanations, such as type of products that was tested, methods to evaluate the results as well as design and duration of the study. How rapid the microbiota changes in response to dietary fibre has not yet been evaluated in a comprehensive way. However, the data available so far indicates that the microbiota responses rapidly to an introduction of fibre and changes in microbiota configuration has been seen already within one day after diet shifts (David et al., 2014; Walker et al., 2011).

Whole grains contain varying quantities of resistant starches, that is, starches that escapes small intestinal digestion. RS starch is fermented by the microbiota, which leads to production of SCFA. Specific species of ruminococci seem to be key species for RS fermentation (Walker et al., 2011), and the fermentation of RS primarily leads to higher concentrations of butyrate in the gut (Nielsen et al., 2014). Butyrate is readily metabolized by the cells lining the colon, which derive about 70% to 90% of their energy from bacterial fermentation products, such as butyrate (Cook and Sellin, 1998). Butyrate is therefore an important regulator of colonic cell growth and differentiation. Specific types of resistant starch (e.g., the chemically modified starches used in the food industry) may be used to manipulate the gut bacteria and their products (including SCFA) so as to optimize health.

15.4 Microbial fermentation end-products and their impact for gut function

The SCFA produced during carbohydrate fermentation are important for the energy supply both for the host and the epithelial cells (Cummings and Englyst, 1987; Williams et al., 2001). SCFA is absorbed from the gut lumen into gut mucosa and blood vessels. The most abundant SCFA are acetate, propionate and butyrate. The type and composition of different carbohydrates is of increasing interest in both human and animal nutrition. To a large extent, this is due to the effects that different dietary polysaccharides have on the intestinal microbiota (Macfarlane and Macfarlane, 2007). Studies in pigs have shown that for wheat-based diets, cellulose is the major carbohydrate entering the large intestine that subsequently stimulates cellulytic bacteria with acetate as the major fermentation end-product. In a rye-based diet, arabinoxylan is the major carbohydrate polymer entering the large intestine stimulating bacterial fermentation with butyrate as the major fermentation end-product (Bach Knudsen et al., 2005).

Besides the nutritional value of SCFA, they also seem to have an important role as signaling molecules. It has repeatedly been shown that SCFA can stimulate receptors in the gut mucosa, such as GPR43 and GLP1 that have an important function for gut permeability and motility (Bolognini et al., 2015). Furthermore, more recently, it was shown that SCFA, in particular butyrate and propionate, have an important role for generation of anti-inflammatory T-regulatory cells, suggesting that these bacterial metabolites mediate communication with the gut associated immune system, and subsequently, affect the balance between pro- and anti-inflammatory mechanisms (Arpaia et al., 2013). In addition, several studies have indicated butyrate as an important signaling molecule regulating the release of hormones, such as insulin and for epigenetic regulation (Arpaia et al., 2013; Canani et al., 2011).

15.5 Microbiome mediated benefits of whole grain consumption

Besides their high content of dietary fibre, whole grains are also a rich source of phytate, phyto-esterogens vitamins and minerals (Slavin, 2003). In most cases, these compounds have been implicated to have an important role for the beneficial effects of whole grain consumption. One example is the impact of dietary lignans. Plant lignans are bioactive compounds found in grains, fruits and vegetables, and among the cereals, rye has the highest content (Smeds et al., 2007). In the gut, plant lignans are converted to enterodiol and enterolactone (commonly referred to as enterolignans) by the gut microbiota, and these compounds are readily absorbed by the intestinal epithelium. Enterolignans have been extensively studied due to their health-promoting effects and has been suggested to contribute to prevention of metabolic and cardiovascular diseases as well as various forms of cancer (Mabrok et al., 2012; Sun et al., 2014; Thompson, 1998). These effects is likely linked to their structural similarity with estrogens, anti-oxidative properties and modulating effects on host enzyme activities (Thompson, 1998). The intake of plant lignans determines blood concentrations of the enterolignans, but this is also dependent on the composition of the colonic microbiota (Clavel et al., 2005). It is well known that treatment with antibiotics has a negative impact on the colonic microbiota, and consequently lowered enterolignan production potentially up to one year after treatment (Kilkkinen et al., 2002). Several bacterial species have been related to enterolignan formation and this function seems to be distributed among different bacterial lineages represented in the gut (Clavel et al., 2005). It is still largely unknown what enzyme systems are involved and how the formation may be affected by different dietary sources, for example, different types of grains.

Several studies have shown that the gut microbiome has an important role for regulation of the metabolism. For example, it has been suggested to regulate glucose homeostasis, lipid metabolism and insulin economy (Bäckhed et al., 2004; Vrieze et al., 2012). There is a large inter-individual variation in the microbial responses to diet (Lampe et al., 2013). It is also apparent that there is a high inter-individual variability in post meal glucose responses. Zeevi and coworkers (2015), monitored the glucose levels in an 800-person cohort for a week and observed large variations in glucose responses between individuals to identical meals. It was recently suggested that the microbiome can be used as a tool to identify subjects that benefit from dietary intervention studies (Korpela et al., 2014; Zeevi et al., 2015). A recent intervention study by Kovatcheva-Datchary and coworkers (2015), tested the effect of a barley kernel-based and white wheat bread on blood glucose, insulin responses and on the microbiome. There were individual variations in how the participants responded to the different breads, but when comparing the responders (i.e., those that got reduced levels of blood glucose and insulin after the barley kernel-based bread) with non-responders, they saw a clear correlation to the microbiome. The responders had significantly more of *Prevotella copri* compared with non-responders and interestingly these results was confirmed when the responder and non-responder microbiome phenotypes were transplanted into germ free mice (Kovatcheva-Datchary et al., 2015). This study highlights the importance of personalized nutrition, and further, the importance of combining both diet and microbiome in studies focusing on metabolism.

15.6 References

Ampatzoglou, A., Atwal, K. K., Maidens, C. M., Williams, C. L., Ross, A. B., Thielecke, F., et al. 2015. Increased whole grain consumption does not affect blood biochemistry, body composition, or gut microbiology in healthy, low-habitual whole grain consumers. *J Nutr*, 145, 215–21.

Arpaia, N., Campbell, C., Fan, X., Dikiy, S., Van Der Veeken, J., Deroos, P., et al. 2013. Metabolites produced by commensal bacteria promote peripheral regulatory T-cell generation. *Nature*, 504, 451–5.

Awati, A., Konstantinov, S. R., Williams, B. A., Akkermans, A. D., Bosch, M. W., Smidt, H., et al. 2005. Effect of substrate adaptation on the microbial fermentation and microbial composition of faecal microbiota of weaning piglets studied in vitro. *Journal of the Science of Food and Agriculture* 85, 1765–72.

Bach Knudsen, K. E. 2001. The nutritional significance of "dietary fibre" analysis. *Animal Feed Science and Technology*, 90, 3–20.

Bach Knudsen, K. E., Serena, A., Kjaer, A. K., Jorgensen, H. & Engberg, R. 2005. Rye bread enhances the production and plasma concentration of butyrate but not the plasma concentrations of glucose and insulin in pigs. *J Nutr*, 135, 1696–704.

Bäckhed, F., Ding, H., Wang, T., Hooper, L. V., Koh, G. Y., Nagy, A., et al. 2004. The gut microbiota as an environmental factor that regulates fat storage. *Proc Natl Acad Sci U S A*, 101, 15718–23.

Benini, L., Castellani, G., Brighenti, F., Heaton, K. W., Brentegani, M. T., Casiraghi, M. C., et al. 1995. Gastric emptying of a solid meal is accelerated by the removal of dietary fibre naturally present in food. *Gut*, 36, 825–30.

Bolognini, D., Tobin, A. B., Milligan, G. & Moss, C. E. 2015. The Pharmacology and Function of Short Chain Fatty Acid Receptors. *Mol Pharmacol*,89, 388–98.

Canani, R. B., Costanzo, M. D., Leone, L., Pedata, M., Meli, R. & Calignano, A. 2011. Potential beneficial effects of butyrate in intestinal and extraintestinal diseases. *World J Gastroenterol*, 17, 1519–28.

Clavel, T., Henderson, G., Alpert, C. A., Philippe, C., Rigottier-Gois, L., Dore, J., et al. 2005. Intestinal bacterial communities that produce active estrogen-like compounds enterodiol and enterolactone in humans. *Appl Environ Microbiol*, 71, 6077–85.

Cook, S. I. & Sellin, J. H. 1998. Review article: Short chain fatty acids in health and disease. *Aliment Pharmacol Ther*, 12, 499–507.

Costabile, A., Klinder, A., Fava, F., Napolitano, A., Fogliano, V., Leonard, C., et al. 2008. Whole-grain wheat breakfast cereal has a prebiotic effect on the human gut microbiota: A double-blind, placebo-controlled, crossover study. *Br J Nutr*, 99, 110–20.

Cummings, J. H. & Englyst, H. N. 1987. Fermentation in the human large intestine and the available substrates. *Am J Clin Nutr*, 45, 1243–55.

David, L. A., Maurice, C. F., Carmody, R. N., Gootenberg, D. B., Button, J. E., Wolfe, B. E., et al. 2014. Diet rapidly and reproducibly alters the human gut microbiome. *Nature*, 505, 559–63.

De Filippo, C., Cavalieri, D., Di Paola, M., Ramazzotti, M., Poullet, J. B., Massart, S., et al. 2010. Impact of diet in shaping gut microbiota revealed by a comparative study in children from Europe and rural Africa. *Proc Natl Acad Sci U S A*, 107, 14691–6.

Gemen, R., De Vries, J. F. & Slavin, J. L. 2011. Relationship between molecular structure of cereal dietary fiber and health effects: Focus on glucose/insulin response and gut health. *Nutr Rev*, 69, 22–33.

Glitso, L. V., Brunsgaard, G., Hojsgaard, S., Sandstrom, B. & Bach Knudsen, K. E. 1998. Intestinal degradation in pigs of rye dietary fibre with different structural characteristics. *Br J Nutr*, 80, 457–68.

Hamaker, B. R. & Tuncil, Y. E. 2014. A perspective on the complexity of dietary fiber structures and their potential effect on the gut microbiota. *J Mol Biol*, 426, 3838–50.

Hartvigsen, M. L., Laerke, H. N., Overgaard, A., Holst, J. J., Bach Knudsen, K. E. & Hermansen, K. 2014. Postprandial effects of test meals including concentrated arabinoxylan and whole grain rye in subjects with the metabolic syndrome: A randomised study. *Eur J Clin Nutr*, 68, 567–74.

Hlebowicz, J., Wickenberg, J., Fahlstrom, R., Bjorgell, O., Almer, L. O. & Darwiche, G. 2007. Effect of commercial breakfast fibre cereals compared with corn flakes on postprandial blood glucose, gastric emptying and satiety in healthy subjects: A randomized blinded crossover trial. *Nutr J*, 6, 22.

Isaksson, H., Fredriksson, H., Andersson, R., Olsson, J. & Åman, P. 2009. Effect of rye bread breakfasts on subjective hunger and satiety: A randomized controlled trial. *Nutr J*, 8, 39.

Ivanov, Ii & Honda, K. 2012. Intestinal commensal microbes as immune modulators. *Cell Host Microbe*, 12, 496–508.

Jacobs, D. R., Jr., Andersen, L. F. & Blomhoff, R. 2007. Whole-grain consumption is associated with a reduced risk of noncardiovascular, noncancer death attributed to inflammatory diseases in the Iowa Women's Health Study. *Am J Clin Nutr*, 85, 1606–14.

Kilkkinen, A., Pietinen, P., Klaukka, T., Virtamo, J., Korhonen, P. & Adlercreutz, H. 2002. Use of oral antimicrobials decreases serum enterolactone concentration. *Am J Epidemiol*, 155, 472–7.

Korpela, K., Flint, H. J., Johnstone, A. M., Lappi, J., Poutanen, K., Dewulf, E., et al. 2014. Gut microbiota signatures predict host and microbiota responses to dietary interventions in obese individuals. *PLoS One*, 9, e90702.

Kovatcheva-Datchary, P., Nilsson, A., Akrami, R., Lee, Y. S., De Vadder, F., Arora, T., et al. 2015. Dietary fiber-induced improvement in glucose metabolism is associated with increased abundance of prevotella. *Cell Metab*, 22, 971–82.

Lampe, J. W., Navarro, S. L., Hullar, M. A. & Shojaie, A. 2013. Inter-individual differences in response to dietary intervention: Integrating omics platforms towards personalised dietary recommendations. *Proc Nutr Soc*, 72, 207–18.

Lappi, J., Salojarvi, J., Kolehmainen, M., Mykkanen, H., Poutanen, K., De Vos, W. M., et al. 2013. Intake of whole-grain and fiber-rich rye bread versus refined wheat bread does not differentiate intestinal microbiota composition in Finnish adults with metabolic syndrome. *J Nutr*, 143, 648–55.

Le Gall, M., Serena, A., Jorgensen, H., Theil, P. K. & Bach Knudsen, K. E. 2009. The role of whole-wheat grain and wheat and rye ingredients on the digestion and fermentation processes in the gut – A model experiment with pigs. *Br J Nutr*, 102, 1590–600.

Lombard, V., Golaconda Ramulu, H., Drula, E., Coutinho, P. M. & Henrissat, B. 2014. The carbohydrate-active enzymes database (CAZy) in 2013. *Nucleic Acids Res*, 42, D490-5.

Lupton, J. R., Morin, J. L. & Robinson, M. C. 1993. Barley bran flour accelerates gastrointestinal transit time. *J Am Diet Assoc*, 93, 881–5.

Mabrok, H. B., Klopfleisch, R., Ghanem, K. Z., Clavel, T., Blaut, M. & Loh, G. 2012. Lignan transformation by gut bacteria lowers tumor burden in a gnotobiotic rat model of breast cancer. *Carcinogenesis*, 33, 203–8.

Macfarlane, G. T. & Macfarlane, S. 2007. Models for intestinal fermentation: association between food components, delivery systems, bioavailability and functional interactions in the gut. *Curr Opin Biotechnol*, 18, 156–62.

Martinez, I., Lattimer, J. M., Hubach, K. L., Case, J. A., Yang, J., Weber, C. G., et al. 2013. Gut microbiome composition is linked to whole grain-induced immunological improvements. *ISME J*, 7, 269–80.

Martinez, I., Stegen, J. C., Maldonado-Gomez, M. X., Eren, A. M., Siba, P. M., Greenhill, A. R., et al. 2015. The gut microbiota of rural papua new guineans: Composition, diversity patterns, and ecological processes. *Cell Rep*, 11, 527–38.

Mcintyre, A., Vincent, R. M., Perkins, A. C. & Spiller, R. C. 1997. Effect of bran, ispaghula, and inert plastic particles on gastric emptying and small bowel transit in humans: The role of physical factors. *Gut*, 40, 223–7.

Metzler-Zebeli, B. U., Hooda, S., Pieper, R., Zijlstra, R. T., Van Kessel, A. G., Mosenthin, R., et al. 2010. Nonstarch polysaccharides modulate bacterial microbiota, pathways for butyrate production, and abundance of pathogenic Escherichia coli in the pig gastrointestinal tract. *Appl Environ Microbiol*, 76, 3692–701.

Neacsu, M., Mcmonagle, J., Fletcher, R. J., Scobbie, L., Duncan, G. J., Cantlay, L., et al. 2013. Bound phytophenols from ready-to-eat cereals: Comparison with other plant-based foods. *Food Chem*, 141, 2880–6.

Nielsen, T. S., Laerke, H. N., Theil, P. K., Sörensen, J. F., Saarinen, M., Forssten, S., et al. 2014. Diets high in resistant starch and arabinoxylan modulate digestion processes and SCFA pool size in the large intestine and faecal microbial composition in pigs. *Br J Nutr*, 112, 1837–49.

Othman, R. A., Moghadasian, M. H. & Jones, P. J. 2011. Cholesterol-lowering effects of oat beta-glucan. *Nutr Rev*, 69, 299–309.

Sekirov, I., Russell, S. L., Antunes, L. C. & Finlay, B. B. 2010. Gut microbiota in health and disease. *Physiol Rev*, 90, 859–904.

Slavin, J. 2003. Why whole grains are protective: Biological mechanisms. *Proc Nutr Soc*, 62, 129–34.

Slavin, J. 2004. Whole grains and human health. *Nutr Res Rev*, 17, 99–110.

Smeds, A. I., Eklund, P. C., Sjöholm, R. E., Willfor, S. M., Nishibe, S., Deyama, T., et al. 2007. Quantification of a broad spectrum of lignans in cereals, oilseeds, and nuts. *J Agric Food Chem*, 55, 1337–46.

Smith, C. E. & Tucker, K. L. 2011. Health benefits of cereal fibre: A review of clinical trials. *Nutr Res Rev*, 24, 118–31.

Sommer, F. & Bäckhed, F. 2013. The gut microbiota-masters of host development and physiology. *Nat Rev Microbiol*, 11, 227-38.

Spiller, G. A., Story, J. A., Wong, L. G., Nunes, J. D., Alton, M., Petro, M. S., et al. 1986. Effect of increasing levels of hard wheat fiber on fecal weight, minerals and steroids and gastrointestinal transit time in healthy young women. *J Nutr*, 116, 778–85.

Sun, Q., Wedick, N. M., Pan, A., Townsend, M. K., Cassidy, A., Franke, A. A., et al. 2014. Gut microbiota metabolites of dietary lignans and risk of type 2 diabetes: A prospective investigation in two cohorts of U.S. women. *Diabetes Care*, 37, 1287–95.

Thompson, L. U. 1998. Experimental studies on lignans and cancer. *Baillieres Clin Endocrinol Metab*, 12, 691–705.

Tosh, S. M. 2013. Review of human studies investigating the post-prandial blood-glucose lowering ability of oat and barley food products. *Eur J Clin Nutr*, 67, 310–7.

Tremaroli, V. & Bäckhed, F. 2012. Functional interactions between the gut microbiota and host metabolism. *Nature*, 489, 242–9.

Trowell, H., Southgate, D. A., Wolever, T. M., Leeds, A. R., Gassull, M. A. & Jenkins, D. J. 1976. Letter: Dietary fibre redefined. *Lancet*, 1, 967.

Walker, A. W., Ince, J., Duncan, S. H., Webster, L. M., Holtrop, G., Ze, X., et al. 2011. Dominant and diet-responsive groups of bacteria within the human colonic microbiota. *ISME J*, 5, 220–30.

Walter, J., Martinez, I. & Rose, D. J. 2013. Holobiont nutrition: Considering the role of the gastrointestinal microbiota in the health benefits of whole grains. *Gut Microbes*, 4, 340–6.

Wilfart, A., Montagne, L., Simmins, H., Noblet, J. & Milgen, J. 2007. Digesta transit in different segments of the gastrointestinal tract of pigs as affected by insoluble fibre supplied by wheat bran. *Br J Nutr*, 98, 54–62.

Williams, B. A., Verstegen, M. W. & Tamminga, S. 2001. Fermentation in the large intestine of single-stomached animals and its relationship to animal health. *Nutr Res Rev*, 14, 207–28.

Vrieze, A., Van Nood, E., Holleman, F., Salojarvi, J., Kootte, R. S., Bartelsman, J. F., et al. 2012. Transfer of intestinal microbiota from lean donors increases insulin sensitivity in individuals with metabolic syndrome. *Gastroenterology, 143*, 913–6 e7.

Zeevi, D., Korem, T., Zmora, N., Israeli, D., Rothschild, D., Weinberger, A., et al. 2015. Personalized nutrition by prediction of glycemic responses. *Cell*, 163, 1079–94.

16 Bioactive Compounds in Whole Grains and Their Implications for Health

Anne-Maria Pajari, Riitta Freese, Susanna Kariluoto, Anna-Maija Lampi, and Vieno Piironen

Department of Food and Nutrition, University of Helsinki, Finland

16.1 Introduction

At population level, consumption of whole grains has been associated with a low incidence of major non-communicable diseases, including cardiovascular diseases, type 2 diabetes and some cancers. Whole grains are rich in essential nutrients, dietary fibre and a number of bioactive molecules of different chemical nature. It is still unclear whether specific components of whole grains, or the whole package is the key in promoting health and preventing disease. This chapter introduces the present knowledge on major bioactive compounds found in whole grain cereals such as wheat, rye, oat and barley (Figure 16.1). So far, the most extensive and systematic analyses on the concentrations of bioactive compounds in cereal grains have been conducted within the European Union funded project "Healthgrain" (FP6; Table 16.1). Bioavailability and metabolism of bioactives in the body as well as their possible health implications are discussed. With regard to health, we have focused on the mechanisms whereby bioactive compounds may decrease the risk for type 2 diabetes, coronary heart disease and cancers.

16.2 Folate

16.2.1 Chemical characteristics

Folate, belonging to the vitamin B group, comprises of 2-amino-4-hydroxy-6-methylpterin (pteridine ring) linked through a methylene bridge to para-aminobenzoate which is conjugated with one or several L-glutamic acid residues with γ-peptide linkage (Figure 16.1). The recommended intake is 400 μg/d for adults (FAO/WHO 2004). The gap between recommended and actual intake has paved the way for mandatory folic acid fortification of cereal products in several countries worldwide, although none in Europe. Cereal products are major dietary sources of folate, contributing to ca. 15–30% of the total intake (Park *et al.* 2012; Helldán *et al.* 2013). Folate in cereals is characterized by a large proportion of formylated vitamers compared to 5-methyltetrahydrofolate (5-methyl-THF) and unsubstituted tetrahydrofolate (THF) (Konings *et al.* 2001; Patring *et al.* 2009; Kariluoto *et al.* 2010; Shewry *et al.* 2010a; Edelmann *et al.* 2012; Edelmann *et al.* 2013; Hefni *et al.* 2018).

Whole Grains and Health, Second Edition. Edited by Rikard Landberg and Nathalie Scheers.

Additional materials available for download online at https://www.wiley.com/en-gb/Whole+Grains+and+Health-p-9781118939437

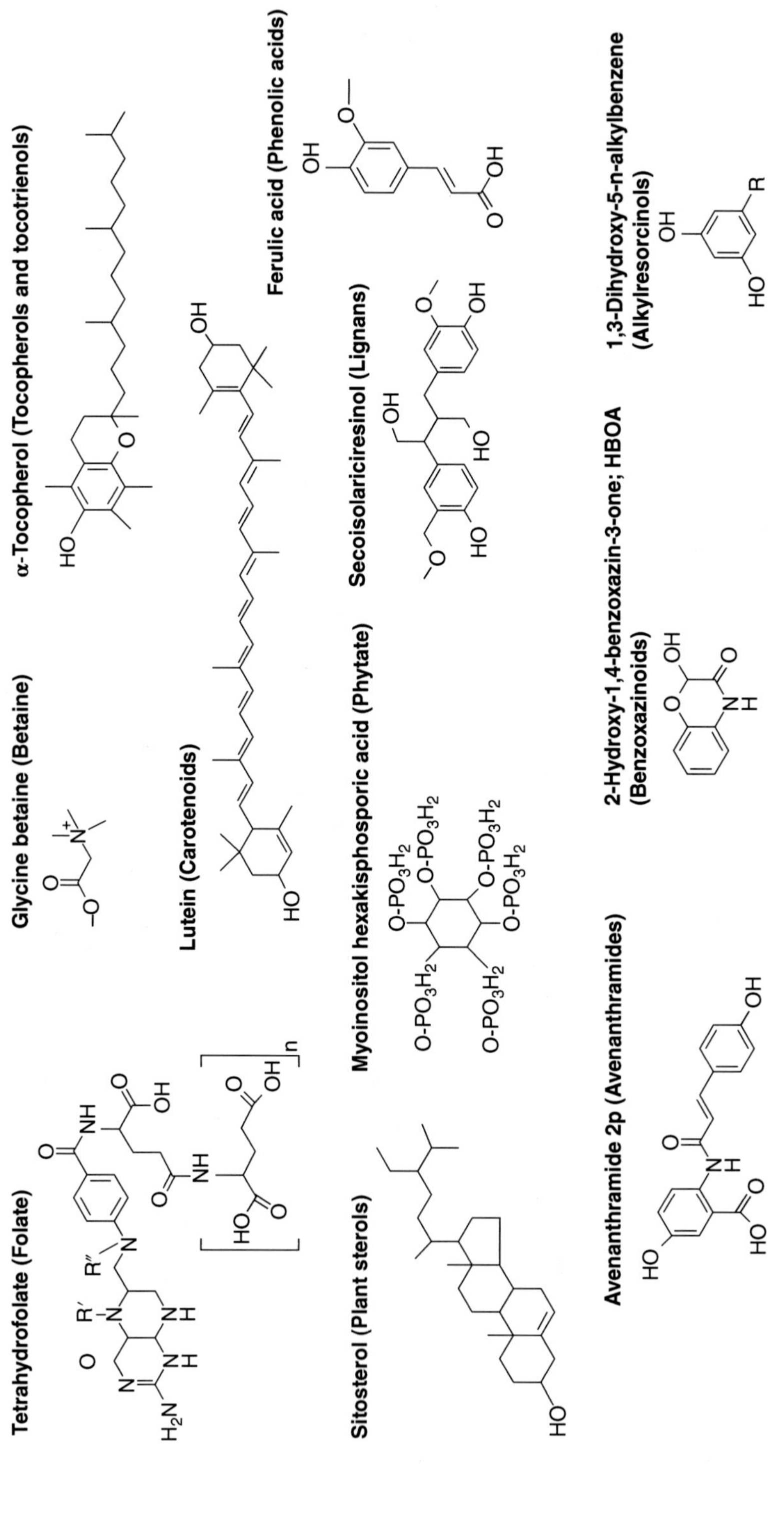

Figure 16.1 Chemical structures of representatives of major bioactive (compound classes) in cereals discussed in this chapter.

Table 16.1 Average contents of folate, tocols, sterols and phenolic acids in wholemeal samples from the Healthgrain Diversity Screen (on dry matter basis; range in parenthesis).

	Number of genotypes	Folate (ng/g dm)	Tocols (μg/g dm)	Sterols (μg/g dm)	Phenolic acids (μg/g dm)
Wheat					
Winter wheat	130	561[a] (364–774)	50[e] (28–80)	841[f] (670–959)	664[g] (326–1171)
Spring wheat	20	551[a] (323–741)	50[e] (36–63)	864[f] (797–949)	612[g] (456–892
Durum wheat	10	741[a] (637–891)	48[e] (40–63)	987[f] (871–1106)	699[g] (536–1086)
Rye	10	693[b] (574–775)	52[b] (44–67)	1228[b] (1098–1420)	685[b] (491–1082)
Oats	5	566[c] (495–604)	26[c] (16–36)	653[c] (618–682)	531[c] (351–873)
Barley	10	657[d] (518–789)	55[d] (46–69)	1048[d] (899–1153)	463[d] (254–675)

[a]Piironen *et al.* 2008.
[b]Nyström *et al.* 2008.
[c]Shewry *et al.* 2008.
[d]Andersson *et al.* 2008a.
[e]Lampi *et al.* 2008.
[f]Nurmi *et al.* 2008.
[g]Li *et al.* 2008.

16.2.2 Folate content in cereals

In the Healthgrain study, folate content of 130 winter wheat cultivars harvested from the same location ranged from 364 to 774 ng/g dm (Table 16.1), and similar values, 336–570 ng/g, have been reported in other studies (Gujska & Kuncewicz 2005; Hefni *et al.* 2018). However, Giordano *et al.* (2016) observed significantly higher folate contents in winter and durum wheat (1024 and 1119 ng/g dm), and folate contents up to 1143 ng/g dm were detected among 12 Australian wheats (Arcot *et al.* 2002). Rye contained more folate than wheat, the average of 10 rye cultivars being 693 ng/g dm (Table 16.1). Kariluoto *et al.* (2001) and Hefni *et al.* (2018) analyzed similar folate contents for 10 rye cultivars grown in Finland (689–853 ng/g dm) and for two Swedish cultivars (660 and 710 ng/g dm). Gujska & Kuncewicz (2005) reported even 1226 and 1349 ng/g dm for two Polish cultivars. However, significantly lower contents, ranging 310–390 ng/g fw, have also been reported (Hefni & Witthöft 2012). Information on folate in oats and barley is limited; however, these two cereals appear to have similar or somewhat higher folate contents compared to wheat. Among oat cultivars, typical folate contents have ranged from 495 to 740 ng/g dm (Table 16.1; Edelmann *et al.* 2012; Hefni *et al.* 2018), but lower values have also been reported (Han *et al.* 2005; Hefni *et al.* 2018). For barley, values have ranged from 520 to 1033 ng/g dm (Andersson *et al.* 2008a; Edelmann *et al.* 2013; Giordano *et al.* 2016; Hefni *et al.* 2018), the highest contents being in hulless barley (Giordano *et al.* 2016; Hefni *et al.* 2018). For other cereals, the data are even more scattered. Dong *et al.* (2011) reported folate contents of 133–1114 ng/g fw among 78 rice germplasms, and a rather low content,

180 ng/g fw, has been reported by Yon & Hyun (2003) for a pooled sample. For maize, folate content ranging from 370 ng/g (Hager *et al.* 2012) to 1290 ng/g fw (Yon & Hyun 2003) have been reported, and for sorghum 770 ng/g fw (Hager *et al.* 2012).

Folate is concentrated to germ and outer layers of the cereal grain. Especially the aleurone fractions are rich in folate (Fenech *et al.* 1999; Buri *et al.* 2004). Wheat bran contains 470–1600 ng/g dm of folate (Konings *et al.* 2001; Arcot *et al.* 2002; Kamal-Eldin *et al.* 2009; Patring *et al.* 2009), which is approximately two-fold more than in native grain. Rye bran has similarly high folate contents (Liukkonen *et al.* 2003; Kamal-Eldin *et al.* 2009). Folate contents in white wheat flours and in sifted rye flours are typically approximately half the contents found in respective whole grain (Patring *et al.* 2009). In a study by Patring *et al.* (2009), commercial oat flakes contained 240–290 ng/g dm of folate and oat bran 300–500 ng/g. Edelmann *et al.* (2012) showed that oat milling produces folate-rich (840–990 ng/g dm) by-products that are normally discarded. In the barley dehulling and pearling processes, 40–60% of the folate was lost (Edelmann *et al.* 2013), and Giordano *et al.* (2016) reported 63–86% folate loss in barley and wheat pearling. In maize, the highest folate content has been found in the germ fraction, and the folate content in the floury endosperm was higher than that in the vitreous endosperm (Blandino *et al.* 2017).

16.2.3 The effect of food processing on folate content

Folate is sensitive to elevated temperatures. The magnitude of losses depends on temperature, time and the presence of oxygen. Autoclaving and puffing of both native and germinated rye grains decreased the folate content by 45% to 54%, whereas in extrusion cooking the folate losses were moderate%, 26% to 28% (Kariluoto *et al.* 2006). Bread baking typically results in losses between 20 and 35% (Arcot *et al.* 2002; Kariluoto *et al.* 2004). However, folate synthesis by yeast is able to compensate folate losses, and as a result, bread can have higher folate content than the flour it is made of (Kariluoto *et al.* 2004). Another example of process-induced enhancement of folate is germination which may lead to a two- to four-fold increase in folate content (Jägerstad *et al.* 2005; Kariluoto *et al.* 2006; Koehler *et al.* 2007). In industrially malted oats, wheat and rye, folate concentration reached 700 ng/g, 1400 ng/g, and 1400–3300 ng/g fw, respectively (Jägerstad *et al.* 2005).

16.2.4 Bioavailability and health implications of folate

The bioavailability of food folate is commonly estimated to be around 50% based on a study by Sauberlich *et al.* (1987). However, this estimate has been questioned as several studies have reported significantly higher (60–98%) bioavailability (Gregory *et al.* 2005). Binding to food matrix and differences in stability affect the bioaccessibility and subsequent bioavailability of folate vitamers. This has implications for their vitamin activity. Folic acid in fortified breads, rice and pasta has been reported to have a high bioavailability (Pfeiffer *et al.* 1997). Interestingly, Vahteristo *et al.* (2002) concluded that natural folate from rye products and orange juice had similar bioavailability as folic acid from fortified white bread. More research is needed to evaluate the bioavailability of folate from cereal products (Öhrvik & Witthöft 2011). Polyglutamyl folates have to be hydrolyzed to monoglutamyl forms before they can be absorbed in the small intestine. In the enterocytes, folates are methylated, transported to the liver and thereafter to peripheral tissues. The major circulating form of folate is 5-methyl-THF-monoglutamate. In the cells, different forms of folate are crucial coenzymes in the metabolism of one-carbon groups, and thus needed for DNA synthesis, amino acid metabolism and methylation reactions. One of the central metabolic routes is the methionine synthase-catalysed methionine cycle where the methyl group is transferred from 5-methyl-THF via vitamin B12 to homocysteine to form methionine and regenerate THF. Folate metabolism is affected by several common polymorphisms, for instance, in the gene of the key enzyme, methylene-THF-reductase (MTHFR). Plasma homocysteine concentrations may be elevated due to multiple causes. Elevated concentration of plasma homocysteine is associated with increased risk of vascular disease (Klatt & Caudill 2019). Suggested mechanisms linking homocysteine to the pathophysiology of coronary heart disease include, for example, endothelial dysfunction, protein modifications and platelet activation (Santilli *et al.* 2016).

16.2.5 Folate and cancer

A role for folate and folic acid in cancer prevention has also been proposed. Dietary intake of folate has been inversely associated with the risk of several cancers in many epidemiological studies (World Cancer Research Fund 2007). However, some studies suggest a U-shape relationship between folate intake and cancer incidence (Chen *et al.* 2014). In line with these observations, a dual and contradicting effect of folic acid on tumor development in the colon has been established in animal studies, showing that folic acid inhibits formation of new, neoplastic foci, but promotes the growth of existing tumors (Mason 2009). Plausible biological mechanisms have been found to explain the role of folate both in inhibiting initiation of cancer and in promoting tumor growth and progression (Smith *et al.* 2008). As folate serves a methyl donor in cells, its deficiency may lead to hypomethylation of DNA, which is an early event in colon carcinogenesis and is associated with genetic instability and increased rate of mutations. On the other hand, proliferating cancer cells need folate for DNA synthesis, and thus an abundant supply of folate may accelerate cancer cell growth (Smith *et al.* 2008). It is noteworthy that the observed adverse effects have been more strongly linked to folic acid, the synthetic form of folate, and its long-term use as supplemental source of folate rather than high folate intake from foods such as whole grains (Kim 2018).

16.3 Glycine betaine, choline and trigonelline

Cereals are also major sources of the methyl donors glycine, betaine, choline and trigonelline. Based on the data obtained in the Healthgrain project, betaine was the dominant methyl donor, with higher contents detected in rye and wheat (2.27 and 1.59 mg/g dm, respectively) than in barley and oats (1.02 and 0.43 mg/g dm, respectively) (Corol *et al.* 2012). Choline contents varied from 0.17 mg/g dm in oats to 0.32 mg/g dm in barley. Oats had the highest trigonelline content, 111.7 μg/g dm, yet very small compared to the other methyl donors. For millet and sorghum, lower betaine contents have been reported, and in maize and rice, betaine contents were negligible (Kojic *et al.* 2017; Servillo *et al.* 2018). Recent studies have shown that methyl donor and distributions vary markedly between species and cultivars (Kojic *et al.* 2017; Hefni *et al.* 2018; Servillo *et al.* 2018). As in the case of folate, betaine and choline in wheat grain are concentrated in the germ and bran fractions (Likes *et al.* 2007). Consequently, whole grain wheat products are better sources of betaine and choline than refined-grain products (Ross *et al.* 2014; Kojic *et al.* 2017).

Betaine is used as a methyl donor by an enzyme system that remethylates homocysteine to methionine in the liver. Betaine can be synthesized from choline. Supplementation with both betaine and choline may decrease circulating homocysteine concentrations. Choline is also needed for phospholipid synthesis and is a precursor for the neurotransmitter acetylcholine (Klatt & Claudill 2019). However, there is evidence that serum concentration of trimethylamine-N-oxide (TMAO), formed from choline by intestinal microbes, is associated with atherosclerosis and the risk of CHD (Zeisel & Warrier 2017). It is questionable whether the association indicates causality. Compounds that have been shown to limit excess lipid deposits in the liver, and thus liver steatosis, are called lipotropes (Fardet & Chardigny 2013). Such compounds may decrease fatty acid synthesis, enhance fatty acid betaoxidation or facilitate triacylglycerol-rich lipoprotein exportation from the liver. Folate, betaine and choline could all be classified as lipotropes. However, there is a great need for human intervention studies to evaluate the effects of lipotropes on non-alcoholic fatty liver disease.

16.4 Tocopherols and tocotrienols

16.4.1 Chemical characteristics, contents in cereals and effects of food processing

Tocopherols (Toc) and tocotrienols (T3), collectively known as tocols, are lipid-soluble compounds with a polar 6-chromanol ring and a hydrophobic isoprenoid side chain. Tocols occur as four natural vitamers (α, β, γ and δ) that differ from each other by the number and position of methyl groups in the ring. The side chain in Toc is saturated and in T3 it contains three double bonds (Kamal-Eldin & Appelqvist 1996). Currently, only 2*R*-α-Toc is regarded to possess vitamin E activity, whereas all tocols are radical scavenging antioxidants (Traber & Stevens 2011). Cereals are seldomly major sources of vitamin E due to their moderate contents of 2R-α-Toc, but they have been calculated to contribute to up to 25% in the average diets in Finland (Helldán *et al.* 2013). However, cereals are more important sources of other tocols, especially of tocotrienols (Tiwari & Cummins 2009; Andersson *et al.* 2014). Tocols contribute markedly to the total antioxidant activity of whole grains (Fardet *et al.* 2008; Fardet 2010). Whole grains are important dietary sources of tocols. Total tocol content of 150 bread wheat genotypes grown under similar conditions, ranged 27.6–79.7 μg/g dm with an average of 50 μg/g dm (Table 16.1) (Lampi *et al.* 2008). Results from several studies fall in the same range (e.g., Panfili *et al.* 2003; Nielsen & Hansen 2008; Abozed *et al.* 2014; Hidalgo *et al.* 2016; Lachman *et al.* 2018). Among other wheat species, the contents in diploid einkorns have been reported to be the highest (Hidalgo *et al.* 2006; Lampi *et al.* 2008; Bradolini *et al.* 2015). Comparable contents of total tocols have been reported in rye being 43.6–67.2 μg/g dm (Ryynänen *et al.* 2004; Nyström *et al.* 2008), and barley grains being 28.4–124.9 μg/g dm (Andersson *et al.* 2008a; Nielsen & Hansen 2008; Temelli *et al.* 2013; Lachman et al. 2018). The contents in oat grains have been indicated to be somewhat lower and ranging 16.1–36.1 μg/g dm (Panfili *et al.* 2003; Shewry *et al.* 2008), whereas in a comprehensive study of 173 accessions the contents ranged 66–94 μg/g dm (Redaelli *et al.* 2016). In wheat, β-T3 was the major vitamer followed by α-Toc, whereas in rye, barley and oats it was α-T3, and the sum of T3 was always greater than that of Toc (Andersson *et al.* 2008a; Lampi *et al.* 2008; Nyström *et al.* 2008; Shewry *et al.* 2008). Both genetic and environmental factors have been shown to have a great impact on tocol contentes in cereals (Shewry *et al.* 2010a, 2010b).

Tocols are unevenly distributed in the grains. In general, tocols are concentrated in the germ, aleurone and bran layers, while the content in the endosperm is lower. Moreover, the germ provides mainly Toc, while T3 are located in the endosperm and bran (Tiwari & Cummins 2009; Andersson *et al.* 2014). For example, there was a three-fold difference in total tocol content of rye bran fraction compared to whole grains (Holasova 1997), and a 35% difference in pearling flours of barley compared to whole grains (Temelli *et al.* 2013), whereas wheat flours consisting mainly of the endosperm contained only ca. 50% of total tocols from that of whole grains (Nielsen & Hansen 2008; Fratianni *et al.* 2013). Although total tocol content of wheat germ was only four- to six-fold of that of whole grain, the difference in α-Toc was 12- to 18-fold (Nielsen & Hansen 2008; Engelsen & Hansen 2009). These examples show that the whole grains and flours containing the bran layers are superior to refined flours as sources of tocols. Since tocols are reactive and easily oxidized in the presence of light, heat and oxidizing lipids, they are also sensitive during food processing and storage. Processes like extrusion and deep-fat frying may be detrimental to tocols, whereas losses during cooking, baking and optimized puffing are smaller (e.g., Liukkonen *et al.* 2003; Leenhardt *et al.* 2006; Tiwar & Cummins 2009; Hidalgo *et al.* 2016). Once lipid oxidation starts in milled grains, tocols are also consumed, which occurs even under storage conditions.

16.4.2 Absorption, distribution, metabolism, excretion and health implications

As tocols are lipid soluble molecules, absorbed tocols are packed into chylomicrons and transported to the systemic blood through the lymph. Tissues may take up tocols during lipolysis of chylomicron triacylglycerols. A small fraction of absorbed tocols may be transported in HDL particles. Main part of tocols is transported to the liver in chylomicron remnants. In the liver, α-Toc transfer protein facilitates the transfer of α-Toc to VLDL for delivery to non-hepatic tissues. Other tocopherols and tocotrienols are largely metabolized in the liver via cytochrome P450-initiated hydroxylation and oxidation followed by oxidation. The resulting hydroxychromanols and carboxychromanols may be further conjugated (sulfated or glucuronidated) (Traber 2013; Jiang 2014) and are mainly excreted in the urine. Tocol bioaccessibility from cereal products is largely unknown and their absolute bioavailability is difficult to estimate due to its lipophilicity. All tocols are scavengers of lipid peroxyl radicals and protect membrane lipids from oxidation. γ-Toc and other tocols with unsubstituted 5-position may trap reactive nitrogen species and thus detoxify, for instance, peroxynitrite. Tocols and their carboxychromanol metabolites have been shown in mechanistic studies to inhibit cyclooxygenase (COX) and 5-lipoxygenase (LOX) catalyzed eicosanoid production and suppress proinflammatory signalling, such as NF-κB and STAT, and may thus protect against inflammation-associated diseases (Jiang 2014). T3 decreases cholesterol synthesis and supplemented doses have been reported to decrease serum cholesterol concentrations in humans (Ahsan *et al.* 2014). Also, other cardioprotective effects have been linked with T3 (Ramanathan *et al.* 2018).

Particularly α-Toc has been intensively studied for its cancer preventive activity during past decades (Ju *et al.* 2010). Even though the relationship between dietary intake of α-Toc/tocols and cancer risk in epidemiological studies has been inconsistent, and at the best suggestive, several large randomized clinical trials with α-Toc supplementation have been carried out since the ATBC trial found that a daily supplementation of a moderate dose of

50 mg α-Toc led to significant reduction in the incidence of prostate cancer in male smokers (Yang *et al.* 2012). However, all the three subsequent large, long-term trials using higher doses of α-Toc failed to show that the supplementations prevented prostate, colon, lung or any other cancers. These results are well in line with a number of earlier animal studies showing that α-Toc had no effect on carcinogenesis of the colon, prostate and lung, only exception being the mammary gland where α-Toc gave protection against tumorigenesis (Ju *et al.* 2010). In recent years, the research focus has sifted to other tocols. It has been reported that a naturally occuring γ-Toc-rich mixture of tocopherols (59.3% γ-Toc, 24.4% δ-Toc, 13.5% α-Toc, 1.6% β-Toc), a by-product of the distillation of vegetable oil, effectively inhibits carcinogenesis and/or tumor formation in animal models of colon, breast and prostate cancers (Ju *et al.* 2010). Furthermore, the effects of different tocoferols on colon (Guan *et al.* 2012), lung (Li *et al.* 2011) and mammary (Smolarek *et al.* 2012) carcinogenesis were compared and it was found that δ-Toc possessed the best anticancer activity, followed by γ-Toc, while α-Toc was without significant effect. δ- and γ-Toc have stronger antinitrative and anti-inflammatory activity than α-Toc. This may explain their anticarcinogenic activity in the colon and lung, where administration of δ- and γ-Toc resulted in decreased oxidative DNA damage, and reduced formation of nitrotyrosine and prostaglandin E_2 (Guan *et al.* 2012, Li *et al.* 2011). In the mammary gland, inhibition of tumorigenesis by δ- and γ-Toc was associated with increased expression of apoptotic proteins, decreased expression of proteins promoting cell survival and proliferation as well as inhibition of estrogen receptor-dependent signalling (Smolarek *et al.* 2012). Thus far, no studies have been reported regarding the effects of whole grain tocols, unique mixtures of tocopherols and tocotrienols.

16.5 Carotenoids

16.5.1 Chemical characteristics, contents in cereals and effects of food processing

Carotenoids are isoprenoids with an extensive system of conjugated double bonds with usually 40 carbon atoms and one or two rings at the end of the molecule. In general, the double bonds exist in *trans* isomers. Carotenoids can be divided into hydrocarbon carotenes and oxygenated xanthophylls. Of the natural carotenoids, β-carotene, α-carotene, and β-cryptoxanthin, have provitamin A activity. Carotenoids are lipid-soluble and contribute to yellow, orange and red colors in the nature. Color derived from carotenoids is an important quality parameter in many cereal foods, especially in pasta. Carotenoids are antioxidants and act mainly by radical scavenging and quenching single oxygen (Fardet *et al.* 2008; Fardet 2010). Whole grains are a good dietary source of carotenoids. Among cereals, corn has the highest average content of total carotenoids (18.2 μg/g) compared to wheat (2.6 μg/g) or barley (3.4 μg/g) (Ndolo & Beta 2013). In corn, zeaxanthin was the major carotenoid species (Panfili *et al.* 2004), whereas in wheat and other cereal grains lutein is the main carotenoid present followed by zeaxanthin and β-carotene (Adom *et al.* 2003; Panfili *et al.* 2004; Fratianni *et al.* 2013; Bradolini *et al.* 2015). Lutein and zeaxanthin belong to the xanthophylls.

There is significant variation in carotenoid contents among wheat species and varieties. For example, total lutein contents of eleven wheat varieties ranged 0.26–1.43 μg/g fw, showing five-fold variation (Adom *et al.* 2003). In other studies, lutein content in bread wheats ranged 0.82–1.14 μg/g fw (Moore *et al.* 2005) and 1.40–2.51 μg/g dw (Hidalgo *et al.* 2006), whereas the contents in durum wheat were higher and ranged 1.96–4.79 μg/g dm (Hidalgo *et al.* 2006). Especially high lutein content of 9.3 μg/g dm was reached in a yellow endosperm wheat variety (Paznocht *et al.* 2018). The total carotenoid contents reported in durum wheat ranged 2.77–6.2 μg/g dm (Fratianni *et al.* 2013; Bradolini *et al.* 2015). Lutein was also the major carotenoid in einkorn wheat accessions (3.92–12.64 μg/g dm), where the overall carotenoid content was 2–4 times higher than in durum and bread wheat (Hidalgo *et al.* 2006). In different types of wheat, lutein was mainly located in the germ, but significant amounts of it occurred in the endosperm and bran of einkorn (Hidalgo & Bradolini 2008). In durum wheat, total carotenoid contents of semolina were comparable to whole grain flours (Fratianni *et al.* 2013). In barley and oats, carotenoids were also concentrated in the germ, whereas in corn, the content in germ was low (Ndolo & Beta 2013). However, the total contribution of carotenoids in endosperm as the major fraction of the kernel was 20.5%–70.6% in wheat, barley and oats (Ndolo & Beta 2013). Since carotenoids are reactive compounds, processing may affect their isomerization and losses. For examples, pasta-making process was reported to cause 27%–80% losses in various wheat types (Fratianni *et al.* 2015) and puffing causes, on average, 54% losses in bread wheat and einkorn (Hidalgo *et al.* 2016). However, after steaming (paraboiling) migration of lutein from the germ to the endosperm in einkorn occurred, which balanced the originally lower content (Hidalgo *et al.* 2008). LOX activity present in cereal grains is known to bleach carotenoids. To avoid losses in bread making, wheat varieties with low LOX activity and high carotenoid content are recommended (Leenhardt *et al.* 2006).

16.5.2 Absorption, distribution, metabolism, excretion and health implications

Carotenoids are absorbed from the small intestine and transported into the body in lipoproteins. Some carotenoids may be enzymatically cleaved into retinal and thus act as provitamin A. Carotenoid bioavailability is largely dependent on their bioaccessibility, for example, the efficiency by which they are released from the food matrix and incorporated into mixed micelles in the small intestine (Yonekura & Nagao 2007; Sy *et al.* 2012). The bioaccessibility of whole grain carotenoids may be affected by grain particle size (Brewer *et al.* 2014) or food preparation methods (Kean *et al.* 2008).

There are several mechanisms by which carotenoids could promote health and prevent degenerative diseases such as coronary heart disease and type 2 diabetes. Carotenoids are scavengers of reactive oxygen species and may function as lipid soluble antioxidants in the body. Carotenoids (or their metabolites) may also function indirectly because they may interact with cellular signalling cascades, such as nuclear factors NF-κB or Nrf2, which are associated with inflammation and oxidative stress (Kaulmann *et al.* 2014). Lutein, the most abundant carotenoid in whole grain cereals, has been associated with decreased intima media thickness and atherosclerosis in animal models (Dwyer *et al.* 2001; Zou *et al.* 2014). Supplementation with lutein has been reported to dose-dependently decrease serum C-reactive protein (CRP) concentrations (Wang *et al.* 2013). More research is needed to clarify the significance of cereal carotenoids on the risk of cardiovascular diseases and diabetes.

β-carotene has been the most studied carotenoid in cancer research, followed by lycopene. Relatively limited data are available on other carotenoids. While dietary intake and plasma concentrations of carotenoids, for example, β-carotene and lutein, have been associated with decreased risk of several cancers (Aune *et al.* 2012; Jung *et al.* 2013), a number of clinical trials with β-carotene supplementation have found no reduction in cancer incidence or have even seen adverse effects of the supplementations (Chatterjee *et al.* 2012). β-carotene has also been extensively studied in animal models of cancer and it has been shown to inhibit carcinogenesis of the mouth, skin, liver, breast, colon and lungs (Chatterjee *et al.* 2012). Lutein has shown anticancer activity against colon, breast and liver carcinogenesis (Raju *et al.* 2005; Park *et al.* 1998, Sindhu *et al.* 2013). The exact mechansims whereby carotenoids prevent tumorigenesis are still under investigation, but they likely involve inhibition of cell proliferation, induction of apoptosis, and modulation of cytochrome P450 and detoxifying enzymes along with its antioxidant activity (Wang & Wang 2011).

16.6 Plant Sterols

16.6.1 Chemical characteristics, contents in cereals and effects of food processing

Plant sterols (PSs) are composed of a tetracyclic cyclopenta-α-phenanthrene ring and a side chain attached at the C-17 atom of the ring structure. They are divided in three groups based on the number of methyl groups at C-4. The most common PSs, named desmethysterols, have no methyl group at C-4. They are a group of compounds differing in the number and location of double bonds in the ring structure and in the structure of the side chain (Piironen *et al.* 2000).

The most common PSs in cereal grains include sitosterol, campesterol, stigmasterol, Δ5-avenasterol, Δ7-avenasterol, and the saturated sterols sitostanol and campestanol. Sitosterol accounts commonly for ca 50% of total PSs (Piironen & Lampi 2004). Stanols are found in significant amounts in rye, wheat and corn. Their proportion ranged 11–29% in wheat and rye cultivars (Nurmi *et al.* 2008; Nyström *et al.* 2008). PSs occur in grains as free sterols and different conjugates, that is, esters with fatty acids or phenolic acids, glycosides and acylated glycosides (Piironen & Lampi 2004).

The reported total PS content varies within and between grain species (Table 16.1). The content ranged 494–1039 μg/g dm in wheat (Nurmi *et al.* 2008; Alignan *et al.* 2009; Iafelice *et al.* 2009; Nurmi *et al.* 2010) and 995–1420 μg/g dm in rye (Nyström *et al.* 2007; Nyström *et al* 2008; Shewry *et al.* 2010a). For barley and oat, the corresponding ranges were 870–1153 μg/g dm and 350–682 μg/g dm, respectively (Määttä *et al.* 1999; Piironen *et al.* 2002; Andersson *et al.* 2008a; Shewry *et al.* 2008). Both genetic and environmental factors affect the content (Nurmi *et al.* 2008; Nurmi *et al.* 2010). High heritability in wheat indicated that increasing PS content could be a realistic target in plant breeding (Shewry *et al.* 2010b).

PSs are unevenly distributed in grains. The total PS content increases in wheat and rye flour fractions as the ash content increases (Piironen *et al.* 2002; Nystöm *et al.* 2007). Among milling products, bran and germ are generally known to be rich PS sources. In 10 studies reviewed by Nurmi (2012), PS content in wheat bran ranged 890–2000 μg/g, while that of wheat bran ranged 2400–4923 μg/g based on results from five studies. Interestingly, grain fractions do not differ only in their PS contents but also in their PS composition. Proportion of stanols is higher in wheat and rye bran than in the inner parts of grains. On the other hand, they are not found in germ (Nyström *et al.* 2007; Nurmi *et al.* 2012). Steryl ferulates are mainly located in the outer layers while glycosides are more evenly distributed (Nyström *et al.* 2007). Nurmi (2012) suggested that steryl ferulates accumulate in the intermediate layer. Rice and corn bran oils are of marked interest as steryl ferulate sources (Liang *et* al. 2014; Sawadikiat & Hongsprabhas 2014).

Cereal products are among the main dietary PS sources if only non-fortified sources are considered. They were shown to be the main PS source both in Finland (42%), the Netherlands (38%) and China (35%) (Normen *et al.* 2001; Valsta *et al.* 2004; Wang *et al.* 2012a). In these studies, the total PS intake for women and men ranged 237–311 md/d and 307–330 mg/d, respectively. As lipids, PSs are prone to oxidation. However, they are fairly stable compounds and their content in cereal foods is mainly determined by the chosen grain fraction used.

16.6.2 Absorption, distribution, metabolism, excretion and health implications

It is well known that unsaturated or saturated plant sterols, or stanols, can decrease serum total- and especially LDL-cholesterol concentrations (Gylling *et al.* 2014). PSs may interfere with the incorporation of cholesterol into mixed micelles, thus decreasing cholesterol absorption from the intestinal lumen. However, also other mechanisms have been suggested (De Smet *et al.* 2012). PS intake of 2 g/d decreases serum LDL-cholesterol up to 10% (Gylling *et al.* 2014). These intakes are not, however, achieved from natural sources. The specific effects of PSs from whole grains have not been intensively studied. In one study, cholesterol absorption after a wheat germ muffin test meal was higher after consumption of muffins containing PS-depleted wheat germ (<6 mg phytosterols) than after the consumption of original wheat germ muffins (328 mg PS) (Ostlund *et al.* 2003). This suggests that endogenous PSs in wheat germ affected cholesterol absorption and metabolism. A naturally PS-rich diet (449 mg PS/2000 kcal, including grain PSs) has been shown to decrease cholesterol absorption and increase fecal cholesterol excretion relative to the PS-poor diet (126 mg phytosterols/2000 kcal) (Lin *et al.* 2010). However, these differences between diets were not reflected in LDL-cholesterol concentrations that were similar after consumption of the diets. PSs have also been studied in relation to cancer in experimental models.

16.6.3 Plant sterols and cancer

β-sitosterol inhibits cell growth in colon, breast and prostate cancer cell lines *In vitro,* possibly by inducing cell cycle arrest through increasing p53 and p21 expression, and by promoting apoptosis through activating Fas-receptor and caspases, affecting Bcl-2 and Bax levels as well as changing ceramide metabolism (Bradford & Awad 2010). In a breast cancer model in PyMT Tg mice, PSs (41% β-sitosterol, 22% stigmasterol, 20% campesterol) given at 0.2% in the diet delayed the onset of tumors and reduced the total tumor burden but only when fed in high-fat context (Llaverias *et al.* 2013).

The effects of PSs on colon tumorigenesis have been investigated in several animal studies with mixed results. An early study by Raich *et al.* (1980) demonstrated that supplementing a chow diet with 0.2% of β-sitosterol (95% β-sitosterol, 4% campesterol, 1% stigmasterol) reduced the incidence and number of colon tumors in carcinogen-treated rats.

In contrast, in the study by Quilliot *et al.* (2001) feeding 24 mg/d of PSs (55% β-sitosterol, 41% campesterol, 4% stigma sterol) as part of either a low- or high-fat diet had no effect on colon tumor formation in carcinogen-treated rats and induced possibly unfavorable effects on gut bacterial activity. In the Min mouse model of colon cancer, plantstanols, and to a lesser extent, sterols at 0.8% of diet enhanced intestinal tumor formation. Enhanced tumorigenesis was accompanied by the activation of the central cancer-promoting pathways, the epidermal growth factor receptor and Wnt pathways, and increased transcriptional activity of beta-catenin in the normal appearing mucosa (Marttinen *et al.* 2013; Marttinen *et al* 2014). The stanol feeding, in particular, resulted in six-fold increase in the amount of cholesterol in caecal contents of stanol-fed mice and affected sterol metabolism and genes of cholesterol synthesis pathway in the mucosa. The results suggest that stanols may disturb colonic cholesterol metabolism, and thereby promote tumor formation (Marttinen *et al.* 2013). While feeding pure plant sterols and stanols at relatively abundant level in a diet, achieved only by supplementation, may accelerate intestinal tumor formation, this is unlikely when PSs come as a part of cereal component in a diet. Indeed, Sang *et al.* (2006) found no effect on the number of intestinal tumors in the Min mouse of a subfraction of wheat bran oil containing PSs.

16.7 Inositol phosphates

16.7.1 Chemical characteristics and abundance of inositol phosphates in cereals

The chemical structure of phytate, or its protonated form phytic acid, is myoinositol (1,2,3,4,5,6) hexakisphosphoric acid (IP6). There are also lower inositol phosphatate salts important for nutrition, myoinositol tri- (IP3), tetra- (IP4) and penta- (IP5) phosphate. In plants, phytate forms complexes that are hydrolysed during germination to release phosphorus and associated minerals for the development of the seedling. Cereals and legumes are the main sources of phytate in diet. According to Schlemmer *et al.* (2009), the daily intake of phytate ranges widely, 180–5577 mg, being low in typical Western diets and high in vegetarian diets. As reviewed by Schlemmer *et al.* (2009), phytate content in wheat varies from 3.9 to 13.5 mg/g. Magallanes-Lopez *et al.* (2017) has recently reported contents within this range for 46 durum wheat varieties (4.62–9.52 mg/g), but even higher contents for durum wheat (14.63–16.78 mg/g) have been reported by Branković *et al.* (2015). In rye, oats and barley, the phytate content typically varies from 3.8 to 14.6 mg/g dm (Schlemmer *et al.* 2009). Higher contents have been observed in maize (7.2–22.2 mg/g dm) and in sorghum (even up to 33.5 mg/g dm), whereas lower in rice (0.6–10.8 mg/g dm) (Schlemmer *et al.* 2009) and pearl millet (1.98–4.10 mg/g) (Boncompagni *et al.* 2018).

16.7.2 Effects of food processing on inositol phosphate content

Studies on food processing effects have been mainly focused on degradation of phytate, leading to improved bioavailability of minerals and subsequent alleviation of mineral deficiency in humans, especially in developing countries. Phytate content can be reduced by endogenous or added phytases, as comprehensively reviewed by Kumar *et al.* (2010). On the other hand, thermal treatments, such as kilning of oats, may inactivate phytases. Soaking increases phytase activity and results in the leakage of water soluble phytate. However, leaching of soluble minerals may counteract the aim to enhance mineral availability (Kruger *et al.* 2014). Germination has been reported to cause approximately 30% phytate reduction in wheat and rye (Schlemmer *et al.* 2009), in white sorghum (Afify *et al.* 2011), and in barley and oats (Hübner *et al.* 2010). However, for barley and oats, smaller decreases (16–17%) have been reported but in optimized conditions almost complete removal of phytate in barley has been achieved (Schlemmer *et al.* 2009). In addition, Azeke *et al.* (2011) reported the germination of rice, maize, millet, sorghum and wheat to reduce phytate 81–88%, with a concurrent increase in phytase activity. However, prolonged germination times were needed to achieve a significant reduction in phytate content

In the baking process of breads, phytate is mostly degraded during the levening of the dough due to phytase activity, rather then the heat treatment in the final baking step. Phytase activity may originate from cereals and associated microbes or be produced by adding microbes or phytases. For instance, in whole meal wheat baking, 60–70% of the initial phytate content was reduced in the dough mixing, and an additional 10–20% reduction was achieved after fermentation with phytase-active yeast (Nor Qhairul Izzreen *et al.* 2017). The extent of phytate hydrolysis depends strongly on the pH (Schlemmer *et al.* 2009; Anson *et al.* 2012). Consequently, sourdough fermentation reduces phytate content more effectively than yeast fermentation only. According to Lopez *et al.* (2003), in sourdough wheat bread phytate reduction was 71% compared to 52% reduction in yeast fermented bread. Buddrick *et al.* (2014) reported a greater phytate reduction in rye bread (86%) compared to wheat and wheat-oat breads (63 and 53%, respectively) due to the acidification of the dough. Combination of food processes may further enhance phytate reduction. For instance, Svanberg *et al.* (1993) showed that germination combined with lactic acid fermentation can yield an almost complete degradation of phytate in white sorghum and maize gruels. Similarly, Baek *et al.* (2014) found a 17% phytate decrease in three-day germinated paddy rice, whereas fermentation of germinated paddy rice led to total of 88% phytate reduction. Soaking and extrusion of whole grain rice could remove 78% of phytate (Albarracin *et al.* 2015), and optimized hydrothermal processing of germinated wheat as much as 95% (Lemmens *et al.* 2018).

16.7.3 Absorption, distribution, metabolism and health implications

Inositol phosphates (especially IP6 and IP5) are antinutrients because they chelate metal ions such as zinc, iron as well as calcium. In addition, these complexes form aggregates, and thereby impair metal absorption in the small intestine. In plant-based diets where cereal foods are the main source of iron and zinc, the decreased bioavailability may contribute to inadequate iron and zinc status. Phytate degradation by phytases (e.g., from *Aspergillus niger*) has been shown to enhance iron bioavailability (Troesch *et al.* 2013). On the other hand, phytate may act as an antioxidant by chelating iron in the intestine (Schlemmer *et al.* 2009). Phytate may decrease starch digestibility in the intestine and modulate postprandial glucose responses (Thompson *et al.* 1987). In the diet of diabetic mice, phytate reduced high blood glucose levels (Lee *et al.* 2006).

Endogenous phytase activity in the human intestine is very small. Phytate may be partly degraded to lower inositol polyphosphates and even unphosphorylated myoinositol in the gastrointestinal tract by food phytases (mainly stomach) and microbial phytases (mainly in the large intestine) (Schlemmer *et al.* 2009). Diet modulates the microbial degradation of phytate (Markiewicz *et al.* 2013). Free myo-inositol is readily absorbed by active transport and incorporated in the body myo-inositol pool (Croze & Soulage 2013). There is some evidence that a small fraction of dietary phytate could be absorbed, probably from the small intestine (Schlemmer *et al.* 2009). However, other authors conclude that absorption of intact IP6 is unlikely (Wilson *et al.* 2015).

16.7.4 Inositol phosphates and cancer

Phytate has been suggested to contribute to the cancer-preventive activity of whole grains in colorectal cancer. Reddy *et al.* (2000) compared the effects of intact wheat bran to those of dephytinized and phytate restored wheat brans, and found that removal or restoration of phytate in wheat bran had no significant effect on tumor multiplicity or volume in the colon of carcinogen-treated rats. Similar results were obtained by Jenab and Thompson (1998) who found that removing phytate and then restoring it to wheat bran had only a marginal effect on colonic aberrant crypt foci formation (ACF) in carcinogen-treated rats even though pure phytic acid at the same concentration was able to reduce the number and size of colon ACFs. In a more recent study, phytate (IP6) extracted from rice bran and administered to carcinogen-treated rats at 0.2% (w/v), 0.5% (w/v), and 1.0% (w/v) via drinking water was shown to reduce both ACF formation and tumor incidence in the colon in a dose-dependent manner (Shafie *et al.* 2013). Inositol phosphates as pure compounds have been reported to inhibit carcinogenesis and tumor formation in several organs, including the skin, lung, breast, prostate and liver, particularly if given via drinking water (Vucenik & Shamsuddin 2006). Some studies with tumor xenograft models have indicated that, in addition to preventing tumor formation, phytate may also possess antimetastatic activity by downregulationg the PI3K/Akt pathway together with diminished cell migration and angiogenesis (Maffucci *et al.* 2005; Vucenik & Shamsuddin 2006). A recent study with BALB/c mice showed that phytate inhibited colorectal cancer metastasis to the liver by modulating tumor microenvironment, for example, by altering expression of extracellular matrix proteins, proteolytic matrix metalloproteinases and several angiogenic and growth factors (Fu *et al.* 2016). This effect may be due to the fact that phytate competes with tumor-promoting iron compunds, such as ferric citrate, which is a common iron fortificant in mouse chow, and thus alleviates the cancer promoting effect (Scheers *et al.*, 2018). In a 1,2-dimethylhydrazine-induced rat colorectal cancer model, phytate was also reported to improve intestinal mucosal barrier damage and to decrease serum concentrations of proinflammatory cytokines (Liu *et al.* 2018).

16.8 Lignans

16.8.1 Chemical characteristics, contents in cereals and effects of food processing

Lignans are diphenolic compounds derived from two phenylpropanoid C6-C3 units coupled via a carbon-carbon single bond at C8 and C8' (Willför *et al.* 2006; Durazzo *et al.* 2013). Some lignans from legumes, flaxseed, wheat, rye and other cereal grains possess phytoestrogenic activity, that is, are converted to the mammalian lignans enterodiol (END) and enterolacton (ENL) in humans. The most common cereal lignans are secoisolariciresinol (SEC), matairesinol (MAT), lariciresinol (LAR), pinoresinol (PIN) and syringaresinol (SYR) (Fardet *et al.* 2008; Durazzo *et al.* 2013; Andersson *et al.* 2014). The number of lignans identified in plants is constantly increasing, for example, by identifying neolignans with alternate bonds between the phenylpropanoid units, and oligomeric lignans. For example, ten novel oligomeric lignans were identified from rye bran (Hanhineva *et al.* 2012). Plant lignans occur as glycosides and aglycones. Lignans are categorized into antioxidants capable of scavenging radicals (Fardet *et al.* 2008; Fardet 2010; Durazzo *et al.* 2013; Andersson *et al.* 2014). Cereals and cereal products contributed to 8.8%–19.9% of total daily lignan intake of 0.8–2.4 mg in 10 countries in Europe, being higher in the non-Mediterranean countries (Zamora-Ros *et al.* 2012). It is difficult to provide comprehensive and reliable profiles and contents of lignans for cereal grains because of large variation in lignan species included in the analysis and differences in methods used, resulting in large variation in reported contents and profiles. As reviewed by Durazzo and co-workers (2013), LAR and SEC were the major lignans in several wheat types and maize, and LAR and PIN in rye, barley and oats. Kuhnle and co-workers (2009), including only MAT, SEC and coumestrol in their study, reported SEC to be the major lignan in oats, barley and wheat. Furthermore, SYR not listed in the review, contributed to 80% of total lignans in wheat and rye, and to 40% in oats (Smeds *et al.* 2009), and was also found as the major one in barley (Peñalvo *et al.* 2005). As an example, the sum of seven lignans in 28 winter rye, 73 spring wheat and 55 spring oat grain samples ranged from 25.0 to 67.0 μg/g, 3.4 to 22.7 μg/g, and from 8.2 to 25.5 μg/g, respectively (Smeds *et al.* 2009). Rye was also considered as the best cereal source of lignans in other studies (Peñalvo *et al.* 2005; Smeds *et al.* 2007; Tetens *et al.* 2013).

Like many other bioactive compounds, lignans are concentrated in the outer layers of the grain. Thus, it has been suggested that lignan contents are highest in the bran fractions and lowest in refined flours (Durazzo *et al.* 2013). Total lignan content of wheat bran was 10-fold higher than that of whole grains, whereas the ratio for rye, oat, barley, and spelt wheat was 2.5- to 4-fold (Smeds *et al.* 2007). In commercial rye and wheat brans, SYR was the major lignan, and the sums of six lignans were 58–70 and 28–36 μg/g fw (Kamal-Eldin *et al.* 2009). The effects of food processing on lignans have not been extensivly studied (Andersson *et al.* 2014). Heating rye flour at 100°C for 40 min did not cause any changes in SYR or LAR, but at 200°C, they started to degrade gradually (Gerstenmeyer *et al.* 2013). Cooking losses of 8% on average, but with a wide range from a loss of 35.5% with oats up to an increase of 13.6% with whole grain durum, were found in whole grain pasta made with different cereals and seeds (Durazzo *et al.* 2013). The effect was greatest for PIN.

16.8.2 Absorption, distribution, metabolism, excretion and health implications

Lignan glycosides are metabolized by intestinal bacteria to lignan aglycones and further to enterolignans (mammalian lignans) enterodiol (END) and enterolactone (ENL). Enterolignans are absorbed from the colon. They are excreted in urine or bile as glucuronides and sulfate esters (Peterson *et al.* 2010). Lignans and enterolignans undergo enterohepatic circulation. A study using purfied secoisolariciresinol-diglycoside (SDG) (Setchell *et al.* 2014) confirmed that SDG is first hydrolyzed to SEC and then metabolized to END and finally ENL. The metabolites are efficiently absorbed (Setchell *et al.* 2014). There is a large inter-individual variation in the production of enterolignans. Factors affecting the conversion include composition and activity of the colonic microbiota, transit time and intestinal redox state (Peterson *et al.* 2010; Landete 2012). The structures of enterolignans resemble that of 17-beta-estradiol. Enterolignans are estrogen receptor ligands and they have been shown to have estrogenic or antiestrogenic effects in various model systems (Landete 2012). The possible cardioprotective effects of lignans have been studied in randomized trials in humans (Peterson *et al.* 2010). There are some indications that lignan supplementation decreases blood pressure, serum cholesterol concentration and systemic inflammation (Frankenfield 2017). However, much more research is needed to confirm whether lignans contribute to the cardioprotective effects of whole grains.

16.8.3 Lignans and cancer

Lignans have been actively studied in the context of cancer prevention, particularly in relation to breast and colorectal cancer in observational studies. Variability and inaccuracy in lignan contents in food databases have hampered epidemiological studies. However, some studies suggest protective role for lignans against cancer, for example, dietary intake of lignans was inversely associated with colorectal cancer risk in a Canadian case-control study (Cotterchio *et al.* 2006) and a Ducth study reported a substantial reduction in colorectal adenoma risk in the subjects with high plasma concentrations of enterodiols (Kuijsten *et al.* 2006). Similarly, in an American study, higher intakes of total lignans as well as LAR and PIN were associated with lower risk of breast cancer and invasive tumors (McCann *et al.* 2012).

Only a limited number of studies have addressed lignans specifically from cereal grains. Davies *et al.* (1999) investigated the effect of rye lignans on colon carcinogenesis in carcinogen-treated rats and reported that rats fed a high-fat diet supplemented with 30% of rye bran had significantly less tumors per animal than rats fed the control diet, which was suggested to be due to rye lignans as the diets were adjusted for their fibre and phytate content. Unfortunately, the same diet failed to show protective effects in the Min mouse model of colon cancer (van Kranen *et al.* 2003). The pure lignans MAT and SEC, the most common cereal lignans, were administered to Min mice at 0.02% (w/w) in diet but neither of them were able to inhibit intestinal tumorigenesis to significant extent even though tumor incidence in the colon of SEC fed mice tended to be lower that in the control mice (Pajari *et al.* 2006). The exact mechanisms whereby lignans may inhibit colon carcinogenesis are not well-defined, but may include inhibition of cell growth by down-regulation of the Wnt/beta-catenin signalling and suppression of inflammatory activity via reduced prostaglandin E_2 and pro-inflammatory cytokine production (Yoo *et al.* 2010; During *et al.* 2012).

Flaxseed is the riches dietary source of lignans, containing particularly high concentrations of SDG that hydrolyzes to SEC in the intestine (Setchell *et al.* 2014). Pure SDG has been extensively studied in animal models of breast cancer and has been found to inhibit chemically induced mammary tumorigenesis and tumor growth as well as regress xenograft tumor growth in atymic mice (Wiggins *et al.* 2013). SDG exerts its effects by inhibiting cell proliferation, inducing apoptosis and reducing the expression of estrogen and growth factor receptors (Chen *et al.* 2009). Pure LAR has also been shown to reduce mammary cancer growth in two different breast cancer models, possible mechanisms involving inhibition of angiogenesis, increased tumor cell apoptosis and increased expression of estrogen receptor β (Saarinen *et al.* 2008). Whether the effects of pure lignans are any indication of those of the same lignas obtained from cereal sources remains to be verified by future studies.

16.9 Phenolic acids

16.9.1 Chemical characteristics, contents in cereals and effects of food processing

Phenolic acids are derivatives of cinnamic or benzoic acids with at least one phenolic hydroxyl group. The most common species in cereal grains are the cinnamic acid derivatives ferulic and p-coumaric acids, and the benzoic acid derivatives syringic and vanillic acids. Phenolic acid may exist in soluble free and conjugated, or insoluble bound forms, and ferulic acid also as di- and trimers. Most phenolic acids are linked with polysaccharides, for example, arabinoxylan and lignin, crosslinking them to support the cell wall structure. They are also involved in the chemical and physical defence systems. Phenolic acids contribute significantly to the antioxidant and other bioactivities of the dietary fibre complex (Fardet *et al.* 2008; Fardet 2010; Stuper-Szablewska & Perkowski 2017). The phenolic hydroxyl groups are essential for their antioxidant activity (e.g., Bondia-Pons *et al.* 2009; Andersson *et al.* 2014). Cereals and cereal products contributed to 4.7%–8.7% of the total daily phenolic acid intake of 289–842 mg in three geographical areas of Europe with the Nothern countries having the highest values (Zamora-Ros *et al.* 2013). Total phenolic acid contents in bread wheats (n=150) grown under similar conditions ranged 326–1171 µg/g dm with an average of 658 µg/g dm (Li *et al.* 2008). Comparable levels have also been found in other studies on wheat cultivars (Guo & Beta 2013; Ndolo & Beta 2014). Contents in barley varied 254–1132 µg/g (Andersson *et al.* 2008a; Guo & Beta 2013; Ndolo & Beta, 2014), in rye 491–1082 µg/g dm (Nyström *et al.* 2008) and in oats 331–873 µg/g (Shewry *et al.* 2008; Guo & Beta 2013; Ndolo & Beta, 2014).

The average proportions of free, soluble conjugated and insoluble bound phenolic acids in wheat were <1%, 22% and 77%, respectively (Li *et al.* 2008). Phenolic acid composition in free acids varied substantially, whereas among bound ones, ferulic acid contributed to 72%–85% of all phenolic acids (Li *et al.* 2008). Other acids present in wheat included p-coumaric, sinapic, vanillic, syringic and isoferulic acids (Li *et al.*, 2008; Ndolo & Beta, 2014). As reviewed by Bondia-Pons *et al.* (2009), ferulic acid contributed to 85%–90%, sinapic acid to 9%–10% and p-coumaric acid to 3%–5% of total phenolic acids in rye. Contents of phenolic acids varied more than of most other bioactive compounds among bread wheat genotypes. Variation was on an average 3.6-fold, whereas that of free acids was even greater, being 9.75-fold (Shewry *et al.* 2013). Yet the ratios of genetic variance to total variance were relatively small, being 28% in total and 6% in free phenolic acids (Shewry *et al.* 2013). Phenolic acids are predominately present in the bran layers making whole grain flours and brans as excellent sources of these compounds (e.g., Stuper-Szablewska & Perkowski 2017). Studies on hand-dissected fractions of germ, pericarp, aleurone and endosperm of wheat, barley and oats showed great differences in contents of individual phenolic acids and their profiles (Ndolo & Beta 2014). The lowest phenolic acid contents were in the endosperm fractions (107–148 µg/g) whereas the highest was found in bran fractions (2910–5138 µg/g). For example, ferulic acid contents in the pericarp and aleurone layers were ca 5-fold higher and in the germ only ca 20 % higher than in the whole grains (Ndolo & Beta 2014), whereas the mean contents in five bread wheat brans were almost 90-fold higher than in the debranned flours (Žilić *et al.* 2012). In more detail, dimers and trimers of ferulic acids were concentrated in the cell walls of pericarp, and free ferulic and p-coumaric acids in cell walls of aleurone (Hemery *et al.* 2011). Phenolic acids are considered as relatively stable compounds during processing (Andersson *et al.* 2014). Free phenolic acids were shown to have a strong impact on the flavor, for example, bitterness, of rye (Heiniö *et al.* 2008). Bioaccesibility of wheat bran phenolic acids in breads was significantly improved by grinding the bran factions into fine powders, however it should be pointed out that only the soluble free and conjugated acids were bioaccesible at all (Hemery *et al.* 2010).

16.9.2 Absorption, distribution, metabolism and health implications

Most data regarding bioactivity of phenolic acids stem from studies having focused on ferulic acid. Only small fraction of ferulic acid in grain foods is free and may be absorbed from the small intestine. Mateo Anson *et al.* (2009) showed that *In vitro* bioaccessibility of ferulic acid from wheat fractions and bread was less than 1%. Food processing (enzymatic treatment, yeast fermentation) has been shown to clearly enhance ferulic acid bioavailability from wheat (Mateo Anson *et al.* 2011) and rye (Lappi *et al.* 2013). Bound ferulic acid may be released and partly metabolized in the colon by microbial fermentation. These products are absorbed mainly by passive absorption. In the liver, ferulic acid is extensively metabolized to various polar metabolites that are excreted in urine. Only small proportion of the ingested ferulic acid dose is excreted unmodified (Mancuso & Santangelo 2014). In a mouse experiment, disintegration of wheat aleurone matrix either enzymatically or physically resulted in different ferulic acid metabolite patterns in urine, indicating that enzymatic processing increased absorption from the small intestine while grinding increased the amount of microbial metabolites (Pekkinen *et al.* 2014).

Ferulic acid has antioxidative and anti-inflammatory effects that could be associated with decreased risk for coronary heart disease and type 2 diabetes. It is of interest as a potential pharmacological agent in treatment and prevention of these chronic diseases (Lillioja *et al.* 2013; Mancuso & Santangelo 2014). Ferulic acid has been reported to decrease blood pressure, prevent arrhythmias, enhance antioxidant enzyme systems and decrease blood glucose concentration (Lillioja *et al.* 2013; Mancuso & Santangelo 2014; Ghosh *et al.* 2017). However, these effects have been mainly shown in in vitro studies or in animal studies with pharmacological ferulic acid doses. Human studies on the physiological effects of ferulic acid are scarce. In a study by Lappi *et al.* (2013), no differences in postprandial glucose responses after ingestion of breads with bioprocessed or native rye bran were observed. Mateo Anson *et al.* (2011) showed that cytokine responses in lipopolysaccharide-stimulated blood samples changed into a more anti-inflammatory direction after the consumption of the bioprocessed bread with higher ferulic acid bioavailability.

16.9.3 Phenolic acids and cancer

A limited number of studies have been carried out on the effects of pure ferulic acid in animal models of cancer, showing that ferulic acid inhibits mammary (Baskaran *et al.* 2010), skin (Huang *et al.* 1988) and oral (Mori *et al.* 1999) carcinogenesis. Ferulic acid also prevented the formation of aberrant crypts (Wargovich *et al.* 2000) and reduced the incidence of tumors (Kawabata *et al.* 2000) in the colon of carcinogen-treated rats. The effect was limited to the initiation phase only, suggesting a moderate protective effect of ferulic acid against colon carcinogenesis. The antitumorigenic effects of ferulic acid were associated with changes in the activity of detoxification enzymes such as gluthatione S-transferase, gluthatione reductase and quinone reductase in both mammary and colon cancer models

(Baskaran *et al.* 2010; Kawabata *et al.* 2000). In cancer cell lines, ferulic acid has been reported to reduce cell proliferation and modulate global gene expresson profile to favor delayed cell cycle progression (Janicke *et al.* 2011). Recent cell culture studies have revealed new anti-carcinogenic mechanisms for ferulic acid such as inhibition of cancer cell migration, down-regulation of growth factor receptors (EGFR), inhibition of telomerase activity and sensitation of cancer cells to cytotoxic effects of chemotherapy drugs (Ghosh *et al.* 2017).

16.10 Avenanthramides

16.10.1 Chemical characteristics, contents in cereals and effects of food processing

Avenanthramides are a group of phenolic compunds with antioxidant properties, unique to oats. They consist of anthranilic acid or hydroxyanthranilic acid linked with an amide bond to one of several possible hydroxycinnamic acids (Collins 2011; Singh *et al.* 2013). More than 40 compounds have been identified in oats (Collins 2011). The three major compounds are derived from 5-hydroxyanthranilic acid and either from p-coumaric acid (named avenanthramide 2p), caffeic acid (2c) or ferulic acid (2f) (Bryngelsson *et al.* 2002a; Dimberg *et al.* 2005; Mattila *et al.* 2005; Shewry *et al.* 2008; Multari *et al.* 2018). New compounds are still identified; 17 novel avenanthramide glucosides were recently reported (Wu *et al.* 2018).

Avenanthramide contents in oat grains vary markedly depending on genetic factors, seed development stage and environmental factors. In grains of five cultivars grown in the same location and year, the total avenanthramide content varied two-fold, ranging 42–91 μg/g dm (Shewry *et al.* 2008), whereas the range was wider, 27-185 μg/g dm, among eight cultivars of husked oats grown also in the same location and growing year (Multari *et al.* 2018). Comparison of 137 oat accessions showed that the effect of environment is highly significant (Redaeli *et al.* 2016). The effect of environment was higher than that of cultivar when 39 cultivars were grown in four locations in the same year (Li *et al.* 2017). Groats contain more avenanthramides than hulls; the mean contents in hand-separated groats and hulls of seven cultivars were 13.7 and 5.9 μg/g dm, respectively (Bryngelsson *et al.* 2002a). Detailed localization of avenanthramides in the grain is, however, not clear. Avenanthramides are suggested to be most likely located in the outer tissues, subaleurone, aleurone and pericarp (Collins 2011).

Processing may either decrease or increase avenanthramide contents. Avenanthramides were not affected by steaming, but drum drying of steamed rolled oats decreased their content markedly (Bryngelsson *et al.* 2002b). On the other hand, steeping of both intact grains and heat-treated grains increased the content due to de novo synthesis or release of bound forms (Bryngelsson *et al.* 2003). Also, germination may increase avenanthramide content (Skoglund *et al.* 2008; Xu *et al.* 2009). Pridal *et al.* (2018) estimated that avenanthramide intake among oat consumers ranges 0.3—2.1 mg/day.

16.10.2 Bioavailability, metabolism and health implications

Avenanthramide bioavailability has been studied in hamsters (Chen *et al.* 2004) and rats (Koening *et al.* 2011) as well as humans (Chen *et al.* 2007). Avenanthramide 2p appears to have the highest bioavailability among the different forms evaluated (Chen *et al.* 2007; Koening *et al.* 2011). In a pharmacokinetic study, 2f had slower elimination rate and longer half-life compared to 2p and 2c (Zhang *et al.* 2017). Avenanthramides have antioxidant and anti-inflammatory effects in vitro (Meydani 2009; Yang *et al.* 2014). The effects include suppressed vascular endothelial cell expression of adhesion molecules, decreased production of inflammatory cytokines, inhibition of smooth muscle cell proliferation and enhanced nitric oxide production. These effects are mediated, for example, through inhibition of *NF-κB* and several cell cycle regulatory proteins (Meydani 2009; Yang *et al.* 2014). There is evidence that avenanthramides may have antioxidative and anti-inflammatory effects also in vivo. In exercised rats, avenanthramide 2c supplementation increased antioxidant enzyme activities in tissues (Ji *et al.* 2003). In humans, one-month supplementation with avenanthramides (3 mg/d) from oats increased serum superoxide dismutase (SOD) activity and the concentration of reduced glutathione compared with placebo treatment (Liu *et al.* 2011). In small parallel studies with 16 postmenopausal (Koenig *et al.* 2014) or young (Koenig *et al.* 2016) women, 8-week consumption of oat cookies (avenanthramides 9.2 mg/d) indicated dereased inflammation in response to physical exercise.

16.10.3 Avenanthramides and cancer

A few studies have been conducted on the role of avenanthramides in cancer and all of them have been in vitro. In human colon cancer cell lines, avenanthramides inhibited cell proliferation, but had no effect on COX-2 activity and prostaglandin E_2 production, the major inflammatory pathway contributing to colorectal cancer (Guo *et al.* 2010). Avenanthramide 2p showed concentration dependent antiproliferative activity and was able to downregulate the canonical Wnt/beta-catenin signalling in human cervical cancer cells (Wang *et al.* 2012b). Dihydroavenanthramide D, a synthetic analog to naturally occurring avenanthramides, reduced MMP-9 mediated cell invasion of MCF-7 human breast cancer cells (Lee *et al.* 2011). Avenanthramides, 2c in particular, were shown to decrease cancer cell viability by inducing apoptosis in breast cancer (Hastings & Keanley 2017) and colon cancer cells (Finetti *et al.* 2018; Scarpa *et al.* 2018). While these studies implicate that avenanthramides may have anti-cancer activity, the effects need to be verified in tumor models *In vivo*.

16.11 Benzoxazinoids

16.11.1 Chemical characteristics, content in cereals and effects of food processing

Benzoxazinoids are plant secondary metabolites, which have been investigated as allochemicals and bioherbicides. They are generally divided into three classes: benzoxazolines (e.g., 2-benzoxazolinone, BOA), lactams (e.g., 2-hydroxy-1,4-benzoxazin-3-one, HBOA) and hydroxamic acids (e.g., 2,4-dihydroxy-7-methoxy-1,4-benzoxazin-3-one, DIMBOA; demethoxylated analogue DIBOA), and they also occur as different glycosides in cereal foods (Andersson *et al.* 2014). However, only limited data is available on their occurrence in grains and cereal foods.

Benzoxazinoids have mostly been studied in rye and wheat (Hanhineva *et al.* 2011; Pedersen *et al.* 2011; Tanwir *et al.* 2013). In wheat and rye, 12 compounds were quantified, and among them, the double-hexose forms were the most abundant compounds (Tanwir *et al.* 2013). Di-hexose of DIBOA followed by di-hexose of HBOA were the main compounds both in wheat and rye. Several double hexoses of DIBOA, HBOA and DIMBOA were for the first time identified by Hanhineva *et al.* (2011). Correspondingly, double-hexose derivatives of DIBOA and HBOA and DIBOA-glucose were shown to be the major forms in commercial cereal foods (Steffensen *et al.* 2017).

Higher benzoxazinoid contents were found in rye than in wheat; the total benzoxazinoid contents in rye and wheat grains were 95 μg/g dm and 4.8 μg/g dm, respectively (Tanwir *et al.* 2013). In wheat, the highest content of the different benzoxazinoids was found in germ (total content 121 μg/g dm). The total content in other fractions was in order fine bran (35 μg/g) > pollard flour (33 μg/g) > coarse bran (6.3 μg/g) > flour (1.6 μg/g). In rye bran and flour, the total benzoxazinoid contents were in this study 434 and 57 μg/g, respectively. Later, clearly higher contents were reported for both wheat and rye milling products (Dihm *et al.* 2017). The contents were in wheat products 409 μg/g dm (whole grain flour) and 71 μg/g dm (refined flour) and in rye product 3200 μg/g dm (coarse flour) and 3570 μg/g dm (fine flour). More quantitative data are thus needed on benzoxazinoids in milling products.

The reporting of benzoxazinoid composition is complicated further due to structural changes during plant development and processing (Pedersen *et al.* 2011; Beckman *et al.* 2013; Tanwir *et al.* 2013; Tanwir *et* al. 2017). Hydrothermal treatment increased contents of all measured 10 benzoxazinoids in durum wheat and rye grains (Pedersen *et al.* 2011). The total content increased from not detected to 4077 nmol/g dm in durum wheat and from 377 to 6079 nmol/g dm and from 160 to 3542 nmol/g dm, respectively, in processing of two rye cultivars. Furthermore, bread contained more benzoxazinoids than expected based on their content in flour. It was concluded that changes associated with hydrothermal processing and baking reflected synthesis of hydroxamic acid glucosides, enzymatic liberation of their aglucones and their subsequent degradation to benzoxazolinones (Pedersen *et al.* 2011). Later studies confirmed that the benzoxazinoid composition and content depend strongly on processing (Tanwir *et al.* 2013; Tanwir *et al.* 2017). As an example, soaking of pearled rye grains decreased di-hexose of DIBOA and HBOA by ca 3-folds, while the contents of other benzoxazinoids increased significantly (Tanwir *et al.* 2013). Upon germination, benzoxazinoid composition changed markedly. It was concluded that the glucosylated compounds release the hexose units to generate agluconic and/or monogluconic compounds (Tanwir *et al.* 2017).

Differences in cereal ingredients and processing lead to high variation in the final consumer products. In 10 Nordic breads, the total benzoxazinoid content ranged from 14 to 3340 μg/g dm (Dihm *et al.* 2017) and in 25 supermarket-available cereal food products from below the detection limit to >500 μg/g dm. The products rich in rye-based ingredients contained >300μg/g dm of these compounds (Steffensen *et al.* 2017). With an intake of 50 g of fresh bread with the highest measured content in the study, the daily intake of bentzoxazinoids was calculated to be ca. 16 mg (Steffensen *et al.* 2017).

16.11.2 Absorption, metabolism and health implications

Bentzoxazinoids are of interest for their pharmaceutical activity and have been studied in various in vitro models (Andersson *et al.* 2014; Adhikari *et al.* 2013). Human studies show that dietary bentzoxazinoids are absorbed and metabolized in humans (Adhikari *et al.* 2013;

Beckmann *et al.* 2013; Hanhineva *et al.* 2014; Jensen *et al.* 2017). Whether bentzoxazinoids contribute to the health effects of whole grains in humans remains still to be shown. Some evidence is available for a role of bentzoxazinoids in cancer prevention and treatment. Bentzoxazinoids and their derivatives have been extensively studied in cancer cell cultures and found to be cytotoxic or able to reduce cell growth in prostate, breast, gastric, lung and pancreatic cancer cell lines (Adhikari *et al.* 2015). A novel benzoxazine derivative also sensitized human colon cancer cells to the effects of a chemotherapeutic drug (Suraj *et al.* 2017). A recent intervention study with prostate cancer patients reported that a week on a high rye diet before radical prostatectomy led to an increase in the concentrations of benzoxazine metabolites in the blood and urine (Steffensen *et al.* 2016). Interestingly, the plasma benzoxazinoids showed a tentative negative correlation with prostate malignant carcinoma, suggesting that further studies with larger number of patients are warranted.

16.12 Alkylresorcinols

16.12.1 Chemical characteristics, contents in cereals and effects of food processing

Alkylresorcinols (ARs) are phenolic lipid-soluble compounds, which are found among cereals especially in rye and wheat. Their structure is composed of a 1,3-dihydroxibenzene (resorcinol) ring and an odd-numbered alk(ne)yl chain attached to carbon 5 of the benzene moiety, that is, they are 1,3-dihydroxy-5-n-alk(en)ylbenzenes (Landberg *et al.* 2014). The side chain may be saturated or contain one or two double bonds. Less frequently, a ketone or hydroxyl group is attached to the chain. In cereals, saturated alkyl chains with 15–25 carbon atoms (C15–C25 ARs) dominate. Because the relative homologue distribution is rather constant for each cereal, the C17/C21 AR ratio may be used as a biomarker to estimate the proportion of wheat and rye consumed (Andersson *et al.* 2014; Landberg *et al.* 2014). However, a total of 29 different compounds were identified in rye, wheat and barley (Knödler *et al.* 2008).

In wheat and rye grains, the AR contents ranged 220–921 μg/g dm (Andersson *et al.* 2008b; Kulawinek *et al.* 2008; Bordiga *et al.* 2016) and 796–1231 μg/g dm (Kulawinek *et al.* 2008; Nyström *et al.* 2008; Shewry *et al.* 2010a), respectively, whereas lower contents, 32–210 μg/g dm, have been reported for barley (Mattila *et al.* 2005; Andersson *et al.* 2008a; Bordiga *et al.* 2016). Both genetic and environmental factors markedly affect AR contents (Andersson *et al.* 2010a). ARs are found only in the outer grain layers, outer cuticle of testa/inner cuticle of pericarp being the exact location (Landberg *et al.* 2008). Because no ARs are found in endosperm or in germ, ARs serve as a selective marker of testa. In a diet, whole grain rye and wheat flour and rye, and wheat bran are the main AR sources. The contents reported for rye bran range 1800–4108 μg/g dm (Mattila *et al.* 2005; Kulawinek *et al.* 2008; Kamal-Eldin *et al.* 2009; Andersson *et al.* 2010b; Pihlava *et al.* 2018), whereas only 90 μg/g dm was found in refined flour (Andersson *et al.* 2010b). The corresponding figures for wheat bran and refined wheat flour were 2400–3625 μg/g and 36–47 μg/g dm, respectively (Mattila *et al.* 2005; Kamal-Eldin *et al.* 2009; Kulawinek *et al.* 2008; Andersson *et al.* 2010b).

ARs are stable throughout food processing (Andersson *et al.* 2010b; Gunenc *et al.* 2013) and the AR content in breads and other products is thus determined by the raw material used. In 159 different cereal products available in Sweden, the AR contents varied from not detectable to 4178 μg/g fw, the majority being less than 500 μg/g fw (Menzel *et al.* 2012). The average daily AR intake, calculated based on food composition data, was in Sweden and UK 23 and 12 mg, respectively (Ross *et al.* 2005).

16.12.2 Absorption, distribution, metabolism and health implications

The bioavailability and bioactivity of ARs has been reviewed by Landberg *et al.* (2014). The absorption and transport of ARs resemble that of tocols. These compounds are absorbed from the small intestine and transported in lipoproteins. Approximately 60% of the dose is absorbed. In the body, ARs are also distributed to erythrocyte membranes and adipose tissue (Landberg *et al.* 2014). The half-life of ARs in circulation is about 5 h. They undergo hepatic metabolism that has similarities with tocopherol metabolism. The main AR metabolites are 3,5-dihydroxy-benzoic acid (DHBA) and 3-(3,5-dihydroxyphenyl)-1-propanoic acid (DHPPA). Also other metabolites have been identified but are minor (Zhu *et al.* 2014). The main excretion route is via kidneys but also biliary route is possible (Landberg *et al.* 2014). The possible bioactivities of ARs have been studied mainly in vitro often using supraphysiological concentrations (Ross *et al.* 2004; Andersson *et al.* 2014; Landberg *et al.* 2014). There are some indications that high AR concentrations could decrease lipolysis. Rye ARs have been shown to inhibit hormone sensitive lipase and decrease lipolysis in adipose cells in vitro; (Andersson *et al.* 2011). In a whole grain intervention study (Ross *et al.* 2012), serum AR concentration was inversely correlated to non-esterified fatty acid concentration in fasting conditions. However, more work is needed to understand whether ARs play a role in inhibiting lipid mobilization in vivo (Ross *et al.* 2012). ARs have been shown to diminish LDL oxidation in vitro (Parikka *et al.* 2006) and ex vivo after a four-week rye bread intervention (Söderholm *et al.* 2012). ARs and their metabolites are currently under investigation as promising biomarkers of whole grain wheat and rye intake (Landberg *et al.* 2014; Landberg *et al.* 2018). In two epidemiological studies, high plasma concentration of total ARs has been associated with reduced risk for distal colorectal cancer (Kyrø *et al.* 2014; Knudsen *et al.* 2014). Whether the association is explained by ARs being good markers for whole grain intake or whether they have an independent effect on carcinogenesis remains as yet unanswered. A number of AR homologues extracted and purified from wheat bran was shown to inhibit growth and proteasome activity (involved in apoptosis regulation) of human colon cancer cells (Zhu *et al.* 2012). ARs isolated from rye bran were reported to possess anti-mutagenic activity (Gasiorowski *et al.* 1996), while another study found that synthetic 5-n-ARs were able to protect against oxidative DNA damage in HT29 colon cancer cells *In vitro* (Parikka *et al.* 2006). These results suggest that ARs may have cancer-preventive properties apart from being just biomarkers of whole grain intake.

16.13 References

Abozed, S.S., Ahmed, Z.S., Rakszegi, M. & Làng, L. (2014) Comparative screening of phytochemicals in Egyptian and Hungarian wheat varieties *International Journal of Agricultural Research* 9, 219–230.

Adhikari, K.B., Laursen, B.B., Gregersen, P.L., Schnoor, H.J., Witten, M., Poulsen, L.K., Jensen, B.M. & Fomsgaard, I.S. (2013) Absorption and metabolic fate of bioactive dietary benzoxazinoids in humans. *Molecular Nutrition & Food Research* 57, 1847–1858.

Adhikari, K.B., Tanwir, F., Gregersen, P.L., Steffensen, S.K., Jensen, B.M., Poulsen, L.K., Nielsen, C.H., Høyer, S., Borre, M. & Fomsgaard, I.S. (2015) Benzoxazinoids: Cereal phytochemicals with putative therapeutic and health-protecting properties. *Molecular Nutrition & Food Research* 59, 1324–38.

Adom, K.K., Sorrells, M.E. & Liu, R.H. (2003) Phytochemical profiles and antioxidant acivity of wheat varieties. *Journal of Agricultural and Food Chemistry* 51, 7825–7834.

Afify, A.M.R., El-Beltagi, H.S., Abd El-Salam, S.M. & Omran, A.A. (2011) Bioavailability of iron, zinc, phytate and phytase activity during soaking and germination of white sorghum varieties. *PLOS ONE* 6, e25512.

Ahsan, H., Ahad, A., Iqbal, J. & Siddiqui, W.A. (2014) Pharmacological potential of tocotrienols: A review. *Nutrition & Metabolism* 11, 52.

Albarracin, M., Gonzalez, R.J. & Drago, S.R. (2015) Soaking and extrusion effects on physicochemical parameters, phytic acid, nutrient content and mineral bio-accessibility of whole rice grain. *International Journal of Food Sciences and Nutrition* 66, 210–215.

Alignan, M., Roche, J., Bouniols, A., Cerny, M., Mouloungui, Z. & Merah, O. (2009) Effects of genotype and sowing date on phytostanol-phytosterol content and agronomic traits in wheat under organic agriculture. *Food Chemistry* 117, 219–225.

Andersson, A.A.M., Åman, P., Wandel, M. & Frolich, W. (2010b) Alkylresorcinols in wheat and rye flour and bread. *Journal of Food Composition and Analysis* 23, 794–801.

Andersson, A.A.M., Dimberg, L., Åman, P. & Landberg, R. (2014) Recent findings on certain bioactive components in whole grain wheat and rye. *Journal of Cereal Science* 59, 249–311.

Andersson, A.A.M., Kamal-Eldin, A., Fras, A., Boros, D. & Åman, P. (2008b). Alkylresorcinols in wheat varieties in the HEALTHGRAIN diversity screen. *Journal of Agricultural and Food Chemistry* 56, 9722-9725.

Andersson, A.M.M., Kamal-Eldin, A. & Åman, P. (2010a). Effects of environment and variety on alkylresorcinols in wheat in the HEALTHGRAIN diversity screen. *Journal of Agricultural and Food Chemistry* 58, 9299–9305.

Andersson, A.A.M., Lampi, A-M, Nyström, L., Piironen, V., Li, L., Ward, J.L., Gebruers, K., Courtin, C.M., Delcour, J.A., Boros, D., Fras, A., Dynkowska, W., Rakszegi, M., Bedő, Z., Shewry, P.R. & Åman, P. (2008a) Phytochemical and dietary fiber components in barley varieties in the Healthgrain diversity screen. *Journal of Agricultural and Food Chemistry* 56, 9767–9776.

Andersson, U., Dey, E.S., Holm, C. & Degerman, E. (2011) Rye bran alkylresorcinols suppress adipocyte lipolysis and hormone-sensitive lipase activity. *Molecular Nutrition & Food Research* 55 Suppl 2, S290–S293.

Anson, N.M., Hemery, Y.M., Bast, A. & Haenen, G.R.M.M. (2012) Optimizing the bioactive potential of wheat bran by processing. *Food & Function* 3, 362–375.

Arcot, J., Wootton, M., Alury, S., Chan, H.Y. & Shrestha, A.K. (2002) Folate levels in twelve Australian wheats and changes during processing into bread. *Food Australia* 54, 18–20.

Aune, D. Chan, D.M.S., Vieira, A.R., Navarro Rosenblatt, D.A., Vieira, R., Greenwood, D.C. & Norat, T. (2012) Dietary compared with blood concentrations of carotenoids and breast cancer risk: A systematic review and meta-analysis of prospective studies. *American Journal of Clinical Nutrition* 96, 356–373.

Azeke, M.A., Egielewa, S.J., Eigbogbo, M.U. & Inegbenose, G.I. (2011) Effect of germination on the phytase activity, phytate and total phosphorus contents of rice (*Oryza sativa*), maize (*Zea mays*), millet (*Panicum miliaceum*), sorghum (*Sorghum bicolor*) and wheat (*Triticum aestivum*). *Journal of Food Science and Technology* 48, 724–729.

Baek, J.E., Lee, E.J. & Koh, B.K. (2014) The effects of germination, fermentation, and fermentation additives on the phytate content of rice flour. *Food Science and Biotechnology* 23, 1447–1451.

Baskaran, N., Manoharan, S., Balakrishnan, S. & Pugalendhi, P. (2010) Chemopreventive potential of ferulic acid in 7,12-dimethylbenz[a]anthracene-induced mammary carcinogenesis in Sprague-Dawley rats. *European Journal of Pharmacology* 637, 22–29.

Beckman, M., Lloyd, A.J., Haldar, S., Seal, C., Brandt, K. & Draper, J. (2013) Hydroxylated phenylacetamides derived from bioactive benzoxazinoids are bioavailable in humans after habitual consumption of whole grain sourdough rye bread. *Molecular Nutrition and Food Research* 57, 1859–1873.

Blandino, M., Alfieri, M., Giordano, D., Vanara, F. & Redaelli, R. (2017) Distribution of bioactive compounds in maize fractions obtained in two different types of large scale milling processes. *Journal of Cereal Science* 77, 251–258.

Boncompagni, E., Orozco-Arroyo, G., Cominelli, E., Gangashetty, P.I., Grando, S., Kwaku Zu, T.T., Daminati, M.G., Nielsen, E. & Sparvoli, F. (2018) Antinutritional factors in pearl millet grains: Phytate and goitrogens content variability and molecular characterization of genes involved in their pathways. *PLOS ONE* 13, 1–30.

Bondia-Pons, I., Aura, A.-M., Vuorela, S., Kolehmainen, M., Mykkänen, H. & Poutanen, K. (2009) Rye phenolics in nutrition and health. *Journal of Cereal Science* 49, 323–336.

Bordiga, M., Locatelli, M., Travaglio, F., Arlorio, M., Reyneri, A., Blandino, M. & Coisson, J.D. (2016). Alkylresorcinol content in whole grains and pearled fractions of wheat and barley. *Journal of Cereal Science* 70, 38–46.

Bradford, P.G. & Awad, A.B. (2010) Modulation of signal transduction in cancer cells by phytosterols. *Biofactors* 36, 241–247.

Bradolini, A., Hidalgo, A., Gabriele, S. & Heun, M. (2015) Chemical composition of wild and feral diploid wheats and their bearing on domesticated wheats. *Journal of Cereal Science* 63, 122–127.

Branković, G., Dragičević, V., Dodig, D., Knežević, D., Kandić, V., Šurlan-Momirović, G. & Sečanski, M. (2015) Phytic acid, inorganic phosphorus, antioxidants in bread and durum wheat and their associations with agronomic traits. *Agricultural and Food Science* 24, 183–194.

Brewer, L.R., Kubola, J., Siriamornpun, S., Herald, T.J. & Shi, Y.C. (2014) Wheat bran particle size influence on phytochemical extractability and antioxidant properties. *Food Chemistry* 152, 483–490.

Bryngelsson, S., Dimberg, L.H. & Kamal-Eldin, A. (2002b) Effect of commercial processing on levels of antioxidants in oats (*Avena sativa* L.). *Journal of Agricultural and Food Chemistry* 50, 1890–1896.

Bryngelsson, S., Ishihara, A. & Dimberg, L.H. (2003) Levels of avenanthramides and activity of hydroxycinnamoyl-CoA: Hydroxyanthranilate N-hydroxycinnamoyl transferase (HHT) in steeped or germinated oat samples. *Cereal Chemistry* 80, 356–360.

Bryngelsson, S., Mannerstedt-Fogelfors, B., Kamal-Eldin, A., Andersson, R. & Dimberg, L.H. (2002a) Lipids and antioxidants in groats and hulls of Swedish oats (*Avena sativa* L). *Journal of Food Science* 82, 606–614.

Buddrick, O., Jones, O.A.H., Cornell, H.J. & Small, D.M. (2014) The influence of fermentation processes and cereal grains in wholegrain bread on reducing phytate content. *Journal of Cereal Science* 59, 3–8.

Buri, R.C., von Reding, W. & Gavin, M.H. (2004) Description and characterization of wheat aleurone. *Cereal Foods World* 49, 274–282.

Chatterjee, M., Roy, K., Janarthan, M., Das, S. & Chatterjee, M. (2012) Biological activity of carotenoids: Its implications in cancer risk and prevention. *Current Pharmaceutical Biotechnology* 13, 180–190.

Chen, C.Y., Milbury, P.E., Collins, F.W. & Blumberg, J.B. (2007) Avenanthramides are bioavailable and have antioxidant activity in humans after acute consumption of an enriched mixture from oats. *Journal of Nutrition* 137, 1375–1382.

Chen, C.Y., Milbury, P.E., Kwak, H.K., Collins, F.W., Samuel, P. & Blumberg, J.B. (2004) Avenanthramides and phenolic acids from oats are bioavailable and act synergistically with vitamin C to enhance hamster and human LDL resistance to oxidation. *Journal of Nutrition* 134, 1459–1466.

Chen, J., Saggar, J.K., Corey, P. & Thompson, L.U. (2009) Flaxseed and pure secoisolaricinol diglucoside, but not flaxseed hull, reduce human breast tumor growth (MCF-7) in athymic mice. *Journal of Nutrition* 139, 2061–2066.

Chen, P., Li, C., Li, X., Li, J., Chu, R. & Wang H. (2014) Higher dietary folate intake reduces the breast cancer risk: A systematic review and meta-analysis. *British Journal of Cancer* 110, 2327–2338.

Collins, F.W. (2011) Oat phenolics: Biochemistry and biological functionality. In: *Oats Chemistry and Technology* (eds. Webster, F.H. & Woods, P.J.). 2nd ed., pp.157–217. AACC International, St. Paul, Minnesota

Corol, D.-I., Ravel, C., Rakszegi, M., Bedo, Z., Charmet, G., Beale, M.H., Shewry, P.R. & Ward, J.L. (2012) Effects of genotype and environment on the contents of betaine, choline, and trigonelline in cereal grains. *Journal of Agricultural and Food Chemistry* 60, 5471–5481.

Cotterchio, M., Boucher, B.A., Manno, M., Gallinger, S., Okey, A. & Harper, P. (2006) Dietary phytoestrogen intake is associated with reduced colorectal cancer risk. *Journal of Nutrition* 136, 3046–3053.

Croze, M.L. & Soulage, C.O. (2013) Potential role and therapeutic interests of myo-inositol in metabolic diseases. *Biochimie* 95, 1811–1827.

Davies, M.J., Bowey, E.A., Adlercreutz, H., Rowland, I.R. & Rumsby, P.C. (1999) Effects of soy or rye supplementation of high-fat diets on colon tumour development in azoxymethane-treated rats. *Carcinogenesis* 20, 927–931.

De Smet, E., Mensink, R.P. & Plat, J. (2012) Effects of plant sterols and stanols on intestinal cholesterol metabolism: Suggested mechanisms from past to present. *Molecular Nutrition & Food Research* 56, 1058–1072.

Dihm, K., Vendelbo Lind, M., Sunden, H., Ross, A. & Savolainen, O. (2017) Quantification of benzoxazinoids and their metabolites in Nordic breads. *Food Chemistry* 235, 7–13.

Dimberg, L.H., Gissen, C. & Nilsson, J. (2005) Phenolic compounds in oat grains (Avena sativa L.) grown in conventional and organic systems. *Ambio* 34, 331–337.

Dong, W., Cheng, Z., Wang, X., Wang, B., Zhang, H., Su, N., Yamamaro, C., Lei, C. & Wang, J. (2011) Determination of folate content in rice germplasm (*Oryza sativa* L.) using tri-enzyme extraction and microbiological assays. *International Journal of Food Sciences and Nutrition* 62, 537–543.

Durazzo, A., Zaccaria, M., Polito, A., Maiani, G. & Carcea, M. (2013) Lignan content in cereals, buckwheat and derived foods. *Foods* 2, 53–63.

During, A., Debouche, C., Raas, T. & Larondelle, Y. (2012) Among plant lignans, pinoresinol has the strongest anti-inflammatory properties in human intestinal Caco-2 cells. *Journal of Nutrition* 142, 1798–1805.

Dwyer, J.H., Navab, M., Dwyer, K.M., Hassan, K., Sun, P., Shircore, A., Hama-Levy, S., Hough, G., Wang, X., Drake, T., Merz, C.N. & Fogelman, A.M. (2001) Oxygenated carotenoid lutein and progression of early atherosclerosis: The Los Angeles atherosclerosis study. *Circulation* 103, 2922–2927.

Edelmann, M., Kariluoto, S., Nyström, L. & Piironen, V. (2012) Folate in oats and its milling fractions. *Food Chemistry* 135, 1938–1947.

Edelmann, M., Kariluoto, S., Nyström, L. & Piironen, V. (2013) Folate in barley grain and fractions. *Journal of Cereal Science* 58, 37–44.

Engelsen, M.M. & Hansen, Å. (2009) Tocopherol and tocotrienol content in commercial wheat mill streams *Cereal Chemistry* 86, 499–502.

FAO/WHO. (2004) Vitamin and mineral requirements in human nutrition. 2nd edition. Joint FAO/WHO expert consultation on human vitamin and mineral requirements (1998: Bangkok, Thailand).

Fardet, A. & Chardigny, J.M. (2013) Plant-based foods as a source of lipotropes for human nutrition: A survey of in vivo studies. *Critical Reviews in Food Science and Nutrition* 53, 535–590.

Fardet, A. 2010. New hypotheses for the health-protective mechanisms of whole-grain cereals: What is beyond fibre? *Nutrition Research Review* 23, 65–134.

Fardet, A., Rock, E. & Rémésy, C. (2008) Is the *in vitro* antioxidant potential of whole-grain cereals and cereal products well reflected *in vivo*? *Journal of Cereal Science* 48, 258–276.

Fenech, M., Noakes, M., Clifton, P. & Topping, D. (1999) Aleurone flour is a rich source of bioavailable folate in humans. *Journal of Nutrition* 129, 1114–1119.

Finetti, F., Moglia, A., Schiavo, I., Donnini, S., Berta, G.N., Di Scipio, F., Perrelli, A., Fornelli, C., Trabalzini, L. & Retta, S.F. (2018) Yeast-derived recombinant avenanthramides inhibit proliferation, migration and epithelial mesenchymal transition of colon cancer cells. *Nutrients* 10, 1159.

Frankenfeld, C.L. (2017) Cardiometabolic risk and gut microbial phytoestrogen metabolite phenotypes. *Molecular Nutrition and Food Research* 61, 1500900.

Fratianni, A., Giuzio, L., Di Criscio, T., Zina, F. & Panfili, G. (2013) Response of carotenoids and tocols of durum wheat in relation to water stress and sulfur fertilization. *Journal of Agricultural and Food Chemistry* 61, 2583–2590.

Fratianni, A., Panfili, G. & Cubadda, R. (2015) Carotenoids, tocols, and retinols during the pasta-making process. In: Processing and Impact on Active Components in Food. (eds. V.R. Preedy), pp. 309–317. Elsevier, Academic Press.

Fu, M., Song, Y., Wen, Z., Lu, X. & Cui, L. (2016) Inositol hexaphosphate and inositol inhibit colorectal cancer metastasis to the liver in BALB/c Mice. *Nutrients* 8, 286.

Gasiorowski, K., Szyba, K., Brokos, B. & Kozubek, A. (1996) Antimutagenic activity of alkylresorcinols from cereal grains. *Cancer Letters* 106, 109–115.

Gerstenmeyer, E., Reimer, S., Berghofer, E., Schwartz, H. & Sontag, G. (2013) Effect of thermal heating on some lignans in flax seeds, sesame seeds and rye. *Food Chemistry* 138, 1847–1855.

Giordano, D., Reyneri, A. & Blandino, M. (2016) Folate distribution in barley (*Hordeum vulgare* L.), common wheat (*Triticum aestivum* L.) and durum wheat (*Triticum turgidum durum* Desf.) pearled fractions. *Journal of the Science of Food and Agriculture* 96, 1709–1715.

Ghosh, S., Basak, P., Dutta, S., Chowdhury, S. & Sil, P.C. (2017) New insights into the ameliorative effects of ferulic acid in pathophysiological conditions. *Food and Chemical Toxicology* 103, 41–55.

Gregory, J.F., Quinlivan, E.P. & Davis, S.R. (2005) Integrating the issues of folate bioavailability, intake and metabolism in the era of fortification. *Trends in Food Science & Technology* 16, 229–240.

Guan, F., Li, G., Liu, A.B., Lee, M.J., Yang, Z., Chen, Y.K., Lin, Y., Shih, W. & Yang, C.S. (2012) δ- and γ-tocopherols, but not α-tocopherol, inhibit colon carcinogenesis in azoxymethane-treated F344 rats. *Cancer Prevention Research* 5, 644–654.

Gujska, E. & Kuncewicz, A. (2005) Determination of folate in some cereals and commercial cereal-grain products consumed in Poland using trienzyme extraction and high-performance liquid chromatography methods. *European Food Research and Technology* 221, 208–213.

Gunenc, A., Tavakoli, H., Seetharaman, K., Mayer, P.M., Fairbanks, D. & Hosseinian, F. (2013) Stability and antioxidant activity of alkylresorcinols in breads enriched with hard and soft wheat brans. *Food Research International* 51, 571–578.

Guo, W. & Beta, T. (2013) Phenolic acid composition and antioxidant potential of insoluble and soluble dietary fibre extracts derived from select whole-grain cereals. *Food Research International* 51, 518–525.

Guo, W., Nie, L., Wu, D., Wise, M.L., Collins, F.W., Meydani, S.N. & Meydani M. (2010) Avenanthramides inhibit proliferation of human colon cancer cell lines in vitro. *Nutrition & Cancer* 62, 1007–1016.

Gylling, H., Plat, J., Turley, S., Ginsberg, H.N., Ellegård, L., Jessup, W., Jones, P.J., Lütjohann, D., Maerz, W., Masana, L., Silbernagel, G., Staels, B., Borén, J., Catapano, A.L., De Backer, G., Deanfield, J., Descamps, O.S., Kovanen, P.T., Riccardi, G., Tokgözoglu, L. & Chapman, M.; European Atherosclerosis Society Consensus Panel on Phytosterols. (2014) Plant sterols and plant stanols in the management of dyslipidaemia and prevention of cardiovascular disease. *Atherosclerosis* 232, 346–360.

Hager, A-S, Wolter, A., Jacob, F., Zannini, E. & Arendt, E.K. (2012) Nutritional properties and ultra-structure of commercial gluten free flours from different botanical sources compared to wheat flours. *Journal of Cereal Science* 56, 239–247.

Han, Y.H., Yon, M. & Hyun, T.H. (2005) Folate intake estimated with an updated database and its association to blood folate and homocysteine in Korean college students. *European Journal of Clinical Nutrition* 59, 246–254.

Hanhineva, K., Keski-Rahkonen, P., Lappi, J., Katina, K., Pekkinen, J., Savolainen, O., Timonen, O., Paananen, J., Mykkänen, H. & Poutanen, K. (2014) The postprandial plasma rye fingerprint includes benzoxazinoid-derived phenylacetamide sulfates. *Journal of Nutrition* 144, 1016–1022.

Hanhineva, K., Rogachev, I., Aura, A.-M., Aharoni, A., Poutanen, K. & Mykkänen, H. (2012) Identification of novel lignans in the whole grain rye bran by non-targeted LC-MS metabolite profileing. *Metabolomics* 8, 399–409.

Hanhineva, K., Rogachev, I., Aura, A.-M., Aharoni, A., Poutanen, K. & Mykkänen, H. (2011) Qualitative characterization of benzoxazinoid derivatives in whole grain rye and wheat by LC-MS metabolite profiling. *Journal of Agricultural and Food Chemistry* 59, 921-927.

Hastings, J. & Kenealey, J. (2017) Avenanthramide-C reduces the viability of MDA-MB-231 breast cancer cells through an apoptotic mechanism. *Cancer Cell International* 17, 93.

Hefni, M. & Witthöft, C.M. (2012) Effect of germination and subsequent oven-drying on folate content in different wheat and rye cultivars. *Journal of Cereal Science* 56, 374–378.

Hefni, M.E., Schaller, F. & Witthöft, C.M. (2018) Betaine, choline and folate content in different cereal genotypes. *Journal of Cereal Science* 80, 72–79.

Heiniö, R.-L., Liukkonen, K.-H., Myllymäki, O., Pihlava, J.-M., Adlercreatz, H., Heinonen, S.-M. & Poutanen, K. (2008) Quantities of phenolic compounds and their impacts on the perceived flavour attributes of rye grain. *Journal of Cereal Science* 47, 566–575.

Helldán, A., Raulio, S., Kosola, M., Tapanainen, H., Ovaskainen, ML. & Virtanen S. (2013) Finravinto 2012 -tutkimus – The National FINDIET 2012 Survey, THL, raportti 16/2013. Helsinki, Finland: The National Institute for Health and Welfare. 187 p.

Hemery, Y., Holopainen, U., Lampi, A.-M., Lehtinen, P., Nurmi, T., Piironen, V., Edelmann, M. & Rouau, X. (2011) Potential of dry fractionation of wheat bran for the development of food ingredients. Part II: Electrostatic separation of particles. *Journal of Cereal Science* 53, 9–18.

Hemery, Y.M., Anson, N.M., Havenaar, B., Haenen, G.R.M.M., Noort, M.W.J. & Rouau, X. (2010) Dry-fractionation of wheat bran increases the bioaccessibility of phenolic acids in breads made from processed bran fractions. *Food Research International* 43, 1429–1439.

Hidalgo, A. & Bradolini, A. (2008) Protein, ash, lutein and tocols distribution in einkorn (*Triticum monococcum* L. subsp. *monococcum*) seed fraction. *Food Chemistry* 107, 444–448.

Hidalgo, A., Bradolini, A. & Gazza, L. (2008) Influence of steaming treatment on chemical and technological characteristics of einkorn (*Triticum monococcum* L. ssp. *monococcum*) wholemeal flour. *Food Chemistry* 111, 549–555.

Hidalgo, A., Bradolini, A., Pompei, C. & Piscozzi, R. (2006) Carotenoids and tocols of einkorn wheat (*Triticum monococcum* ssp. *monococcum* L.) *Journal of Cereal Science* 44, 182–193.

Hidalgo, A., Scuppa, S. & Bradolini, A. (2016) Technological quality and chemical composition of puffed grains from einkorn (*Triticum monococcum* L. subsp. *monococcum*) and bread wheat (*Triticum aestivum* L. subsp. *aestivum*). *Food Science and Technology* 68, 541–548.

Holasova, M. (1997) Distribution of tocopherols and tocotrienols in the main products of wheat and rye milling. *Potravinarske Vedy* 15, 343–350.

Huang, M.T., Smart, R.C., Wong, C.Q. & Conney, A.H. (1988) Inhibitory effect of curcumin, chlorogenic acid, caffeic acid, and ferulic acid on promotion in mouse skin by 12-O-Tetradecanoylphorbol-13-acetate. *Cancer Research* 48, 5941–5946.

Hübner, F., O'Neil, T., Cashman, K.D. & Arendt, E.K. (2010) The influence of germination conditions on beta-glucan, dietary fibre and phytate during the germination of oats and barley. *European Food Research and Technology* 231, 27–35.

Iafelice, G., Verardo, V., Marconi, M. & Caboni, E.F (2009) Characterization of total, free and esterified phytosterols in tetraploid and hexaploid wheats. *Journal of Agricultural and Food Chemistry* 57, 2267–2273.

Jägerstad, M., Piironen, V., Walker, C., Ros, G., Carnovale, E., Holasova, M. & Nau, H. (2005) Increasing natural food folates through bioprocessing and biotechnology. *Trends in Food Science & Technology* 16, 298–306.

Janicke, B., Hegardt, C., Krogh, M., Önning, G., Åkesson, B., Cirenajwis, H.M. & Ordesson, M. (2011) The antiproliferative effect of dietary fiber phenolic compounds ferulic acid and p-coumaric acid on the cell cycle of Caco-2 cells. *Nutrition & Cancer* 63, 611–622.

Jenab, M. & Thompson, L. (1998) The influence of phytic acid in wheat bran on early biomarkers of colon carcinogenesis. *Carcinogenesis* 19, 1087–1092.

Jensen, B.M., Adhikari, K.B., Schnoor, H.J., Juel-Berg, N., Fomsgaard, I.S. & Poulsen, L.K. (2017) Quantitative analysis of absorption, metabolism, and excretion of benzoxazinoids in humans after the consumption of high- and low-benzoxazinoid diets with similar contents of cereal dietary fibres: A crossover study. *European Journal of Nutrition* 56, 387–397.

Jensen, B.M., Poulsen, L.L., Nielsen, C.H., Borre, M., Borre, M., Hoyer, S. & Fomsgaard, I.S. (2017) Bioactive small molecules in commercially available cereal food: Benzoxazinoids. *Journal of Food Composition and Analysis* 64, 213–222.

Ji, L.L., Lay, D., Chung, L.E., Fuy, Y. & Peterson, D.M. (2003) Effects of avenanthramides on oxidant generation and antioxidant enzyme activity in exercised rats. *Nutrition Research* 23, 1579–1590.

Jiang, Q. (2014) Natural forms of vitamin E: Metabolism, antioxidant, and anti-inflammatory activities and their role in disease prevention and therapy. *Free Radical Biology and Medicine* 72, 76–90.

Ju, J., Picinich, S.C., Yang, Z., Zhao, Y., Suh, N., Kong, A.N. & Yang, C.S. (2010) Cancer-preventive activities of tocopherols and tocotrienols. *Carcinogenesis* 31, 533–542.

Jung, S., Wu, K., Giovannucci, E., Spiegelman, D., Willett, W.C. & Smith-Warner, S.A. (2013) Carotenoid intake and risk of colorectal adenomas in a cohort of male health professionals. *Cancer Causes Control* 24, 705–717.

Kamal-Eldin, A. & Appelqvist, L. 1996. The chemistry and antioxidant properties of tocopherols and tocotrienols. *Lipids* 31, 671–701.

Kamal-Eldin, A., Lærke, H., Bach Knudsen, K., Lampi, A-M, Piironen, V., Adlercreutz, H., Katina, K., Poutanen, K. & Åman, P. (2009) Physical, microscopic and chemical characterisation of industrial rye and wheat brans from the Nordic countries. *Food & Nutrition Research,* 53, 10.3402/fnr.v53i0.1912.

Kariluoto, M.S., Vahteristo, L.T. & Piironen, V.I. (2001) Applicability of microbiological assay and affinity chromatography purification followed by high-performance liquid chromatography (HPLC) in studying folate contents in rye. *Journal of the Science of Food and Agriculture* 81, 938–942.

Kariluoto, S., Edelmann, M. & Piironen, V. (2010) Effects of environment and genotype on folate contents in wheat in the HEALTHGRAIN diversity screen. *Journal of Agricultural and Food Chemistry* 58, 9324–9331.

Kariluoto, S., Liukkonen, K-H, Myllymäki, O., Vahteristo, L., Kaukovirta-Norja, A. & Piironen, V. (2006) Effect of germination and thermal treatments on folates in rye. *Journal of Agricultural and Food Chemistry* 54, 9522–9528.

Kariluoto, S., Vahteristo, L., Salovaara, H., Katina, K., Liukkonen, K. & Piironen, V. (2004) Effect of baking method and fermentation on folate content of rye and wheat breads. *Cereal Chemistry* 81, 134–139.

Kaulmann, A. & Bohn, T. (2014) Carotenoids, inflammation, and oxidative stress-implications of cellular signaling pathways and relation to chronic disease prevention. *Nutrition Research* 34, 907–929.

Kawabata, K., Yamamoto, T., Hara, A., Shimizu, M., Yamada, Y., Matsunaga, K., Tanaka, T. & Mori, H. (2000) Modifying effects of ferulic acid on azoxymethane-induced colon carcinogenesis in F344 rats. *Cancer Letter* 31, 15–21.

Kean, E.G., Hamaker, B.R. & Ferruzzi, M.G. (2008) Carotenoid bioaccessibility from whole grain and degermed maize meal products. *Journal of Agricultural and Food Chemistry* 56, 9918–9926.

Kim, Y.I. (2018) Folate and cancer: A tale of Dr. Jekyll and Mr. Hyde? *American Journal of Clinical Nutrition* 107, 139–142.

Klatt, K.C. & Caudill, M.A. (2019). Folate, choline, vitamin B12 and vitamin B6. In: Stipanuk, M. & Caudill, M.A., eds. Biochemical, Physiological, and Molecular Aspects of Human Nutrition. 4th ed. Elsevier, St. Louis, MO.

Knudsen, M.D., Kyrø, C., Olsen, A., Dragsted, L.O., Skeie, G., Lund, E., Aman, P., Nilsson, L.M., Bueno-de-Mesquita, H.B., Tjønneland, A., Landberg, R. (2014) Self-reported whole-grain intake and plasma alkylresorcinol concentrations in combination in relation to the incidence of colorectal cancer. *American Journal of Epidemiology* 179, 1188–1196.

Knödler, M. , Kaiser, A., Carle, R. & Schieber, A. (2008) Profiling of Alk(en)ylresorcinols in cereals by HPLC-DAD-APcI-MSn. *Analytical and Bioanalytical Chemistry* 391, 221–228.

Koehler, P., Hartmann. G., Wieser, H. & Rychlik, M. (2007) Changes of folate, dietary fiber, and proteins in wheat as affected by germination. *Journal of Agricultural and Food Chemistry* 55, 4678–4683.

Koenig, R., Dickman, J.R., Kang, C., Zhang, T., Chu, Y.F. & Ji, L.L. (2014) Avenanthramide supplementation attenuates exercise-induced inflammation in postmenopausal women. *Nutrition Journal* 13, 21.

Koenig, R.T., Dickman, J.R., Wise, M.L. & Ji, L.L. (2011) Avenanthramides are bioavailable and accumulate in hepatic, cardiac, and skeletal muscle tissue following oral gavage in rats. *Journal of Agricultural and Food Chemistry* 59, 6438–6443.

Koenig, R.T., Dickman, J.R., Kang, C.H., Zhang, T., Chu, Y.F. & Ji L.L. (2016) Avenanthramide supplementation attenuates eccentric exercise-inflicted blood inflammatory markers in women. *European Journal of Applied Physiology* 116, 67–76.

Kojic, J., Krulj, J., Ilic, N., Loncar, E., Pezo, L., Mandic, A. & Bodroža Solarov, M. (2017) Analysis of betaine levels in cereals, pseudocereals and their products. *Journal of Functional Foods* 37, 157–163.

Konings, E.J.M., Roomans, H.H.S., Dorant, E., Goldbohm, R.A., Saris, W.H.M. & Van den Brandt, P.A. (2001) Folate intake of the Dutch population according to newly established liquid chromatography data for foods. *American Journal of Clinical Nutrition* 73, 765–776.

Kruger, J., Oelofse, A. & Taylor, J.R. (2014) Effects of aqueous soaking on the phytate and mineral contents and phytate: Mineral ratios of wholegrain normal sorghum and maize and low phytate sorghum. *International Journal of Food Sciences and Nutrition* 65, 539–546.

Kuhnle, G.G.C., Dell'Aquila, C., Aspinall, S.M., Runswich, S.A., Mulligan, A.A. & Bingham, S.A. (2009) Phytoestrogen content of cereals and cereal-based foods consumed in the UK. *Nutrition and Cancer* 61, 302–309.

Kuijsten, A., Arts, I.C., Hollman, P.C., vant't Veer, P. & Kampman, E. (2006) Plasma enterolignans are associated with lower colorectal adenoma risk. *Cancer Epidemiology Biomarkers Prevention* 15, 1132–1136.

Kulawinek, M., Jaromin, A., Kozubek, A. & Zarnowsky, R. (2008) Alkylresorcinols in selected Polish rye and wheat cereals and whole-grain cereal products. *Journal of Agricultural and Food Chemistry* 56, 7236–7242.

Kumar, V., Sinha, A.S., Makkar, H.P.S. & Becker, K. (2010). Dietary roles of phytate and phytase in human nutrition: A review. *Food Chemistry* 120, 345–959.

Kyrø, C., Olsen, A., Landberg, R., Skeie, G., Loft, S., Åman, P., Leenders, M., Dik, V.K., Siersema, P.D., Pischon, T., Christensen, J., Overvad, K., Boutron-Ruault, M.-C., Fagherazzi, G., Cottet, V., Kuhn, T., Kühn, T., Chang-Claude, J., Boeing, H., Trichopoulou, A., Bamia, C., Trichopoulos, D., Palli, D., Krogh, V., Tumino, R., Vineis, P., Panico, S., Peeters, P.H., Weiderpass, E., Bakken, T., Åsli, L.A., Argüelles, M., Jakszyn, P., Sánchez, M.J., Amiano, P., Huerta, J.M., Barricarte, A., Ljuslinder, I., Palmqvist, R., Khaw, K.T., Wareham, N., Key, T.J., Travis, R.C., Ferrari, P., Freisling, H., Jenab, M., Gunter, M.J., Murphy, N., Riboli, E., Tjønneland, A. & Bueno-de-Mesquita, H.B. (2014) Plasma alkylresorcinols, biomarkers of whole-grain wheat and rye intake, and incidence of colorectal cancer. *Journal of National Cancer Institute* 106, djt352.

Lachman, J., Hejtmánková, A., Orsák, M., Popov, M. & Martinek, P. (2018) Tocotrienols and tocopherols in colored-grain wheat, tritordeum and barley. *Food Chemistry* 249, 725–735.

Lampi, A.-M., Nurmi, T., Ollilainen, V. & Piironen, V. (2008) Tocopherols and tocotrienols in wheat genotypes in the HEALTHGRAIN diversity screen. *Journal of Agricultural and Food Chemistry* 56, 9716–9721.

Landberg, R., Kamal-Eldin, A., Salmenkallio-Marttila, M., Rouau, X. & Åman, P. (2008) Localization of alkylresorcinols in wheat, rye and barley kernels. *Journal of Cereal Science* 48, 401–406.

Landberg, R., Marklund, M., Kamal-Eldin, A. & Åman, P. (2014) An update on alkylresorcinols – occurrence, bioavailability, bioactivity and utility as biomarkers. *Journal of Functional Foods* 7, 77–89.

Landberg, R., Wierzbicka, R., Shi, L., Nybacka, S., Kamal-Eldin, A., Hedblad, B., Lindroos, A.K., Winkvist, A. & Forslund, H. (2018) New alkylresorcinol metabolites in spot urine as biomarkers of whole grain wheat and rye intake in a Swedish middle-aged population. *European Journal of Clinical Nutrition* 72, 1439–1446.

Landete, J.M. (2012) Plant and mammalian lignans: A review of source, intake, metabolism, intestinal bacteria and health. *Food Research International* 46, 410–424.

Lappi, J., Aura, A.M., Katina, K., Nordlund, E., Kolehmainen, M., Mykkänen, H. & Poutanen, K. (2013) Comparison of postprandial phenolic acid excretions and glucose responses after ingestion of breads with bioprocessed or native rye bran. *Food & Function* 4, 972–981.

Lee, S.H., Park, H.J., Chun, H.K., Cho, S.Y., Cho, S.M. & Likkehoj, H.S. (2006) Dietary phytic acid lowers the blood glucose level in diabetic KK mice. *Nutrition Research* 26, 474–479.

Lee, Y.R., Noh, E.M., Oh, H.J., Hur, H., Kim, J.M., Han, J.H., Hwang, J.K., Park, B.H., Park, J.W., Youn, H.J., Jung, S.H., Kim, B.S., Jung, J.Y., Lee, S.H., Park, C.S. & Kim JS. (2011) Dihydroavenanthramide D inhibits human breast cancer cell invasion through suppression of MMP-9 expression. *Biochemical and Biophysical Research Communications* 405, 552–527.

Leenhardt, F., Lyan, B., Rock, E., Boussard, A., Potus, J., Chanliaud, E. & Remesy, C. (2006) Wheat lipoxygenase activity induces greater loss of carotenoids than vitamin E during breadmaking *Journal of Agricultural and Food Chemistry* 54, 1710–1715.

Lemmens, E., De Brier, N., Spiers, K.M., Ryan, C., Garrevoet, J., Falkenberg, G., Goos, P., Smolders, E. & Delcour, J.A. (2018) The impact of steeping, germination and hydrothermal processing of wheat (*Triticum aestivum* L.) grains on phytate hydrolysis and the distribution, speciation and bio-accessibility of iron and zinc elements. *Food Chemistry* 264, 367–376.

Li, G.X., Lee, M.J., Liu, A.B., Yang, Z., Lin, Y., Shih, W.J. & Yang, C.S. (2011) δ-tocopherol is more active than α- or γ-tocopherol in inhibiting lung tumorigenesis *in vivo*. *Cancer Prevention Research* 4, 404–413.

Li, L., Schewry, P.R. & Ward, J.L. (2008) Phenolic acids in wheat varieties in the HEALTHGRAIN diversity screen. *Journal of Agricultural and Food Chemistry* 56, 9732–9739.

Li, X.-P., Li, M.-Y., Ling, A-J., Hu, Xin-Z., Ma, Z., Liu, L. & Li, Y.-X. (2017) Effects of genotype and environment on avenanthramides and antioxidant activity of oats grown in northwestern China. *Journal of Cereal Science* 73, 130–137.

Liang, Y., Gao, Y., Lin, Q., Luo, F., Wu, W., Lu, Q. & Liu, Y. (2014) A review of the research progress on the bioactive ingredients and physiological activities of rice bran oil. *European Food Research and Technology* 238, 169–176.

Likes, R., Madl, R.L., Zeisel, S.H. & Craig, S.A.S. (2007) The betaine and choline content of a whole wheat flour compared to other mill streams. *Journal of Cereal Science* 46, 93–95.

Lillioja, S., Neal, A.L., Tapsell, L. & Jacobs, D.R. Jr. (2013) Whole grains, type 2 diabetes, coronary heart disease, and hypertension: Links to the aleurone preferred over indigestible fiber. *Biofactors* 39, 242–258.

Lin, X., Racette, S.B., Lefevre, M., Spearie, C.A., Most, M., Ma, L. & Ostlund, R.E. Jr. (2010) The effects of phytosterols present in natural food matrices on cholesterol metabolism and LDL-cholesterol: A controlled feeding trial. *European Journal of Clinical Nutrition* 64, 1481–1487.

Liu, C., Chen, C., Yang, F., Li, X., Cheng, L. & Song, Y. (2018) Phytic acid improves intestinal mucosal barrier damage and reduces serum levels of proinflammatory cytokines in a 1,2-dimethylhydrazine-induced rat colorectal cancer model. *British Journal of Nutrition* 120, 121–130.

Liu, S., Yang, N., Hou, Z.-H., Yao, Y., *et al.* (2011) Antioxidant effects of oats avenanthramides on human serum. *Agricultural Sciences in China* 10, 1301–1305.

Liukkonen, K-H, Katina, K., Wilhelmsson, A., Myllymäki, O., Lampi, A-M, Kariluoto, S., Piironen, V., Heinonen, S-M, Nurmi, T., Adlercreutz, H., Peltoketo, A., Pihlava, J-M, Hietaniemi, V. & Poutanen, K. (2003) Process-induced changes on bioactive compounds in whole grain rye. *Proceedings of the Nutrition Society* 62, 117–122.

Llaverias, G., Escolà-Gil, J.C., Lerma, E., Julve, J., Pons, C., Cabré, A., Cofán, M., Ros, E., Sánchez-Quesada, J.L. & Blanco-Vaca, F. (2013) Phytosterols inhibit the tumor growth and lipoprotein oxidizability induced by a high-fat diet in mice with inherited breast cancer. *Journal of Nutritional Biochemistry* 24, 39–48.

Lopez, H.W., Duclos, V., Coudray, C., Krespine, V., Feillet-Coudray, C., Messager, A., Demigné, C. & Rémésy, C. (2003) Making bread with sourdough improves mineral bioavailability from reconstituted whole wheat flour in rats. *Nutrition* 19, 524–530.

Määttä, K., Lampi, A.-M., Petterson, J., Fogelfors, B.M., Piironen, V. & Kamal-Eldin, A. (1999) Phytosterol content in seven oat cultivars grown at three locations in Sweden. *Journal of the Science of Food and Agriculture* 79, 1021–1027.

Maffucci, T., Piccolo, E., Cumashi, A., Iezzi, M., Riley, A.M., Saiardi, A.Godage, H.J., Rossi, C. & Broggini, M., S., Potter, B.V.L., Innocenti, P. & Falasca, M. (2005) Inhibition of the phosphatidylinositol 3-kinase/Akt pathway by inositol pentakisphosphate results in antiangiogenic and antitumor effects. *Cancer Research* 65, 8339–8349.

Magallanes-Lopez, A.M., Hernandez-Espinosa, N., Velu, G., Posadas-Romano, G., Ordoñez-Villegas, V.M.G., Crossa, J., Ammar, K. & Guzmán, C. (2017) Variability in iron, zinc and phytic acid content in a worldwide collection of commercial durum wheat cultivars and the effect of reduced irrigation on these traits. *Food Chemistry* 237, 499–505.

Mancuso, C. & Santangelo, R. (2014) Ferulic acid: Pharmacological and toxicological aspects. *Food and Chemical Toxicology* 65, 185–195.

Markiewicz, L.H., Honke, J., Haros, M., Świątecka, D. & Wróblewska, B. (2013) Diet shapes the ability of human intestinal microbiota to degrade phytate--in vitro studies. *Journal of Applied Microbiology* 115, 247–259.

Marttinen, M., Päivärinta, E., Storvik, M., Huikko, L., Luoma-Halkola, H., Piironen, V., Pajari, A.M. & Mutanen, M. (2013) Plant stanols induce intestinal tumor formation by up-regulating Wnt and EGFR signaling in Apc Min mice. *Journal of Nutritional Biochemistry* 24, 343–352.

Marttinen, M., Pajari, A.M., Päivärinta, E., Storvik, M., Marttinen, P., Nurmi, T., Niku, M., Piironen, V. & Mutanen, M. (2014) Plant sterol feeding induces tumor formation and alters sterol metabolism in the intestine of Apc(Min) mice. *Nutrition & Cancer* 66, 259–269.

Mason, J.B. (2009) Folate, cancer risk, and the Greek god, Proteus: A tale of two chameleons. *Nutrition Reviews* 67, 206–212.

Mateo Anson, N., Aura, A.M., Selinheimo, E., Mattila, I., Poutanen, K., van den Berg, R., Havenaar, R., Bast, A. & Haenen, G.R. (2011) Bioprocessing of wheat bran in whole wheat bread increases the bioavailability of phenolic acids in men and exerts antiinflammatory effects ex vivo. *Journal of Nutrition* 141, 137–143.

Mateo Anson, N., van den Berg, R., Havenaar, R., Bast, A. & Haenen, G.R.M.M. (2009) Bioavailability of ferulic acid is determined by its bioaccessibility. *Journal of Cereal Science* 49, 296–300.

Mattila, P., Pihlava, J.-M. & Hellström, J. (2005) Contents of phenolic acids, alkyl- and alkenylresorcinols, and avenanthramides in commercial grain products. *Journal of Agricultural and Food Chemistry* 53, 8920–8295.

McCann, S.E., Hootman, K.C., Weaver, A.M., Thompson, L.U., Morrison, C., Hwang, H., Edge, S.B., Ambrosone, C.B., Horvath, P.J. & Kulkarni, S.A. (2012) Dietary intakes of total and specific lignans are associated with clinical breast tumor characteristics. *Journal of Nutrition* 142, 91–98.

Menzel, C., Kamal-Eldin, A., Marklund, M., Andersson, A., Åman, P. & Landberg, R. (2012) Alkylresorcinols in Swedish cereal food products. *Journal of Food Composition and Analysis* 28, 119–125.

Meydani, M. (2009) Potential health benefits of avenanthramides of oats. *Nutrition Reviews* 67, 731–735.

Moore, J., Hao, Z., Zhou, K., Luther, M., Costa, J. & Yu, L. (2005) Carotenoid, tocopherol, phenolic acid, and antioxidant properties of Maryland-grown soft wheat. *Journal of Agricultural and Food Chemistry* 53, 6649–6657.

Mori, H., Kawabata, K., Yoshimi, N., Tanaka, T., Murakami, T., Okada, T. & Murai, H. (1999) Chemopreventive effects of ferulic acid on oral and rice germ on large bowel carcinogenesis. *Anticancer Research* 19, 3775–3778.

Multari, S., Pihlava, J.-M., Ollennu-Chuasam, P., Hietaniemi, V., Yang, B. & Suomela, J.-P. (2018) Identification and quantification of avenanthramides and free and bound phenolic acids in eight cultivars of husked oat (Avene sativa L). *Journal of Agricultural and Food Chemistry* 66, 2900–2908.

Ndolo, V.U. & Beta, T. (2013) Distribution of carotenoids in endosperm, germ, and aleurone fractions of cereal grain kernels. *Food Chemistry* 139, 663–671.

Ndolo, V.U. & Beta, T. (2014) Comparative studies on composition and distribution of phenolic acids in cereal grain botanical fractions. *Cereal Chemistry* 91, 522–530.

Nielsen, M.M. & Hansen, Å. (2008) Rapid high-performance liquid chromatography determination of tocopherols and tocotrienols in cereals *Cereal Chemistry* 85, 248–251.

Nor Qhairul Izzreen, M. N., Nuobariene, L., Rasmussen, S.K., Arneborg, N. & Hansen, Å.S. (2017) Changes in phytate content in whole meal wheat dough and bread fermented with phytase-active yeasts. *Cereal Chemistry* 94, 922–927.

Normen, A. L., Brants, H. A. M., Voorrips, L. E., Andersson, H. A., Van den Brandt, P. A. & Goldbohm, R. A. (2001) Plant sterol intakes and colorectal cancer risk in the Netherlands cohort study on diet and cancer. *American Journal of Clinical Nutrition* 74, 141–148.

Nurmi, T. (2012) Variation of phytosterols and steryl ferulates in wheat grains and fractions (dissertation). *EKT-series 1576*. University of Helsinki, Finland. http://ethesis.helsinki.fi

Nurmi, T., Lampi, A.-M., Nyström, L. & Piironen, V. (2010) Effects of environment and genotype on phytosterols in wheat in the HEALTHGRAIN diversity screen. *Journal of Agricultural and Food Chemistry* 58, 9314–9323.

Nurmi, T., Lampi, A. M., Nyström, L., Hemery, Y., Rouau, X. & Piironen, V. (2012) Distribution and composition of phytosterols and steryl ferulates in wheat grain and bran fractions. *Journal of Cereal Science* 56, 379–388.

Nurmi, T., Nyström, L., Edelmann, M., Lampi, A.-M., & Piironen, V. (2008) Phytosterols in wheat genotypes in the HEALTHGRAIN diversity screen. *Journal of Agricultural and Food Chemistry* 56, 9710–9715.

Nyström, L., Lampi, A-M, Andersson, A.A.M., Kamal-Eldin, A., Gebruers, K., Courtin, C.M., Delcour, J.A., Li, L., Ward, J.L., Fras, A., Boros, D., Rakszegi, M., Bedő, Z., Shewry, P.R. & Piironen, V. (2008) Phytochemicals and dietary fiber components in rye varieties in the Healthgrain diversity screen. *Journal of Agricultural and Food Chemistry* 56, 9758–9766.

Nyström, L., Paasonen, A., Lampi, A.-M. &Piironen, V. (2007). Total plant sterols, steryl ferulates and steryl glycosides in milling fractions of wheat and rye. *Journal of Cereal Science* 45, 106–115.

Öhrvik, V.E. & Witthöft, C.M. (2011) Human folate bioavailability. *Nutrients* 3, 475–490.

Ostlund, R.E. Jr, Racette, S.B. & Stenson, W.F. (2003) Inhibition of cholesterol absorption by phytosterol-replete wheat germ compared with phytosterol-depleted wheat germ. *American Journal of Clinical Nutrition* 77, 1385–1389.

Pajari, A.-M., Smeds, A.I., Oikarinen, S.I., Eklund, P.C., Sjöholm, R.E. & Mutanen M. (2006) The plant lignans matairesinol and secoisolariciresinol administered to Min mice do not protect against intestinal tumor formation. *Cancer Letters* 233, 309–314.

Panfili, G., Fratianni, A. & Irano, M. (2003) Normal phase high-performance liquid chromatography method for the determination of tocopherols and tocotrienols in cereals *Journal of Agricultural and Food Chemistry* 51, 3940-3944.

Panfili, G., Fratianni, A. & Irano, M. (2004) Improved normal-phase high-performance liquid chromatography procedure for the determination of carotenoids in cereals. *Journal of Agricultural and Food Chemistry* 52, 6373–6377.

Parikka, K., Rowland, I.R., Welch, R.W. & Wähälä, K. (2006) In vitro antioxidant activity and antigenotoxicity of 5-n-alkylresorcinols. *Journal of Agricultural and Food Chemistry* 54, 1646–1650.

Park, J.S., Chew, B.P. (1998) Dietary lutein from maricold extract inhibits mammary tumor development in BALB/c mice. *Journal of Nutrition* 128, 1650–1656.

Park, J.Y., Nicolas, G., Freisling, H., Biessy, C., Scalbert, A., Romieu, I., Chajès, V., Chuang, S.C., Ericson, U., Wallström, P., Ros, M.M., Peeters, P.H., Mattiello, A., Palli, D., María Huerta, J., Amiano, P., Halkjær, J., Dahm, C.C., Trichopoulou, A., Orfanos, P., Teucher, B., Feller, S., Skeie, G., Engeset, D., Boutron-Ruault, M.C., Clavel-Chapelon, F., Crowe, F., Khaw, K.T., Vineis, P. & Slimani, N. (2012) Comparison of standardised dietary folate intake across ten countries participating in the European Prospective Investigation into Cancer and Nutrition. *British Journal of Nutrition* 108, 552–569.

Patring, J., Wandel, M., Jägerstad, M. & Frølich, W. (2009) Folate content of Norwegian and Swedish flours and bread analysed by use of liquid chromatography-mass spectrometry. *Journal of Food Composition and Analysis* 22, 649–656.

Paznocht, L., Kotíková, Z., Šulc, M., Lachman, J., Orsák, M., Eliášová, M. & Martinek, P. (2018) Free and esterified carotenoids in pigmented wheat, tritordeum and barley grains. *Food Chemistry* 240, 670–678.

Pedersen, H.A., Laursen, B., Mortensen, A. & Fomsgaard, I.S. (2011) Bread from common cereal cultivars contains an important array of negletted bioactive benzoxazinoids. *Food Chemistry* 127, 1814–1820.

Pekkinen, J., Rosa, N.N., Savolainen, O.I., Keski-Rahkonen, P., Mykkänen, H., Poutanen, K., Micard, V. & Hanhineva, K. (2014) Disintegration of wheat aleurone structure has an impact on the bioavailability of phenolic compounds and other phytochemicals as evidenced by altered urinary metabolite profile of diet-induced obese mice. *Nutrition & Metabolism (London)* 11, 1.

Peñalvo, J.L., Haajanen, K.M., Botting, N. & Adlercreutz, H. (2005) Quantification of lignans in food using isotope dilution gas chromatography/mass spectrometry. *Journal of Agricultural and Food Chemistry,* 53, 9342–9347.

Peterson, J., Dwyer, J., Adlercreutz, H., Scalbert, A., Jacques, P. & McCullough, M.L. (2010) Dietary lignans: Physiology and potential for cardiovascular disease risk reduction. *Nutrition Reviews* 68, 571–603.

Pfeiffer, C.M., Rogers, L.M. & Gregory, J.F. (1997) Determination of folate in cereal-grain food products using trienzyme extraction and combined affinity and reversed-phase liquid chromatography. *Journal of Agricultural and Food Chemistry* 45, 407–413.

Pihlava, J.-M., Hellström, J., Kurtelius, T. & Mattila, P. (2018) Flavonoids, anthocyanins, benzoxazinoids, lignans and alkylresorcinols in rye (Secale cereale) and some rye propoducts. *Journal of Cereal Science* 79, 183-192.

Piironen, V & Lampi, A.-M. (2004) Occurrence and levels of phytosterols in foods. In: Phytosterols as Functional Food Components and Nutraceuticals. (eds. P.C. Dutta), pp. 1–32. Marcel Dekker, Inc, New York;.

Piironen, V., Edelmann, M., Kariluoto, S. & Bedo, Z. (2008) Folate in wheat genotypes in the HEALTHGRAIN diversity screen *Journal of Agricultural and Food Chemistry* 56, 9726–9731.

Piironen, V., Lindsay, D. G., Miettinen, T. A., Toivo, J. & Lampi, A. (2000) Plant sterols: Biosynthesis, biological function and their importance to human nutrition. *Journal of the Science of Food and Agriculture* 80, 939–966.

Piironen, V., Toivo, J. & Lampi, A. M. (2002) Plant sterols in cereals and cereal products. *Cereal Chemistry* 79, 148–154.

Pridal, A.A., Böttger, W. & Ross, A.B. (2018) Analysis of avenanthramides in oat products and estimation of avenanthramide intake in humans. *Food Chemistry* 253, 93-100.

Quilliot, D., Boman, F., Creton, C., Pelletier, X., Floquet, J. & Debry, G. (2001) Phytosterols have an unfavourable effect on bacterial activity and no evident protective effect on colon carcinogenesis. *European Journal of Cancer Prevention* 10, 237–243.

Redaelli, R., Dimberg, L., Germeier, C.H., Berardo, N., Locatelli, S. & Guerrini, L. (2016) Variability of tocopherols, tocotrienols and avenanthramides contents in European oat germplasm. *Euphytica* 207, 273–292.

Raicht, R.F., Cohen, B.I., Fazzini, E.P., Sarwal, A.N., Takahashi, M. (1980) Protective effect of plant sterols against chemically induced colon tumors in rats. *Cancer Research* 40, 403–405.

Raju, J., Swamy, M.V., Cooma, I., Patlolla, J.M., Pittman, B., Reddy, B.S., Steele, V.E. & Rao, C.V. (2005) Low doses of beta-carotene and lutein inhibited AOM-induced rat colonic ACF formation but high doses augment ACF incidence. *International Journal of Cancer* 113, 798–802.

Ramanathan, N., Tan, E., Loh, L.J., Soh, B.S. & Yap, W.N. (2018) Tocotrienol is a cardioprotective agent against ageing-associated cardiovascular disease and its associated morbidities. *Nutrition & Metabolism* 15, 6.

Reddy, B.S., Hirose, Y., Cohen, L.A., Simi, B., Cooma, I. & Rao, C.V. (2000) Preventive potential of wheat bran fractions against experimental colon carcinogenesis: Implications for human colon cancer prevention. *Cancer Research* 60, 4792–4797.

Ross, A.B., Becker, W., Chen, Y., Kamal-Eldin, A. & Åman, P. (2005). Intake of alkylresorcinols from wheat and rye in the United Kingdom and Sweden. *British Journal of Nutrition* 94, 496–499.

Ross, A.B., Bourgeois, A., Macharia, H.N., Kochhar, S., Jebb, S.A., Brownlee, I.A. & Seal, C.J. (2012). Plasma alkylresorcinols as a biomarker of whole-grain food consumption in a large population: Results from the WHOLEheart Intervention Study. *American Journal of Clinical Nutrition* 95, 204–211.

Ross, A.B., Kamal-Eldin, A. & Aman, P. (2004). Dietary alkylresorcinols: Absorption, bioactivities, and possible use as biomarkers of whole-grain wheat- and rye-rich foods. *Nutrition Reviews* 62, 81–95.

Ross, A.B., Zangger, A. & Guiraud, S.P. (2014) Cereal foods are the major source of betaine in the Western diet – Analysis of betaine and free choline in cereal foods and updated assessments of betaine intake. *Food Chemistry* 145, 859–865.

Ryynänen, M., Lampi, A., Salo-Väänänen, P., Ollilainen, V. & Piironen, V. (2004) A small-scale sample preparation method with HPLC analysis for determination of tocopherols and tocotrienols in cereals *Journal of Food Composition and Analysis* 17, 749–765.

Saarinen, N.M., Wärri, A., Dings, R.P.M., Airio, M., Smeds, A.I. & Mäkelä, S. (2008) Dietary lariciresinol attenuates mammary tumor growth and reduces blood vessel density in human MCF-7 breast cancer xenografts and carcinogen-induced mammary tumors in rats. *International Journal of Cancer* 123, 1196–1204.

Sang, S., Ju, J., Lambert, J.D., Lin, Y., Hong, J., Bose, M., Wang, S., Bai, N., He, K., Reddy, B.S., Ho C.-T., Li, F. & Yang C.S. (2006) Wheat bran oil and its fractions inhibit human colon cancer cell growth and intestinal tumorigenesis in $Apc^{min/+}$ mice. *Journal of Agricultural and Food Chemistry* 54, 9792–9797.

Santilli, F., Davì, G. & Patrono, C. (2016) Homocysteine, methylenetetrahydrofolate reductase, folate status and atherothrombosis: A mechanistic and clinical perspective. *Vascular Pharmacology* 78, 1–9.

Sauberlich, H.E., Kretsch, M.J., Skala, J.H., Johnson, H.L. & Taylor, P.C. (1987) Folate requirement and metabolism in nonpregnant women. *American Journal of Clinical Nutrition* 46, 1016–1028.

Sawadikiat, P. & Hongsprabhas, P. (2014) Phytosterols and μ-oryzanol in rice bran oils and distillates from physical refining process. *International Journal of Food Science & Technology* 49, 2030–2036.

Scarpa, E.S., Mari, M., Antonini, E., Palma, F. & Ninfali, P. (2018) Natural and synthetic avenanthramides activate caspases 2, 8, 3 and downregulate hTERT, MDR1 and COX-2 genes in CaCo-2 and Hep3B cancer cells. *Food & Function* 9, 2913–2921.

Scheers, N.M., Pereira, D.I.A., Faria, N., Powell, J.J. (2018) Ferric citrate and ferric EDTA but not ferrous sulfate drive amphiregulin-mediated activation of the MAP kinase ERK in gut epithelial cancer cells. *Oncotarget* 9 (24), 17066–17077

Schlemmer, U., Frølich, W., Prieto, R.M. & Grases, F. (2009) Phytate in foods and significance for humans: Food sources, intake, processing, bioavailability, protective role and analysis. *Molecular Nutrition & Food Research* 53 Suppl 2, S330–S375.

Servillo, L., D'Onofrio, N., Giovane, A., Casale, R., Cautela, D., Ferrari, G., Castaldo, D. & Balestrieri, M.L. (2018) The betaine profile of cereal flours unveils new and uncommon betaines. *Food Chemistry* 239, 234–241.

Setchell, K.D., Brown, N.M., Zimmer-Nechemias, L., Wolfe, B., Jha, P. & Heubi, J.E. (2014) Metabolism of secoisolariciresinol-diglycoside the dietary precursor to the intestinally derived lignan enterolactone in humans. *Food & Function* 25, 491–501.

Shafie, N.H., Esa, N.M., Ithinin, H., Akim, A.M., Saad, N. & Pandurangan, A.K. (2013) Preventive inositol hexaphosphate extract from rice bran inhibits colorectal cancer through involvement of Wnt/β-catenin and COX-2 pathways. *BioMed Research International*, ID681027

Shewry, P.R., Hawkesford, M.J., Piironen, V., Lampi, A.-M., Gebruesrs, K., Boros, D., Andersson, A.A.M., Åman, P., Rakszegi, M., Bedo, Z. & Ward, J.L. (2013) Natural variation in grain composition of wheat and related cereals. *Journal of Agricultural and Food Chemistry* 61, 8295–8303.

Shewry, P.R., Piironen, V., Lampi, A-M, Edelmann, M., Kariluoto, S., Nurmi, T., Fernandez-Orozco, R., Andersson, A.A.M., Åman, P., Fras´, A., Boros, D., Gebruers, K., Dornez, E., Courtin, C.M., Delcour, J. A., Ravel, C., Charmet, G., Rakszegi, M., Bedo, Z. & Ward, J. L. (2010a) Effects of genotype and environment on the content and composition of phytochemicals and dietary fiber components in rye in the HEALTHGRAIN diversity screen. *Journal of Agricultural and Food Chemistry* 58, 9372–9383.

Shewry, P.R., Piironen, V., Lampi, A-M, Nyström, L., Li, L., Rakszegi, M., Fras, A., Boros, D., Gebruers, K., Courtin, C.M., Delcour, J.A., Andersson, A.A.M., Dimberg, L., Bedő, Z. & Ward, J.L. (2008) Phytochemical and fiber components in oat varieties in the Healthgrain diversity screen. *Journal of Agricultural and Food Chemistry* 56, 9777–9784.

Shewry, P.R., Piironen, V., Lampi, A-M., Edelman, M., Kariluoto, S., Nurmi, T., Fernandez-Orozco, R., Ravel, C., Charmet, G., Andersson, A.A.M, Åman, P., Boros, D., Gebruers, K., Dornez, E., Courtin, M. C., Delcour, J.A., Rakszegi, M, Bedo, Z. & Ward, J.L. (2010b) The HEALTHGRAIN wheat diversity screen: Effects of genotype and environment on phytochemicals and dietary fiber components. *Journal of Agricultural and Food Chemistry* 58, 9291–9298.

Singh, R., De, S. & Belkheir, A. (2013) *Avena sativa* (oat), a potential nutraceutical and therapeutic agent: an overview. *Critical Review of Food Science and Nutrition* 53, 126–144.

Sinhdu, E.R., Firdous, A.P., Ramnath, V. & Kuttan, R. (2013) Effect of carotenoid lutein on N-nitrosodiethylamine-induced hepatocellular carcinoma and its mechanism of action. *European Journal of Cancer Prevention* 22, 320–327.

Skoglund, M., Peterson, D.M., Andersson, R., Nilsson, J. & Dimberg, L.H. (2008) Avenanthramide content and related enzyme activities in oats as affected by steeping and germination. *Journal of Cereal Science* 48, 294–303.

Smeds, A.I., Eklund, P.C., Sjöholm, R.E., Willför, S.M., Nishibe, S., Deyama, T. & Holmbom, B.R. (2007) Quantification of a broad spectrum of lignans in cereals, oilseeds, and nuts. *Journal of Agricultural and Food Chemistry* 55, 1337–1346.

Smeds, A.I., Jauhiainen, L., Tuomola, E. & Peltonen-Sainio, P. (2009) Characterization of variation in the lignan content and composition of winter rye, spring wheat, and spring oat. *Journal of Agricultural and Food Chemistry* 57, 5837–5842.

Smith, A.D., Kim, Y.-I. & Refsum, H. (2008) Is folic acid good for everyone? *American Journal of Clinical Nutrition* 87, 517–533.

Smolarek, A.K., So, J.Y., Burgess, B., Kong, A.-N.K., Reuhl, K., Lin, Y., Shih, W.J., Li, G., Lee, M.-J., Chen, Y.-K., Yang, C.S. & Suh, N. (2012) Dietary administration of δ- and γ-tocopherol inhibits tumorigenesis in the animal model of estrogen receptor-positive, but not HER-2 breast cancer. *Cancer Prevention Research* 5, 1310–1320.

Söderholm, P.P., Alfthan, G., Tikkanen, M.J. & Adlercreutz, H. (2012) Rye bread intake improves oxidation resistance of LDL in healthy humans. *Atherosclerosis* 221, 583–586.

Steffensen, S.K., Adhikari, K.B., Laursen, B.B., Jensen, C., Gregersen, P.L., Bhattarai, B., Martin Marais, L., Schnorr, H.,Tanwir, F., Dionisio, G., Adhikari, K.B., Fomsgaard, I. S. & Gregersen, P.L. (2017) Biosynthesis and chemical transformation of benzoxazinoids in rye during germination and the identification of a rye Bx6-like gene. *Phytochemistry* 140, 95–107.

Steffensen, S.K., Pedersen, H.A., Adhikari, K.B., Laursen, B.B., Jensen, C., Høyer, S., Borre, M., Pedersen, H.H., Borre, M., Edwards, D. & Fomsgaard, I.S. (2016) Benzoxazinoids in prostate cancer patients after a rye-intensive diet: Methods and initial results. *Journal of Agricultural and Food Chemistry* 64, 8235–8245.

Stevenson, L., Phillips, F., O'Sullivan, K. & Walton, J. (2012). Wheat bran: Its composition and benefits to health, a European perspective. *International Journal of Food Science and Nutrition* 63, 1001–1013.

Stuper-Szablewska, K. & Perkowski, J. (2017) Phenolic acids in cereal grain: Occurrence, biosynthesis, metabolism and role in living organisms. *Critical Reviews in Food Science and Nutrition.*

Suraj, R., Radhamani, S., Meehan-Andrews, T. & Bradley, C. (2017) Role of a novel benzoxazine derivative in the chemosensitization of colon cancer. *Apoptosis* 22, 988–1000.

Svanberg, U., Lorri, W. & Sandberg, A. S. (1993) Lactic fermentation of non-tannin and high-tannin cereals: Effects on in vitro estimation of iron availability and phytate hydrolysis. *Journal of Food Science* 58, 408–412.

Sy, C., Gleize, B., Dangles, O., Landrier, J.F., Veyrat, C.C. & Borel, P. (2012) Effects of physicochemical properties of carotenoids on their bioaccessibility, intestinal cell uptake, and blood and tissue concentrations. *Molecular Nutrition & Food Research* 56, 1385–1397.

Tanwir, F., Fredholm, M., Gregersen, P.L. & Fomsgaard, I.S. (2013) Comparison of the levels of bioactive benzoxazinoids in different wheat and rye fractions and the transformation of these compounds in homemade foods. *Food Chemistry* 141, 444–450.

Temelli, F., Stobbe, K., Rezaei, K. & Vasanthan, T. (2013) Tocol composition and supercritical carbon dioxide extraction of lipids from barley pearling flour. *Journal of Food Science* 78, 1643–1650.

Tetens, I., Turrini, A., Tapanainen, H., Christensen, T., Lampe, J.W., Fagt, S., Håkansson, N., Lundquist, A., Hallund, J., Valsta, L.M. & The Phytohealth WP1 working group. (2013) Dietary intake and main sources of plant lignans in five European countries. *Food & Nutrition Research* 57, 19805 - http://dx.doi.org/10.3402/fnr.v57i0.19805

Thompson, L.U., Button, C.L. & Jenkins, D.J. (1987) Phytic acid and calcium affect the in vitro rate of navy bean starch digestion and blood glucose response in humans. *American Journal of Clinical Nutrition* 46, 467–473.

Tiwari, U. & Cummins, E. (2009) Nutritional importance and effect of processing on tocols in cereals. *Trends in Food Science and Technology* 20, 511–520.

Traber, M.G. (2013) Mechanisms for the prevention of vitamin E excess. *Journal of Lipid Research* 54, 2295–2306.

Traber, M.G. & Stevens, J.F. (2011) Vitamins C and E: Beneficial effects from a mechanistic perspective *Free Radical Biology & Medicine* 51, 1000-1013.

Troesch, B., Jing, H., Laillou, A. & Fowler, A. (2013) Absorption studies show that phytase from *Aspergillus niger* significantly increases iron and zinc bioavailability from phytate-rich foods. *Food and Nutrition Bulletin* 34(2 Suppl), S90–101.

Vahteristo, L., Kariluoto, S., Bärlund, S., Kärkkäinen, M., Lamberg-Allardt, C., Salovaara H. & Piironen, V. (2002) Functionality of endogenous folates from rye and orange juice using human in vivo model. *European Journal of Nutrition* 41, 271–278.

Valsta, L. M., Lemström, A., Ovaskainen, M. L., Lampi, A. M., Toivo, J., Korhonen, T. & Piironen, V. (2004) Estimation of plant sterol and cholesterol intake in Finland: Quality of new values and their effect on intake. *British Journal of Nutrition* 92, 671–678.

van Kranen, H.J., Mortensen, A., Sorensen, I.K., van den Berg-Wijnands, J., Beems, R., Nurmi, T., Adlercreutz, H. & van Kreijl, C.F. (2003) Lignan precursors from flaxseed or rye bran do not protect against the development of intestinal neoplasis in ApcMin mice. *Nutrition & Cancer* 45, 203–210.

Vucenik, I. & Shamsuddin, M. (2006) Protection against cancer by dietary IP_6 and inositol. *Nutrition & Cancer* 55, 109–125.

Wang, D., Wise, M.L., Li, F. & Dey, M. (2012b) Phytochemicals attenuating aberrant activation of β-catenin in cancer cells. *PLoS One* 7, e50508.

Wang, M.X., Jiao, J.H., Li, Z.Y., Liu, R.R., Shi, Q. & Ma, L. (2013) Lutein supplementation reduces plasma lipid peroxidation and C-reactive protein in healthy nonsmokers. *Atherosclerosis* 227, 380–385.

Wang, P., Chen, Y.-M., He, L.-P., Chen, C.G., Zhang, B., Xue, W.-Q. & Su, Y.-Xi. (2012a) Association of natural intake of dietary plant sterols with carotid intima-media thickness and blood lipids in Chinese adults: A cross-section study. *PLoS One* 7, e32736.

Wang, Y. & Wang, X.-D. (2011) β-Carotene and other carotenoids in cancer prevention. In: Vegetables, Whole Grains, and Their Derivatives in Cancer Prevention. (eds. M. Mutanen & A.-M. Pajari) pp. 67–89. Springer Science+Bussiness Media.

Wargovich, M.J., Jimenez, A., McKee, K., Steele, V.E., Velasco, M., Woods, J., Price, R., Gray, K. & Kellof, G.J. (2000) Efficacy of potential chemopreventive agents on rat colon aberrant crypt formation and progression. *Carcinogenesis* 21, 1149–1155.

Wiggins, A.K., Mason, J.K. & Thompson, L.U. (2013) Beneficial influence of diets enriched with flaxseed and flaxseed oil on cancer. In: *Cancer Chemoprevention and Treatment by Diet Theraphy.* (ed. W.S.S. Cho), pp. 55–89. Springer Science+Business Media, Dordrecht.

Willför, S.M., Smeds, A.I. & Holmbom, B.R. (2006) Chromatographic analysis of lignans. *Journal of Chromatography A* 1112, 64–77.

Wilson, M.S., Bulley, S.J., Pisani, F., Irvine, R.F. & Saiardi, A. (2015) A novel method for the purification of inositol phosphates from biological samples reveals that no phytate is present in human plasma or urine. *Open Biology* 5, 150014.

World Cancer Research Fund/American Institute for Cancer Research. (2007) *Food, nutrition, physical activity, and the prevention of cancer: A global perspective*. AICR, Washington, DC.

Wu, W., Tang, Y., Yang, J., Idehen, E. & Sang, S. (2018) Avenanthramide aglycones and glucosides in oat bran: Chemical profile, levels in commercial oat products, and cytotoxicity to human colon cancer cells. *Journal of Agricultural and Food Chemistry* 66, 8005–8014.

Xu, J.G., Tian, C.R., Hu, Q.P., Luo, J.Y., Wang, X.D. & Tian, X.D. (2009) Dynamic changes in phenolic compounds and antioxidant activity in oats (Avena nuda L.) during steeping and germination. *Journal of Agricultural and Food Chemistry* 57, 10392–10398.

Yang, C.S., Suh, N. & Kong, A.N. (2012) Does vitamin E prevent or promote cancer? *Cancer Prevention Research* 5, 701–705.

Yang, J., Ou, B., Wise, M.L. & Chu, Y. (2014). in vitro total antioxidant capacity and anti-inflammatory activity of three common oat-derived avenanthramides. *Food Chemistry* 160, 338–345.

Yon, M. & Hyun, T.H. (2003) Folate content of foods commonly consumed in Korea measured after trienzyme extraction. *Nutrition Research* 23, 735–746.

Yonekura, L. & Nagao, A. (2007) Intestinal absorption of dietary carotenoids. *Molecular Nutrition & Food Research* 51, 107–115.

Yoo, J.H., Lee, H.J., Kang, K., Jho, E.H., Kim, C.Y., Baturen, D., Tunsaq, J. & Nho, C.W. (2010) Lignans inhibit cell growth via regulation of Wnt/beta-catenin signaling. *Food Chemistry and Toxicology* 48, 2247–2252.

Zamora-Ros, R., Knaze, V., Luján-Barroso, L., Kuhnle, G.G.C., Mulligan, A.A., Touillaud, M., Slimani, N., Romieu, I., Powell, N., Tumino, R., Peeters, P.H.M., de Magistris, M.S., Ricceri, F., Sonestedt, E., Drake, I., E Sonestedt, E., Drake, I., Hjartåker, A., Skie, G., Mouw, T., Wark, P.A., Romaguera, D., Bueno-de-Mesquita, H.B., Ros, M., Molina, E., Sieri, S., Quiros, J.R., Huesta, J.M., Tjønneland, A., Halkjær, J., Masala, G., Teucher, B., Kaas, R., Travis, R.C., Dilis, V., Benetou, V., Trichopoulou, A., Amiano, P., Ardanaz, E., Boeing, H., Förster, J., Clavel-Chapelon, F., Fagherazzi, G., Perquier, F., Johansson, G., Johansson, I., Cassidy, A., Overvade, K. & González, C. A. (2012) Dietary intakes and food sources of phytoestrogens in the European Prospective Investigation into Cancer and Nutrition (EPIC) 24-hour dietary recall cohort. *European Journal of Clinical Nutrition* 66, 932–941.

Zamora-Ros, R., Rothwell, J. A., Scalbert, A., Knaze, V., Romieu, I., Slimani, N., Fagherazzi, G., Perquier, F., Touillaud, M., Molina-Montes, E., Huerta, J.M., Barricarte, A., Amiano, P., Menéndez, V., Tumino, R., de Magistris, M.S., Palli, D., Ricceri, F., Sieri, S., Crowe, F.L., Khaw, K.-T., Wareham, N.J., Grote, V., Li, K., Boeing, H., Förster, J., Trichopoulou, A., Benetou, V., Tsiotas, K., Bueno-de-Mesquita, H.B., Ros, M., Peeters, P.H.M., Tjønneland, A., Halkjær, J., Overvad, K., Ericson, U., Wallström, P., Johansson, I., Landberg, R., Weiderpass, E., Engeset, D., Skeie, G., Wark, P., Riboli, E. & Gonzalez, C. A. (2013). Dietary intakes and food sources of phenolic acids in the European Prospective Investigation into Cancer and Nutrition (EPIC) study. *British Journal of Nutrition*, 110, 1500–1511.

Zeisel, S.H. & Warrier, M. (2017) Trimethylamine N-oxide, the microbiome, and heart and kidney disease. *Annual Review of Nutrition* 37, 157–181.

Zhang, T., Shao, J., Gao, Y., Chen, C., Yao, D., Chu, Y.F., Johnson, J., Kang, C., Yeo, D. & Ji, LL. (2017) Absorption and elimination of oat avenanthramides in humans after acute consumption of oat cookies. *Oxidative Medicine and Cellular Longevity* 2017, 2056705.

Zhu Y, Soroka DN, Sang S. (2012) Synthesis and inhibitory activities against colon cancer cell growth and proteasome of alkylresorcinols. *Journal of Agricultural and Food Chemistry* 60, 8624–8631.

Zhu, Y., Shurlknight, K.L., Chen, X. & Sang, S. (2014) Identification and pharmacokinetics of novel alkylresorcinol metabolites in human urine, new candidate biomarkers for whole-grain wheat and rye intake. *Journal of Nutrition* 144, 114–122.

Žilić, S., Serpen, A., Akillioğu, G., Janković, M. & Gökmen, V. (2012) Distributions of phenolic compounds, yellow pigments and oxidative enzymes in wheat grains and their relation to antioxidant capacity of bran and debranned flour. *Journal of Cereal Science* 56, 652–658.

Zou, Z.Y., Xu, X.R., Lin, X.M., Zhang, H.B., Xiao, X., Ouyang, L., Huang, Y.M., Wang, X. & Liu, Y.Q. (2014) Effects of lutein and lycopene on carotid intima-media thickness in Chinese subjects with subclinical atherosclerosis: A randomised, double-blind, placebo-controlled trial. *British Journal of Nutrition* 111, 474–480.

17 Potential Negative Effects of Whole grain Consumption

Afaf Kamal-Eldin[1], Agneta Åkesson[2], Maria Kippler[3], Karl-Erik Hellenäs[4], Nathalie Scheers[5], and Ann-Sofie Sandberg[5]

[1]Department of Food Science. College of Food & Agriculture, United Arab Emirates University, Al-Ain, UAE
[2]Nutritional Epidemiology Unit, Institute of Environmental Medicine, Karolinska Institutet, Stockholm, Sweden
[3]Metals and Health, Institute of Environmental Medicine, Karolinska Institutet, Stockholm, Sweden
[4]The National Food Agency, Uppsala, Sweden
[5]Division of Food and Nutrition Science, Department of Biology and Biological Engineering, Chalmers University of Technology, Gothenburg, Sweden

17.1 Introduction

Cereal grains contain some anti-nutritional factors, contaminants or environmental pollutants that may reach levels that are high enough to pose risk for the general population, segments within population, or the environment (Nadeem *et al.* 2010). The possible adverse effects related to whole grain consumption are important to consider with increased consumption of whole grains and especially bran-rich fractions. It has also been argued that the consumption of cereal grains has dominated only in the last 10 000 years of human evolution, following the agricultural revolution, and that this change in human diet may be associated with the development of different diseases related to increased energy consumption, for example, overweight, obesity and diabetes (Cordain 1999). Besides easily accessible energy, several naturally occurring and process-generated compounds have been identified in whole grain cereals and food products thereof. Some of the cereal proteins may provoke immune responses causing allergies or trigger autoimmune responses leading to food sensitivity in genetically predisposed individuals. Besides these proteins, there are several other cereal components that may cause different adverse effects depending on the consumption pattern of different whole grain products. Examples of these include naturally occurring or anthropogenic compounds such as the heavy metal cadmium, the iron absorption inhibitor phytate, phenolic compounds involved in oxidative stress (often called antioxidants) and heat-generated compounds such as acrylamide. The potential adverse effects of some components of whole grain cereal are summarized in Table 17.1.

Whole Grains and Health, Second Edition. Edited by Rikard Landberg and Nathalie Scheers.

Additional materials available for download online at https://www.wiley.com/en-gb/Whole+Grains+and+Health-p-9781118939437

Table 17.1 Classes and examples of components of whole grains with possible adverse effects on human health.

Class	Example compounds	Occurrence in whole grain cereals
Allergenic proteins	1) Albumin, globulins, α-amylase inhibitors, and non-specific lipid transfer proteins. 2) Cysteine-rich albumin and globulin proteins from the endosperm are weak trypsin inhibitors. 3) Lectins are high molecular weight proteins concentrated in the germ (e.g., wheat germ agglutinin)	Wheat, rye, barley, oats, rice and sorghum
Autoimmune sensitizing proteins	Gluten (glutamin and prolamin-rich protein such as gliadin in wheat, hordeins in barley and secalins in rye).	Wheat, rye and barley
Phytate	*Myo*-inositol hexaphosphate-storage form of phosphorus located in the germ and aleurone layer	All cereal grains
Heavy metals	Cadmium	All cereal grains
Phenolic compounds, especially tannins	Low levels in non-pigmented and very high levels in pigmented cereals	All cereals, but especially the bran fractions of colored cultivars sorghum, millet, barley and rice
Heat induced toxicants	Acrylamide	All cereals, but formation potential higher in rye than wheat and oats, which are higher than corn and rice

17.2 Allergies associated with grain intake

The human immune system consists of specialized cells designed to respond both to foreign antigens and damaged or defect cells of domestic origin, with the mission to dispose of debris and to remember the encounter. Central to the response are T cells (T lymphocytes), which are polarized or differentiated into specific subsets when presented with an antigen (Kidd 2003). The outcome of this process is diverse, but a simplified version may state that if the trigger is an intracellular antigen such as a virus or if the cell is defect, the T cells differentiate into a Th1 type of T cells classified according to the cytokines they secrete. If extracellular antigens, including systemic infections or agents, acquired from the environment such as allergens activate the T cells, they polarize into a Th2 type subset of T cells. Th1 cells secrete interferon γ as the major cytokine and are pro-inflammatory, while Th2 cells preferentially secrete IL-4, which are associated with the promotion of the specific antibodies (Ig E) causing allergic manifestations. To summarize in a simplistic way, there is an ongoing struggle between Th1 and Th2 T cell populations, and the balance between these is determined by external triggers and physiological needs. An illustrative example of this is the state of pregnancy in which the T-cell population is dominated by Th2 cells (Reinhard *et al.* 1998). This imbalance is physiologically important since it diminishes the risk of recognizing the fetus as non-self (Th1 response), which would lead to a rejection of the fetus (spontaneous abortion). In addition, pregnant rheumatoid arthritis (Th1 mediated disease) patients experience a decline or total loss of symptoms during the pregnancy with a relapse of symptoms about six months postpartum. With this background in mind, we may now start to discuss the immunological responses that are associated with cereals. To date, there are no indications that whole grain products would be more immunogenic than refined grains since the reacting agents are mostly proteins or short peptides, which are present in all parts of the grain.

Some common proteins in wheat, such as albumin, globulins, α-amylase inhibitors, and non-specific lipid transfer proteins (nsLTPS), are observed to elicit allergic reactions due to Th2 driven production of specific antibodies (immunoglobulin E; Ig E) in allergic individuals. The allergic reaction is often manifested by hay fever or nettle rash (hives), which are caused by the release of histamine, an organic nitrogenous compound, in the affected tissues. Histamine increases the permeability of capillaries, facilitating the invasion of immune cells and causes the tissue swelling associated with rhinitis and watery eyes. There are a few different types of wheat allergy slightly differing in reactivity and symptoms (Mittag *et al.* 2004). Baker's asthma is an occupational disease caused by the inhalation of wheat flour in which albumin, globulins, α-amylase/trypsin inhibitors are the major allergens. The very same allergens seem to be involved in Ig E mediated food allergy after ingestion of wheat products in sensitized individuals. Another wheat allergy is wheat-dependent exercise-induced anaphylaxis (WDEIA) caused by the ingestion of ω_5 type gliadin. The symptoms may range from urticaria to more severe allergic reactions. The prevalence of wheat allergy differs geographically, but is approximately 0–0.5%.

17.3 Non-allergic conditions associated with wheat, barley and rye intake

Gluten proteins, which is a collective name for glutamin and prolamin-rich proteins (such as gliadin in wheat, hordeins in barley and secalins in rye), may trigger celiac disease in genetically predisposed individuals carrying, for example, the HLA-DQ8 and/or HLA-DQ2 genotypes. Gluten is present throughout the kernel and is therefore toxic for celiacs independent of the extent of grain refinement. Celiac disease (also referred to as gluten-sensitive enteropathy or gluten intolerance) is a Th1-mediated autoimmune disorder in which gluten-derived peptides cause inflammation of the gastrointestinal lining manifested as, for example, intestinal pain and malnutrition. In celiac disease, deamidation of gluten-derived peptides in the small intestine by the enzyme tissue transglutaminase 2 (TG2) produces charged long-lived intermediaries, which may cause a Th1-driven immune response associated with the production of Ig A type antibodies directed against gluten components but also towards TG2 belonging to self; hence, celiac disease is an autoimmune disorder. Research is in progress to develop a food additive that interferes with the deamidation of gluten peptides by TG2 (Engström *et al.* 2017) in order to prevent gluten to become toxic during the passage through the gastrointestinal tract in affected individuals.

Dermatitis herpetiformis (DH) is a very similar condition to celiac disease, but is distinguished by a skin rash not observed in celiacs. The genetic profiles of the diseases are analogous except for an increased frequency of the DR7 allele in celiacs, while the DR2 allele is increased in DH patients (Sachs *et al.* 1986). The prevalence of dermatitis herpetiformis is approximately about a tenth of that of celiac disease, which is typically around 1% worldwide, but is higher in northern countries such as Finland and Sweden.

17.4 The heavy metal cadmium

Cadmium is a toxic metal with no known biological function in man, but which mimics other metals that are essential to diverse biological functions. Cadmium accumulates and remains in the body, especially in the renal cortex, for an extended period of time. Renal tubular damage is generally considered the first adverse effect that occurs as a result of too high exposure. While exposure to cadmium has long been recognized as a health hazard in industrial workers and in populations with very high environmental exposure, the awareness of the widespread low-level cadmium contamination of agricultural soil has increased the concern. Because cadmium is easily taken up by crops, the exposure from food may be high enough in many areas of the world to be of importance to human health. Even the cadmium exposure present in the general population has been shown to be associated with several other adverse effects (on bone, including increased risk of osteoporosis and fractures, and increased risk of cardiovascular diseases and hormone-related cancers) adding further concern (Akesson *et al.* 2014). Cadmium occurs in nature mainly in conjunction with zinc and also to some extent with lead and copper, and is thus an inescapable by-product of the metallurgy of these metals. The discovery of its usefulness in various applications, for example, as stabilizer, color pigment, cathode, anticorrosive agent and so on increased the industrial use during the early 1900s. Because of its high toxicity, dispersive use of cadmium was later restricted by law in many countries, but the content in the top layers of arable land had already increased and the metal had been introduced into the food chain. The current release of cadmium and its compounds to arable land originates mainly from atmospheric deposition (e.g., metal smelting, combustion of fossil fuels, and waste incineration), and from the use of cadmium-containing phosphate fertilizers and sewage sludge. Cadmium may also occur naturally in certain areas. Compared to other metals, cadmium and cadmium compounds are relatively water soluble in soil, and are therefore more bioavailable and tend to bio-accumulate in different organisms.

The diet is the main source of cadmium exposure. Smokers are additionally exposed through inhalation of smoke from the cadmium-accumulating tobacco plant. The dietary exposure to cadmium is influenced both by the cadmium concentrations in different foods and by the consumption pattern. The metal is present in virtually all foods. The highest concentrations are present in mollusks, crustaceans, offal products, oil seeds, cocoa beans and in certain wild mushrooms, but due to a general low consumption of these foods, they are not so important for the overall dietary exposure in most populations. Instead, plant foods such as cereals and vegetables, including root vegetables, are the main contributors to dietary exposure and estimated to contribute to about 70–80% of the total exposure. When comparing different cereal products, the highest concentrations are found in wheat, in particular whole grain products of wheat origin (Table 17.2). In certain contaminated areas of Asia, rice has been shown to contain very high concentrations of cadmium. In European and North American countries, the average dietary cadmium intake is estimated to 10–20 μg/day.

The bioavailability of cadmium from food is an important determinant when considering the potential risk of adverse health effects. In general, the gastrointestinal uptake of cadmium is low, usually a few percent. Cross-sectional human studies have shown that individuals with low iron stores and iron deficiency have increased cadmium concentrations in blood, urine and kidney (Barregard *et al.* 2010; Berglund *et al.* 1994), which is supported by experimental studies showing that dietary cadmium is absorbed via iron transporters (Ryu

Table 17.2 Cadmium content in different whole grain products.

Whole grain product	Range mean (mg/kg)	Max (mg/kg)
Wheat (non-specified)	0.009–0.0647	0.390
Wheat (bran and germ)*	0.0647	0.2200
Wheat grains and flour†	0.0300	0.1580
Barley	0.017	-
Oats	0.003–0.021	0.096
Rye	0.015–0.016	0.067
Rice	0.004–0.0253	0.510
Corn	0.003	0.008

*Only bran and germ when explicitly reported.
†Mainly data from wheat grain testing, which includes the wheat bran, and the flour category includes whole grain flour.
(Sources: EFSA [2009]; JECFA [2011]; USFDA [2014]).

et al. 2004). Also, in experimental studies, marginal deficiencies of zinc and calcium have been shown to increase the gastrointestinal absorption, organ accumulation and retention of dietary cadmium (Reeves and Chaney 2008). The gastrointestinal absorption of cadmium also appears to be inhibited by fibre and phytate (Lind *et al.* 1998), suggesting that diets with a high content of natural fibres may decrease the gastrointestinal absorption of cadmium despite the fact that fibre-rich foods contain more cadmium than food with low fibre content. In two large prospective cohort studies that estimated the dietary cadmium exposure from food in relation to incidence of breast cancer and fractures (Julin *et al.* 2012; Thomas *et al.* 2011), they attempted to disentangle if the harmful effect of cadmium is reduced by being exposed through whole grains and vegetables rather than from foods considered less healthy. Indeed, some support for this was observed as the highest risks were observed in those with the highest dietary cadmium exposure that at the same time had the lowest consumption of whole grains and vegetables. The average urinary excretion of cadmium, which reflects the kidney cadmium accumulation, is 0.5–1.0 μg/g creatinine. The average blood concentration is approximately 0.5–1.0 μg/L in nonsmokers, and it is twice as high in smokers. The available information shows that associations with negative health effects occur in population strata with a fairly low dietary cadmium intake, corresponding to urinary cadmium excretion as low as 0.5–2 μg/g creatinine. Thus, there is an urgent need to reduce the cadmium exposure as much as possible. Foremost, it is highly important to reduce the dispersion of cadmium into the environment and to decrease the contamination of cadmium on arable land. Alternative ways to reduce the exposure could include the development of cereal types that do not take up and accumulate cadmium from soil.

17.5 The mineral absorption inhibitor phytate

Phytate (*myo*-inositol hexaphosphate; $InsP_6$) is the principal storage form of phosphorus in plants. The phytate molecule has high affinity for divalent cations such as Fe^{2+}, Zn^{2+}, Ca^{2+}, Mg^{2+} because it is negatively charged. In plants, phytate occurs as metal complexes, for example, potassium, magnesium, calcium and iron complexes. These complexes are soluble at the acidic conditions of the stomach. In the small intestine at the site of mineral absorption (pH 6-7), phytate carries seven to eight out of twelve negative charges. As a consequence, insoluble complexes with essential dietary minerals are formed that renders the minerals unavailable for absorption. Furthermore, phytate salts easily form insoluble aggregates and also protein digestibility can be reduced (Reddy *et al.* 1982). Phytate occurs in all plant foods, but the main sources are cereals, legumes, oilseeds and nuts where phytate constitutes 1–3%. The content of phytate is much lower in vegetables, roots and tubers. In cereals phytate is located in the germ and the aleurone layer, while in legume seeds, phytate is present in protein bodies of the endosperm or the cotyledon (Reddy *et al.* 1982). Food preparation and processing can influence phytate content. In unprocessed food, almost only the hexa phosphate form ($InsP_6$) occurs. During food processing, there is a formation of lower inositol phosphates. Application of biological food processing techniques is a means to degrade phytate by action of endogenous plant phytase, addition of phytase or phytase-producing microorganisms. Preparation and processing at conditions that are favorable for the phytase activity is therefore an option to degrade phytate. Thus, soaking, germination, hydrothermal treatment, malting, fermentation and addition of exogenous phytase at such conditions have been demonstrated to substantially degrade phytate (Sandberg and Svanberg 1991; Svanberg *et al.* 1993; Fredlund *et al.* 1997; Larsson and Sandberg 1995; Türk and Sandberg 1992). On the other hand, heat treatment has very little influence on phytate content in foods as phytate shows high stability under practical conditions of boiling and heat treatment (Pontoppidan *et al.* 2007).

As phytate is prone to form insoluble complexes with metals at physiological pH, the site and degree of phytate hydrolyses in the gut has nutritional implications. No degradation of phytate occurs in the stomach and small intestine of humans unless there is an active dietary phytase. This was demonstrated in ileostomy subjects where a phytate degradation of 55–66% was found through the stomach and small intestine when the diet contained active phytase (Sandberg *et al.* 1987, 1988). In contrast, when the cereal phytase in the diet was deactivated by heat treatment or extrusion cooking dietary phytate was almost completely recovered in the intestinal contents. That no hydrolysis products of phytate was found also supported that no degradation occurred (Sandberg *et al.* 2002). Microbial phytases are more stable at the acidic conditions of the stomach and are active in a broader pH area than plant phytases, and are therefore more effective to degrade phytate in the gut. Indirect evidence for phytate hydrolysis by *A. niger* phytase in the human stomach was reported by Sandberg *et al.* (1996) in a single meal iron absorption study. Addition of *A. niger* phytase to a high-phytate meal was markedly improving iron absorption. Using a pig model and adding microbial phytase (*Citrobacter Braakii*), it was shown that the main phytate degradation took place in the stomach (Pontoppidan *et al.* 2012). Degradation of phytate by microbial phytase in the colon can be expected considering the large number of microorganisms present. This degradation has been shown to be extensive and inversely related to the calcium content of the diet (Cruickshank *et al.* 1945; Walker *et al.* 1948; Sandberg *et al.* 1993).

It has been assumed that phytate cannot be absorbed due to its high negative charge, and that almost all phytate from the diet is recovered in terminal ileum. However, recent studies in cell lines, animals and humans, suggest that $InsP_6$ may be absorbed as it has been detected in human plasma and urine and correlated to the dietary intake (Schlemmer *et al.* 2009). The mechanism for absorption is not known. For human nutrition, phytate constitutes a problem in terms of mineral supply. Low iron and zinc absorption from plant-based diets is considered a major factor in the etiology of iron and zinc deficiency. This is a severe problem in low-income countries where the diet is based on staple foods especially cereals and legumes. Phytate is a major inhibitor of iron and zinc absorption and the inhibiting effect has been shown to be dose-dependent and for iron absorption occurring already at very low concentrations (Hallberg *et al.* 1989; Hurrell 2004; Fredlund *et al.* 2006). Some of the degradation products of phytate (inositol penta phosphates) were also identified as inhibitors of iron and zinc absorption, and inositol tetra and tri phosphates were found to contribute to the negative effect in processed foods (Sandberg *et al.* 1999; Sandström and Sandberg 1992). Controlled degradation of inositol hexaphosphates to triphosphates was shown to substantially increase human iron and zinc absorption from single meals (Sandberg 1991; Brune *et al.* 1992; Hurrell *et al.* 1992). The preparation/processing has to be optimized and removal of phytate has to be extensive to improve zinc absorption and virtually complete to improve iron absorption. For high-tannin cereals, the iron-binding polyphenols also has to be removed to increase absorption (Hurrell 2004). Also, the combination with milk, as often is the case in infant formulas in industrialized countries, will have a strong negative effect on iron absorption despite dephytinization (Davidsson *et al.* 1997). Combining dephytinization with enrichment strategies adding promoters of absorption, that is, animal protein, ascorbic acid and biofortification will be needed to improve iron and zinc nutrition in low-income countries. In an attempt to turn the inhibitory properties of phytate to our benefit, we have recently developed an iron fortificant that uses the strong binding capacity of phytate to make an iron-amino acid complex into a bioavailable iron fortificant of condiments such as bouillons (Gupta *et. al*, 2020; Dold *et.al.* 2020).

Potential anti-cancer activity of phytate would be one of the most beneficial health effects. Phytate inhibition of carcinoma development has been demonstrated in carcinogen-induced cancer models in animals (Liao *et al.* 2007), but the significance for humans needs further evaluation. Antioxidative effects of phytate has also been demonstrated in vitro, including inhibition of the hydroxyl radical formation by iron binding, but not so far shown in vivo.

17.6 Anti-nutrient properties of phenolic compounds

The types of phenolic compounds and their levels in different cereals have already been discussed in detail in previous chapters. The phenolic compounds in cereals include compounds belonging to several groups, for example, phenolic acids, flavonoids, stilbenes, coumarins, anthocyanins, proanthocyanidins, tannins, klason lignin and cutin/subrin. Most of the discussion about dietary phenolic compounds refers to them as antioxidants providing nutritional benefits as free radical scavengers and as signaling molecules. In this section, we discuss the other side of the double-sword nature of dietary phenolic compounds and focus on the anti-nutritional effects associated with them. The main phenolic compounds in non-pigmented cereal grains are phenolic acids, which have less anti-nutritional effects compared to the polyphenolic compounds belonging to the different classes of flavonoids. Table 17.3 provides approximate data on the content of phenolic acids in the common varieties of wheat, rye, oats, barley, corn and rice (Irakli *et al.* 2012). Small portions of these phenolic

Table 17.3 Estimated phenolic acid content in selected whole grain cereals (mg/kg).

Phenolc acid	Wheat	Rye	Oats	Barley	Corn	Rice
Ferulic acid	255	220	1045	325	955	67
p-coumaric acid	14	30	608	77	96	23
Sinapic acid	46	51	107	43	79	24
Caffeic acid	0.5	12	10	7	6	1
Vanillic acid	3.5	16	21	6	6	4
Syringic acid	4	6	20	6	5	5
Gallic acid	6	8	2	7	1	6
4-hydroxybenzoic acid	5	8	8	6	5	5
Trans-cinnamic acid	6	5	8	7	7	5
Procatechuic acid	-	4	1	6	-	-
Total acids	340	360	1830	490	1160	140
Percent acids bound	98	87.5	97	97.5	99.5	92

Data approximated from Irakli *et al.* (2012).

compounds are present in free form, while the majority is found in bound forms. Among these cereal grains, oats and corn seem to have much more phenolic acids. The main phenolic acids are ferulic and p-coumaric acids.

Observations on domestic animals showed that phenolic compounds can act as antinutritional factors through their chelation of transition metal ions or their complexation with proteins. Thus, it was suggested that large intake of dietary flavonoids may reduce the nutritional value of foods by reducing mineral bioavailability and affecting the digestibility of proteins and carbohydrates (Carmona *et al.* 1996). Of special significance is the presence of tannins (galic acid oligomers/polymers) and proanthocyanidins (oligomers of flavan-3-ols called condensed tannins) in the bran fraction of some cereal grains, especially those of colored varieties of sorghum, millet, rice and corn. Dietary tannins may decrease the nutritional value of food by forming protein complexes that inactivate digestive enzymes, reduce protein digestibility, damage the mucosal lining of the gastrointestinal tract and may also chelate and inhibit iron absorption (Butler and Rogler 1992). The tannin contents of cereals and legume,s and their effects on protein and mineral digestibility can be reduced by dehulling, fermentation, germination and cooking (Reddy and Pierson 1994).

17.7 The heat-induced toxicant acrylamide

Acrylamide (2-propenamide, C_2H_5NO) falls under the category "processing contaminants," together with, for example, heterocyclic amines, polyaromatic hydrocarbons, furans and chloropropane diols. Heat-induced formation of acrylamide in food was unknown until first reported by Swedish scientists (Tareke *et al.* 2002). Acrylamide had then been used for long as an industrial volume chemical with well documented toxicity, both as a neurotoxic agent and potential human carcinogen as classified by the International agency for research on cancer (IARC 1994). The risks associated with acrylamide exposure from the consumption of heat-processed foods have been evaluated in international quantitative risk assessments (WHO/FAO 2006, 2011; EFSA 2014). The evaluations concordantly concluded that acrylamide in cooked foods is of concern to human health in respect to increased risk for cancer. The risk estimation was based mainly on results from cancer studies made with experimental animals. Studies in humans have so far not been able to provide conclusive evidence of increased cancer risk. Risk management and control of heat-induced toxicants is complicated by the fact that they are formed through similar mechanisms as desirable chemicals and properties, for example, color, taste, smell and crispiness. Other effects of heating are beneficial for food safety and nutrition, for example, killing of microorganism and preventing their growth by lowering the water content as well as formation of antioxidants from the Maillard reaction. A risk-benefit dilemma specifically related to cereal products and acrylamide is that whole grain products are normally significantly higher in acrylamide than white flour products.

Acrylamide is typically found in vegetable foods that have been heated enough to develop a fairly dry and brown/yellow surface, that is, foods prepared by cooking methods such as deep frying, oven baking and roasting. There are three major food sources for intake of acrylamide: potato products, cereal-based foods and coffee. These three groups are all significant exposure contributors. Their relative importance varies strongly depending on dietary habits and preferences in different age groups and regions. The mean total dietary acrylamide exposure was estimated to vary from 0.3 to 1.9 μg/kg body weight per day for different European dietary surveys and age groups (EFSA 2014). An overview of acrylamide contents of different food groups and intake estimates is given in Table 17.4. The most important cereal products for acrylamide intake among the general population include soft bread, crisp bread, breakfast cereals, and biscuits and cookies. Biscuits, gruel and porridge are of major importance for children. The level of whole grain consumption is likely to be an important determinant for intake from cereal foods, that is, countries

Table 17.4 Acrylamide levels in different food groups and their relative contribution to the acrylamide exposure from food in adult European populations.

	Acrylamide concentration (μg/kg)		Intake (% of total)
Food group	Mean (μg/kg)	95th percentile (μg/kg)	Min – max[1]
Soft bread	42	156	9.2–22
Wheat	38	120	
Other	57	240	
Breakfast cereals	161	552	1–11
Bran & whole grain	211	716	
Wheat & rye	170	410	
Other grains	102	403	
Bisciuts, crisp bread	265	1048	1.3–17
French fries	308	909	9.6–49
Potato crisps	389	932	0.6–6.6
Coffee	249	543	3.2–27

Data from EFSA (2014).

[1]Lowest and highest intake percentage based on 17 surveys representing 15 different EU countries.

where white bread from wheat dominates are likely to have lower acrylamide exposure in relation to regions where more dark bread and whole grain and rye products are consumed.

Table 17.4 illustrates that the contribution from a food group to the acrylamide exposure, and thus cancer risk is not given by the acrylamide concentration alone. As an example, soft bread has the lowest acrylamide levels among the cereal food groups, but is at the same time the main contributor to exposure due to a relatively high consumption. Soft bread must therefore not be overlooked when mitigation efforts are considered. Heat-induced acrylamide formation in food is part of the Maillard reaction cascade in which amino acids react with sugars and other carbonyl compounds. Acrylamide is formed from one specific amino acid, asparagine, through complex reaction pathways, including mainly the reducing sugars fructose and glucose. Other formation mechanisms, for example, pyrolytic formation from wheat gluten has been reported but is believed to be of minor general importance. Significant acrylamide formation requires temperatures above 120°C. The formation accelerates during the final phases of the cooking process, when the moisture content falls low enough to allow the temperature to rise to the critical temperature range. In normal bread baking, for example, this happens only at the surface of a bread loaf, meaning that acrylamide is formed mainly in the crust of soft bread. Besides thermal input, the availability of free asparagine, rather than sugars, in the raw material is the single most important determinant of acrylamide formation in cereal products (Postles 2013). This is in contrast to potatoes, where acrylamide formation strongly correlated to levels of glucose and fructose in the tubers. In cereals, asparagine is mainly localized to the outer parts of the grain, that is, bran and germ (Mustafa 2007; Curtis 2010). Whole flour products are thus higher in acrylamide compared to products from refined flours. Rye is higher in asparagine, thus giving more acrylamide than wheat and oats, which are, in turn, higher than corn and rice (Elmore *et al.* 2005; Curtis 2014).

Numerous research reports on formation factors and mitigation methods have been published since the discovery of acrylamide as a heat-induced toxicant in 2002. Most studies were made on laboratory or pilot scale, and some of these have been reported to have been successfully applied in full-scale production. The "Acrylamide toolbox," produced and updated at regular intervals by the industry organization FoodDrinkEurope, in collaboration with the European Commission, gives an overview of different mitigation tools (FoodDrinkEurope 2014). The tools are categorized under the headings Commercial application, Development, and Research. Based on the "toolbox," a series of very short branch-specific brochures are available in 22 EU languages. Also, a code of practice for acrylamide was adopted by the WHO/FAO Codex Alimentarius (WHO/FAO 2009) and guidance for the industry was recently presented by the Food and Drug Administration in the USA (FDA 2013). Many mitigation methods for cereal products are aimed at limiting the available amount of the critical precursor asparagine. Most efficiently this can be achieved by treatment of the dough prior to baking with the enzyme asparaginase, commercially available for this purpose. To some extent, it can also be achieved by prolonged fermentation time since baker's yeast consumes asparagine. Selection of raw materials naturally low in asparagine may be a feasible option, but more research concerning the impact of agronomical practices and cereal varieties on the asparagine level is needed. Sulfur fertilization can be applied to the soil in areas where sulfur depravation otherwise causes excessive asparagine levels in the grain.

Reducing and optimizing the thermal input to avoid overcooking is an obvious mitigation method. Final moisture content and color may be used as control parameters and as indirect indicators of acrylamide formation. Longer baking time at lower temperature, without changing the final moisture, can also be effective for some products. Options related to recipe modifications include replacing ammonium bicarbonate with other raising agents, adding calcium salts and replacing fructose by glucose. Lowering the whole grain content will lower the acrylamide content but also the nutritional value, and is therefore not recommendable from a balanced risk-benefit perspective.

17.8 Conclusion and future perspectives

With the recommendations that humans may benefit from increasing their consumption of whole grain cereals and bran-rich fractions, it is important to consider some possible adverse effects of certain constituents. In this chapter, we have discussed the acclaimed adverse effects of some constituents of whole grain cereals and their bran, including allergenic proteins and proteins that provoke food sensitivity; toxic effects of the heavy metal cadmium; phytate and phenolic compounds for their chelation of iron; and acrylamide, which is a heat-generated class II carcinogen. The presence of cereal ingredients containing potential hazardous proteins needs to be declared on the food packages to aid individuals with allergies or food sensitivities to avoid foods with adverse effects. For acrylamide, current risk assessments have identified exposure from heat-treated foods as a potential concern for human health. The scientific community and the food sector need to continue developing and implementing methods that can reduce the acrylamide levels, without at the same time comprising other food safety and nutritional or health-promoting aspects such as those beneficial effects associated with whole grain cereals. As for the other compounds, research is needed to better identify the levels that may contribute negative effects on long-term consumption.

17.9 References

Akesson, A, Barregard, L, Bergdahl, IA, *et al.* (2014) Non-renal effects and the risk assessment of environmental cadmium exposure. *Environmental Health Perspectives* 122, 431–438.

Barregard, L, Fabricius-Lagging, E, Lundh ,T, Mölne, J, Wallin, M, Olausson, M, Modigh, C, Sallsten, G. (2010) Cadmium, mercury, and lead in kidney cortext of living kidney donors: Impact of different exposure sources. *Environ. Res. January*, 110(1), 47–54. doi:10.1016/j.envres.2009.10.010

Brune, M, Rossander-Hulthén, L, Hallberg, L, Gleerup, A, Sandberg, A-S. (1992) Human iron absorption from bread: Inhibiting effects of cereal fibre, phytate and inositol phosphates with different numbers of phosphate groups. *J. Nutr.* 122, 442–449.

Butler, LG, Rogler, JC. (1992) Biochemical mechanisms of the antinutritional effects of tannins, Chapter 23, In *Phenolic Compounds in Food and Their Effects on Health 1 – Analysis, Occurrence, and Chemistry,* Chi-Tang Ho, Chang Y. Lee, Mou-Tuan Huang (Eds.), *ACS Symposium series* vol. 506, pp. 298–304.

Carmona, A, Borgudd, L, Borges, G, Levy-Benshimol, A. (1996) Effect of black bean tannins on *in vitro* carbohydrate digestion and absorption. *Nutr. Biochem.* 7, 445–450.

Cordain, L. (1999) Cereal grains: Humanity's double-edged sword, In Simopoulos AP (ed.): *Evolutionary Aspects of Nutrition and Health (Diet, Exercise, Genetics and Chronic Disease), World Rev. Nutr. Diet. Basel, Karger,* vol. 84, pp. 19–73.

Cruickshank, EWH, Duckworth J, Kosterlitz HW, Warnock GM. (1945) The digestibility of the phytase-P of oatmeal in adult man. *J. Physiol.* 104, 41–46.

Curtis TY, Powers SJ, Balagiannis D, Elmore JS, Mottram DS, Parry MAJ, Rakszegi M, Bedö Z, Shewry PR, Halford NG. (2010) Free amino acids and sugars in rye grain: Implications for acrylamide formation. *J. Agric. Food Chem.* 58, 1959–1969.

Curtis TY, Postles J, Halford NG. (2014) Reducing the potential for processing contaminant formation in cereal products. *Journal of Cereal Science* 59, 382–392.

Davidsson L, Galan P, Cherouvrier F, Kastenmayer P, Juillerat MA, Hercberg S, Hurrell RF. (1997) Bioavailability in infants of iron from infant cereals: Effect of dephytinization. *Am. J. Clin. Nutr* 65, 916–920.

Dold S, Zimmermann MB, Jeroense F, Zeder C, Habeych E, Galaffu N, Grathwohl D, Tayeri Forman J, Merinat S, Rey B, Sabatier M, Moretti D. (2020) Iron bioavailability from bouillon fortified with a novel ferric phytate compound: A stable iron isotope study in healthy women (part II). *Scientific Reports*, 10, 5339. doi.org/10.1038/s41598-020-62307-1

EFSA. (2009) Scientific opinion of the panel on contaminants in the food chain on a request from the European Commission on cadmium in food. *The EFSA Journal* 980, 1–139.

EFSA. (2014) Draft Scientific Opinion on Acrylamide in Food, EFSA Panel on Contaminants in the Food Chain (CONTAM), European Food Safety Authority (EFSA), Parma, Italy. http://www.efsa.europa.eu/en/consultations/call/140701.pdf

Elmore JS, Koutsidis G, Dodson AT, Mottram DS, Wedzicha BL. (2005) Measurement of acrylamide and its precursors in potato, wheat, and rye model systems. *J. Agric. Food Chem.* 53, 1286–1293.

Engström N, Saenz-Mendez P, Scheers J, Scheers N. (2017) Towards Celiac-safe foods: Decreasing the affinity of transglutaminase 2 for gliadin by addition of ascorbyl palmitate and $ZnCl_2$ as detoxifeiers. *Sci. Rep.* 7, 77.

FDA. (2013) Guidance for industry, *Acrylamide in foods, Draft guidance* Nov. 2013. http://www.fda.gov/downloads/Food/GuidanceRegulation/GuidanceDocumentsRegulatoryInformation/ChemicalContaminantsMetalsNaturalToxinsPesticides/UCM374534.pdf

FoodDrinkEurope. (2014) Acrylamide Toolbox, last update 10 January 2014. http://www.fooddrinkeurope.eu/publications/category/toolkits/

Fredlund K, Asp N-G, Larsson M, Marklinder I, Sandberg A-S. (1997). Phytate reduction in whole grains of wheat, rye, barley and oats during hydrothermal treatment. *J. Cereal Sci.* 25, 83–91.

Fredlund K, Isaksson M, Rossander-Hulthén L, Almgren A, Sandberg AS. (2006). Absorption of zinc and retention of calcium: Dose-dependent inhibition by phytate. *J. Trace Elements in Med. Biol.* 20, 49–57.

IARC (International Agency for Research on Cancer). (1994) IARC Monographs on the Evaluations of Carcinogenic Risks to Humans. Volume 60. Some Industrial Chemicals. Acrylamide. Summary of data reported and Evaluation. IARC, *Lyon.*

Irakli, MN, Samanidou, VF, Biliaderis, CG, Papadoyannis, IN. (2012) Development and validation of an HPLC-method for determination of free and bound phenolic acids in cereals after solid-phase extraction. *Food Chemistry* 134, 1624–1632.

Gupta S, Habeych E, Scheers N, Merinat S, Rey B, Gallafu N, Sandberg A-S. (2020) The development of a novel ferric phytate compound for iron fortification of bouillons (part I). *Scientific Reports* 10, 5340. doi:10.1038/s41598-020-61833-2

Hallberg L, Brune M, Rossander L. (1989) Iron absorption in man: Ascorbic acid and dose-dependent inhibition by phytate. *Am. J. Clin. Nutr.* 49, 140–144.

Hurrell RF. (2004) Phytic acid degradation as a means of improving iron absorption. *Int. J. Vitam. Nutr. Res.* 74, 445–452.

Hurrell RF, Juillerat MA, Reddy MB, Lynch SR, Dassenko SA, Cook JD. (1992) Soy protein, phytatem and iron absorption in humans. *Am. J. Clin. Nutr.* 56, 573–578.

JECFA. (2011) Safety evaluation of certain food additives and contaminants. (WHO FOOD ADDITIVES SERIES).World Health Organization, Geneva.

Järup, L, Åkesson, A. (2009) Current status of cadmium as an environmental health problem. *Toxicology and Applied Pharmacology* 238, 201–208.

Julin, B, Wolk, A, Bergkvist, L, Bottai, M, Akesson, A. (2012) Dietary cadmium exposure and risk of postmenopausal breast cancer: A population-based prospective cohort study. *Cancer Research* 72, 1459–1466.

Kidd, P. (2003) Th1/Th2 balance: The hypothesis, its limitations, and implcations for health and disease. *Alternative Medicine Review* 8: 223–246.

Larsson M, Sandberg A-S. (1995) Malting of oats in a pilot plant process: Effects of heat treatment, storage and soaking conditions on phytate reduction. *J. Cereal Sci.* 21, 87–95.

Liao J, Seril DN, Yang AL, Lu GG, Yang G-Y. (2007) Inhibition of chronic ulcerative colitis associated adenocarcinoma development in mice by inositol compounds. *Carcinogenesis* 28, 446–454.

Lind, Y, Engman, J, Jorhem, L, Glynn, AW. (1998) Accumulation of cadmium from wheat bran, sugar-beet fibre, carrots and cadmium chloride in the liver and kidneys of mice. *British Journal of Nutrition* 80, 205–211.

Mittag, D, Niggemann, B, Sander, I, Reese, I, Fiedler, EM, Worm, M, Vieths, S, Reese, G. (2004) Immunoglobulin E-reactivity of wheat-allergic subjects (baker's asthma, food allergy, wheat-dependent, exercise-induced anaphylaxis) to wheat protein fractions with different solubility and digestibility. *Molecular Nutrition & Food Research* 48(5), 380–389.

Mustafa A, Åman P, Andersson R, Kamal-Eldin A. (2007) Analysis of free amino acids in cereal products. *Food Chemistry* 105, 317–324.

Nadeem, M, Anjum, FM, Rai Amir, M, Khan, MR, Hussain, S, Javed, MS. (2010) An overview of anti-nutritional factors in cereal grains with special reference to wheat – A review, *Pak. J. Food Sci.* 20, 54–61.

Pontoppidan K, Glitsoe V, Guggenbuhl P, Piñón Quintana A, Simões Nunes C, Pettersson D, Sandberg A-S. (2012) *in vitro* and *in vivo* degradation of myo-inositol hexakisphosphate by a phytase from *Citrobacter braaki*. *Arch. Animal Nutr.* 66, 431–444.

Pontoppidan K, Pettersson D, Sandberg AS. (2007) The level of thermal feed treatment influences the inositol phosphate composition. *Animal Feed Sci. and Techn.* 132, 137–147.

Postles J, Powers SJ, Elmore JS, Mottram DS, Halford NG. (2013) Effects of variety and nutrient availability on the acrylamide-forming potential of rye grain. *Journal of Cereal Science* 57, 463–470.

Reddy NR, Sathe SK, Salunkhe DK. (1982) Phytates in legumes and cereals. *Advances in Food Research* 28, 1–92.

Reddy NR, Pierson MD. (1994) Reduction in antinutritional and toxic components in plant food by fermentation. *Food Res. Int.* 27, 281–290.

Reeves, PG, Chaney, RL. (2008) Bioavailability as an issue in risk assessment and management of food cadmium: A review. *Science of the Total Environment* 398, 13–19.

Reinhard, G, Noll, A, Schlebusch, H., Mallmann, P, Ruecker, AV. (1998) Shifts in the TH1/TH2 Balance during Human Pregnancy Correlate with Apoptotic Changes. *Biochemical and Biophysical Research Communications* 245(3), 933–938.

Ryu, DY, Lee, SJ, Park, DW, *et al.* (2004) Dietary iron regulates intestinal cadmium absorption through iron transporters in rats. *Toxicology Letters* 152, 19–25.

Sachs, JA, Awad, J, McCloskey, D, Navarrete, C, Festenstein, H, Elliot, E, Walker-Smith, JA, Griffiths, CE, Leonard, JN, Fry, L. (1986) Different HLA associated gene combinations contribute to susceptibility for coeliac disease and dermatitis herpetiformis. *Gut.* 27(5), pp. 515–520.

Sandberg, A-S. (1991) The effect of food processing on phytate hydrolysis and availability of iron and zinc. (Symposium on nutritional and toxicological consequences of food processing, 1990 Washington DC). In *Advances in Experimental Medicine and Biology*, 289, pp. 499–508.

Sandberg, A-S, Andlid, T. (2002) Phytogenic and microbial phytases in human nutrition. *Inst. J. Food Sci. Techn.* 37, 823–833.

Sandberg, A-S, Andersson, H. (1988). The effect of dietary phytase on the digestion of phytate in the stomach and small intestine of humans. *J. Nutr.* 118, 469–473.

Sandberg, A-S, Svanberg, U. (1991) Phytate hydrolysis by phytase in cereals: Effects on *in vitro* estimation of iron availability. *J. Food Sci.* 56, 1330–1333.

Sandberg, A-S, Andersson, H, Carlsson, N-G, Sandström, B. (1987) Degradation products of bran phytate formed during digestion in the human small intestine: Effect of extrusion cooking on digestibility. *J. Nutr.* 117, 2061–2065.

Sandberg, A-S, Brune, M, Carlsson, N-G, Hallberg, L, Skoglund, E, Rossander-Hulthén, L. (1999). Inositol phosphates with different number of phosphate groups influence iron absorption in humans. *Am. Clin. Nutr.* 70, 240–246.

Sandberg, A-S, Larsen, T, Sandström, B. (1993) High dietary calcium level decreases colonic phytate degradation in pigs fed a rapeseed diet. *J. Nut.r* 123, 559–566.

Sandberg, A-S, Rossander-Hulthén, L, Türk, M. (1996) Dietary *Aspergillus niger* phytase increases iron absorption in humans. *J. Nutr.* 126**,** 476–480.

Sandström, B, Sandberg, A-S. (1992) Inhibitory effects of isolated inositol phosphates on zinc absorption in humans. *J. Trace Elements and Electrolytes in Health and Disease* 6, 99–103.

Schlemmer, U, Frølich, W, Prieto, RM, Grases, F. (2009) Phytate in foods and significance for humans: Food sources, intake, processing, bioavailability, protective role and analysis. *Mol. Nutr. Food Res.* 53, S330–S375.

Svanberg, U, Lorri, W, Sandberg, A-S. (1993) Lactic fermentation of non-tannin and high-tannin cereals: Effects on *in vitro* estimation of iron availability and phytate hydrolysis. *J. Food Sci.* 58, 408–412.

Tareke, E, Rydberg P, and Karlsson, P. (2002). Analysis of Acrylamide: A Carcinogen formed in heated foodstuffs. *Journal of Agricultural and Food Chemistry* 50, 4998–5006.

Thomas, LD, Michaelsson, K, Julin, B, Wolk, A, Akesson, A. (2011) Dietary cadmium exposure and fracture incidence among men: A population-based prospective cohort study. *Journal of Bone and Mineral Research* 26, 1601–1608.

Türk M, Sandberg, A-S. (1992). Phytate hydrolysis during bread-making: Effect of phytase addition. *J. Cereal Sci.* 15, 281–294.

USFDA. (2014) *Total diet study*, [Online], Available: http://www.fda.gov/downloads/Food/FoodScienceResearch/TotalDietStudy/UCM184301.pdf (accessed Nov. 11, 2014].

Walker, ARP, Fox, FW, Irving, KT. (1948). Studies in human mineral metabolism. 1. The effect of bread rich in phytate-phosphorous on the metabolism of certain mineral salts with special reference to calcium. *Biochem J.* 42, 452–462.

WHO/FAO. (2006) Safety evaluation of certain contaminants in food, In Ed M Scheffer, WHO Food Additives series 55 (ISBN 92-4-166055-4)/FAO Food and nutrition paper 32 (ISBN 92-5-105426-6), pp. 1–156, WHO/FAO, Geneva/Rome.

WHO/FAO. (2009) Code of Practice for the Reduction of Acrylamide in Foods. *CAC/RCP* 67-2009. http://www.codexalimentarius.org/input/download/standards/11258/CXP_067e.pdf

WHO/FAO. (2011) Safety evaluation of certain contaminants in food. In Ed M Scheffer, WHO Food Additives series 63 (ISBN 978 92 4 166063 1)/FAO JECFA monographs 8 (ISBN 978-92-5-106736-9), pp. 1–152, WHO/FAO, Geneva/Rome.

18 Application of Metabolomics for the Assessment of Process-induced Changes in Whole Grain Foods

Amanda J. Lloyd, Kathleen Tailliart, Manfred Beckmann, and John Draper

Institute of Biological, Environmental and Rural Sciences, Aberystwyth University, Aberystwyth, UK

18.1 Introduction

Whole grain cereals are staple foods providing major sources of carbohydrates, proteins, vitamins and minerals for the world's population. They also contain a range of bioactive compounds that have health promoting effects (Kris-Etherton *et al.* 2002). These bioactives vary between and with cereal species. Furthermore, food processing may affect the quantity, composition and structure of bioactives in cereal products, making it difficult to elucidate the bioactivity of individual compounds, but on the other hand, makes it possible to optimize the content of specific compounds in foods (as reviewed by Andersson *et al.* 2010).

The impact of food processing methodology on the chemical composition of whole grain foods can be investigated through metabolomics (as reviewed by Khakimov *et al.* 2014). Metabolomics can be described as the application of high-throughput analytical chemistry technologies directed at characterizing the metabolome, with its development following that of genomics, transcriptomics and proteomics. Rather than being limited to targeting only one or a few compounds at a time, new metabolomic technologies allow researchers to investigate hundreds, or even thousands of metabolites at a time (as reviewed by Scalbert *et al.* 2014).

18.2 Targeted versus untargeted approaches

Knowing the bioactive chemical content of grain or processed food products made of whole grains is a requirement for investigating the bioavailability and biochemical impact of any particular metabolite. Metabolomics experiments can be conducted using two basic approaches: untargeted and targeted (Wishart 2008; Scalbert *et al.* 2014). Targeted metabolomic approaches aim at measuring defined groups of previously identified metabolites that are biochemically relevant, with optimized methods for specific chemical classes. Quantitative data is generated by using internal standards and reference compounds to confirm the structure and absolute concentrations of specific compounds. However, the combination of several targeted methods can only cover a modest proportion of the known

Whole Grains and Health, Second Edition. Edited by Rikard Landberg and Nathalie Scheers.

Additional materials available for download online at https://www.wiley.com/en-gb/Whole+Grains+and+Health-p-9781118939437

metabolome, but will fail to detect the chemistry that has yet to be fully characterized and novel chemical conversions induced by specific food-processing methods.

In contrast to targeted approaches, untargeted metabolomics technologies offer the possibility for comprehensive metabolite characterization of a single sample without preconception of the relation of individual metabolites to the research hypotheses. Metabolic fingerprinting approaches are hypothesis-generating, since there is no preconception of what is expected to be found. Such approaches generate information without any pre-separation of molecules in a sample and can be used to rapidly survey on metabolite content, without any chemical bias (no separation and no targeting of specific chemical group). Untargeted profiling is an alternative hypothesis-driven metabolomics approach in which chemical classes of metabolites in a complex sample are separated prior to measurement such as using chromatographic methods. Putative identification of new components can be performed by looking at the correlation of signals, as well as the detailed comparison of the fragmentation patterns of chromatographic peaks with the behavior of available standard compounds (Beckmann *et al.* 2013; Bondia-Pons *et al.* 2013; Johansson-Persson *et al.* 2013; Lee, *et al.* 2013; Hanhineva *et al.* 2014). This type of annotation is required for untargeted assays in metabolite-rich matrices, in which the verification of identity with authentic standards for each detected metabolite is normally not possible. It is likely that knowledge regarding the phytochemical diversity in dietary plant-based food products will increase dramatically in the near future with the use of data-driven, untargeted fingerprinting and profiling metabolomic investigations. Unfortunately, in both fingerprinting and profiling, bias is formed from the choice of instrument used and the instrumental conditions, as no instrument can fully detect a "global" chemical fingerprint/profile as yet.

Such untargeted methods provide ideal discovery tools to investigate whole grain food composition at different stages of processing or to study the fate of bioactives after ingestion of a whole grain-rich diet (O'Gorman *et al.* 2013; Scalbert et *al.* 2014). The multivariate data from fingerprinting is analyzed in an unbiased manner by application of statistical approaches (chemometrics) to find "explanatory" metabolites that discriminate between sample classes or that can predict, for example, Whole grain exposure. If statistical validation is not performed correctly, then there will be severe bias in terms of overfitting to the samples and/or variables. This is one of the main pitfalls in metabolomics. Correlation analysis of such key "explanatory" metabolites between sample groups can aid in understanding both the structure and metabolic relationships between any unknown, "novel" metabolites, as potential derivatives, conjugates and break-down products of a parent metabolite (as reviewed by Scalbert *et al.* 2014). However, this method can be limited by the capacity, accuracy and resolution of the analytical instrument detecting them. Nuclear Magnetic Resonance spectroscopy (NMR) and Mass Spectrometry (MS) coupled with either Gas (GC) or Liquid Chromatography (LC) are currently the most widely used technologies for metabolomic analysis of whole grains and whole grain-derived foods. They each have their own advantages and disadvantages (Table 18.1). A single platform that combines global identification as well as quantification of the whole metabolome does not yet exist. Thus, a selection or combination of multiple technology platforms is often necessary. The selection of analytical instrumentation depends on the goals of the study and the choice is usually a compromise between sensitivity, selectivity and speed (O'Gorman *et al.* 2013; Claus *et al.* 2014; Wishart 2008; Zhang *et al.* 2012; Scalbert *et al.* 2009; Scalbert *et al.* 2014; Khakimov *et al.* 2014). There is a complementary relationship between untargeted metabolomics and targeted chemical analysis approaches: An untargeted

Table 18.1 Widely used technologies for metabolomic analysis of whole grains and whole grain–derived foods.

Metabolomics tool	Advantages	Disadvantages
NMR	Little or no pre-treatment needed prior to analysis Quantitative Non-destructive (samples can be re-used) Fast (2-3 min/sample) Requires no derivatization Requires no prior separation Detects all organic classes in the μmolar range High reproducibility/low experimental error Compatible with liquids and solids High throughput capacity and automated analyses Provides structural information of unknown compounds Good for untargeted profiling of primary metabolism	Poor sensitivity vs MS techniques Cannot detect low abundance metabolites Cannot detect or ID salts and inorganic ions Cannot detect non-protonated compounds Requires larger (0.5 mL) samples Large degree of spectral overlap in the resonances of complex biological samples Expensive instrumentation Large instrument footprint
Direct MS	High throughput (no chromatographic peaks to align) Robust Little sample preparation required No separation prior to MS Signals may be annotated directly by atomic mass information Wide chemical diversity Semi-quantitative	Ion suppression Isomers cannot be differentiated Measured *m/z* signals may be mistakenly related to noise or instrument artifacts Analytes must dissolve in a solvent

(continued)

Table 18.1 Widely used technologies for metabolomic analysis of whole grains and whole grain–derived foods. (*continued*)

Metabolomics tool	Advantages	Disadvantages
GC-MS	Robust, mature technology	Sample not recoverable
	Relatively inexpensive	Requires sample derivatization for detection of polar and non-volatile metabolites
	Quantitative (with calibration)	Derivatized product not stable (e.g. amino acids)
	Modest sample size requirement	
	High sensitivity, good dynamic range	Derivatization introduces variability
	Greater sensitivity towards non-polar and volatiles compared to LC-MS	Can produce derivatization artifacts
	Greater sensitivity towards non-polar and volatiles compared to LC-MS	Requires separation
	Large body of software and databases for metabolite ID	Relatively slow scan rates (20-30 min/sample)
	High resolution	Cannot be used in imaging
	Reproducible chromatographic separation and retention times	Narrower range of metabolites can be detected compared to LC-MS
	High separation efficiency	
	Detects most organic and some inorganic molecules	Requires volatile and thermally stable analytes for non derivatization
	Detects volatile and non-volatile compounds with derivatisation	Requires volatile and thermally stable analytes for non derivatization
	Detects medium polar to polar compounds	
	Can separate structurally similar metabolites (i.e. cis and trans stereoisomers)	
LC-MS	Superb sensitivity towards polar/easily ionized metabolites	Sample not recoverable
	Very flexible technology	Sensitivity towards polar/easily ionized metabolites
	Detects most organic and some inorganic molecules without derivatization	Only semi-quantitative for untargeted analytes
	Minimal sample size requirement	Expensive instrumentation
	Can be used in metabolite imaging (MALDI)	Can be slow (7-60 min/sample)
		Poor chromatographic resolution and reproducibility vs. GC
		Less robust instrumentation than NMR or GC-MS
	Has potential for detecting largest portion of metabolome	Limited body of software and databases for metabolite ID
	Can analyze trace components in complex mixtures	Novel compound ID is difficult
	No requirements for metabolites to be volatile	Ion suppression
	High mass accuracy combined with databases allow identification of unknowns	Low chromatographic resolution of structurally similar metabolites
	MS/MS provides structural information	Difficult to ionize volatile metabolites

(Source: Wishart 2008; Scalbert *et al.* 2009; Zhang *et al.* 2012; Claus and Swann 2013; O'Gorman *et al.* 2013; Khakimov *et al.* 2014; Scalbert *et al.* 2014.)

analysis is often performed first to detect differences in the set of analytes in the samples under investigation and hypothesis-generating. If novel biotransformations, for example, are hypothesized from such untargeted comparisons, a targeted method is then required to specifically identify and quantify of the compounds under investigation. An overview of such an approach is shown in Figure 18.1.

18.3 Bioactive compounds present in whole grain cereals

In addition to dietary fibre, whole grains contain a wide range of bioactive compounds, that are, extra-nutritional elements that typically occur in small quantities. These substances are of interest as a result of their impact (often beneficial) on human health (Kris-Etherton *et al.* 2002). Common bioactive compounds present in whole grain wheat and rye include alkylresorcinols, benzoxazinoids, phenolic compounds, lignans, phytosterols and tocols. Other bioactive compounds in whole grain cereals include phytic acid, γ-oryzanols, avenanthramides, carotenoids, inositols and betaine (reviewed by Gani *et al.* 2012). Food processing followed by reconstitution, using techniques such milling and thermal processing, can alter the concentrations of the bioactives as well as changing their bioaccessibility, and ultimately, affecting their potential health effects upon absorption.

Alkylresorcinols (ARs), homologues of the 1,3-dihydroxy-5-alkylbenzene with odd-numbered alkyl side chains containing from C15:0 to C25:0 as well as unsaturated alkyl side chains, are phenolic lipids that are abundant in the outer layers of rye, wheat and triticale kernels, found in low amounts in barley, maize and peas, and absent in highly refined white flour (Ross *et al.* 2003; Ross *et al.* 2004a) and oats (Kozubek and Tyman 1999).

Benzoxazinoids are found mainly in cereals, including wheat, rye and maize (Pedersen *et al.* 2011; Adhikari *et al.* 2012b). These secondary metabolites are divided into three groups based on their structural differences: benzoxazolinones, such as 2-benzoxazolinone (BOA) and 6-methoxy-2-benzoxazolinone (MBOA); lactams, including 2-hydroxy-1, 4-benzoxazin-3-one (HBOA), 2-hydroxy-7-methoxy-1, 4-benzoxazin-3-one (HMBOA) and their respective 2-β-D glucosides; and hydroxamic acids, such as 2, 4-dihydroxy-1, 4-benzoxazin-3-one (DIBOA), 2, 4-dihydroxy-7-methoxy-1, 4-benzoxazin-3-one (DIMBOA), and their corresponding glucosides.

Phenolic compounds possess one or more aromatic rings with one or more hydroxyl groups and generally are categorized as phenolic acids, flavonoids, stilbenes, coumarins and tannins. The most common phenolic compounds found in grains are flavonoids and phenolic acids. They are present in cereals in free and/or conjugated forms. Flavonoids have a basic C_6-C_3-C_6 skeleton that consists of two aromatic rings joined by a three carbon link; they include anthocyanins, flavonols, flavones, flavanone and flavonols. Cereals have only small quantities of flavonoids, except for barley, which contains small amounts of catechin and some di- and tri- pro-cyanidins (McMurough and Baert 1994). Phenolic acids are derivatives of benzoic and cinnamic acids and are present in all cereals. Phenolic acids can be subdivided into two major groups, hydroxybenzoic acids and hydroxylcinnamic acid derivatives. Hydroxybenzoic acid derivatives include p-hydroxybenzoic, protocatechuic, gallic, syringic and vanillic acids. Hydroxycinnamic acid derivatives comprise p-coumaric, caffeic, ferulic, and sinapic acids. The major phenolic acids in cereals are ferulic acids and p-coumaric acid (coumaric acids are hydroxyl derivatives of cinnamic acid) (Adom and Liu 2002; Holtekjølen *et al.* 2006)

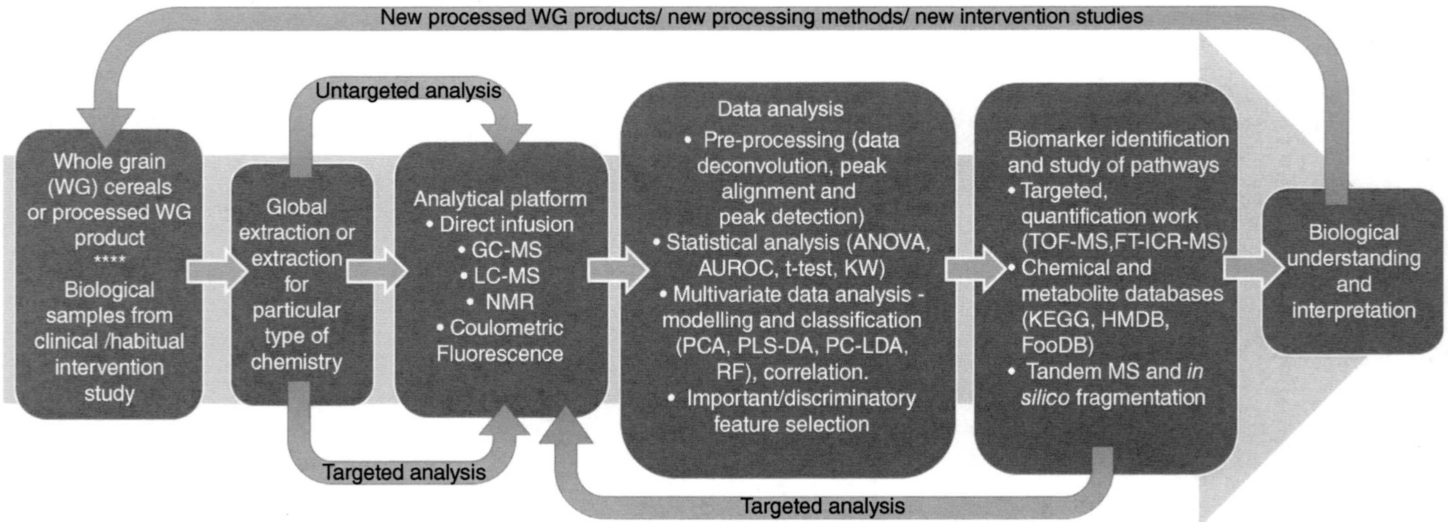

Figure 18.1 Overview of integrated metabolomics experiment. WG, Whole grain; MS, Mass spectrometry; GC, Gas chromatography; LC, liquid chromatography; NMR, nuclear magnetic resonance; AUROC, Area Under the ROC (receiver operating characteristic) curve; KW, Krustal-Wallis; PCA, principal component analysis; PLS-DA , partial least squares discriminant analysis; LDA, linear discriminant analysis; RF, Random Forest; TOF, time-of-flight; HMDB , Human Metabolome Database; FooDB, Food Component Database (Wishart 2008; Draper *et al*. 2009; Wishart *et al*. 2013; Scalbert *et al*. 2014).

Lignans are formed from monolignols (cinnamic alcohols) by dimerization of two cinnamic acid residues and are characterized by oxy-substitutions in the aromatic rings. Plant lignans occur both as aglycones and glycosides. The common plant lignans in the human diet includes secoisolariciresinol, matairesinol, lariciresinol, pinoresinol and syringaresinol. Whole grain rye is the richest cereal source of lignans and quantitatively the most abundant lignans in rye have been reported to be syringaresinol and pinoresinol (Smeds *et al.* 2007).

Phytosterols are a collective term for plant sterols and stanols. All sterols contain the fused four-ring system of 1,2-cyclopentanoperhydrophenantrene with a hydroxyl group attached in position C3. This system can also contain an unsaturated, double bond, mostly between C5 and C6 or between C7 and C8. Stanols do not contain double bonds in the ring. In cereals, plant sterols occur as free sterols, steryl esters with fatty acids, or phenolic acids, steryl glycosides and acylated steryl glycosides (Nyström *et al.* 2007). The most abundant sterols in cereal grains are sitosterol, campesterol, stigmasterol and brassicasterol (Piironen *et al.* 2002). The largest amounts of phytosterols are found in rye grains, and their contents in grains of wheat, barley and oat are much lower (Piironen *et al.* 2002).

Tocopherols and tocotrienols, commonly named tocols, are chemical compounds known as vitamin E. Tocols differ in the number of methyl groups attached to the ring of 6-chromanol. Investigations by Zielinski *et al.* (2001) revealed that the richest sources of tocols were grains of wheat and rye, while barley and oat grains contained lesser quantities of these compounds.

Avenanthramides are a group of hydroxycinnamoylanthranilate alkaloids that occur in oats (Mattila *et al.* 2005). They are substituted cinnamic acid amides of anthranilic acids and there are at least 25 distinct entities. The three major aventhramides reported in oats are aventhramide-1, 3 and 4, which are also known as aventhramides B, C and A, respectively.

Carotenoids are classified into hydrocarbons (carotenes) and their oxygenated derivatives (xanthophylls). Carotenoids commonly found in whole grain cereals are lutein, zeaxanthin, beta-cryptoxanthin, beta carotene and alpha carotene (Adom *et al.* 2003). Carotenoids are more evenly distributed within the grain, with significant quantities within endosperm, in contrast to other most bioactives (Konopka *et al.* 2004).

18.4 Processing of grains

Processing is a prerequisite for the consumption of whole grains by humans. The range of cereal foods is wide, from bakery products to breakfast cereals and porridges, from drinks to meal accompaniments and snacks. Despite the growing consumer interest in health aspects of food, good sensory properties, availability of products, ease of use, price and consumer acceptability remain key priorities among consumers. Food processing has an important effect on the nutrient profile of cereal food items, and ultimately, the health effects of these foods. Food processing followed by reconstitution, using techniques such milling and thermal processing, can modify the bioavailability of carbohydrates, such as delaying the glycemic responses (Björck *et al.* 1994) or enhancing the solubility and fermentability of dietary fibre components (Beer *et al.* 1997). Additionally, processing can alter the concentrations and stability of whole grain bioactives as well as changing their bioaccessibility and ultimately affecting their potential health effects on absorption (as reviewed by Gani *et al.* 2012). To improve health benefits from grain consumption, it is critical to understand the bioactive ingredients and their distributions in whole grains, as well as the effects of food formula, food processing and cooking on the availability of these

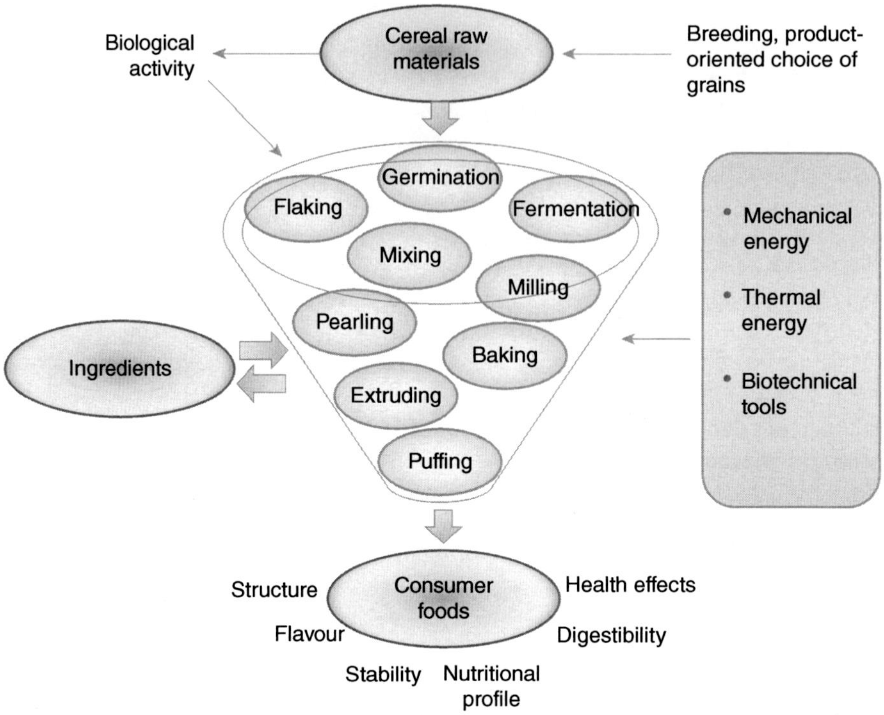

Figure 18.2 Factors influencing cereal product quality. With kind permission from Poutanen *et al*. 2014.

largely beneficial components. Manufacturing of whole grain foods demands knowledge of process-induced changes in these bioactives. The choice of cereal recipe and processing method is crucial in preserving health-enhancing properties of cereal products. Figure 18.2 illustrates the complexity in producing healthy tailored whole grain products desirable for human consumption (kindly taken from Poutanen *et al.* 2014).

18.5 Milling

Milling is the transformation of raw grains into finer primary products for secondary processing into consumer products. Milling of whole grains (such as wheat and rye) separates the outer bran and germ from the starchy endosperm to produce bran and refined white flours for use in bakery products or milled to make a granular product called semolina for pasta production. The bran in whole grain flours is not separated/fractioned, thus it tends to contain more of the health-promoting chemical components that are important for human health (Liukkonen *et al.* 2003; Mattila *et al.* 2005; Heiniö *et al.* 2008; Mateo Anson *et al.* 2008). Oat is generally used as whole grain after the hull is removed to make oat flakes, flours and groats. Oat kernels are always heated prior to milling to inactivate enzymes and prolong shelf life due to the high content of oil in oat. Corn is fractionated into its components by either dry or wet milling, where dry milling separates the different fractions to make flour and wet milling separate corn into largely chemical constituents (starch, protein, fibre and oil). Sorghum grains are milled into three fractions, gross, medium and fine. The fine fraction is used as gluten-free flour for making products for celiac patients.

Targeted methods have been used in various combinations of chromatography and MS to quantitate previously identified either single metabolites of interest or defined groups in a particular chemical class. Using such approaches, the outer fraction of milled grains has been shown to contain much higher levels of bioactive compounds such as phenolic compounds, phytosterols, tocols- tocopherols, and tocotrienols, lignans and carotenoids than the inner parts (Liukkonen *et al.* 2003; Ross *et al.* 2003; Mattila *et al.* 2005; Heiniö *et al.* 2008; Mateo Anson *et al.* 2008; Beckmann *et al.* 2013). ARs have been found in wheat, rye, triticale and barley, but not in rice, oats, maize, sorghum or millet (Ross *et al.* 2003) It has been demonstrated in multiple studies that for whole grain wheat and rye, the fractioned bran contains the highest amount of total AR content, followed by whole grain flours and last refined flours (Liukkonen *et al.* 2003; Andersson *et al.* 2010; Menzel *et al.* 2012). Unlike most cereals, the majority of bioactive compounds in buckwheat are present in free form distributed throughout the entire grain (Quettier-Deleu *et al.* 2000; Hung and Morita 2008).

A large number of targeted methods are available for the analysis of intact ARs in cereals. To date, GC has been found to be the method of choice for analysis and identification of cereal ARs, after extraction with hydrophobic solvents such as acetone, ethyl acetate, methanol or ethanol (as reviewed by Ross et al., 2004b), either in their native form or after derivatization (Ross *et al.* 2001; Ross *et al.* 2003; Konopka *et al.* 2004; Andersson *et al.* 2010; Menzel *et al.* 2012) or by colorimetry (Landberg *et al.* 2009; Sampietro *et al.* 2009). Different methods of detection have also been used, including coularray electrochemical detection (CAED) (Ross and Kochhar 2009), diode array detector (DAD) (Mattila *et al.* 2005; Knödler *et al.* 2010), ultraviolet and or fluorescence detection (Ross, 2012). Using targeted approaches, the calculated ratio of the homologues C17:0 and C21:0, has been reported to distinguish between different whole grain species (Chen *et al.* 2004; Landberg *et al.* 2009; Knödler *et al.* 2010). It has been demonstrated recently that the profile of ARs in cereal grains is even more complex than previously thought by using a highly optimized and targeted method of LC-DAD-MS (Knödler *et al.* 2008). After solid-phase extraction of ARs from rye, wheat, spelt and barley, Knödler *et al.* (2008) detected 29 ARs that had characteristic AR UV spectral behavior and MS/MS fragmentation patterns, 5 of which had been characterized for the first time.

Metabolomics experiments profiling certain chemical classes have been conducted to determine the profiles of different grain fractions. Chandrasekara and Shahidi (2011) used high performance liquid chromatography LC equipped with both UV-DAD and LC-MS/MS detection to profile over 50 phenolic compounds and flavonoids in milled millet grains after extraction specifically for soluble phenolics. Compounds were identified by comparing their relative retention times as well as UV and MS/MS spectra with authentic compounds. Unknown compounds present in the extracts were tentatively identified using additional literature and quantified as equivalents of the closely related available standards. Chandrasekara and Shahidi (2011) suggested a high concentration of phenolic compounds in the outermost bran fractions layers; however, the contents and distribution of the range of phenolic compounds varied among fractions as well as the millet genotype. The power of metabolomics profiling using untargeted, data driven methodology was demonstrated in a qualitative approach by Hanhineva *et al.* (2012) with rye bran samples, specifically enriched for phenolics. In addition to the most abundant lignans in whole grain rye, syringaresinol and pinoresinol (Smeds *et al.* 2007) as well as novel buddlenol-derivatives were identified in whole grain rye bran by UPLC-qTOF-MS. Putative identification of lignan components in the bran was performed by combining MS/MS of available standard compounds belonging to different lignan types with the fragmentation data obtained from unknown metabolites in the samples (Hanhineva *et al.* 2011; Hanhineva *et al.* 2012).

Beckmann *et al.* (2013) used a semi-quantitative, targeted direct infusion accurate mass analysis approach for the analysis of three key benzoxazinoids BOA, HPAA and DIBOA di-glycoside in bran-rich and low-bran content rye flour. All benzoxazinoids were shown to be increased in high bran flour when compared with low bran rye flour. This was confirmed by Tanwir *et al.* (2013), who used a Q Trap LC-MS/MS to target and quantify 12 known benzoxazinoid compounds in rye whole grain, flour and fractioned bran, showing that the total benzoxazinoid concentration was highly increased in bran, which contained the majority of the germ. The benzoxazinoids mainly causing this increase were the glycosides and hexose sugar derivatives of HBOA, HMBOA and DIBOA. These results also showed considerably higher concentrations of benzoxazinoids in rye than in wheat, which is in accordance with previous findings (Hanhineva *et al.* 2011; Pedersen *et al.* 2011). In wheat, the germ fraction contained the highest amount of benzoxazinoids, followed by the bran and pollard flour (aleurone layer: layer beneath the bran) as the second most benzoxazinoid-enriched fractions (Tanwir *et al.* 2013). It was suggested that during seed development the germ (the living part of the seed) is continually producing these metabolites that are transported to the seed coat and aleurone layers, potentially as protection against pathogen attack. Barley and oat have been shown not to contain any of the signals for benzoxazinoid metabolites (Hanhineva *et al.* 2011).

Recently a semi-untargeted metabolite profiling approach was used to determine the biochemical composition of global methanol extracts on whole grain corn, oat and wheat after milling on global methanol extracts (Lee *et al.* 2013). A multi-platform approach using GC-MS after derivatization and UPLC-MS/MS was used to provide broad coverage of the diverse small molecules present in the grains. This global analysis identified 325 metabolites belonging to diverse chemical classes including carbohydrates, antioxidants, vitamins, amino acids as well as secondary metabolites including flavanoids, phytosterols, phenylpropanoids and terpenoids. Differences in secondary metabolites were observed between the grain types, and many of these nutrients were altered in concentration in the bran fractions. This pilot study only provided a glimpse into distinct profiles of different grains and their fractions; however, it demonstrates that grain components can be usefully evaluated using an untargeted metabolomics approach.

18.6 Germination and malting

The major application of germination has been in the malting of barley for beer production. A traditional malting process can be divided into steeping/soaking, which increases the moisture content of the kernel, germination and kilning (drying), thereby allowing the endogenous enzymes to modify the grain constituents. In addition to producing raw materials, malting thus has the potential to improve nutritional properties of grain by enhancing the content, stability and bioavailability of bioactives (as reviewed by Hübner and Arendt 2013; Kaukovirta-Norja *et al.* 2004). Many targeted analyses have been used to demonstrate the effects of germination on phytochemical concentrations. The processes of steeping and germination in a controlled malting system were shown to result in increased levels of avenanthramides in oat when compared to raw grains (Skoglund *et al.* 2008). Germination of wheat has been shown to double the content of α-tocopherol (Ozturk *et al.* 2012). Another targeted chemical analysis was performed by (Liukkonen *et al.* 2003) who showed an increase in lignans after rye grains had germinated compared with native grains, using an optimized isotope dilution GC-MS method. Germination increased the level of lignins in whole grain rye nearly two-fold, but fermentation of germinated rye increased the levels by over three-fold in comparison with untreated rye (Katina *et al.* 2007), measured using targeted GC-MS. Additionally targeted methods were used to demonstrate an increase of phytosterols and benzoxazinoids (LC–DAD–MS) after germination, but no change in ARs (methanol extraction by HPLC: Katina *et al.* 2007). Free, esterified, glycosidic and bound phenolic acids measured by HPLC-UV increased after germination (Katina *et al.* 2007), which agreed with the findings of Liukkonen *et al.* (2003), who used the same technique to show an increase in the easily-extractable phenolic compounds after germination of rye grains.

A targeted profiling method using HPLC -DAD was used by Hithamani and Srinivasan (2014) to profile individual phenolic compounds in two types of millet after soaking and germination. Similarities between the polyphenolic profile of native finger and pearl millet were revealed – protocatechuic acid, syringic acid, p-coumaric acid, ferulic acid, sinapic acid, salicylic acid and t-cinnamic acid. Additionally, gallic acid, p-hydroxy benzoic acid, gentisic acid and caffeic acid were identified in finger millet. The total concentration of phenolic compounds increased in finger millet and decreased in pearl millet after germination; however, salicylic acid increased in both varieties. Caffeic acid and protocatechiuc acid decreased in finger millet after germination, and ferulic acid increased, which matched that of Subba Rao and Muralikrishna (2002), who used similar extraction methods and HPLC analyses but different run-conditions after malting finger millet. The HPLC profile of the bioaccessible polyphenols (dialyzate) of both millets revealed that not all compounds were bioavailable (Hithamani and Srinivasan 2014). However, of those available, an increase was observed in both finger and pearl millet as a result of germination.

UPLC-DAD was used to assess the phenolic profiles of Canadian wheat while germinating (Hung *et al.* 2011). Seven phenolic acids were detected including 4-hydroxybezoic, vanillic, caffeic, syringic, p-coumaric, ferulic and sinapic acid. During the germination, syringic acid increased with increasing duration of germination, resulting in the increase in total phenolic content of the sprouted wheat flours. In another study, an untargeted GC-MS and GC-FID (flame ionization detection) method was used to profile barley over a period of micro-malting procedure involving steeping, germination and kiln-drying (Frank *et al.* 2011). Investigation of the obtained fractions by GC resulted in the detection of 587 distinct peaks of which 173 were identified by means of MS. A range of fatty acid methyl esters, hydrocarbons and minor lipids were found in the non-polar extract plus bioactive metabolites: 2 phenolics (methyl-cinnamate, methyl-ferulate, 14 sterols (including sitosterol, campesterol, stigmasterol) and 2 tocopherols. Using unsupervized multivariate modeling on these data, it was shown that these non-polar metabolites appeared to increase as the malting process progressed, particularly sitosterol and campestanol.

18.7 Soaking/hydrothermal processing of grains

Conditioning of grain with water (soaking) and water/heat (hydrothermal processing: HTP) before grinding can improve milling qualities of the grain by decreasing toughness of the endosperm. Quantitative benzoxazinoid profiling using targeted LC-MS/MS methods has been performed using rye and wheat bread after HTP to analyze their effects on the levels of benzoxazinoids (Pedersen *et al.* 2011; Tanwir *et al.* 2013). Pedersen *et al.* (2011) showed increases in benzoxazinoid composition of durum wheat, commercial rye and an old Nordic rye landrace on HTP, particularly hydroxamic acids and benzoxazolinones. Tanwir *et al.* (2013) noted that soaking and boiling of pearled rye resulted in the conversion of di-glucosylated hydroxamic acids into mono-glucosylated hydroxamic acids and free aglycones, indicating that these compounds may be used as storage molecules. Soaking resulted in greater changes in the benzoxazinoid concentrations than boiling, which may be due to the enzymatic hydrolysis of the di-hexoses into mono-hexoses. Changes associated with hydrothermal processing reflected the synthesis of hydroxamic acid glucosides, the enzymatic liberation of their aglycones and their subsequent degradation to benzoxazolinones (Pedersen *et al.* 2011; Tanwir *et al.* 2013).

18.8 Baking and roasting

Baking is a common process used to increase the nutritional value and acceptability of processed cereals. Whole grain bakery products are expected to be better sources of phenolic compounds compared with refined flour products due to the concentration of phenolic compounds in the outer layers of the grains. For bread baking, the major challenges are to increase the content of whole grain and dietary fibre to improve the nutritional value, while retaining the desired texture and shelf life for consumer appeal and to improve the glycemic profile.

In heat processed foods, AR form starch-lipid complexes, which must be broken down to allow accurate quantification. Typically, a hot 1-propanol extraction method (Ross *et al.* 2003) or an accelerated solvent extraction has been used (Holt *et al.* 2012). The AR content remains stable in the matrix throughout food processing, including baking (Ross *et al.* 2003; Gunenc *et al.* 2013) and pasta manufacturing and cooking (Landberg *et al.* 2006). A good correlation between AR measured content in ingredients and in final products has been reported (Chen *et al.* 2004; Andersson *et al.* 2010). In cereal-based foods, the AR content and relative homologue composition vary considerably in different whole grain wheat and rye products due to the different proportions of whole grain and bran in the products (Ross *et al.* 2003; Chen *et al.* 2004; Kulawinek *et al.* 2008; Andersson *et al.* 2010; Menzel *et al.* 2012). It is possible to estimate the whole grain wheat and/or rye content as well as the relative proportion between these cereals in a given cereal derived product on the basis of AR content and C17:0/C21:0 ratio. The AR content has therefore been suggested for use as a marker to authenticate the whole grain wheat and rye content of cereal food products (Ross *et al.* 2003; Chen *et al.* 2004; Andersson *et al.* 2010). Following on from this, multivariate unsupervised cluster analysis has been used to group whole-rye and whole-wheat products, and mixed cereal products prepared from rye and wheat and their bran or flour on the basis of targeted measurements of AR homologues by HPLC-DAD (Kulawinek *et al.* 2008) Targeted metabolomic analyses accompanied by the use of appropriate statistical algorithms offers an objective way to evaluate the quality of whole grain rye and/or wheat and their derived products. This could be a valuable tool for issues related to the evaluation of the quality and subsequent labeling of whole grain rye and wheat-derived foods.

Pedersen *et al.* (2011) quantified the benzoxazinoid content of the baked bread using conventional flour from durum wheat, commercial of rye and an old Nordic rye landrace and flour from HTP grains using a LC-MS/MS method. Total benzoxazinoids concentrations increased after baking using all three conventional whole grain flours with the rye flours, showing a greater increase than wheat. Control "blank" wheat flour showed undetectable benzoxazinoids in neither the flour nor the bread. When HTP flour was used, there was an increased concentration of benzoxazinoids compared to bread made with convention flour, due to elevated benzoxazolinone in HTP bread. Additionally, in the bread baked with HTP flour, the concentration of hydroxamic acids, hydroxamic acid glucosides, lactams and lactam glucosides all decreased. These observations are consistent with the known chemical degradation of hydroxamic acids to benzoxazolinones in aqueous solution (Bravo and Niemeyer 1985; Sicker *et al.* 2000). The elevated content of benzoxazolinones is consistent with the chemical degradation of hydroxamic acids occurring as the principal conversion during baking, with the biosynthesis of hydroxamic acids having occurred largely during the HTP treatment.

Total carotenoids, tocopherol and tocotrienol were shown to decrease after bread making when compared with the starting wheat flour (Leenhardt *et al.* 2006), using HPLC. The major carotenoid and tocol losses occurred during kneading. This was agreed by Hidalgo and Brandolini (2010), who used the same approach demonstrating a decrease α-tocopherol, α-tocotrienol and β-tocotrienol content in different wheat varieties during bread baking and biscuit making. Degradation was highest during dough mixing, while dough leavening and oven baking had almost no effect. Changes in free and bound ferulic, caffeic, sinapinic, vanillic and p-coumaric acids during baking in whole grain wheat bread, cookie and muffin were investigated using HPLC–UV (Abdel-Aal and Rabalski 2013). Baking resulted in significantly increased amounts of free phenolic acids and lower amounts of bound phenolic acids compared with whole grain flour suggesting liberation of bound phenolic acids, increasing their bioavailability. In addition, phenolic acids and their derivatives were less accessible to oxidation and less degradable in high-fat bakery products (muffin and cookie), as compared to low-fat bread. When phenolic profiles (using HPLC–DAD) of finger millet and pearl millet were considered, roasting significantly released phenolic acids from the food matrix and made them more bioaccessible, in particular, syringic acid (Hithamani and Srinivasan 2014). Roasting seemed to cause the largest increase on total phenolic compounds in finger millet, predominately caused by an increase of vanillic acid, salicylic acid, p-coumaric and t-cinnamic acid, and marginally ferulate, while caffeic acid totally disappeared on roasting. In pearl, millet roasting caused the same increase in vanillic acid, salicylic acid and t-cinnamic acid (marginally) but not p-coumaric. An increase in p-hydroxy benzoic was also observed. Open-pan boiling, pressure cooking and microwaving generally decreased the concentrations of phenolic compounds or caused no change in two types of millet. Pressure cooking and microwave heating provided lesser amounts of bioaccessible polyphenols when compared to the native finger millet; however, the opposite was seen in pearl millet. Open-pan boiling increased the total concentration of bioaccessible polyphenols in both millet varieties. The different cooking methods altered the phenolic profiles in different ways, and the two types of millet grains showed differences too.

Recently, a targeted analysis of lignans found in rye grains and flour after heating using HPLC–UV has been performed (Gerstenmeyer *et al.* 2013). Heating rye flour and grains at 100°C caused an increase of the concentrations of lariciresinol, pinoresinol and syringaresinol with increasing time. Roasting rye flour or grains at 250 °C resulted in a complete degradation of these three lignans. The content of lignans in home-baked breads was lower than in the flour, especially in the bread crust. The effect of cooking on lignan content in whole grain pasta has also been examined (Durazzo *et al.* 2013). After cooking, total lignans losses were observed in oat, rye and rice-added pastas, whereas increases were observed in barley-added and whole durum wheat pastas. These differences between the whole grains were due to differences in lignan profile, where lariciresinol increased in barley-added and whole durum wheat pastas after cooking, while decreasing in oat, rye and rice-added pastas. Additionally, the concentration of pinoresinol and secoisolariciresinol decreased in most of the pastas after cooking (Durazzo *et al.* 2013).

18.9 Pasta processing and extrusion cooking

Extrusion cooking is simultaneous actions of temperature, pressure and shear; their intensities and interactions vary enormously depending on feed ingredients, extruder configuration and the desired characteristics of end-products. Such whole grain food products include pasta, some breads, breakfast cereals and ready-to-eat snacks. During pasta preparation the α-tocopherol, α-tocotrienol and β-tocotrienol content was found to decrease in different wheat varieties, measured using HPLC (Hidalgo and Brandolini 2010). Degradation was highest during the kneading phase of pasta production, with additional losses during pasta extrusion under no vacuum. This was in accordance with Fratianni *et al.* (2012), who reported a total loss of tocopherols and tocotrienols during egg pasta production, confirming that the degradation was mostly limited to the kneading phase. Additionally, Fratianni *et al.* (2012) demonstrated that carotenoids (α + β-carotene, lutein, zeaxanthinand b-criptoxanthin) decreased during the kneading step.

Extrusion cooking of grains caused a significant decrease in tocopherols and tocotrienols in wheat, barley, rye and oat whole grains (Zielinski *et al.* 2001). The least resistant to HTP was α-tocopherol and α-tocotrienol. The remaining tocopherols were more stable; however, the degree of their degradation was up to 50%. In a study by Bryngelsson *et al.* (2002), steaming (and flaking) was shown to cause a decrease in total tocotrienols and drum drying (of steamed rolled oats) caused a decrease in tocotrienols and tocopherols. However, autoclaving (of grains) caused an increase of total tocols. It has been previously shown that the outer layer of grains have been shown to contain much higher levels of tocols than the inner parts (Liukkonen *et al.* 2003), thus flaking (before steaming) and rolling (before drum drying) would cause a decrease of the outer grain layers compared to whole oats (after autoclaving). Avenanthramides were seen to decrease after exposure to all methods of HTP, suggesting they are unstable during these processing methods (Bryngelsson *et al.* 2002).

The effect of cooking on the phenolic acids profile of wheat pasta samples enriched with debranning fractions was investigated using HPLC (Fares *et al.* 2010). The main effect of processing semolina into pasta (uncooked) was a decrease of the free phenolic acids fraction, due to loss of p-hydroxybenzoic acid, in the control and all of the enriched samples. Conversely, the bound fraction did not change. The observed reduction in the content of phenolic acids during pasta processing may be due to the combined impact of the addition of water and oxygen during kneading. Cooking using low temperature-long duration drying conditions affected almost of all the bound fraction of phenolic acids, which showed a consistent increase in all samples while free phenolic acid levels did not vary. Only the pasta samples enriched highly with bran showed an increase in free ferulic acid. Free and bound phenolics of whole grain wheat pasta samples manufactured using low temperature-long time and high temperature-short time drying conditions were compared by West *et al.* (2013) using HPLC–UV. High temperature-short time drying conditions increased the amount of free protocatechuic acid in different whole grain flour blend pasta samples compared with low temperature-long-time conditions. Free syringic and ferulic acid increased with low temperature-long-time drying conditions, while p-hydroxybenzoic acid showed no difference, demonstrating that phenolic acids have different susceptibilities to thermal processing. Very few bound phenolics were detected in pasta samples after either of the drying methods.

Significant increases in free and ester-bound vanillic, syringic, coumaric and ferulic acids in wheat, barley, rye and oat after extrusion (at different temperatures), such as for making breakfast cereals, were noted by Zielinski *et al.* (2001), using HPLC. The changes in free phenolic acids were more pronounced when compared to the bound ones, indicating that HTP of cereal grains may liberate phenolic acids and their derivatives from the wall cells. Bryngelsson *et al.* (2002) used HPLC to show that various hydrothermal processes such as steaming (and flaking) and autoclaving applied to oats were effective in increasing the assayable phenolic contents, particularly ferulic and p-coumaric acids and vanillin, which could be released by hydrolysis from their bound forms. Losses of caffeic acid were observed possibly due to it being heat liable.

An untargeted profiling approach using GC-MS and LCMS was used to describe the modifications induced during the industrial process of semolina into different kinds of pasta (Beleggia *et al.* 2011). In total, 76 chemical entities were detected in semolina (66 common to all semolina samples), 75 in extruded pasta (59 present in all pasta samples) and 74 were detected in dried pasta (55 common to all types of pasta). A range of chemistry was observed, including amino acids, sugars, fatty acids and the bioactives: tocopherols, phytosterols and carotenoids. Data demonstrated that the pasta manufacturing process had a global effect on the composition of the metabolites, at each processing step with reducing tocopherols and phytosterols from semolina – dried pasta – extruded pasta and a reduction in carotenoids (lutein and cantaxanthin) from extruded to dried pasta. This suggested that thermal degradation may be occurring during processing, so temperature adjustments may help maintain the content of tocopherols and phytosterols in pasta. The carotenoids degradation levels could be due to the kneading and enzymatic activity of the semolina. Additionally, in each processing step wholemeal products were significantly different from the other types of pasta, containing the highest amount of most measured analytes, including the bioactives tocopherols, phytosterols and carotenoids.

18.10 Fermentation and bioprocessing

During sourdough baking, particularly, many biochemical changes happen that may affect bread texture. Sourdough baking usually involves four steps; 1) preparation of the sourdough by mixing wholemeal flour, yeast and *Lactobacillus* cultures and fermenting; 2) addition of fresh wholemeal flour; 3) proofing; and 4) baking the bread. Pizza dough samples were analyzed for their soluble-free, soluble-conjugated, and insoluble bound ferulic acid concentrations using HPLC (Moore *et al.* 2009). The soluble-free ferulic acid contents of two wheat varieties increased significantly as result of fermentation, and decreased either soluble-conjugated or insoluble-bound ferulic acid. Free and total phenolic acids were analyzed by Menga *et al.* (2009) using HPLC–DAD in wheat flour, wheat flour with added bran and fermented baked bread. When compared with the respective flours, free ferulic acid increased and p-hydroxybenzoic decreased in baked bread (Menga *et al.* 2009). A significant increase of free phenolic acids was shown after fermentation of barley and oat groat with a specific lactic acid bacteria strain, thereby improving their bioavailability (HPLC–DAD; Hole *et al.* 2012). Additionally, yeast fermentation of rice bran can differentially alter bioactive compounds compared to non-fermented rice bran (Ryan *et al.* 2011). Using GC-MS untargeted and targeted metabolite analyses, fermentation was shown to reduce the quantity of p-coumaric acid and increase ferulic acid, however little change was observed for sterols and tocopherols (Ryan *et al.* 2011). Bread baked using bran bioprocessed with yeast fermentation contained increased the levels of free ferulic acid, p-coumaric acid and sinapic acid (HPLC–DAD) and by using bioprocessed bran in combination with cell wall hydrolytic enzymes increased the content of ferulic acid further (Mateo Anson *et al.* 2009). Food processing may affect the uptake of these compounds. A study showed that the uptake of phenolic acids was higher from bread with bioprocessed bran included than from control bread with native bran (Mateo Anson *et al.* 2011). The changes in phenolic acid composition during fermentation and bioprocessing could potentially be a result of enzymatic hydrolysis of insoluble bound or soluble conjugated forms by enzymes produced from yeast or other microorganisms and enzymes present.

Chemical approaches using GC-MS and HPLC showed that the fermentation phase during sourdough rye baking decreased the levels of tocopherols and tocotrienols and did not seem to alter sterols, ARs, lignans and phenolic acids (Liukkonen *et al.* 2003). After baking, the amount of all measured bioactive compounds, except tocopherols and tocotrienols, were at the same or slightly higher than those of the wholemeal flour. Benzoxazinoids were not measured. An increase in benzoxazinoids was observed after fermentation of native rye meal with yeast, lactic acid bacteria by Katina *et al.* (2007) but no increase of sterols, lignans or ARs. Increased benzoxazinoids, ARs, sterols, lignans were observed when yeast fermentation followed germination, suggesting differences in the stability and fluctuations in bioactive compounds during fermentation.

Biomarker-leads from an untargeted MS metabolomics investigation suggesting benzoxazinoid derivatives as important signals discriminating between high and low sourdough rye bread consumers initiated targeted accurate mass analysis to semi-quantify aglycones and glycoside derivatives of urinary metabolites in the bread (Beckmann *et al.* 2013). DIBOA diglycoside, DIBOA glucoside, BOA and HBOA were detected and semi-quantified in sourdough rye bread and the two flours used in the bread manufacturing: bran rich and low bran rye flour. DIBOA-diglucosides were abundant prior to fermentation, with higher concentrations evident in the bran-rich flour than the low-bran flour. After fermentation and baking, the main benzoxazinoid present in whole grain sourdough rye bread was BOA, together elevated concentrations of HPAA compared with the flour and a small amount of DIBOA-glucoside. The fermentation and baking process caused the formation of BOA from the unstable DIBOA aglycone (Beckmann *et al.* 2013). Hanhineva *et al.* (2014) showed that after, BOA was also detected in rye 100% whole grain sourdough baked rye bread and white wheat bread enriched with rye bran, however hexose-conjugated DIBOA was the main benzoxazinoid detected. White wheat bread enriched with rye bran bioprocessed with hemicelluloltic enzymes and yeast fermentation induced the conversion of hexose-conjugated DIBOA into BOA. This bioprocessing technique partially hydrolyzes and solubilizes the cell walls, similar to what happens in sourdough baking (Hanhineva *et al.* 2014)

BOA can be further metabolized into the phenylacetamide HPAA, indicating that the bioprocess involving yeast fermentation and fermentation in sourdough breads can cause the biotransformation of benzoxazinoids (Beckmann *et al.* 2013; Hanhineva *et al.* 2014).

Another transformation route for the DIBOA is the formation of HHPAA via the HBOA intermediate, which has been found in wheat breads containing rye bran and bioprocessed rye bran (Hanhineva *et al.* 2014). However, HHPAA has not been found in sourdough rye bread (Beckmann *et al.* 2013; Hanhineva *et al.* 2014) perhaps due to the acidic conditions during the sourdough baking process. Food processing appears to cause significant transformation of native benzoxazinoid structures, but it is yet unclear to what extent bioactivity can be attributed to such compounds.

18.11 Bioactives in human intervention studies

The food metabolome is affected by the way bioactives are metabolized and absorbed in the human body. Bioactive compounds within human biofluids predominantly occur as phase I and phase II bio-transformed glucuronides or sulfate conjugates or as derivatives, conjugates and microbiota breakdown products. Within biofluids, often researchers include pre-treatment steps to liberate the free aglycones by acid or enzymatic hydrolysis. Recently, studies have putatively identified new and related components by the detailed comparison of MS/MS fragmentation of the unknown metabolites with the behavior of available standard compounds in that chemical class as well as chromatographic retention times of molecules with similar chemistry. Correlation analysis of key explanatory metabolites between sample groups will aid in understanding derivatives, conjugates and break-down products of a parent metabolite. The discovery of new bioactives and their derivatives within biofluids is hindered by lack of commercially available standards and metabolite databases. An important challenge for the future will be to extend existing databases, increase standard synthesis and ultimate availability and develop novel software tools and databases allowing the in silico prediction of the metabolic fate of food constituents.

Recently, untargeted, data driven metabolite fingerprinting and profiling studies have been employed to determine types and amounts of compounds taken up and excreted in the course of human whole grain consumption (Beckmann *et al.* 2013; Bondia-Pons *et al.* 2013; Johansson-Persson *et al.* 2013; Hanhineva *et al.* 2014). Beckmann *et al.* (2013) used FIE-MS fingerprinting coupled with multivariate modeling and feature selection (Random Forest) to show 10–22 signals were responsible for the discrimination of urine samples from participants who reported high habitual whole grain sourdough rye bread consumption. In contrast, urine samples from participants who reported high habitual intakes of rye flakes, rye pasta or total whol- grain rye products could not be discriminated adequately from their wash-out samples with this method (Beckmann *et al.* 2013). The plasma profiles of individuals up to 24 hours after consuming a meal containing whole grain sourdough rye bread, white wheat bread enriched with unprocessed rye bran or with bioprocessed rye bran were investigated to find key discriminatory rye-specific metabolites (Hanhineva *et al.* 2014). Fasting and postprandial samples were analyzed by an untargeted metabolomic approach using LC–MS, which suggested (using paired t-tests) that 9 of the 2097 detected metabolites were rye bread specific.

The same untargeted LC-MS approach was used to discover 20 discriminatory features in plasma between participants on high-fibre and low-fibre diets for 5 weeks (Johansson-Persson *et al.* 2013). Additionally, HPLC followed by data processing was implemented to discover 14 discriminatory signals associated with whole grain rye bread consumption after a 4-week intervention, 7 of which were nitrogen containing compounds (Bondia-Pons *et al.* 2013). Garcia-Aloy *et al.* (2014) applied untargeted HPLC and multivariate analysis methods on urine from free living volunteer that were stratified by habitual bread consumption into non-consumers, white-bread and whole grain bread consumers, identifying 18 features associated with bread consumption.

Conjugated HHPAA with a sulfate or glucuronide has been shown to be an abundant hydroxylated phenylacetamide metabolite in plasma and urine samples after sourdough rye bread consumption (Beckmann *et al.* 2013; Hanhineva *et al.* 2014). However, the HHPAA aglycone has not been detected in the sourdough rye bread, strongly suggesting that it was metabolized endogenously, potentially from the hexose-conjugated DIBOA precursor, which was very abundant in the bread. Bondia-Pons *et al.* (2013) detected this sulfonated benzoxazinoid precursor DIBOA as a discriminating benzoxazinoid after consumption of a whole grain rye bread compared with a refined-wheat bread diet. HMBOA glucuronide and HMBOA were higher in bread consumers than the non-bread consumers (Garcia-Aloy *et al.* 2014). Hanhineva *et al.* (2014) showed that another hydroxylated phenylacetamide HPAA sulfate was observed at the highest concentration in the plasma samples collected after a diet of white wheat bread enriched with bioprocessed rye. This was in agreement with Beckmann *et al.* (2013), who also showed HPAA sulfate elevation after sourdough rye bread consumption. Garcia-Aloy *et al.* (2014) demonstrated that HPAA and HPAA glucuronide was higher in the urine of bread consumers than the non-bread consumers. Additionally, using untargeted metabolite fingerprinting it was discovered that a HBOA glucuronide was strongly discriminatory of habitual whole grain sourdough rye bread exposure in humans (Beckmann *et al.* 2013). This is in agreement with Garcia-Aloy *et al.* (2014), who showed HBOA glycoside increased after bread consumption in a free-living population. A commonly reported pathway for the degradation of HBOA and BOA involves transformation to phenoxazinones via a highly unstable 2-aminophenol (2-AP) intermediate. AP sulfate has been identified as a discriminatory signal in a free-living population after consumption of a whole grain rye bread compared with a refined-wheat bread diet or no bread (Bondia-Pons *et al.* 2013; Garcia-Aloy *et al.* 2014). Johansson-Persson *et al.* (2013) also showed that 2-AP increased after a high-fibre diet. In summary, a wider than previously thought range of potentially bioactive benzoxazinoids are bioavailable in humans consuming whole grain products.

As for alkylresorcinols in human intervention studies, Bondia-Pons *et al.* (2013) showed that AR metabolites are excreted in urine as polar conjugates (e.g., glucuronide or sulfate conjugates) after phase II metabolism. They identified a sulfate derivative of DHPPA as the most discriminatory urine metabolite after the cereal intervention, which was excreted to a higher extent after rye bread than a refined-wheat bread diet. Both sulfate and glucuronide forms of DHPPA were seen as discriminatory, importantly without any need of a previous derivatization or purification steps. Additionally, it was suggested compounds annotated as 3,5-dihydroxycinnamic acid sulfate and 3,5-dihydroxyphenylethanol sulfate may also be AR metabolites, which would not have been detected if a targeted approach had been used (Bondia-Pons *et al.* 2013). Very recently, it was shown after the consumption of whole grain bread in a free-living population, there appeared to increased levels of DHPPA glucuronide, the microbial–derived 3,5-dihydroxyphenylethanol sulfate and 5-(3,5-dihydroxyphenyl)pentanoic acid (DHPPTA) sulfate (Garcia-Aloy *et al.* 2014). In a data-driven metabolomics approach utilizing HPLC-coulometric electrode array detection, Zhu *et al.* (2014) identified 10 alkylresorcinol metabolites in mice and in humans, including 3 phenolic acids and 7 of their phase II conjugates, including DHPPTA (confirmed by analyzing the ^{1}H and ^{13}C NMR spectra). It has been suggested that DHPPTA and DHBA-glycine may be used in combination with DHBA and DHPPA as potential biomarkers to increase the accuracy of recording WG wheat and rye intake in epidemiologic studies.

Feruloylgycine sulfate and a group of correlated signals were shown as discriminatory after sourdough rye bread consumption (Beckmann *et al.* 2013). A significant postprandial rise in the concentration of the common phenolic acid derivative, ferulic acid-4-O-sulfate was also observed by Bondia-Pons *et al.* (2013) after rye bread consumption. An increase of dihydroferulic acid sulfate and another microbial derived metabolite hydroxybenzoic acid glucuronide was observed after bread consumption (Garcia-Aloy *et al.* 2014). It was suggested that the feruloylglycine and correlated compounds, ferulic acid-4-O-sulfate and dihydroferulic acid sulfate may arise from the metabolism/transformation of ferulates found in whole grain products (Beckmann *et al.* 2013; Bondia-Pons *et al.* 2013; Garcia-Aloy *et al.* 2014).

When ingested, lignans, including secoisolariciresnol and matairesinol, are converted into the mammalian lignans enterodiol and enterolactone, respectively, by microbial enzymes in the colon and are detectable in urine (Bondia-Pons *et al.* 2013; Garcia-Aloy *et al.* 2014) plasma (Johnsen *et al.* 2004) or serum (Knust *et al.* 2006). The measurements of the main metabolic end-product of lignan metabolism, enterodiol and enterolactone may be considered to reflect the total lignan intake. Enterodiol and enterolactone can be further transformed into glucuronides and sulfated conjugates for their enterohepatic and blood circulation, and finally, being excreted via urine and blood (Knust *et al.* 2006; Bondia-Pons *et al.* 2009; Garcia-Aloy *et al.* 2014). Untargeted metabolomic approaches have been used to show that the glucuronide form of enterolactone is a discriminatory signal after rye bread and whole grain bread consumption (Bondia-Pons *et al.* 2009; Garcia-Aloy *et al.* 2014)

18.12 Conclusion

Bioactives have been shown to have some health benefits (Kris-Etherton *et al.* 2002); however, a bioactive is not consumed in isolation and in one single form. Food processing can help or impede the release of these bioactive compounds from the fibre matrix of the cereal or alter their form or concentration, effecting downstream absorption and metabolism after ingestion. Attention has to be paid during the milling process regarding the removal of the outer layers of cereal grains. This would help in reducing the loss of bioactive compounds and increasing the health benefits of the final products. All processing steps alter the nutritional properties of the grains and may be used to improve the nutrition value in food products. Processes such as germination, malting, soaking and hydrothermal processing of grains all appear to increase the concentration and bioavailability of a wide variety of bioactives in whole grains. On the other hand, baking and roasting appears to generally cause a decrease in bioactives, particularly during dough mixing. Such processes have been seen to increase the amounts of free phenolic acids and lower amounts of bound phenolic acids compared with whole grain flour, suggesting liberation of bound phenolic acids increasing their bioavailability. Open-pan boiling, pressure cooking and microwaving generally decreased the concentrations of bioactive compounds. During extrusion cooking, many bioactives have been observed to decrease, particularly during the kneading and extrusion phases. However, extrusion at different temperatures and durations can significantly affect the bound and free fraction of phenolic acids, suggesting thermal degradation may be occurring during processing. Fermentation has been seen to both increase and change bioactives compared with non-fermented products, potentially being a result of enzymatic hydrolysis of insoluble bound or soluble conjugated bioactives. Specific processing approaches could be a good means to improve bioavailability of bioactives in whole grain products. Processing of whole grain products needs to be tailored to promote maximum bioactives within the food matrix and in a form which are readily absorbed and are bio-accessible, enhancing their health effects. The grain variety, bran content, and the food processing methodology and digestion appear to greatly influence specific bioactive content; great care will need to be taken to distinguish between different sources.

Traditional and classical investigations of whole grain bioactives have focused on specific molecules and chemical type, failing to detect many of the novel chemical conversions induced by specific food processing methods. There are now a large number of different metabolomics technologies and combined instrumentation methods for the analysis of intact bioactives in cereals and food matrices. Monitoring the metabolic changes associated with processing by untargeted metabolomic profiling/fingerprinting hypothesis-generating approaches rather than targeted methods can be used to identify more "global" process-related alterations. These methods can provide feedback to guide towards production of food with increased positive/beneficial health properties. The same type of feedback loop can also be used to identify parameters (metabolites) indicative of good processing performance or sensory attributes. Future high throughput, untargeted metabolomics will allow investigations in deciphering the bioactive compounds in whole grain cereals as part of studies aiming at elucidating the health benefits of these products. In addition, by utilizing untargeted, more "global" metabolomic profiling and fingerprinting coupled with targeted quantification, the ingestion, absorption and excretion of whole grains and products can be explored over the wider metabolome level.

18.13 References

Abdel-Aal, E.-S. M. & Rabalski, I. (2013). Effect of baking on free and bound phenolic acids in wholegrain bakery products. *Journal of Cereal Science*, 57, 312–318.

Adhikari, K. B., Laursen, B. B., Laerke, H. N. & Fomsgaard, I. S. (2012b). Bioactive benzoxazinoids in rye bread are absorbed and metabolized in pigs. *Journal of Agricultural and Food Chemistry*, 60, 2497–2506.

Adom, K. K. & Liu, R. H. (2002). Antioxidant activity of grains. *Journal of Agricultural and Food Chemistry*, 50, 6182–6187.

Adom, K. K., Sorrells, M. E. & Liu, R. H. (2003). Phytochemical profiles and antioxidant activity of wheat varieties. *Journal of Agricultural and Food Chemistry*, 51, 7825–7834.

Andersson, A. A. M., Åman, P., Wandel, M. & Frølich, W. (2010). Alkylresorcinols in wheat and rye flour and bread. *Journal of Food Composition and Analysis*, 23, 794–801.

Beckmann, M., Lloyd, A. J., Haldar, S. *et al.* (2013). Hydroxylated phenylacetamides derived from bioactive benzoxazinoids are bioavailable in humans after habitual consumption of whole grain sourdough rye bread. *Molecular Nutrition and Food Research*, 57, 1859–1873.

Beer, M. U., Wood, P. J., Weisz, J. & Pillion, N. (1997). Effect of cooking and storage on the amount and molecular weight of (1-3)(1-4)-β-D-glucan extracted from oat products by an in vitro digestion system. *Cereal Chemistry*, 74, 705 – 709.

Beleggia, R., Platani, C., Papa, R. *et al.* (2011). Metabolomics and food processing: From semolina to pasta. *Journal of Agricultural and Food Chemistry*, 59, 9366–9377.

Björck, I., Granfeldt, Y., Liljeberg, H., Tovar, J. & Asp, N.-G. (1994). Food properties affecting the digestion and absorption of carbohydrates. *The American Journal of Clinical Nutrition*, 59, 699S–705S.

Bondia-Pons, I., Aura, A.-M., Vuorela, S. *et al.* (2009). Rye phenolics in nutrition and health. *Journal of Cereal Science*, 49, 323–336.

Bondia-Pons, I., Barri, T., Hanhineva, K. *et al.* (2013). UPLC-QTOF/MS metabolic profiling unveils urinary changes in humans after a whole grain rye versus refined wheat bread intervention. *Molecular Nutrition and Food Research*, 57, 412–422.

Bravo, H. R. & Niemeyer, H. M. (1985). Decomposition in aprotic solvents of 2, 4-dihydroxy-7-methoxy-1, 4-benzoxazin-3-one, a hydroxamic acid from cereals. *Tetrahedron*, 41, 4983–4986.

Bryngelsson, S., Dimberg, L. H. & Kamal-Eldin, A. (2002). Effects of commercial processing on levels of antioxidants in oats (Avena sativa L.). *Journal of Agricultural and Food Chemistry*, 50, 1890–1896.

Chandrasekara, A. & Shahidi, F. (2011). Determination of antioxidant activity in free and hydrolyzed fractions of millet grains and characterization of their phenolic profiles by HPLC-DAD-ESI-MSN. *Journal of Functional Foods*, 3, 144–158.

Chen, Y., Ross, A. B., Åman, P. & Kamal-Eldin, A. (2004). Alkylresorcinols as markers of whole grain wheat and rye in cereal products. *Journal of Agricultural and Food Chemistry*, 52, 8242–8246.

Claus, S. P. & Swann, J. R. (2013). Nutrimetabonomics: applications for nutritional sciences, with specific reference to gut microbial interactions. *Annual review of food science and technology*, 4, 381–399.

Draper, J., Enot, D. P., Parker, D. *et al.* (2009). Metabolite signal identification in accurate mass metabolomics data with MZedDB, an interactive m/z annotation tool utilising predicted ionisation behaviour 'rules' *BMC Bioinformatics*, 10.

Durazzo, A., Zaccaria, M., Polito, A., Maiani, G. & Carcea, M. (2013). Lignan content in cereals, buckwheat and derived foods. *Foods*, 2, 53–63.

Fares, C., Platani, C., Baiano, A. & Menga, V. (2010). Effect of processing and cooking on phenolic acid profile and antioxidant capacity of durum wheat pasta enriched with debranning fractions of wheat. *Food Chemistry*, 119, 1023–1029.

Frank, T., Scholz, B., Peter, S. & Engel, K.-H. (2011). Metabolite profiling of barley: Influence of the malting process. *Food Chemistry*, 124, 948–957.

Fratianni, A., Criscio, T. D., Mignogna, R. & Panfili, G. (2012). Carotenoids, tocols and retinols evolution during egg pasta-making processes. *Food Chemistry*, 131, 590–595.

Gani, A., Wani, S. M., Masoodi, F. A. & Hameed, G. (2012). Whole-grain cereal bioactive compounds and their health benefits: A review. *Journal of Food Processing & Technology*, 3.

Garcia-Aloy, M., Llorach, R., Urpi-Sarda, M. *et al.* (2014). Nutrimetabolomics fingerprinting to identify biomarkers of bread exposure in a free-living population from the PREDIMED study cohort. *Metabolomics.*

Gerstenmeyer, E., Reimer, S., Berghofer, E., Schwartz, H. & Sontag, G. (2013). Effect of thermal heating on some lignans in flax seeds, sesame seeds and rye. *Food Chemistry*, 138, 1847–1855.

Gunenc, A., Tavakoli, H., Seetharaman, K. *et al.* (2013). Stability and antioxidant activity of alkyresorcinols in breads enriched with hard and soft wheat brans. *Food Research International*, 51, 571–578.

Hanhineva, K., Keski-Rahkonen, P., Lappi, J. *et al.* (2014). The postprandial plasma rye fingerprint includes benzoxazinoid-derived phenylacetamide sulfates. *Journal of Nutrition*, 144, 1016–1022.

Hanhineva, K., Rogachev, I., Aura, A.-M. *et al.* (2012). Identification of novel lignans in the whole grain rye bran by non-targeted LC–MS metabolite profiling. *Metabolomics*, 8, 399–409.

Hanhineva, K., Rogachev, I., Aura, A. M. *et al.* (2011). Qualitative characterization of benzoxazinoid derivatives in whole grain rye and wheat by LC-MS metabolite profiling. *Journal of Agricultural and Food Chemistry*, 59, 921–927.

Heiniö, R.-L., Liukkonen, K.-H., Myllymäki, O. *et al.* (2008). Quantities of phenolic compounds and their impacts on the perceived flavour attributes of rye grain. *Journal of Cereal Science*, 47, 566–575.

Hidalgo, A. & Brandolini, A. (2010). Tocols stability during bread, water biscuit and pasta processing from wheat flours. *Journal of Cereal Science*, 52, 254–259.

Hithamani, G. & Srinivasan, K. (2014). Effect of domestic processing on the polyphenol content and bioaccessibility in finger millet (*Eleusine coracana*) and pearl millet (*Pennisetum glaucum*). *Food Chemistry*, 164, 55–62.

Hole, A. S., Rud, I., Grimmer, S. *et al.* (2012). Improved bioavailability of dietary phenolic acids in whole grain barley and oat groat following fermentation with probiotic *Lactobacillus acidophilus* , *Lactobacillus johnsonii*, and *Lactobacillus reuteri*. *Journal of Agricultural and Food Chemistry*, 60, 6369–6375.

Holt, M. D., Moreau, R. A., DerMarderosian, A., McKeown, N. & Jacques, P. F. (2012). Accelerated solvent extraction of alkylresorcinols in food products containing uncooked and cooked wheat. *Journal of Agricultural and Food Chemistry*, 60, 4799–4802.

Holtekjølen, A. K., Kinitz, C. & Knutsen, S. H. (2006). Flavanol and bound phenolic acid contents in different barley varieties. *Journal of Agricultural and Food Chemistry*, 54, 2253–2260.

Hübner, F. & Arendt, E. K. (2013). Germination of cereal grains as a way to improve the nutritional value: A review. *Critical Reviews in Food Science & Nutrition*, 53, 853–861.

Hung, P. & Morita, N. (2008). Distribution of phenolic compounds in the graded flours milled from whole buckwheat grains and their antioxidant capacities. *Food Chemistry*, 109, 325–331.

Hung, P. V., Hatcher, D. W. & Barker, W. (2011). Phenolic acid composition of sprouted wheats by ultra-performance liquid chromatography (UPLC) and their antioxidant activities. *Food Chemistry*, 126, 1896–1901.

Johansson-Persson, A., Barri, T., Ulmius, M., Onning, G. & Dragsted, L. O. (2013). LC-QTOF/MS metabolomic profiles in human plasma after a 5-week high dietary fiber intake. *Analytical and Bioanalytical Chemistry*, 405, 4799–4809.

Johnsen, N. F., Hausner, H., Olsen, A. *et al.* (2004). Intake of whole grains and vegetables determines the plasma enterolactone concentration of Danish women. *Journal of Nutrition*, 134, 2691–2697.

Katina, K., Laitila, A., Juvonen, R. *et al.* (2007). Bran fermentation as a means to enhance technological properties and bioactivity of rye. *Food Microbiology*, 24, 175–186.

Kaukovirta-Norja, A., Wilhelmson, A. & Poutanen, K. (2004). Germination: A means to improve the functionality of oat. *Agricultural and Food Science*, 13, 100–112.

Khakimov, B., Bak, S. & Engelsen, S. B. (2014). High-throughput cereal metabolomics: Current analytical technologies, challenges and perspectives. *Journal of Cereal Science*, 59, 393–418.

Knödler, M., Kaiser, A., Carle, R. & Schieber, A. (2008). Profiling of Alk(en)ylresorcinols in cereals by HPLC-DAD-APcI-MSn. *Analytical and Bioanalytical Chemistry*, 391, 221–228.

Knödler, M., Most, M., Schieber, A. & Carle, R. (2010). A novel approach to authenticity control of whole grain durum wheat (Triticum durum Desf.) flour and pasta, based on analysis of alkylresorcinol composition. *Food Chemistry*, 118, 177–181.

Knust, U., Hull, W. E., Spiegelhalder, B. *et al.* (2006). Analysis of enterolignan glucuronides in serum and urine by HPLC-ESI-MS. *Food and Chemical Toxicology*, 44, 1038–1049.

Konopka, I., Kozirok, W. & Rotkiewicz, D. (2004). Lipids and carotenoids of wheat grain and flour and attempt of correlating them with digital image analysis of kernel surface and cross-sections. *Food Res Int*, 37, 429–438.

Kozubek, A. & Tyman, J. H. (1999). Resorcinolic lipids, the natural non-isoprenoid phenolic amphiphiles and their biological activity. *Chem Reviews*, 99, 1–26.

Kris-Etherton, P. M., Hecker, K. D., Bonanome, A. *et al.* (2002). Bioactive compounds in foods: their role in the prevention of cardiovascular disease and cancer. *The American Journal of Medicine*, 113, 71–88.

Kulawinek, M., Jaromin, A., Kozubek, A. & Zarnowski, R. (2008). Alkylresorcinols in selected polish rye and wheat cereals and whole-grain cereal products. *Journal of Food and Agricultural Chemistry*, 56, 7236–7242.

Kulawinek, M., Jaromin, A., Kozubek, A. & Zarnowski, R. (2008). Alkylresorcinols in selected Polish rye and wheat cereals and whole-grain cereal products. *Journal of Agricultural and Food Chemistry*, 56, 7236–7242.

Landberg, R., Andersson, A. A. M., Åman, P. & Kamal-Eldin, A. (2009). Comparison of GC and colorimetry for the determination of alkylresorcinol homologues in cereal grains and products. *Food Chemistry*, 113, 1363–1369.

Landberg, R., Linko, A., M., A., K.-E. *et al.* (2006). Human plasma kinetics and relative bioavailability of alkylresorcinols after intake of rye bran. *Journal of Nutrition*, 136, 2760–2765.

Lee, D. P., Alexander, D. & Jonnalgadda, S. S. (2013). Diversity of nutrient content in grains – A pilot metabolomics analysis. *Journal of Nutrition amd Food Science*, 3, (2).

Leenhardt, F., Lyan, B., Rock, E. *et al.* (2006). Wheat lipoxygenase activity induces greater loss of carotenoids than vitamin E during breadmaking. *Journal of Agricultural and Food Chemistry*, 54, 1710–1715.

Liukkonen, K.-H., Katina, K., Wilhelmsson, A. *et al.* (2003). Process-induced changes on bioactive compounds in whole grain rye. *Proceedings of the Nutrition Society*, 62, 117–122.

Mateo Anson, N., Aura, A. M., Selinheimo, E. *et al.* (2011). Bioprocessing of wheat bran in whole wheat bread increases the bioavailability of phenolic acids in men and exerts antiinflammatory effects ex vivo. *Journal of Nutrition*, 141, 137–143.

Mateo Anson, N., Selinheimo, E., Havenaar, R. *et al.* (2009). Bioprocessing of wheat bran improves in vitro bioaccessibility and colonic metabolism of phenolic compounds. *Journal of Agricultural and Food Chemistry*, 57, 6148–6155.

Mateo Anson, N., Van den Berg, R., Havenaar, R., Bast, A. & Haenen, G. R. M. M. (2008). Ferulic acid from aleurone determines the antioxidant potency of wheat grain (*Triticum aestivum* L.). *Journal of Agricultural and Food Chemistry*, 56.

Mattila, P., Pihlava, J.-m. & Hellström, J. (2005). Contents of phenolic acids, alkyl-and alkenylresorcinols, and avenanthramides in commercial grain products. *Journal of Agricultural and Food Chemistry*, 53, 8290–8295.

McMurough, I. & Baert, T. (1994). Identification of proanthocyanidins in Beer and their direct measurement with a dual electrode electrochemical detector. *Journal of the Institute of Brewing*, 100, 409–414.

Menga, V., Fares, C., Troccoli, A., Cattivelli, L. & Baiano, A. (2009). Effects of genotype, location and baking on the phenolic content and some antioxidant properties of cereal species. *International Journal of Food Science & Technology*, 45, 7–16.

Menzel, C., Kamal-Eldin, A., Marklund, M. *et al.* (2012). Alkylresorcinols in Swedish cereal food products. *Journal of Food Composition and Analysis*, 28, 119–125.

Moore, J., Luther, M., Cheng, Z. & Yu, L. (2009). Effects of baking conditions, dough fermentation, and bran particle size on antioxidant properties of whole-wheat pizza crusts. *Journal of Agricultural and Food Chemistry*, 57, 832–839.

Nyström, L., Paasonen, A., Lampi, A.-M. & Piironen, V. (2007). Total plant sterols, steryl ferulates and steryl glycosides in milling fractions of wheat and rye. *Journal of Cereal Science*, 45, 106–115.

O'Gorman, A., Gibbons, H. & Brennan, L. (2013). Metabolomics in the identification of biomarkers of dietary intake. *Computational and structural biotechnology journal*, 4.

Ozturk, I., Sagdic, O., Hayta, M. & Yetim, H. (2012). Alteration in α-tocopherol, some minerals, and fatty acid contents of wheat through sprouting. *Chemistry of Natural Compounds*, 47, 876–879.

Pedersen, H. A., Laursen, B., Mortensen, A. & Fomsgaard, I. S. (2011). Bread from common cereal cultivars contains an important array of neglected bioactive benzoxazinoids. *Food Chemistry*, 127, 1814–1820.

Piironen, V., Toivo, J. & Lampi, A.-M. (2002). Plant sterols in cereals and cereal products. *Cereal Chemistry*, 79, 148–154.

Poutanen, K., Sozer, N. & Della Valle, G. (2014). How can technology help to deliver more of grain in cereal foods for a healthy diet? *Journal of Cereal Science*, 59, 327–336.

Quettier-Deleu, C., Gressier, B., Vasseur, J. *et al.* (2000). Phenolic compounds and antioxidant activities of buckwheat (*Fagopyrum esculentum* Moench) hulls and flour. *Ethnopharma*, 72.

Ross, A., Shepherd, M., Schupphaus, M. *et al.* (2003). Alkylresorcinols in cereals and cereal products. *Journal of Agricultural and Food Chemistry*, 51, 4111–4118.

Ross, A. B., Åman, P. Andersson, R and Kamal-Eldin. A. (2004a). Chromatographic analysis of alkylresorcinols and their metabolites. *Journal of Chromatography A* 1054,(1): 157-164.

Ross, A. B., Kamal-Eldin, A. & Åman, P. (2004b). Dietary alkylresorcinols: absorption, bioactivities, and possible use as biomarkers of whole-grain wheat- and rye-rich products. *Nutrition Reviews*, 62, 81–68.

Ross, A. B., Kamal-Eldin, A., Jung, C., Shepherd, M. J. & Åman, P. (2001). Gas chromatographic analysis of alkylresorcinols in rye (Secale cereale L) grains. *Journal of the Science of Food and Agriculture*, 81, 1405–1411.

Ross, A. B. & Kochhar, S. (2009). Rapid and sensitive analysis of alkylresorcinols from cereal grains and products using HPLC–coularray-based electrochemical detection. *Journal of Agricultural and Food Chemistry*, 57, 5187–5193.

Ryan, E. P., Heuberger, A. L., Weir, T. L. *et al.* (2011). Rice bran fermented with saccharomyces boulardii generates novel metabolite profiles with bioactivity. *Journal of Agricultural and Food Chemistry*, 59, 1862–1870.

Sampietro, D. A., Vattuone, M. A. & Catalán, C. A. N. (2009). A new colorimetric method for determination of alkylresorcinols in ground and whole-cereal grains using the diazonium salt Fast Blue RR. *Food Chemistry*, 115, 1170–1174.

Scalbert, A., Brennan, L., Fiehn, O. *et al.* (2009). Mass-spectrometry-based metabolomics: Limitations and recommendations for future progress with particular focus on nutrition research. *Metabolomics*, 5, 435–458.

Scalbert, A., Brennan, L., Manach, C. *et al.* (2014). The food metabolome: A window over dietary exposure. *The American Journal of Clinical Nutrition*, 99, 1286–1308.

Sicker, D., Frey, M., Schulz, M. & Gierl, A. (2000). Role of natural benzoxazinones in the survival strategy of plants. *International review of cytology*, 198, 319–346.

Skoglund, M., Peterson, D. M., Andersson, R., Nilsson, J. & Dimberg, L. H. (2008). Avenanthramide content and related enzyme activities in oats as affected by steeping and germination. *Journal of Cereal Science*, 48, 294–303.

Smeds, A. I., Eklund, P. C., Sjöholm, R. E. *et al.* (2007). Quantification of a broad spectrum of lignans in cereals, oilseeds, and nuts. *Journal of Agricultural and Food Chemistry*, 55, 1337–1346.

Subba Rao, M. V. & Muralikrishna, G. (2002). Evaluation of the antioxidant properties of free and bound phenolic acids from native and malted finger millet (ragi, Eleusine coracana Indaf-15). *Journal of Agricultural and Food Chemistry*, 50 889–892.

Tanwir, F., Fredholm, M., Gregersen, P. L. & Fomsgaard, I. S. (2013). Comparison of the levels of bioactive benzoxazinoids in different wheat and rye fractions and the transformation of these compounds in homemade foods. *Food Chemistry*, 141, 444–450.

West, R., Seetharaman, K. & Duizer, L. M. (2013). Effect of drying profile and whole grain content on flavour and texture of pasta. *Journal of Cereal Science*, 58, 82–88.

Wishart, D. S. (2008). Metabolomics: Applications to food science and nutrition research. *Trends in Food Science & Technology*, 19, 482-493.

Wishart, D. S., Jewison, T., Guo, A. *et al.* (2013). HMDB 3.0 — The human metabolome database in 2013. *Nucleic Acids Research*, 41, D801–D807.

Zhang, A., Sun, H., Wang, P., Han, Y. & Wang, X. (2012). Modern analytical techniques in metabolomics analysis. *Analyst*, 137, 293–300.

Zhu, Y., Shurlknight, K. L., Chen, X. & Sang, S. (2014). Identification and pharmacokinetics of novel alkylresorcinol metabolites in human urine, new candidate biomarkers for whole-grain wheat and rye intake. *Journal of Nutrition*, 144, 114–22.

Zielinski, H., Kozlowska, H. & Lewczuk, B. (2001). Bioactive compounds in the cereal grains before and after hydrothermal processing. *Innovative Food Science & Emerging Technologies*, 2, 159–169.

19 Application of Metabolomics for the Assessment of Health Effects of Whole grain Foods

Kati Hanhineva[1,2,3]

[1]University of Turku, Department of Biochemistry, Food Chemistry and Food Development Unit, Turun yliopisto, Finland
[2]Chalmers University of Technology, Department of Biology and Biological Engineering, Division of Food and Nutrition Science, Gothenburg, Sweden
[3]University of Eastern Finland, School of Medicine, Department of Public Health and Clinical Nutrition, Kuopio, Finland

19.1 Introduction

The improvements in analytical technologies within the past decade have enabled the development of the metabolomics analytics that can provide accurate, sensitive and high-throughput approaches to explore the content of metabolites, that is, small molecules present in virtually any biological material. The greatest advantage of metabolomics lies within the ability to address thousands of analytes concomitantly from minimal sample material in untargeted metabolite profiling setups (Patti et al. 2012). Such approaches are typically conducted on samples representing different treatment groups, and the metabolite alterations caused by the perturbations are revealed with statistical and chemometrical evaluations. This untargeted approach enables finding of unexpected changes that are neglected in traditional hypothesis driven targeted analyses focusing on a predetermined set of clinical biomarkers, and therefore are typically applied for the purpose of exploring novel biomarker candidates or events in cellular metabolism. Furthermore, the constant analytical development providing for improved sensitivity and accuracy within the mass spectrometry technologies accompanied with development of the data-analytical approaches, including the identification of metabolites, will ensure yet deeper insight to metabolic networks involved in the response of our body to different dietary regimens.

The untargeted metabolite profiling approaches enable the measurement of a priori unknown constituents in the biological sample. This property is a distinct advantage when addressing research questions involving myriad chemical species, like in the case of investigation of the impact of whole grain consumption on endogenous metabolism and its possible relation to metabolic health: When compared to refined grain controls, the untargeted metabolite profiling enables addressing the bioavailability and kinetics semi-quantitatively of dietary whole grain–derived phytochemicals, which

Whole Grains and Health, Second Edition. Edited by Rikard Landberg and Nathalie Scheers.

Additional materials available for download online at https://www.wiley.com/en-gb/Whole+Grains+and+Health-p-9781118939437

have been proposed as candidates behind the beneficial effect on health beyond the simple provision of energy and nutrients (Fardet 2010; Borneo and Leon 2012). Metabolomics techniques also offer the possibility to semi-quantitatively examine a wide scale of endogenous metabolites potentially affected by the consumption of WG. Likewise, the role of gut microbiota in modulating the composition of WG phytochemicals and their bioavailability in the gut greatly benefits from metabolite profiling approaches. Such indications of affected endogenous metabolism can then be subject to detailed inspection with targeted analytical techniques.

The utilization of metabolomics has increased remarkably within whole grain cereals research, similarly to life science research in general. Various metabolite analysis applications, including both mass spectrometry and NMR-based technology, have been utilized in this research field. Metabolite profiling analyses have been exploited in the examination of the phytochemical composition of different whole grain species as well as to investigate changes in phytochemical composition during food manufacturing processes (Chapter 20). This chapter focuses on the published metabolomics research regarding endogenous metabolic changes observed in studies involving whole grain consumption and impact on health.

19.2 Study designs

The evidence from prospective, observational studies on the impact of whole grains on human health is convincing as high consumption has been associated with reduced risk of major chronic diseases including cardiovascular diseases (Anderson 200; Jensen et al. 2004; Mellen et al. 2008; Harris and Kris-Etherton 2010), type 2 diabetes (Aune et al. 2013; de Munter et al. 2007) and certain cancers (Aune et al. 2011; Jacobs et al. 1998). However, results from short-term intervention studies evaluating the impact of whole grain food intake on risk factors of such conditions have shown mixed results. Many studies have evaluated the impact of various foods on postprandial glycemic and insulinemic responses. Surprisingly few metabolomics studies have so far been performed in acute post-prandial studies involving high intake of whole grains (Hanhineva et al. 2014; Moazzami et al. 2014; Shi 2016; Neacsu et al., 2017). The majority of the so far published metabolomics investigations in this field are from longer term dietary interventions involving various different study setups with varying dietary schemes, encompassing both analysis of fasting plasma or serum (Moazzami et al. 2011; Ross et al. 2013; Johansson-Persson et al. 2013; Hanhineva et al. 2015; Moazzami et al. 2012; Lankinen et al. 2014; Lankinen et al. 2010; Lankinen et al. 2011) as well as urine samples (Bondia-Pons et al. 2013; Ross et al. 2013; Beckmann et al. 2013; Garcia-Aloy et al. 2014). Only few studies with dietary information of whole grain consumption have been analyzed with targeted metabolite biomarker panel kits (Bouchard-Mercier et al. 2013; Floegel et al. 2013), and one study is reporting the plasma biomarker candidates (metabolomics analysis by Metabolon) related to dietary patterns, including whole grains (Playdon et al. 2017). Additionally, several studies utilizing metabolomics approaches of animal models in whole grain research have been published including pig (Nielsen et al. 2014; Bertram et al. 2006; Bertram et al. 2009; Norskov et al. 2013; Norskov et al. 2013; Yde et al. 2012; Krog Ingerslev et al. 2015) and rodents (Pekkinen et al. 2014; Fardet et al. 2007) studies. Publications reporting metabolomics analysis within whole grain research are listed in Table 19.1.

Table 19.1 Metabolomics applications investigating the impact of a whole grain rich diet on endogenous metabolism.

Study participants	Study design	Sampling	Test product	Analytical method	Reference
human and pig	randomized crossover	postprandial blood	white wheat bread, rye bread with whole-rye kernels, 2 white-wheat breads supplemented with either arabinoxylan or oat beta-glucan	LC-MS	Nielsen et al. 2014
postmenopausal women with elevated serum cholesterol and BMI	randomized crossover, 8-wk intervention separated by 8-wk washout period	fasting serum	whole grain rye bread and refined-wheat bread	NMR	Moazzami et al. 2012
pig	parallel, 3-wk washout followed by 9.5-wk experimental diet period	24h urine, postprandial blood	whole grain rye bread enriched with rye bran and refined-wheat bread with cellulose-rich wheat fibre	LC-MS	Norskov et al. 2013
individuals with metabolic syndrome	parallel, 4-wk baseline and 12-wk intervention	fasting serum	oat and wheat bread and potato group, and rye bread and pasta group	LC-MS, GC-MS	Lankinen et al. 2010
prostate cancer patients	randomized crossover, 2-wk washout followed by 6-wk intervention	fasting plasma	diet rich in whole grain rye and rye-bran products or refined-grain products with added cellulose	NMR	Moazzami et al. 2011
healthy adult volunteers	4-wk washout, 2 x 4-wk intervention with increasing consumption of test products	24h urine at the end of each test period	diet rich in whole grain rye foods	FIE-MS	Beckmann et al. 2013
postmenopausal women	randomized crossover, 8-wk interventions separated by 8-wk washout period	fasting plasma	whole grain rye bread and refined-wheat bread	LC-MS, GC-MS	Lankinen et al. 2010
healthy adult volunteers	randomized crossover, 5-wk interventions separated by 3-wk washout period	fasting plasma	high-fibre diet with oat bran, rye bran and sugarbeet fibre and low-fibre diet with similar test products but without fibre enrichment	LC-MS	Johansson-Persson et al. 2013
rat	crossover, 2-wk test diet periods	plasma, urine, liver	diets enriched with whole grain wheat or refined-wheat flour	NMR	Fardet et al. 2007

(continued)

Table 19.1 Metabolomics applications investigating the impact of a whole grain rich diet on endogenous metabolism. (*continued*)

Study participants	Study design	Sampling	Test product	Analytical method	Reference
pig	crossover, 1-wk test diet periods	plasma	whole grain rye bread or refined-wheat bread	NMR	Bertram et al. 2006
healthy adult volunteers with slightly elevated serum cholesterol levels	randomized crossover, 4-wk interventions separated by 4-wk washout period	24h urine	wholemeal-rye bread or refined-wheat bread	LC-MS	Bondia-Pons et al. 2013
healthy adult volunteers	randomized crossover	postprandial plasma	whole grain rye, refined-wheat bread enriched with rye bran or bioprocessed rye bran, or refined-wheat bread	LC-MS	Hanhineva et al. 2014
obese mice	parallel, 8-wk feeding periods	urine	High fat feeds enriched with four differentially processed aleurone preparations or pure ferulic acid	LC-MS	Pekkinen et al. 2014
adults with features of metabolic syndrome	parallel, 12-wk interventions	fasting plasma	whole grain enriched diet, healthy diet with similar intake in whole grains, or control diet with reduced intake of whole grains	LC-MS	Hanhineva et al. 2014
healthy adult volunteers	randomized crossover, 3-wk interventions separated by 2-wk washout	faeces, 24h urine, fasting plasma	whole grain wheat breakfast cereals or placebo cereals	targeted GC-MS and LC-MS	Costabile et al. 2008
human	EPIC-Potsdam	(fasting?) serum	whole grain bread	targeted LC-MS	Floegel et al. 2014

19.2.1 Acute postprandial interventions

NMR investigation on postprandial plasma samples after intake of whole grain rye and refined rye bread was done with refined wheat as control (Moazzami et al. 2014). A clear difference was observed between the postprandial insulin response accompanied by increased levels of two branched chain amino acids (BCAA), leucine and isoleucine, after the refined wheat bread as compared to the rye breads. Higher fasting plasma levels of BCAA have been related to increased risk of type 2 diabetes, although it is presently being discussed whether they reflect the insulin-resistant status triggered by dietary or other factors, or if they per se induce metabolic dysregulation, thus leading to insulin resistance (Lynch 2014; Manders et al. 2012). The authors suggest that differences in dietary protein content and metabolism between refined and whole grain diets could lead to the increased circulating levels of insulinogenic amino acids after consumption of refined wheat products, thereby increasing postprandial insulin levels (Moazzami et al. 2014). Interestingly, isoleucine levels were also increased in fasting serum after 8 weeks dietary intervention with refined wheat products compared to whole grain rye (Moazzami et al. 2012), and also in fasting plasma after an intervention with refined cereal compared to endosperm rye bread consumption (Lankinen et al. 2010). However, in the latter case, the increase in BCAA was merely suggested to be related to the increased daily protein intake observed in the group consuming refined products (Lankinen et al. 2010).

The postprandial response to whole grain products has been investigated also in a study involving both humans and pigs consuming the same test breads, including commercial white wheat bread as control, and rye bread with whole rye kernels as well as two customized breads enriched with arabinoxylan and beta-glucan (Nielsen et al. 2014). One of the main conclusions from the study was that pigs are suitable as a model for humans in a dietary study setting since the metabolic responses were very similar in both species. The observed differences in the response between the white wheat and rye kernel bread included mainly lipid species, as, for example, PC(38:4) and PC(36:4) as well as LysoPC(18:1) were statistically significantly increased after the meal with rye kernel bread when compared to the white wheat bread (Nielsen et al. 2014). Another study examining the postprandial plasma metabolite content after different breads focused only on such compounds that were present in circulation after a meal containing rye bran but not after white wheat (Hanhinevan et al. 2014). Surprisingly few compounds fell in this category, and the key tentatively identified compounds included phenylacetamides, metabolized forms of benzoxazinoids. These compounds are reported for various different bioactivities, and therefore their potential role in the metabolic response to whole grain products should be taken into consideration, although has not been so far addressed. The same compounds were observed also in urine samples alongside several other potential benzoxazinoid and alkylresorcinol derivatives, when whole grain diet was compared against refined grain consumption (Zhu et al., 2016).

One of the shortcomings of these studies is that they report only a relatively narrow range of metabolites, which clearly demonstrates the variability of results obtainable by different analytical platforms. Large-scale, comprehensive metabolite profiling demonstrating postprandial metabolic responses across a wider array of metabolite classes is yet to come. This is of particular interest in the case of whole grain rye, since the untargeted approach, being free from a priori hypothesis of metabolic regulations, is open for wider detection and interpretation of the observed phenomenon of decreased postprandial insulin response.

19.2.2 Short- to medium-term interventions

Samples from several dietary interventions have been analyzed by both NMR and MS-based metabolomics analyses. One of the most frequently discussed findings in terms of impact of whole grains on health is the elevated level of betaine in plasma. This has been reported in two NMR metabolomics investigations on various study setups: after diet rich in whole grain rye products versus refined-cereal products in prostate cancer patients (Moazzami 2011), after whole grain rye versus refined wheat diet in postmenopausal women with elevated serum total cholesterol levels (Moazzami et al. 2012), as well as by targeted analytical methods after a 2-week intervention diet based on either whole grain or refined-grain–based foods (Ross et al. 2011). Analogous findings have also been reported in animal studies on pigs (Bertram et al. 2009; Bertram et al. 2006) and rats (Fardet et al. 2007). Whole grain rye is one of the most important dietary sources of betaine (Ross et al. 2014), and therefore the elevated plasma betaine levels observed in several studies are most likely directly linked to the increased dietary intake. Betaine is an important methyl donor in endogenous metabolism, and additionally, one of its main roles is in the metabolic conversion of homocysteine to methionine releasing dimethylglycine (Moazzami et al. 2011). The production of methionine from homocysteine is partially controlled by insulin, and therefore the decreased homocysteine levels, favorable for reduced risk of cardiovascular diseases, could be related to the lower levels of inhibiting insulin, although the methionine levels in this study were not reported. Interestingly, a recent LC-MS metabolomics study reported increase in several betaine compounds including pipecolic acid betaine, γ-butyrobetaine and several unknown betaine signals after whole grain rich diet, but not glycine betaine (generally termed in literature as betaine) (Hanhineva et al. 2015). This finding indicates that there might be more complicated metabolism of betaine related compounds involved in the impact of whole grain products on health than suggested earlier.

One of the most common alterations in (fasting) plasma metabolite composition in dietary interventions include changes in the lipid pool (Lankinen et al. 2011; O'Gorman et al. 2014; Nielsen et. al. 2014). In the case of whole grain intake, the modifications observed for lipids are not as pronounced as in the case for example dietary fish intake (Lankinen et al. 2011), as several studies report rather individual, relatively mild alterations on lipid composition in terms of whole grain intake. Lankinen et al. (2010) analyzed the serum lipidomic profile after a diet rich in oat and wheat bread (high insulin response), and another diet enriched with endosperm rye bread (low insulin response). A major observation included the diminished level of two diacylglycerols (DG(40:1) and DG(36:1)) as well as increase in docosahexaenoic acid (DHA 22:6n-3) during the rye bread intervention. The oat and wheat based diet, on the other hand, caused significant increase is several LysoPC species, including LysoPC(16:0) sn-1, LysoPC(18:0) sn-1, and LysoPC(18:2e). The increase in serum DHA after the rye-based diet was an interesting observation as grains do not contain DHA; however, it may have been processed via endogenous desaturation and elongation of α-linolenic acid, which is abundant in rye bread. Also, a potential source could have been in other dietary items like fish, although this was not apparent based on the dietary records from the participants (Lankinen et al. 2010).

One of the most thoroughly investigated dietary interventions involving increased intake of whole grain products is the SYSDIMET study, which was investigated by both NMR metabolomics (Lankinen et al. 2014), LC-MS lipidomics (Lankinen et al. 2011) and non-targeted LC-MS metabolite profiling (Hanhineva et al. 2015). This study involved three arms: one enriched with fish, bilberries and whole grain products (the healthy diet); and another with the similar whole grain products, but no fish or bilberries allowed in diet (the whole grain diet). The control diet consisted of mainly refined grain products with limitations on the intake of fish and bilberries. While several metabolic changes related to the healthy diet were reported by all of the metabolomics approaches, there were no metabolic changes detected in the whole grain enriched group when analyzed by NMR, and only mild alterations were observed with the lipidomics platform, namely, slight increase in PC(40:7), and lipid assigned as either PE(38:4) or PC(35:4). The non-targeted LC-MS profiling reported an increase in two compounds tentatively identified as glucuronidated alkylresorcinols in both the healthy diet group as well as the group consuming whole grain products.

Additionally, the ketone bodies 3-hydroxybutyric acid and acetone were shown to increase with whole grain consumption in prostate cancer patients (Moazzami et al. 2011). The ketone bodies are formed from free fatty acids in the liver, thus indicating increased catabolic metabolism in the whole grain rye group. It was suggested that the lower postprandial insulin secretion in the whole grain rye group leads to lower glucose distribution in peripheral tissues, eventually evoking the catabolic metabolism typically occurring under starvation. This interesting finding, however, has not been replicated in other studies, and may reflect population, disease state, gender or diet-specific differences among studies. A somewhat contrasting result was received in a dietary intervention on healthy adults, in which lower urinary excretion of carnitine and acetylcarnitine was detected in participants having high consumption of whole grain products (Ross et al. 2013). Since high urinary excretion of acetylcarnitine is associated with fasting status, the authors suggested that a diet rich in whole grains may decrease fat oxidation during fasting. Notably, these two studies represent very different diets, participants and sample material, and therefore a direct comparison is probably not relevant.

LC-MS based metabolomics has been applied also on a study investigating the alterations of plasma metabolite profiles after high-fibre diet consisting of oat bran, rye bran and sugar beet, together with low-fibre control diet containing no added fibre (Johansson-Persson et al. 2013). In this study, major metabolic alterations were observed in the fibre-derived phytochemical phase II metabolic compounds, including benzoxazionoid, alkylresorcinol, and potential derivatives of saponins related to the consumption of oat bran and sugarbeet. This study, however, did not record any changes in endogenous compounds. A non-targeted LC-MS metabolite profiling approach was applied in a dietary crossover intervention comparing the metabolic changes caused by a diet rich in whole grain rye and control diet based on refined wheat in a study population consisting of postmenopausal women (Bondia-Pons et al. 2013). Increased excretion of several phenolic compounds, including both alkylresorcinol-derived metabolites and phenolic acid derivatives, was observed as well as several benzoxazinoid-derived, endogenously metabolized compounds. An interesting finding in this study was the increase of urinary levels of indolyl-3-acryloylglycine in the participants consuming high amounts of whole grain rye. This metabolite is produced by the colonic microbiota from dietary tryptophan. The fasting plasma samples from the same intervention study were also analyzed by lipidomics and CG-MS metabolomics

(Lankinen et al. 2011). In this study, another microbial breakdown product of tryptophan was found elevated after the rye-rich diet, namely, indoleacetic acid. Additionally, ribitol and ribonic acid, pecursors of tryptohan, were also found at increased levels in the rye diet group, confirming the dietary-induced alteration in tryptophan metabolism in this study population. The authors suggested that this might have a link with reducing appetite and food intake as tryptophan is precursor for the hormone serotonin that participates in depressing hunger.

Another metabolomics investigation utilizing flow infusion electrospray ionization MS on fasting plasma samples collected from an 8-week intervention on whole grain rye foods identified several endogenously processed phytochemical derivatives mainly from benzoxazinoid and ferulic acid origin, like phenylacetylglutamine derivative and N-feruloylglycine-sulfate (Beckmann et al. 2013). This study did not report any particular endogenous compounds that would have been affected with the intervention. A recent publication reported yet another group of endogenous metabolites that were altered between consumers of whole grain and refined-grain diets, namely, bile acids (Ginos et al., 2018). The authors discussed that the observed changes could be related to beneficial effects on glucose homeostasis.

19.3 Metabolomics in epidemiological studies on whole grains and health

Until today, very few metabolomics approaches have been undertaken on epidemiological studies involving examination of dietary intake of whole grain products. A sub-cohort including 2380 participants from the EPIC Potsdam Study was assessed by targeted metabolomics analysis combined with statistical evaluation in terms of dietary pattern analysis (Floegel et al. 2013). While the purpose of the study was to link certain dietary patterns with serum metabolic profiles and not necessarily with single food items, the consumption of whole grain products was contributing to inverse association with diacylphosphatidylcholines C(36:1), C(32:1) and C(40:4), which have been linked to a higher risk of type 2 diabetes in the same population (Floegel et al. 2014). Interestingly, one of the mentioned phosphatidylcholines has the same distribution of carbon atoms and double bonds in the fatty acids as the acylglycerols reported by Lankinen et al. (2010). However, the exact structure of the fatty acids was not reported in either of the studies. Also several acyl-alkylphosphatidylcholines (C(34:0, C36:1, C34:1, C30:0) were associated with low intake of whole grain bread, and similarly also with acylcarnitines C14, C2 and C18. Additionally, plasma hexose levels were linked with a dietary pattern characterized with high intake of non-whole grain bread and low intake of whole grain bread (Floegel et al. 2013).

Another epidemiological investigation utilizing the same targeted metabolite profiling kit focused on analysis between Western dietary pattern characterized by higher intakes of refined-grain products, desserts, sweets and processed meats, whereas the contrasting dietary pattern termed as prudent diet was associated with high intake of vegetables, fruits, whole grain products and non-hydrogenated fats (Bouchard-Mercier et al. 2013). This analysis mainly indicated several metabolites linked with the Western diet, but did not report any particular compounds that would have been associated particularly in terms of the dietary intake levels of whole grain products. A nested case-control study within the Finnish cohort "Alpha-Tocopherol, Beta-Carotene Cancer Prevention Study" reported several unknown compounds that were related to whole grain intake (Playdon et al., 2017). Aminophenol sulphate, a metabolite derived from benzoxazinoids, was one of the few identified metabolites related to whole grain intake. This finding is confirming results from earlier studies reporting the same compound from dietary intervention studies (Bondia-Pons et al. 2013; Zhu et al., 2016).

Garcia-Aloy et al. (2014) investigated the urinary metabolite changes related to habitual bread consumption in altogether 155 participants. Unlike majority of the other studies within the field of whole grain research, this study had, in addition to the whole grain and refined-grain bread groups, a group without any consumption of bread. As typical for studies investigating urine samples, the majority of the findings were related to the phytochemicals derived from the bread consumption. Several benzoxazinoid compounds were, for example, excreted in higher amounts on bread consumption, but interestingly, no difference was observed between the two bread groups (Garcia-Aloy et al. 2014). Among the few endogenous metabolites significantly different between the study groups, 2,8-dihydroxyquinoline-β-D-glucuronide (2,8-DHQ glucuronide) was increased on whole grain bread consumption. A suggested link with improved lipid profile and impact on cardiovascular health was proposed via peroxisome proliferator-activated receptor (PPARα) agonist, as 2,8-DHQ-glucuronide has been proposed as a potential urinary biomarker of PPAR agonist function. N-α-Acetylcitrulline, which is part of the arginine biosynthetic pathway, was the sole metabolite with elevated levels in the group without bread in their diet. However, a causal relationship between whole grain bread consumption and its urinary levels was difficult to postulate.

19.4 Whole grain research on animal models utilizing metabolomics

While plasma and urine are the predominant sample materials available from human studies, animal trials are often necessitated in order to find out more detailed information on the perturbations caused by the dietary differences on cellular metabolism. The information obtainable from the organs is particularly important since the metabolite composition in the peripheral organs is expected to better reflect endogenous metabolism than (fasting) plasma, in which organ-specific perturbations are effectively diluted. However, as for human studies, animal trials in whole grain research employing metabolomics techniques are so far relatively few.

High whole grain wheat consumption in comparison to refined grain has been associated with increased urinary excretion of aromatic amino acids such as tryptophan, phenylalanine, tyrosine, hippurate, creatine, citrate and fumarate in a rat feeding trial (Fardet et al. 2007). A recent investigation in a rodent model with a diet enriched with wheat aleurone demonstrated a large variety of phytochemical derivatives with differential accumulation depending on the processing degree of the aleurone preparations (Pekkinen, et al. 2014).

Several metabolomics investigations have been published on a dietary animal model utilizing cathedrized pigs (Bertram et al. 2006; Yde et al. 2012; Norskov et al. 2013; Norskov et al. 2013; Bertram et al. 2009; Nielsen et al. 2014; Krog Ingerslev et al., 2015). One of the most important findings that these studies have brought to light is the difference in plasma and urine levels of various oxylipins after whole grain rich feeding when compared to refined products.

Oxylipins are oxygenated fatty acids suggested to be located in the lipid-rich germ (Norskov et al. 2013). The authors evaluated the levels of oxylipins after a diet rich in whole grain rye versus refined wheat, and had results showing the qualitative difference between the oxylipins associated with the two of the diets: The pigs fed with whole grain rye had a higher level of arachidonic acid derived from oxylipins, whereas several oxylipins derived from linoleic acid were increased after the diet based on refined wheat (Norskov et al. 2013). This may link directly to the differential fatty acid composition of the bread products used in the study, but the authors suggest that endogenous metabolism via lipoxygenase may be involved in the differential response between the diets. While the importance of diet-derived oxylipins is not known, the discussion involves at least their potential role in promoting epithelial cell growth (Norskov et al. 2013).

19.5 Conclusion and future prospects

The utilization of metabolomics within whole grain research focusing on health implications has so far produced highly variable results in terms of endogenous metabolic perturbations. It has been demonstrated that the main metabolic differences associated with consumption of whole grain products are related to certain grain-derived phytochemical classes including alkylresorcinols, benzoxazinoids, phenolic acids and lignans. However, there is yet no such similar prevailing realization on the modifications whole grain consumption has on the endogenous metabolism and therefore no consensus picture on the mechanisms for beneficial health effects of whole grain consumption. So far, indications exist that the metabolism involving betaine compounds is affected by whole grain, and that some alterations in lipid profiles are encountered by whole grain. The interpretation of the findings is hindered also by the lack of standardization in the reporting of metabolite identifications, especially the lipids that may be reported with varying levels of structural detail. Additionally, various microbial processed metabolites potentially related to protein and amino acid metabolism are reported in separate studies, and the involvement of microbiota in the response to whole grain products is very likely taken into fact that many phytochemicals of whole grains are embedded in the bran/fibre matrix that is transported for the digestion to colon.

As for whole grain research in general, the large variability in consumed products, grain varieties and differences in consumed levels are likely some of the most important factors behind the variability in results. Whole grains are a rich source of phytochemicals, and varying compositions of those may have synergistic and/or antagonistic effects via different metabolic mechanisms. Similarly, different approaches in sample collection, metabolite extraction and choice of analytical platform can clearly increase the variability in results. For example, many of the important metabolites may be in very low concentration range, and therefore utilization of state-of-the-art methodology and instrumentation is thus necessitated.

Until now, there is no study that has combined investigation of both postprandial and fasting plasma samples collected from clinical interventions, and observational epidemiological studies, with the most advanced metabolomics technologies. While such an approach would require a remarkable analytical effort, it is perceived to be essential in the elucidation of the metabolic link between whole grain intake and beneficial outcomes reported in epidemiological investigations. With the important caveat that organ and tissue metabolism in animal models may differ from human metabolism, animal trials with access to organ samples are similarly yet to be better exploited, as they offer great potential to untangle the underlying biochemical events and pathways affected by whole grain consumption. The hypothesis-generating approaches in untargeted metabolite profiling will have an important role in addressing such research question by involving a wider range of potentially important metabolites.

19.6 References

ANDERSEN, M.B., RINNAN, A., MANACH, C., POULSEN, S.K., PUJOS-GUILLOT, E., LARSEN, T.M., ASTRUP, A. and DRAGSTED, L.O., 2014. Untargeted metabolomics as a screening tool for estimating compliance to a dietary pattern. *Journal of Proteome Research,* 13(3), pp. 1405–1418.

ANDERSON, J.W., 2003. Whole grains protect against atherosclerotic cardiovascular disease. *The Proceedings of the Nutrition Society,* 62(1), pp. 135–142.

AUNE, D., CHAN, D.S., LAU, R., VIEIRA, R., GREENWOOD, D.C., KAMPMAN, E. and NORAT, T., 2011. Dietary fibre, whole grains, and risk of colorectal cancer: Systematic review and dose-response meta-analysis of prospective studies. *BMJ (Clinical Research Ed.),* 343, p. d6617.

AUNE, D., NORAT, T., ROMUNDSTAD, P. and VATTEN, L.J., 2013. Whole grain and refined grain consumption and the risk of type 2 diabetes: a systematic review and dose-response meta-analysis of cohort studies. *European Journal of Epidemiology,* 28(11), pp. 845–858.

BECKMANN, M., LLOYD, A.J., HALDAR, S., SEAL, C., BRANDT, K. and DRAPER, J., 2013. Hydroxylated phenylacetamides derived from bioactive benzoxazinoids are bioavailable in humans after habitual consumption of whole grain sourdough rye bread. *Molecular Nutrition & Food Research,* 57(10), pp. 1859–1873.

BERTRAM, H.C., BACH KNUDSEN, K.E., SERENA, A., MALMENDAL, A., NIELSEN, N.C., FRETTE, X.C. and ANDERSEN, H.J., 2006. NMR-based metabonomic studies reveal changes in the biochemical profile of plasma and urine from pigs fed high-fibre rye bread. *The BritishJjournal of Nutrition,* 95(5), pp. 955–962.

BERTRAM, H.C., MALMENDAL, A., NIELSEN, N.C., STRAADT, I.K., LARSEN, T., KNUDSEN, K.E. and LAERKE, H.N., 2009. NMR-based metabonomics reveals that plasma betaine increases upon intake of high-fiber rye buns in hypercholesterolemic pigs. *Molecular Nutrition & food Research,* 53(8), pp. 1055–1062.

BONDIA-PONS, I., BARRI, T., HANHINEVA, K., JUNTUNEN, K., DRAGSTED, L.O., MYKKANEN, H. and POUTANEN, K., 2013. UPLC-QTOF/MS metabolic profiling unveils urinary changes in humans after a whole grain rye versus refined wheat bread intervention. *Molecular Nutrition & Food Research,* 57(3), 412–22.

BORNEO, R. and LEON, A.E., 2012. Whole grain cereals: Functional components and health benefits. *Food & Function,* 3(2), pp. 110–119.

BOUCHARD-MERCIER, A., RUDKOWSKA, I., LEMIEUX, S., COUTURE, P. and VOHL, M.C., 2013. The metabolic signature associated with the Western dietary pattern: A cross-sectional study. *Nutrition Journal,* 12, p. 158.

E MUNTER, J.S., HU, F.B., SPIEGELMAN, D., FRANZ, M. and VAN DAM, R.M., 2007. Whole grain, bran, and germ intake and risk of type 2 diabetes: A prospective cohort study and systematic review. *PLoS Medicine,* 4(8), p. e261.

FARDET, A., 2010. New hypotheses for the health-protective mechanisms of whole-grain cereals: What is beyond fibre? *Nutrition Research Reviews,* 23(1), pp. 65–134.

FARDET, A., CANLET, C., GOTTARDI, G., LYAN, B., LLORACH, R., REMESY, C., MAZUR, A., PARIS, A. and SCALBERT, A., 2007. Whole-grain and refined wheat flours show distinct metabolic profiles in rats as assessed by a 1H NMR-based metabonomic approach. *The Journal of Nutrition,* 137(4), pp. 923–929.

FLOEGEL, A., VON RUESTEN, A., DROGAN, D., SCHULZE, M.B., PREHN, C., ADAMSKI, J., PISCHON, T. and BOEING, H., 2013. Variation of serum metabolites related to habitual diet: A targeted metabolomic approach in EPIC-Potsdam. *European Journal of Clinical Nutrition,* 67(10), pp. 1100–1108.

FLOEGEL, A., WIENTZEK, A., BACHLECHNER, U., JACOBS, S., DROGAN, D., PREHN, C., ADAMSKI, J., KRUMSIEK, J., SCHULZE, M.B., PISCHON, T. and BOEING, H., 2014. Linking diet, physical activity, cardiorespiratory fitness and obesity to serum metabolite networks: Findings from a population-based study. *International Journal of Obesity (2005),* 38(11), pp. 1388–1396.

GARCIA-ALOY, M., LLORACH, R., URPI-SARDA, M., TULIPANI, S., SALAS-SALVADÃ³, J., MARTÃNEZ-GONZÃ¡LEZ, M., CORELLA, D., FITÃ³, M., ESTRUCH, R., SERRA-MAJEM, L. and ANDRES-LACUEVA, C., 2014. Nutrimetabolomics fingerprinting to identify biomarkers of bread exposure in a free-living population from the PREDIMED study cohort. *Metabolomics,* pp. 1–11.

Ginos, B.N.R., Navarro, S.L., Schwarz, Y., Gu, H., Wang, D., Randolph, T.W., Shojaie, A., Hullar, M.A.J., Lampe, P.D., KRATZ, M., NEUHOUSER, M.L., RAFTERY, D. AND LAMPE, J.W., 2018. Circulating bile acids in healthy adults respond differently to a dietary pattern characterized by whole grains, legumes and fruits and vegetables compared to a diet high in refined grains and added sugars: A randomized, controlled, crossover feeding study. *Metabolism Clinical and Experimental,* 83, pp. 197–204.

HANHINEVA, K., KESKI-RAHKONEN, P., LAPPI, J., KATINA, K., PEKKINEN, J., SAVOLAINEN, O., TIMONEN, O., PAANANEN, J., MYKKÄNEN, H. and POUTANEN, K., 2014. The postprandial plasma rye fingerprint includes benzoxazioid-eerived phenylacetamide sulfates. *J. Nutr.,* 144, pp. 1–7.

HANHINEVA, K., LANKINEN, M.A., PEDRET, A., SCHWAB, U., KOLEHMAINEN, M., PAANANEN, J., DE MELLO, V., SOLA, R., LEHTONEN, M., POUTANEN, K., UUSITUPA, M. and MYKKÄNEN, H., 2015. Nontargeted metabolite profiling discriminates diet-specific biomarkers for consumption of whole grains, fatty fish, and bilberries in a randomized controlled trial. *The Journal of Nutrition,* 145(1), pp. 7–17.

HARRIS, K.A. and KRIS-ETHERTON, P.M., 2010. Effects of whole grains on coronary heart disease risk. *Current Atherosclerosis Reports,* 12(6), pp. 368–376.

JACOBS, D.R.,Jr, MARQUART, L., SLAVIN, J. and KUSHI, L.H., 1998. Whole-grain intake and cancer: An expanded review and meta-analysis. *Nutrition and Cancer,* 30(2), pp. 85–96.

JENSEN, M.K., KOH-BANERJEE, P., HU, F.B., FRANZ, M., SAMPSON, L., GRONBAEK, M. and RIMM, E.B., 2004. Intakes of whole grains, bran, and germ and the risk of coronary heart disease in men. *The American Journal of Clinical Nutrition,* 80(6), pp. 1492–1499.

JOHANSSON-PERSSON, A., BARRI, T., ULMIUS, M., Ã–NNING, G. and DRAGSTED, L., 2013. LC-QTOF/MS metabolomic profiles in human plasma after a 5-week high dietary fiber intake. *Analytical and Bioanalytical Chemistry,* 405(14), pp. 4799–4809.

JUNTUNEN, K.S., LAAKSONEN, D.E., POUTANEN, K.S., NISKANEN, L.K. and MYKKANEN, H.M., 2003. High-fiber rye bread and insulin secretion and sensitivity in healthy postmenopausal women. *The American Journal of Clinical Nutrition,* 77(2), pp. 385–391.

KALLIO, P., KOLEHMAINEN, M., LAAKSONEN, D.E., PULKKINEN, L., ATALAY, M., MYKKANEN, H., UUSITUPA, M., POUTANEN, K. and NISKANEN, L., 2008. Inflammation markers are modulated by responses to diets differing in postprandial insulin responses in individuals with the metabolic syndrome. *The American Journal of Clinical Nutrition,* 87(5), pp. 1497–1503.

KROG INGERSLEV, A., KARAMAN, I., BAGCTOGLU, M., KOHLER, A., KAPPEL THEIL, P., BACH KNUDSEN, K.E. AND SKOU HEDEMANN, M., 2015. Whole grain consumption increases gastrointestinal content of sulfate-conjugated oxylipins in pigs – A multicompartmental metabolomics study. *Journal of Proteome Research*, 14, pp. 3095–3110.

LANKINEN, M., KOLEHMAINEN, M., JAASKELAINEN, T., PAANANEN, J., JOUKAMO, L., KANGAS, A.J., SOININEN, P., POUTANEN, K., MYKKANEN, H., GYLLING, H., ORESIC, M., JAUHIAINEN, M., ALA-KORPELA, M., UUSITUPA, M. and SCHWAB, U., 2014. Effects of whole grain, fish and bilberries on serum metabolic profile and lipid transfer protein activities: A randomized trial (Sysdimet). *PloS One,* 9(2), p. e90352.

LANKINEN, M., SCHWAB, U., GOPALACHARYULU, P.V., SEPPANEN-LAAKSO, T., YETUKURI, L., SYSI-AHO, M., KALLIO, P., SUORTTI, T., LAAKSONEN, D.E., GYLLING, H., POUTANEN, K., KOLEHMAINEN, M. and ORESIC, M., 2010. Dietary carbohydrate modification alters serum metabolic profiles in individuals with the metabolic syndrome. *Nutrition, Metabolism, and Cardiovascular Diseases: NMCD,* 20(4), pp. 249–257.

LANKINEN, M., SCHWAB, U., KOLEHMAINEN, M., PAANANEN, J., POUTANEN, K., MYKKANEN, H., SEPPANEN-LAAKSO, T., GYLLING, H., UUSITUPA, M. and ORESIC, M., 2011. Whole grain products, fish and bilberries alter glucose and lipid metabolism in a randomized, controlled trial: The Sysdimet study. *PloS One,* 6(8), p. e22646.

LANKINEN, M., SCHWAB, U., SEPPANEN-LAAKSO, T., MATTILA, I., JUNTUNEN, K., MYKKANEN, H., POUTANEN, K., GYLLING, H. and ORESIC, M., 2011. Metabolomic analysis of plasma metabolites that may mediate effects of rye bread on satiety and weight maintenance in postmenopausal women. *The Journal of Nutrition,* 141(1), pp. 31–36.

LAPPI, J., MYKKANEN, H., BACH KNUDSEN, K.E., KIRJAVAINEN, P., KATINA, K., PIHLAJAMAKI, J., POUTANEN, K. and KOLEHMAINEN, M., 2014. Postprandial glucose metabolism and SCFA after consuming wholegrain rye bread and wheat bread enriched with bioprocessed rye bran in individuals with mild gastrointestinal symptoms. *Nutrition Journal,* 13(1), pp. 13, p. 104.

LEINONEN, K., LIUKKONEN, K., POUTANEN, K., UUSITUPA, M. and MYKKANEN, H., 1999. Rye bread decreases postprandial insulin response but does not alter glucose response in healthy Finnish subjects. *European Journal of Clinical Nutrition,* 53(4), pp. 262–267.

LYNCH, C.J. and ADAMS, S.H., 2014. Branched-chain amino acids in metabolic signalling and insulin resistance. *Nature Reviews: Endocrinology,* 10(12), pp. 723–736.

MANDERS, R.J., LITTLE, J.P., FORBES, S.C. and CANDOW, D.G., 2012. Insulinotropic and muscle protein synthetic effects of branched-chain amino acids: Potential therapy for type 2 diabetes and sarcopenia. *Nutrients,* 4(11), pp. 1664–1678.

MELLEN, P.B., WALSH, T.F. and HERRINGTON, D.M., 2008. Whole grain intake and cardiovascular disease: A meta-analysis. *Nutrition, Metabolism, and Cardiovascular Diseases: NMCD,* 18(4), pp. 283–290.

MOAZZAMI, A.A., BONDIA-PONS, I., HANHINEVA, K., JUNTUNEN, K., ANTL, N., POUTANEN, K. and MYKKANEN, H., 2012. Metabolomics reveals the metabolic shifts following an intervention with rye bread in postmenopausal women – A randomized control trial. *Nutrition Journal,* 11**,** p. 88.

MOAZZAMI, A.A., SHRESTHA, A., MORRISON, D.A., POUTANEN, K. and MYKKANEN, H., 2014. Metabolomics reveals differences in postprandial responses to breads and fasting metabolic characteristics associated with postprandial insulin demand in postmenopausal women. *The Journal of Nutrition,* 144(6), pp. 807–814.

MOAZZAMI, A.A., ZHANG, J.X., KAMAL-ELDIN, A., AMAN, P., HALLMANS, G., JOHANSSON, J.E. and ANDERSSON, S.O., 2011. Nuclear magnetic resonance-based metabolomics enable detection of the effects of a whole grain rye and rye bran diet on the metabolic profile of plasma in prostate cancer patients. *The Journal of Nutrition,* 141(12), pp. 2126–2132.

NEACSU, M., MCMONAGLE, J., FLETCHER, R.J., HULSHOF, T., DUNCAN, S.H., SCOBBIE, L., DUNCAN, G.J., CANTLAY, L., HORGAN, G., DE ROOS, B., DUTHIE, G.G. AND RUSSELL, W.R., 2017. Availability and dose response of phytophenols from a wheat bran rich cereal product in healthy human volunteers. *Molecular Nutrition and Food Research,* 61(3), p. 1600202.

NIELSEN, K.L., HARTVIGSEN, M.L., HEDEMANN, M.S., LAERKE, H.N., HERMANSEN, K. and BACH KNUDSEN, K.E., 2014. Similar metabolic responses in pigs and humans to breads with different contents and compositions of dietary fibers: A metabolomics study. *The American Journal of Clinical Nutrition,* 99(4), pp. 941–949.

NORSKOV, N., HEDEMANN, M., THEIL, P. and KNUDSEN, K., 2013. Oxylipins discriminate between whole grain wheat and wheat aleurone intake: A metabolomics study on pig plasma. *Metabolomics,* 9(2), pp. 464–479.

NORSKOV, N.P., HEDEMANN, M.S., LAERKE, H.N. and KNUDSEN, K.E., 2013. Multicompartmental non-targeted LC-MS metabolomics: explorative study on the metabolic responses of rye fiber versus refined wheat fiber intake in plasma and urine of hypercholesterolemic pigs. *Journal of Proteome Research,* 12(6), pp. 2818–2832.

O'GORMAN, A., MORRIS, C., RYAN, M., O'GRADA, C.M., ROCHE, H.M., GIBNEY, E.R., GIBNEY, M.J. and BRENNAN, L., 2014. Habitual dietary intake impacts on the lipidomic profile. *Journal of Chromatography.B, Analytical Technologies in the Biomedical and Life Sciences,* 966, pp. 140–146.

PATTI, G.J., YANES, O. and SIUZDAK, G., 2012. Innovation: Metabolomics: The apogee of the omics trilogy. *Nature Reviews: Molecular Cell Biology,* 13(4), pp. 263–269.

PEKKINEN, J., ROSA, N.N., SAVOLAINEN, O.I., KESKI-RAHKONEN, P., MYKKANEN, H., POUTANEN, K., MICARD, V. and HANHINEVA, K., 2014. Disintegration of wheat aleurone structure has an impact on the bioavailability of phenolic compounds and other phytochemicals as evidenced by altered urinary metabolite profile of diet-induced obese mice. *Nutrition & Metabolism,* 11(1), p. 1.

PLAYDON, M.C., MOORE, S.C., DERKACH, A., REEDY, J., SUBAR, A.F., SAMPSON, J.N., ALBANES, D., GU, F., KONTTO, J., LASSALE, C., LIAO, L.M., MÄNNISTÖ, S., MONDUL, A.M., WEINSTEIN, S.J., IRWIN, M.L., MAYNE, S.T. AND STOLZENBERG-SOLOMON, R., 2017. Identifying biomarkers of dietary patterns by using metabolomics. *American Journal of Clinical Nutrition,* 105, pp. 450–465.

ROSS, A.B., BRUCE, S.J., BLONDEL-LUBRANO, A., OGUEY-ARAYMON, S., BEAUMONT, M., BOURGEOIS, A., NIELSEN-MOENNOZ, C., VIGO, M., FAY, L.B., KOCHHAR, S., BIBILONI, R., PITTET, A.C., EMADY-AZAR, S., GRATHWOHL, D. and REZZI, S., 2011. A whole-grain cereal-rich diet increases plasma betaine, and tends to decrease total and LDL-cholesterol compared with a refined-grain diet in healthy subjects. *The British Journal of Nutrition,* 105(10), pp. 1492–1502.

ROSS, A.B., PERE-TREPAT, E., MONTOLIU, I., MARTIN, F.P., COLLINO, S., MOCO, S., GODIN, J.P., CLEROUX, M., GUY, P.A., BRETON, I., BIBILONI, R., THORIMBERT, A., TAVAZZI, I., TORNIER, L., BEBUIS, A., BRUCE, S.J., BEAUMONT, M., FAY, L.B. and KOCHHAR, S., 2013. A whole-grain-rich diet reduces urinary excretion of markers of protein catabolism and gut microbiota metabolism in healthy men after one week. *The Journal of Nutrition,* 143(6), pp. 766–773.

ROSS, A.B., ZANGGER, A. and GUIRAUD, S.P., 2014. Cereal foods are the major source of betaine in the Western diet – Analysis of betaine and free choline in cereal foods and updated assessments of betaine intake. *Food Chemistry,* 145, pp. 859–865.

SHI, L., BRUNIUS, C., LINDELÖF, M., SHAMEH, S.A., WU, H., LEE, I., LANDBERG, R. AND MOAZZAMI, A.A., 2017. Targeted metabolomics reveals differences in the extended postprandial plasma metabolome of healthy subjects after intake of whole-grain rye porridges versus refined wheat bread. *Molecular Nutrition and Food Research,* 61(7), p. 1600924.

YDE, C.C., WESTERHUIS, J.A., BERTRAM, H.C. and BACH KNUDSEN, K.E., 2012. Application of NMR-based metabonomics suggests a relationship between betaine absorption and elevated creatine plasma concentrations in catheterised sows. *The British Journal of Nutrition,* 107(11), pp. 1603–1615.

ZHU, Y., WANG, P., SHA, W. AND SANG, S., 2016. Urinary biomarkers of whole grain wheat intake identified by non-targeted and targeted metabolomics approaches. *Scientific Reports*, 6, p. 36278.

20 Using Transcriptomics and RNA Sequencing to Assess Health Effects of Whole Grains

Marjukka Kolehmainen

University of Eastern Finland, Institute of Public Health and Clinical Nutrition, Kuopio, Finland

20.1 Introduction

Omics tools are regarded as powerful methodologies for studying health effects of whole diets, foods and their components. They are applied with special benefit if there is no prior knowledge or literature available of the effect of a certain food due to the high throughput of the methods. This chapter concentrates on transcriptomics and its later advances, such as RNA sequencing. Transcriptomics is a tool to study the whole genome-wide gene expression (output is RNA transcripts) within the specific tissue, such as, for example, adipose tissue. It is important to note that the transcriptome, that is, the whole genome-wide RNA transcripts, are always tissue specific since the metabolism differs among the tissues with their different physiological tasks. For example, the basic task of adipose tissue is to store and release fatty acids depending on the energy balance in the human body that will determine part of the genetic pathways that respond to dietary intake. Before the omics-revolution, single-gene experiments were only based on already known metabolic pathways that made it difficult to see the full picture. For example, when transcriptomics were used in human studies, it was revealed that the effect of weight loss on the whole genome-wide gene expression, showed that many unexpected and unknown gene transcripts or genetic pathways were increased/decreased while the "main" genetic pathways did not seem to respond, or responded surprisingly little as a result of the intervention.

20.2 Transcriptomics and RNA sequencing

Transcriptomics is a chip-technology that demands a general good knowledge of the genome and its activated genes. As we know today, the regulation of gene expression is complex and we have just now learned that there are activities such as epigenetics, that is, regulation of expression by methylation of DNA, which may change our view on health effects of the diet. In addition, the transcriptome of cells and tissues is meta stabile and is continuously modified in response to circadian rhythm, lifestyle, diet and so on. In this respect, transcriptomics may be viewed as quite limiting technology, which has resulted in development of other methods for studying gene expression, such as RNA sequencing (2).

Whole Grains and Health, Second Edition. Edited by Rikard Landberg and Nathalie Scheers.

Additional materials available for download online at https://www.wiley.com/en-gb/Whole+Grains+and+Health-p-9781118939437

Applying RNA sequencing, it is possible to study alternative splicing of certain genes, post-transcriptional modifications and various RNA populations such as microRNAs. However, RNA sequencing is not yet very much used in clinical dietary interventions, although the quality of diet will have an effect also on RNA splicing. Alternative splicing of RNA is a cellular mechanism where different RNA transcripts are produced within the cells depending on the conditions in the cell or tissue. It has been speculated that 95–100% of human exones maybe spliced during the process (3). This potentially has important health effects that may have not been known before. As an example, there are studies using single gene approaches to study the effect of weight loss on the splicing within tissues (4). The results indicate that the expression of the gene related to glucose metabolism, namely, INSR and especially its variant INS-B mRNA, was found to increase after weight loss and it was negatively correlated with the circulating insulin concentration (4).

To this end, it is evident that studying the effects of whole grains on gene expression and genetic activity would greatly complement our view of health effects of cereal products. Especially the effect on epigenetic activity (5) has huge potential for example of examining the effects of whole grain consumption in humans, from uterus until late ages. However, the studies investigating the health effects of whole grain at the genetic level are scarce, and thus far have mostly applied transcriptomics with microarray technology as the only method. One has to keep in mind, that if effects of dietary factors are studied along with weight reduction, the effects contributed by the diet is hard, maybe even impossible, to dissect among the effects due to weight reduction (6, 7). Thus, genetic and other effects caused by the diet should be studied in subjects on isocaloric diets.

20.3 Effects of whole grains on gene expression

The main interest in studies concerning the genetic response to the diet in humans, has been in the effects of the various dietary fatty acids or diets used to lose weight. To the best of my knowledge, there is only one study that has applied the transcriptomic approach to study the effects of whole grain and refined-rye products on the gene expression in adipose tissue (8). Adipose tissue is an interesting target tissue to be studied within dietary interventions due to its active role in glucose and lipid metabolism as well as in the development of low-grade inflammation preceding chronic diseases such as cardiovascular disease, type 2 diabetes and certain cancers. Adipose tissue is also one of the peripheral insulin sensitive tissues, where insulin regulates its basic function: storing the fatty acids. Moreover, adipose tissue as such is relatively easy to obtain during the dietary interventions, since subcutaneous adipose tissue samples are easy to gather by needle biopsy before and after the intervention. Another tissue, widely used in dietary interventions, and lately, also in postprandial studies, is peripheral blood mononuclear cells. However, this cell population has not yet been studied in the context of health effects of whole grains.

Kallio et al. (8) performed a study where rye (25% of the energy intake) and pasta (5% of the energy intake) containing diets were compared to wheat (25% of the energy intake) and potato (5% of the energy intake) containing diets in a 12-week long isocaloric dietary intervention in participants with symptoms associated with the metabolic syndrome. The biopsies of subcutaneous adipose tissue samples were collected during fasting conditions in the beginning and in the end of the intervention. It was found that the first phase insulin secretion was decreased, in participants with decreased glucose tolerance, after a 12-week rye and pasta diet. This improvement is especially important as it reduces the risk of progressing into type 2 diabetes within this particular risk group. Along with this finding it was shown that the expression of the genes related to insulin signaling and apoptosis were down-regulated in response to the rye and pasta containing diet. The reduction in expression of apoptosis-related genes has been reported to be mainly an effect of weight reduction (9). However, in the here discussed study, waist circumference of the same group decreased without weight loss during the intervention, thus supporting a rye-specific effect on apoptosis-related genes.

Regarding the down-regulated expression of insulin signaling related genes, it was speculated that this finding was based on the improved first phase insulin secretion due to repeated lower postprandial insulin responses caused by the rye containing diet. The gene TCF7L2, known as bearer of a strong risk variant for type 2 diabetes, and the insulin receptor gene were down-regulated in the adipose tissue along the rye containing diet. The beneficial postprandial glucose metabolism may have decreased the demand for receptor binding, and thereby a down-regulation of the insulin receptor and TCF7L2 expression. The intervention diet may have improved the insulin sensitivity within the adipose tissue, partly resulting in the decrease in the expression of these genes. Marked changes in the expression of genes were found also in the group on wheat and potato diets (8). It was observed that the expression of inflammation-related genes was increased. It was speculated that the large postprandial fluctuations in the glucose and insulin concentration may have caused increase acute inflammation after the meals that may have induced the increase of these genes in this group. These findings lead to further analyses of the inflammation response (10). It was found that the concentrations of free fatty acids and adrenaline increased postprandially probably due to a dramatic decrease in glucose concentration. Moreover, the increase of low-grade inflammation in the wheat and potato containing diet group was also confirmed by the increase of the circulating interleukin 6 and interleukin 10, the latter indicating also the physiological need for compensation of the inflammation via anti-inflammatory activity (10).

20.4 Conclusion

The main findings of the studies (8, 10) showed that the diet rich in rye improved the first phase insulin secretion along the beneficial changes in the genetic function within adipose tissue, which most probably was due to the beneficial changes in the postprandial metabolism. On the other hand, the study showed new, unexpected effects of the diet rich in wheat that increased inflammatory gene expression at the tissue and body level, which again, was most probably due to the changes in the postprandial metabolism. These findings were based on genetic effects of diets rich in cereals in a population with high risk of chronic diseases and underlines the great potential of applying transcriptomics when studying the health effects of cereal diets, exposing both beneficial and non-beneficial effects. More advanced techniques such as RNA sequencing may potentially add value to clinical dietary interventions based on transcriptomics, but may require combined efforts in large international consortia to overcome the high costs.

20.5 References

1 Cancello R, Henegar C, Viguerie N, Taleb S, Poitou C, Rouault C, Coupaye M, Pelloux V, Hugol D, Bouillot JL, et al. Reduction of macrophage infiltration and chemoattractant gene expression changes in white adipose tissue of morbidly obese subjects after surgery-induced weight loss. *Diabetes* 2005;54:2277–86.

2 Martin JA, Wang Z. Next-generation transcriptome assembly. *Nat Rev Genet* 2011;12:671–82.
3 Kaminska D, Pihlajamaki J. Regulation of alternative splicing in obesity and weight loss. *Adipocyte* 2013;2:143–7.
4 Kaminska D, Hamalainen M, Cederberg H, Kakela P, Venesmaa S, Miettinen P, Ilves I, Herzig KH, Kolehmainen M, Karhunen L, et al. Adipose tissue INSR splicing in humans associates with fasting insulin level and is regulated by weight loss. *Diabetologia* 2014;57:347–51.
5 de Mello VD, Pulkkinen L, Lalli M, Kolehmainen M, Pihlajamaki J, Uusitupa M. DNA methylation in obesity and type 2 diabetes. *Ann Med* 2014;46:103–13.
6 Dahlman I, Forsgren M, Sjogren A, Nordstrom EA, Kaaman M, Naslund E, Attersand A, Arner P. Downregulation of electron transport chain genes in visceral adipose tissue in type 2 diabetes independent of obesity and possibly involving tumor necrosis factor-alpha. *Diabetes* 2006;55:1792–9.
7 Harris Jackson K, West SG, Vanden Heuvel JP, Jonnalagadda SS, Ross AB, Hill AM, Grieger JA, Lemieux SK, Kris-Etherton PM. Effects of whole and refined grains in a weight-loss diet on markers of metabolic syndrome in individuals with increased waist circumference: a randomized controlled-feeding trial. *Am J Clin Nutr* 2014;100:577–86.
8 Kallio P, Kolehmainen M, Laaksonen DE, Kekalainen J, Salopuro T, Sivenius K, Pulkkinen L, Mykkanen HM, Niskanen L, Uusitupa M, et al. Dietary carbohydrate modification induces alterations in gene expression in abdominal subcutaneous adipose tissue in persons with the metabolic syndrome: the FUNGENUT Study. *Am J Clin Nutr* 2007;85:1417–27.
9 Kolehmainen M, Salopuro T, Schwab US, Kekalainen J, Kallio P, Laaksonen DE, Pulkkinen L, Lindi VI, Sivenius K, Mager U, et al. Weight reduction modulates expression of genes involved in extracellular matrix and cell death: the GENOBIN study. *Int J Obes (Lond)* 2008;32:292–303.
10 Kallio P, Kolehmainen M, Laaksonen DE, Pulkkinen L, Atalay M, Mykkanen H, Uusitupa M, Poutanen K, Niskanen L. Inflammation markers are modulated by responses to diets differing in postprandial insulin responses in individuals with the metabolic syndrome. *Am J Clin Nutr* 2008;87:1497–503.

21 Whole Grains from an Industry Perspective

Frank Thielecke[1] and Wolfgang Bindzus[2]

[1]Thielecke Consulting, Bettenstrasse, Allschwil, Switzerland
[2]Cereal Partners Worldwide S.A., Orbe, Switzerland

21.1 Introduction

Until the nineteenth century, grains were commonly eaten as whole grains. Advances in the milling and processing of grains allowed large-scale separation and removal of the bran and germ, resulting in refined flour that consists primarily of the endosperm, which offers advantages with regard to processing and stability [1]. At that time, refined flours were the preferred choice among consumers. In more recent years, food manufacturers have developed an increasing number of new food products and reformulated existing products with increased levels of whole grains to meet increasing consumer demands for healthy products. For example, a recent survey has shown that 43% of consumers in the United Kingdom say they look to buy food that contains whole grain. Further, in Brazil, 25% of consumers state that they would like to eat more products containing whole grain (Mintel report 2018). A recent survey conducted by the Swedish Bread institute confirms these trends (United Minds 2017), as half (51%) of the 1015 respondents replied to intent to eat more whole grain products in order to eat healthier. Further, on average, 66% agreed with the claim that whole grains increase saturation, 76% of older people agreed that whole grains improve bowel health. These data show that consumers look to whole grain foods as more nutritious and healthy choice of eating and also make certain associations with health benefits of whole grains.

21.2 Whole grains in foods

Over the last decades, evidence from nutrition research suggests that consuming whole grains is associated with several health benefits. In addition, sustainable diets have gained considerable attention in food and nutrition debates, finding, for example, its way into a report from the advisory committee of the 2015 Dietary guideline for Americans. The guideline states that

> meeting current and future food needs will depend on two concurrent approaches: altering individual and population dietary choices and patterns and developing agricultural and production practices that reduce environmental impacts and conserve resources, while still meeting food and nutrition needs.

Globally, grains are the most important food source, providing about 50% of the total energy consumed [2]. Plant-based diets featuring whole grains are widely recognized as sustainable, certain grains like millet and teff use less water, whole grains support better

Whole Grains and Health, Second Edition. Edited by Rikard Landberg and Nathalie Scheers.

Additional materials available for download online at https://www.wiley.com/en-gb/Whole+Grains+and+Health-p-9781118939437

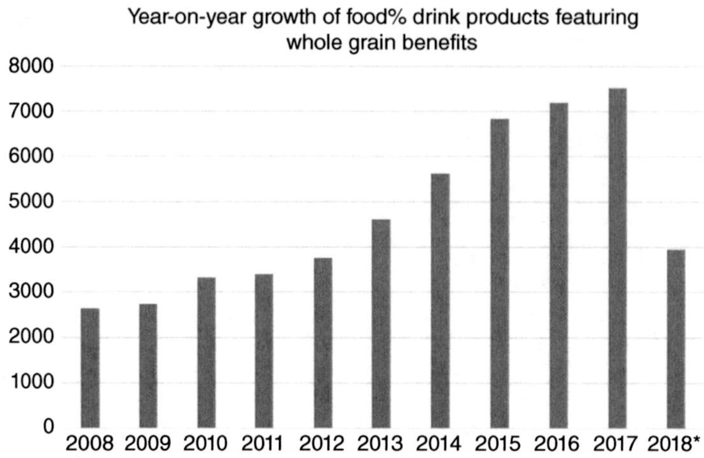

Figure 21.1 Growth of food and drink products featuring whole grain benefits. (Source: Mintel GNPD). *Data until July 2018.

land use and result in more food compared to refined grain [3]. The preceding information and the desire to offer healthy food products motivate food manufacturers to increase the use whole grain in grain-based food products. Consequently, there appears to be a continuing trend to add whole grain claims to product labels globally, as indicated by the increase in the number of new-product launches over time (see Figure 21.1).

When taking a closer look at, for example, the year 2014, the growth in food products featuring whole grains was mainly driven by bakery (1970 product launches) and breakfast cereals (1691 product launches) followed by snacks (864 product launches) and side dishes (512 product launches). While the average growth in terms of new-product launches with whole grain claims during the 2012–2014 period globally was 8.61%, the emerging markets picked up on the trend; they now lead the growth in launches ranging from 20% in India to 190% in Indonesia (Mintel GNPD). In principle, this trend continued over the following years, slightly alleviated in its trend line. Further, retail sales of whole grain products in many markets outperformed their refined grain alternatives. Mintel estimated for the United States, the sales of whole grain bakery and breakfast cereals products demonstrate consistently higher sales as refined-grain counterparts. Similar developments are seen in Europe, where the development of whole grain new-product lines contributes significantly to retail sales (see Table 21.1).

The constantly rising number of food products containing whole grain with consistently improving quality has been enabled by a combination of innovations and new discoveries in the grain breeding and milling industries, food recipe development and manufacturing as well as in food and nutrition sciences. These innovative solutions lead to whole grain food products with improved eating quality, shelf stability, food safety and nutritional value. In this chapter, we categorize whole grain containing foods in those with long established history, for example, whole grain breads or staple whole grain breakfast cereals and in those where whole grain is either a new raw material in the recipe, for example, pasta or where the whole grain content is significantly increased, for example, breakfast cereals. In whole grain foods with an established history, the manufacturing processes are well developed, and product identity and

Table 21.1 Average weekly sales (AWS) of bakery and breakfast cereals new launches* (Data: 2015 to July 2018).

Country	All products AWS	All products SKUs	Whole grain AWS	Whole grain SKUs
Spain	€5,438	656	€9,852	80
France	€8,277	883	€14,153	103
Italy	€7,325	704	€17,234	90
Germany	€7,947	940	€10,074	108
Netherlands	€3,664	355	€7,038	76

*New products and new variants only.
Source: Mintel Iris.

product benefits are well known and accepted by consumers. This is not necessarily the case for foods where whole grains are new ingredients in the recipe, in most cases, replacing previously used refined flours. Hence, the discussion about opportunities and challenges for using whole grains in manufactured foods will primarily focus on this second category.

The replacement of refined grains with whole grains in existing recipes or the development of innovative new whole grain foods introduces a number of challenges. The main ones are:

1. Product quality changes;
2. Product consistency; and
3. Production efficiency.

For example, challenges in product quality may include undesired off-flavors, undesired texture attributes or a potential reduction in shelf life. Although the challenges in whole grain food manufacturing may appear complex, we discuss examples that aim to illustrate how advancements in food science, food technology development and product innovation have established, and continue to develop, a diverse range of applicable solutions. These solutions may be based on whole grain selection, whole grain processing and pre-treatments, recipe modulations, process design changes, process parameter adjustments or a combination thereof. The predominant angle of this review focuses on the breakfast cereals category, but the underlying principles are likely to be applicable to various food categories.

21.3 Whole grain raw materials

Whole grains, as defined by AACCI and HealthGrain Forum contain a common group of macro components, namely, starch, protein, fibre and lipids [4, 5]. In addition, whole grains contain a number of bioactive compounds such as vitamins, minerals and a range of phytochemicals [6]. It is important to note that different whole grains show significant differences in composition of these macro and micro components, and understanding these differences is important for food manufacturing, food quality and nutrition compositions for foods containing whole grains. For example, whole grains may show significant differences in the relative proportions of these macro components as well as significant structural differences in any of the macro compositions, in particular, in the starch and protein fractions. The starch composition in whole grains hold different ratios of amylose and amylopectin, and the starch granule itself exhibits morphological differences in size and shape as well as differences in type and level of crystallinity. These differences in composition and structure were subject to extensive research in wheat, maize, rice, oat, barley and rye, but are less well understood for ancient whole grains such as amaranth, quinoa, millet and others. The traditional research approach has looked at compositional analysis, structure analysis and structure models as well as links to functional properties. Modern analysis establishes links between grain genome and grain composition [7]. Table 21.2 illustrates the variability in the chemical composition of grains.

In this context, it is important to highlight that these are average values, and that actual values for individual whole grain varieties may differ significantly. This is, in particular, the case for varieties that are developed through breeding programs with targets of, for example, high levels of protein or high levels of fibre. Moreover, a certain level of variability is inherent to any grain and is influenced by genetic factors and a number of environmental factors [10]. Environmental factors include soil quality, use and type of fertilizer as well as weather conditions during growth and time of harvest. Furthermore, storage conditions before and after milling may impact changes in composition due to enzyme activity in grains and presence of microorganisms. The inherent variability in whole grains is an important consideration for food manufacturers as it may impact processability of the recipe, quality of the manufactured food, and also it's nutritional value. As food manufacturers continue to develop and manufacture more products with whole grain all across the world, it is important to continue to build knowledge that helps to control the impact of whole grain variability in food processing and on food product attributes. A significant contribution to understanding variability of macro- and micro components in whole grains came from the Diversity Screen research that was conducted within the frame of the EU HealthGrain project [11, 12]. This data helps to estimate the impact of genetic versus environmental factors on variability in grain composition and, in particular, on variability in a range of selected bioactive compounds in grains. Based on the wide diversity in grain composition and structural differences in the macro components, whole grains behave differently in food processing and show significant variety in functional and nutritional properties in finished foods. However, in order to simplify, we review the functional properties of whole grains in manufactured foods by focusing on the main structural changes,

Table 21.2 Composition of cereal grains (g/100 g, average values).

	Wheat	Rye	Corn	Barley	Oats	Rice
Moisture	12.6	13.6	11.3	12.1	13.1	13.0
Protein (Nx6.25)	11.3	9.4	8.8	11.1	10.8	7.7
Lipids	1.8	1.7	3.8	2.1	7.2	2.2
Available carbohydrates	59.4	60.3	65.0	62.7	56.2	73.7
Fibres	13.2	13.1	9.8	9.7	9.8	2.2
Minerals	1.7	1.9	1.3	2.3	2.9	1.2

Sources: [8, 9].

which happen as a result of common processing conditions. The main structural and chemical changes in grain compositions include:

- Starch gelatinization;
- Protein denaturing;
- Maillard reactions;
- Lipid oxidations; and
- Molecular degradation in starch or protein polymers (under certain high-shear conditions).

The extent of these structural and chemical changes depends on properties of the grain composition, recipe parameters and process conditions. For example, starch gelatinization is mainly driven by process temperature and water level in the recipe, but also depends on the inherent starch gelatinization temperature in the grain type and on recipe ingredients that impact the availability of free water. Such ingredients are fibre, sugar or added proteins. While each food recipe and food process design has its unique set of crucial parameters that influence these structural changes, it is of general importance to consider the impact of available moisture and thermal exposure because both parameters have direct or indirect impact on essentially all structural changes previously listed.

21.3.1 Dry milling

In addition to the assessment of the whole grain composition, it is also important to look at grain dry milling and how this process impacts whole grain raw material properties and their functionality in food processing and finished products. The dry milling industry has developed a number of different methods to produce milled whole grain products.

As shown in Table 21.3 for dry milled products from wheat, a milled whole grain product may be classified by its particle size range. Dry-milled wheat products range from large particle size products such as *cracked wheat* (>1 mm) to small particle size products such as *whole grain flour*, which has typically a particle size below 0.018 mm, or even *ultra-fine whole grain flour* with even smaller particle size. In addition to describing milled whole grain products by their particle size, we like to mention that there are alternative ways to describe milled whole grain products. Examples are to describe or identify milled whole grain products by its milling method with consumer-focused descriptions such as *stone milled whole grain flour* or technical descriptions such as *roller milled and heat-stabilized whole grain flour*.

Table 21.3 Particle size of dry-milled product produced from wheat.

Product	Particle Size (μm)
Groats	>1000
Semolina, coarse	600–1000
Semolina, fine	300–600
Flour	< 180

Source [13].

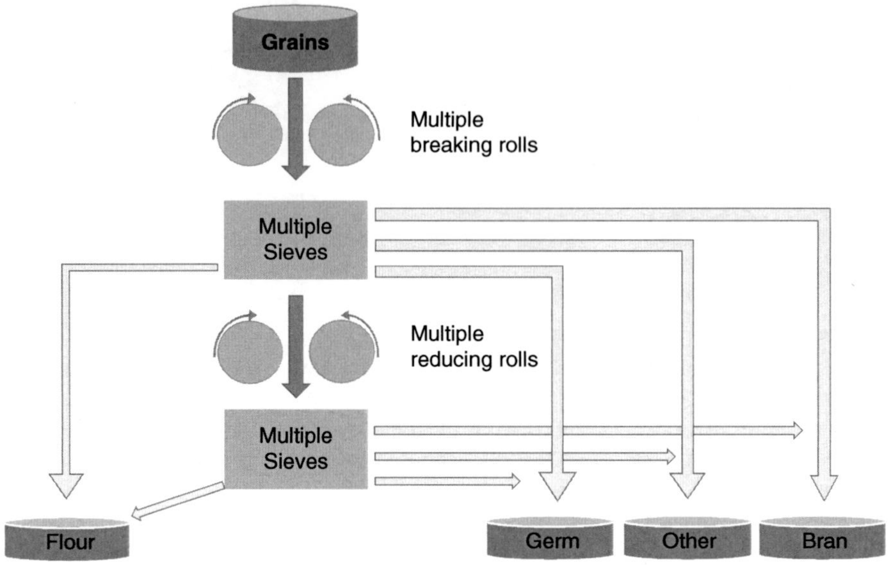

Figure 21.2 Simplified diagram of the Roller milling process.

21.3.2 Milling techniques

The most common dry milling methods for whole grains are roller milling, hammer milling or traditional stone milling. Over many decades, the dry milling industry has developed and optimized roller milling process designs for the production of refined dry-milled grain products, but the process is also suitable for the production of milled whole grain products, provided the milled grain portions are re-combined.

Based on worldwide available milling capacity, roller milling (see Figure 21.2) represents today the main process used for dry milling of whole grain flours [14]. This milling technique enables control of grain fraction separation and particle size control, therefore it became the preferred method to produce refined flours and milling side stream fractions (bran, germ) with the highest purity and greatest control of particle size.

The roller milling process design consists of multiple milling and separation stages. In a simplified view, each stage consists of pairs of milling rolls followed by a separation steps, mainly based on particle size or density. The separated fractions flow to downstream milling and separation stages or are re-introduced in upstream process steps. The process design and flow enable stepwise reductions in particle size and controlled separation as well as re-combination of individual milling streams in the overall process flow. Furthermore, the milling process between two counter-rotating rolls offers a high degree of control via various process parameters. The roller surface designs (see Figure 21.3) can be tailored to favor mechanical actions of pressure, shear or cut, the distance between the rolls can be varied and the speed or differential speed between the rolls can be controlled [14].

Compared to the traditional stone milling process or the alternative, more modern, hammer milling process, the roller milling process design offers the highest level of control in terms of particle size distribution and energy input into the milled-grain particles. In addition, this process separates and re-combines milling streams along the process flow and enables, if needed, additional treatments of selected milling streams. For example, it is

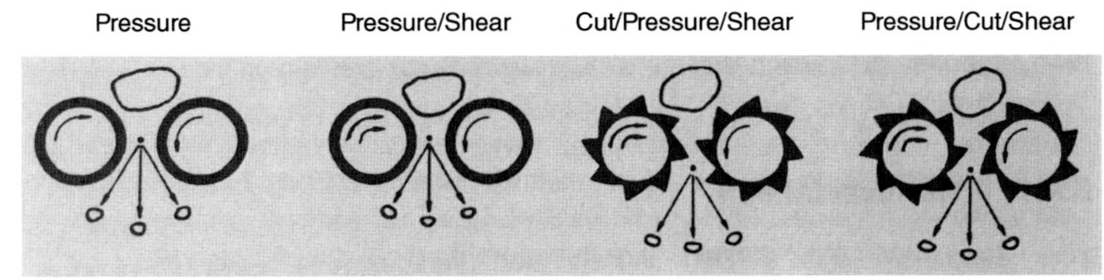

Figure 21.3 Mechanical actions in roller milling as functions of roller surface design and speed.

possible to treat the bran-rich milling stream with additional milling steps and achieve a product with small particle size fibre [15, 16]. Another example would be to apply a heat treatment to the germ-rich milling stream to achieve whole grain flour with increased stability. The stone milling process represents one of the oldest methods of whole grain flour milling (see Figure 21.4). In this process, the grain is milled in one passage between one fixed and one revolving stone. The main process and product quality control parameters are the gap between the stones, the speed of the rotating stone and the grain throughput.

Compared to roller milling process designs, the stone milling process has the disadvantages to mill grains at much lower throughput and to produce a milled product with wider particle size distribution and less uniform treatment. This introduces higher risk of heat-induced damage to fractions of the flour that may impact flour quality criteria. The hammer milling process is a more modern process that also mills grain kernels in one passage without separation. In this process, particle size is mainly controlled by the size of the screen in the hammer mill, but also impacted by other process parameters such as mill speed and throughput. The size as well as the uniformity in particle size are important parameters that impact the behavior of the raw material in food processes as well as functionality in finished food products. For example, the size and hardness of a flour particle impacts its hydration kinetics during food processing, which, in turn, influences the kinetics of structural changes of starch gelatinization and protein denaturation. Starch gelatinization and protein denaturation are important for quality and consistency in any grain containing

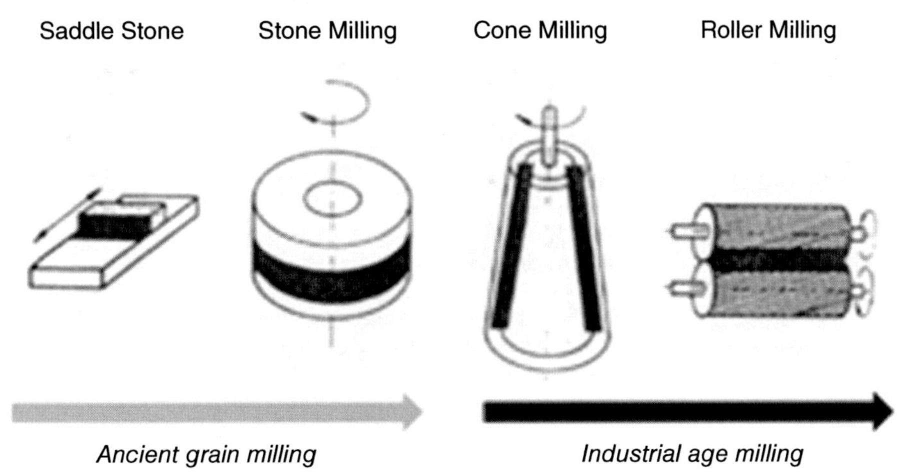

Figure 21.4 History of milling technology.

dough-based product. In general, an increase in particle size and particle hardness results in slower hydration kinetics. Further, a wider particle size distribution leads to a less uniform hydration of the milled grain with small particles having higher hydration and larger particles having less. As the availability of water impacts starch gelatinization, the uniformity of water distribution in the milled grain impacts the degree of gelatinization and uniformity of gelatinization in processed grain products, such as batch-cooked or extruded whole grain breakfast cereals. In most cases, process conditions can be adjusted to the particle size of the flour, but it is more difficult to adjust to and compensate for a wider particle size distribution in milled grains.

In food manufacturing, other important quality criteria are the stability of the whole grain flour during storage and the impact of the flour on the shelf life stability of whole grain–containing foods. In the intact kernels, lipids are predominantly present and protected in the germ, but are also present to a much smaller extend in the bran layers and the endosperm. Milled whole grain products, in particular those with smaller particle size such as whole grain flour have a higher risk of accelerated lipid oxidation through enzymatic or non-enzymatic pathways compared to refined flour. This is because whole grain flours have higher levels of lipids and higher levels of enzyme activity [17]. The milling industry has developed a variety of methods that utilize thermal treatments or combined heat-moisture treatments to minimize enzyme activity, and therefore enhance shelf life stability of milled whole grain flours [18, 19]. However, it is important to point out that the process conditions need to consider secondary effects of the heat or heat/moisture treatment, which could result in partial denaturation of grain proteins or partial gelatinization of the starch fraction in grains. The presence and extend of these structural changes may impact the behavior and performance of whole grain flours in food processing and in finished foods. For example, if the heat treatment leads to partial denaturation of gluten protein in whole grain wheat flour, this would negatively impact the baking quality of the flour. Further, partial starch gelatinization would impact the behavior of flour during cooking processes and may lead to product quality changes.

Whole grain foods contain milled whole grain from various milling processes. Criteria for selecting milled whole grain from a certain milling process for a food recipe include required whole grain flour quality, cost, consumer requirements or availability. For example, if a defined particle size range is required, it may be most suitable to use flour from a roller milling process. An example for how consumer requirements impact the choice of flour may be a product positioned for "traditional food preparation" on the basis of using stone-milled whole grain flour. Regardless of the dry milling method selected, it is important that the method of milling and the process design considers the proposed and accepted definition of whole grain products.

21.4 Whole grains in manufactured foods

In the following section, we describe opportunities and challenges in reformulated foods where whole grains replace traditional use of refined grains in food products or where whole grains are introduced as new ingredient into food recipes. This review considers perspectives from product development, manufacturing and food science. For selective areas, we branch out to emerging developments in research and technology, and attempt an outlook to future opportunities or anticipated challenges that would benefit from future research or cross-functional solutions. In this, we realize that consensus for what defines and qualifies as whole grain food is still under debate. A recent proposal from the

Healthgrain Forum defines *whole grain food products* as food that contains at least 30% whole grain ingredients in the overall product, while the whole grain content must exceed the total amount of refined grains on a dry weight basis. [20] The motivation for this definition was to provide more clarity on whole grain content in food for both consumers as well as manufacturers. As to the latter, it also encourages food manufacturers to replace more refined grains with whole grain ingredients. With respect to the consumers' perception, the labeling and health-related communication presents a significant challenge. A recent survey in Sweden identified potential pitfalls in consumer evaluation of bread [21]. While 844 out of 1134 respondents perceived bread as healthy, this was mainly associated with attributes such "coarse," "whole grain," "fibre-rich," "sourdough" and "rye" to name a few; the authors also described the difficulties of the consumers in identifying healthy breads. This was especially true for consumers with a lower education level.

Over recent years, food manufacturers have identified many opportunities to introduce whole grain–containing foods based on reformulations of products that already exist in the market. These include bread, ready-to-eat breakfast cereals (RTEC), pasta and frozen meals. In most of these cases, whole grains replace refined grains in the respective recipes. The approach for successful reformulation of such products requires at least two fundamental considerations prior to defining a product reformulation strategy:

1. Intended benefit of using whole grain in the food product; and
2. Product quality attributes that are valued by the consumer target group.

The answers to these questions will frame the product reformulation approach, but will also guide the choice of whole grain that can be considered. For example, the desired product benefit could be positioning for a specific health benefit, a specific grain taste or for the use of a locally recognized grain. Another factor that guides, and at the same time, restricts the whole grain choice is an existing standard of identity for a particular food. Food examples *Corn Flakes* breakfast cereals, *Maize Tortilla Chips* or *Rye Bread*. One may assume that the use of a specific type of whole grain may limit the options of a food manufacturer to modify and control desired product attributes. However, based on current knowledge and experience in food science, process technology advancements coupled with an evolving understanding of the behavior of whole grains in various recipe frameworks, a food manufacturer can turn to a number of potential solutions. These include grain variety selection, milling and pre-treatment of the grain, recipe modifications, or changes in process design and process parameters. Examples for pre-treatments of whole grains are to apply a heat treatment to increase the stability of milled grains or germination to change the nutritional profile and taste attributes of grains [22]

21.4.1 Whole grains in traditional breakfast cereals

Corn Flakes are traditionally produced from maize flaking grits that represent a refined part of the maize kernel obtained from the dry milling process. In the traditional *Corn Flakes* process, maize flaking grits are cooked in batch cookers, dried and tempered to a desired moisture that makes the grits suitable for flaking on flaking rolls, followed by toasting and optional coating and drying [23]. The reformulation to a recipe with whole grain corn as the main ingredient is associated with various constraints. First, the traditional batch-cooking process is not well designed for the cooking of whole-maize kernels or a uniform blend of milled whole grain maize. Further, cooked whole-maize kernels are

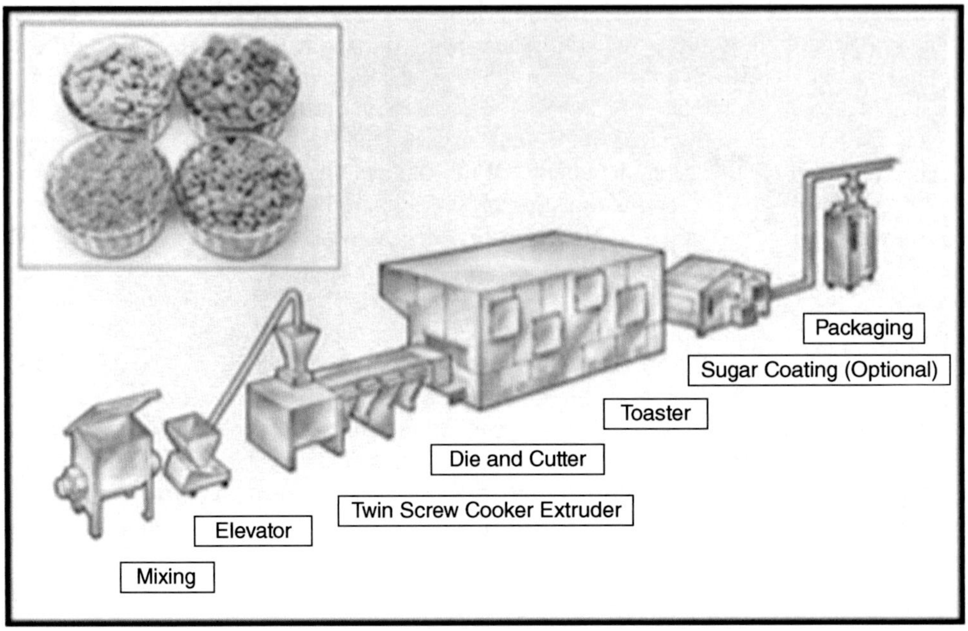

Figure 21.5 Process line for extruded breakfast cereals.

difficult to flake and would produce a product with significantly different appearance, texture and taste when compared to the standard product on the market. A feasible solution is offered by turning to an alternative process design. The breakfast cereal manufacturer can replace the batch-cooking process by extrusion cooking (see Figure 21.5).

This process design change enables the manufacturer to use whole grain corn flour or whole grain corn semolina. The extrusion process forms the cooked dough into pellets that can then be treated similar to batch-cooked flaking grits in the down-stream process of flaking and toasting. In the context of this discussion, we would like to note that process design changes are typically capital intensive, and it is desired to turn first to solutions that utilize grain properties, recipe changes or process parameter adjustments. A secondary challenge in the reformulation of a product with refined-corn flour to a product with whole grain maize is the oil content in the maize kernels. The higher oil content introduces reduced oxidative stability that results in higher rancidity risks, and therefore risk for reduced product shelf life. The manufacturer has at least two common solutions for this. One solution consists of a pre-treatment of the whole grain flour. A heat treatment process can be applied directly after dry milling to minimize enzyme activity in the whole grain maize flour, which, in turn, increases product stability [18, 19]. A second solution is recipe-based. In this case, antioxidants such as tocopherols, citric acid and rosaminic acid can be added to the recipe to minimize fat oxidation in the finished product. Polyphenols that are present in the whole grain, but not or in much lower content in refined grain can potentially increase the stability in the final product. The use of type and levels of antioxidants in a food recipe depends on technical functionality to achieve the desired result as well as food regulations that govern the selected market for the product.

21.5 Whole grains in extruded products

In the following, the relationship between grain compositions and product-quality parameters are discussed for extruded grain-based foods as this platform is a good example for a food manufacturing process that enables the use of a combination of different grains. The process of extrusion cooking of grains and grain components has been studied extensively [24, 25]. A study from Pfaller [26] used a systems-analytical approach to understand the behavior of wheat flours with different degree of milling in the extrusion process and the impact on finished product quality. It was observed that a change from highly refined-wheat flour to a less refined-wheat flour impacts the ability to introduce mechanical energy into the plasticized dough in the extruder. This was attributed to the effects of the flour composition on reduced viscosity in the extruder that is in direct relation to higher fat content and reduced starch content. Furthermore, for the same level of energy input as defined by specific mechanical energy input (SME) and product temperature (PT) into the plasticized dough in the extruder, a change from refined-wheat flour to less refined-flour resulted in reduced expansion and more color development. The expansion behavior of whole grain recipes in extrusion is highly impacted by fibre content and type of fibre [25, 27, 28]. For example, insoluble fibre particles, as present in milled whole grains, reduce expansion and create an expanded foam structure with higher number of small cells and thinner cell walls. This foam structure leads also to a softer texture of the expanded product.

Moreover, the impact of proteins needs to be evaluated, in particular, if the use of whole grains contributes to a significant protein increase in a given recipe. The majority of fibre in grain is classified as insoluble fibre. This is important in this discussion as insoluble and soluble fibre impact expansion and texture properties of extruded foods in different ways [27]. Insoluble fibres such as wheat and maize bran tend to reduce volumetric expansion, reduce bubble size in expanded food structures and increase its bulk density. The reduction in bubble size may go along with a larger number of bubbles in the foam structure and a more uniform bubble size distribution. It is argued that insoluble fibre particles act as nucleation agents and impact the expanded foam structure in the described ways. In most cases, reduced volumetric expansion and higher bulk density result in a harder product texture. However, certain studies observed opposite effects. A study on an extruded cornmeal recipe reported reduced expansion and softer texture with increasing levels of wheat bran [29]. Different findings underline the necessity to assess effects of whole grain compositions on finished product properties in the context of process conditions and other recipe parameters. Therefore, more research is required to fully understand the mechanisms of various fibre types in an extruded direct-expanded dough matrix, in particular, for more complex recipes. The observations from various studies about extrusion cooking of whole grain flours can be put in context to the compositional data shown in Table 21.2 and one can create representative scenarios that illustrate the impact of whole grains and combinations thereof on product quality of extruded foods. For example, whole grain maize has, on average, a higher starch content and lower protein and fibre content as whole grain wheat or whole grain oats. Due to lower fibre and protein levels, an extruded whole grain maize product exhibits a high level of expansion, a foam structure with larger bubbles and more irregular bubble size distribution as well as typically a harder texture. In contrast, an extruded whole grain wheat product compared to whole grain maize, higher fibre levels exhibit a foam structure with smaller bubbles, a more uniform bubble size distribution and usually a softer texture. If these two "extremes" are undesirable product attributes for a consumer, one can assess an optimized blend of these two whole grains that give the desired combination of product attributes. Another important difference between whole grains listed in Table 21.2 is the level of fat content. The level of fat may also impact the foam structure and texture development in extruded whole grain formulations, maybe more importantly, impact risk of rancidity on shelf life of the product. In line with the strategy previously described, one could reduce the shelf life risks in a whole grain oats recipe with partial replacement of whole grain oats with a whole grain with lower fat content. In summary, the examples illustrate that the knowledge about relationships between whole grain compositions and food product attributes can be used to optimize functional properties of whole grain foods through the use of blends of whole grains. In this context, we would like to highlight that this approach has certain limitations if, for example, the objective of using whole grains in a certain food is linked to specific health promoting benefits, obtained from an individual whole grain.

21.6 Sensory characteristics

The sensory attributes of foods, mainly described by taste, texture and appearance, are critical food quality criteria as they influence food choices and consumer purchase decisions. When foods containing refined flours are reformulated with whole grains, one can generally observe that the reformulation to whole grain causes a change in all three sensory dimensions.

Dependent on the taste attributes valued by the consumer target group, the use of whole grains may enhance a desired taste profile or introduce undesired off flavors. Whole grains contain a number of components that contribute directly or indirectly to flavor and taste development in foods. The main components are volatile compounds, phenolic compounds, free amino acids, small peptides and sugars [30]. In addition, lipids and their reaction products, obtained from oxidative and enzyme-catalyzed pathways, contribute to flavor development [31]. For manufactured whole grain–containing foods, it is important to realize that certain taste attributes are impacted directly by flavor components present in whole grains such as aldehydes, alcohols and ketones and other taste attributes are influenced indirectly by flavor precursors that react during food process conditions. These pre-cursors are amino acids, fatty acids, phenolic compounds and reducing sugars [32]. For the class of precursors, the intensity of contributions to flavor development in foods is predominantly driven by Maillard reaction pathways and respective reaction conditions. From a food processing perspective, this means that the flavor development depends predominantly on recipe parameters, exposure to thermal energy and on the level of moisture at respective food-processing steps. For example, conditions used in baking or toasting of foods tend to result in significant flavor development, whereas short-time processing conditions as found in extrusion cooking tend to provide little flavor development.

Whole grain compositions may also introduce undesired flavors. One of the main off-flavors associated with grains is bitterness. It has been shown that the bitter taste is linked to phenolic compounds that are present in grains [32]. For example, in rye, the main phenolic compounds that may contribute to bitter taste are alcylrecorcinols and phenolic acids with the majority being ferulic acid and sinapic acids [32]. These components are primarily located in the bran layers of grain kernels. Recent research on bitterness markers in whole grain wheat bread suggests that processing induced pathways in fermentation and Maillard reaction had significant impact on bitterness-related off-taste in the finished products [33].

Although significant advancements have been made in identification of off-flavor compositions and understanding of reaction pathways, further research is required to understand the complexity of interactions between grain compositions, recipe parameters and food processing as well as the complexity in the interactions between individual flavor compositions in a given food matrix. In addition, processing steps, such as fermentation, and Maillard reaction pathways that contribute to flavor development also play a role in the creation or release of bioactive compounds with potentially health-promoting benefits. Therefore, we suggest that any strategy that aims to optimize taste attributes of whole grains or whole grain foods should take a holistic view and should also assess the impact on bioactive compounds, and, on the contrary, any risks for the creation of process contaminants.

21.7 Whole grains and food safety

Another aspect of manufacturing food, including whole grain foods, is food safety. Potential food safety hazards associated with grains can be classified in physical, chemical and biological hazards [34]. Physical hazards include primarily earth, stones, metal or any other non-edible components that could be introduced to grain batches during harvest, transport or storage prior to milling or food processing. Grain cleaning procedures are designed to minimize these hazards. Chemical hazards in grains are primarily pesticide residues, heavy metals or other chemical compounds absorbed during growth from the soil or environment and mycotoxins that may occur due to presence of fungi on the grain surface. Biological hazards are linked to the presence of bacteria and other microorganisms. There are five mycotoxin types relevant for grains: Deoxynivalenol, zearalenone, ochratoxin, fumonisins and aflatoxins. Most mycotoxins are heat stable, and therefore not inactivated by most food-processing methods. Strategies to minimize risks include good agricultural and manufacturing practices such as dry grain storage and avoidance of grain damage. Furthermore, efforts in grain breeding aim to achieve enhanced fungi resistance [35]. The *whole grain* definition by HealthGrain Forum in the European Union allows removing up to 10% of the outer bran layers from grain kernels. This offers the opportunity to reduce biological or chemical food-safety risks associated with residue, fungi growth or contaminations on the grain surface. As mycotoxins are primarily located on the surface of grain kernels, this may open an opportunity to reduce the mycotoxin risks in whole grains by applying grain-peeling methods that remove the outer bran layers. Regulations ensure that all potential safety hazards are within legal limits.

21.8 Outlook and research needs

We finish this chapter with an outlook on future challenges and opportunities where research and science may help to continue to advance and grow the potential for whole grains in foods and nutritious diets. These areas of future research should focus on enhancing the nutritional value as well as improving the eating quality of whole grain foods, but also tackle questions of sustainability and ensuring high quality supply in grain agriculture.

The nutritional value of whole grain foods is impacted by the whole grain composition, the food recipe ingredients and the manufacturing process. Today, the diverse range of whole grain–containing foods is mirrored by an equally wide range of food-processing platforms. They differ considerably in exposure of whole grain compositions to process conditions described by temperature, pressure, shear and time as well as in key recipe parameters such as moisture and pH. During processing of whole grain–containing recipes, the possible structural changes may impact the macro structure of the grain composition, the polymer structures or even molecular structures. Studies have shown that these food-processing–induced structural changes typically cause a shift from slowly digestible starch to more rapidly digestible starch [36, 37] and also show that food processes with higher energy input increase bioavailability of micronutrients through energy-induced release from a bound, not-bioavailable, structure [38, 39]. In addition, it is known that Maillard reaction pathways lead to diverse range of reaction products, with some of them showing antioxidative properties [40, 41]. These examples illustrate that, dependent on the food manufacturing process and recipe used, whole grain foods may have significantly different properties with different nutrition value and potential health impact. Future research may lead to advanced insights that describe the impact of food processing on nutrition value of whole grain foods and may lead to whole grain food products with optimized nutrition.

It is foundational to the success of any food-product development that these products meet consumer expectations, hence provide superior and consumer accepted sensory properties. We discussed in this review that whole grains may introduce off-tastes such as bitterness, but we believe the full extent of how whole grains impact changes is food taste profiles is not well enough understood. Enhanced understanding about the relationships between processing of whole grain foods and occurrence of off-flavor compounds may enable the development of whole grain foods with more superior taste profiles. Another field with significant potential for nutrition and taste benefits in whole grain foods is the use of "ancient grains." Compared to commonly used grains in food manufacturing, the structural features of ancient grains, their behavior in milling and food processing as well as their properties in finished foods are not well enough known and understood. From a manufacturing perspective, this also includes basic aspects of sourcing, optimum growing conditions and variability of composition and quality criteria in ancient grains. The area of grain agriculture ranging from grain breeding to farming will face significant challenges in the future with needs for sustainable farming practices, or, specifically, the consumer demand for organically grown grains. Further, more visible changes in climate and weather conditions during grain growing cycles are likely to put higher demands on grain breeding and farming practices for consistent quality and yield to meet future demands.

In conclusion, we believe that the collaborative efforts among academia, the grain and food industry as well as food regulatory authorities have and will continue to enable advancements in offering a growing range of healthy and nutritious whole grain food choices to consumers.

21.9 References

1 Cordain, L., et al., *Origins and evolution of the Western diet: Health implications for the 21st century. Am J Clin Nutr*, 2005. 81(2): pp. 341–54.

2 FAO. *Wheat – The largest primary commodity*. 2018. 30.08.2018]; Available from: http://www.fao.org/resources/infographics/infographics-details/en/c/240943/?utm_source=facebook&utm_medium=social+media&utm_campaign=fao+facebook

3 Wholegrainscouncil. *Whole grains: A sustainable food*. 2016. 30.08.2018]; Available from: https://wholegrainscouncil.org/sites/default/files/atoms/files/WG_SustainableFood_infographic.pdf

4 van der Kamp, J.W., et al., *The HealthGrain definition of "whole grain." Food Nutr Res*, 2014. 58.

5 AACCInternational. Whole grains. 29.08.2018]; Available from: http://www.aaccnet.org/initiatives/definitions/pages/wholegrain.aspx

6 Frolich, W., P. Aman, and I. Tetens, *Whole grain foods and health – A Scandinavian perspective. Food Nutr Res*, 2013. 57.

7 Eversole, K., et al., *Slicing the wheat genome. Science*, 2014. 345(6194): pp. 285–7.

8 Souci, S.W.F., W.; Kraut, H., Food Composition and Nutrition Tables, 7th revised and completed edition. 7 ed. 2008. MedPharm Scientific Publishers.

9 Belitz, H.-D.G., W.; Schieberle, P., Cereals and Cereal Products. 2009. Berlin Springer.

10 Shewry, P.R., et al., *Natural variation in grain composition of wheat and related cereals. Journal of Agricultural and Food Chemistry*, 2013. 61(35): pp. 8295–303.

11 Shewry, P.R., et al., *The HealthGrain Wheat Diversity Screen: Effects of genotype and environment on phytochemicals and dietary fiber components. Journal of Agricultural and Food Chemistry*, 2010. 58(17): pp. 9291–8.

12 Ward, J.L., et al., *The HealthGrain Cereal Diversity Screen: Concept, results, and prospects. J Agric Food Chem*, 2008. 56(21): pp. 9699–709.

13 Klingler, R.W., *Grundlagen der Getreidetechnologie*. 2 ed. 2010. Hamburg: Behr's Verlag. 356.

14 Doblado-Maldonado, A.F.P., O.A.; Sweley, J.C.; Rose, D.J., *Key issues and challenges in whole wheat flour milling and storage*. Journal of Cereal Science, 2012. 56(2): pp. 119–26.

15 Mingus, J.W., R; Cox, S.; Schlueter, D.; Woodling, S. *Recombined whole grain having visually indistinguishable particulate matter and related baked products*. US Patents 2006 17.08.2018]; Available from: https://patents.google.com/patent/US20070269579

16 Täufel, A., *Wheat Flour Milling VIII and 341* Food / Nahrung, ed. E.S.H. Posner, A. N. . Vol. 41. 1997. St. Paul, Minnesota, USA: American Association of Cereal Chemistry, Inc. 341.

17 Deora, N.S., *Whole wheat flour stability: An insight. Acta Scientific Nutritional Health*, 2018. 2(3): pp. 8–18.

18 Rose, D.J., et al., *Enhanced lipid stability in whole wheat flour by lipase inactivation and antioxidant retention. Cereal Chemistry*, 2008. 85(2): pp. 218–23.

19 Haynes, L.C., *Production of Stabilized Whole Grain Wheat Flour and Products Thereof*, U. Patent, Editor. 2016. *Kraft Foods Group Inc.: USA.*

20 Ross, A.B., et al., *Perspective: A definition for whole-grain food products – Recommendations from the Healthgrain Forum. Adv Nutr*, 2017. 8(4): pp. 525–31.

21 Sandvik, P., et al., *Consumers' health-related perceptions of bread – Implications for labeling and health communication. Appetite*, 2018. 121: pp. 285–93.

22 Nelson, K., et al., *Germinated grains: A superior whole grain functional food? Can J Physiol Pharmacol*, 2013. 91(6): pp. 429–41.

23 Tegge, G., *Breakfast Cereals and How They Are Made*. Edited by Robert B. Fast and Elwood F. Caldwell. St. Paul, Minnesota (U.S.A.) 1990. 372 pages; 110 illustrations. Hardcover ~79 U.S. Order from American Association of Cereal Chemists, 3340 Pilot Knob Road, St. Paul, Minnesota, 55121, U.S.A. Starch-Stärke, 1990. 42(8): pp. 325–325.

24 Guy, R., Extrusion Cooking. 2001, Cambridge England: Woodhead Publishing Limited.

25 Lue, S.H., F.; Huff, H.E., *Extrusion cooking of corn meal and sugar beet fiber: Effects on expansion properties, starch gelatinization, and dietary fiber content. Cereal Chemistry*, 1991. 68: pp. 227–34.

26 Pfaller, W., *Einfluss der Zusammensetzung von Getreidemahlerzeugnissen und ausgewählten Rezepturen auf das Kochextrusionsverhalten und die Extrudateigenschaften*. 1987. Technical University Berlin: Berlin.27. Robin, F., H.P. Schuchmann, and S. Palzer, *Dietary fiber in extruded cereals: Limitations and opportunities*. Trends in Food Science & Technology, 2012. **28**(1): pp. 23–32.

28 Brennan, M.A., J.A. Monro, and C.S. Brennan, *Effect of inclusion of soluble and insoluble fibres into extruded breakfast cereal products made with reverse screw configuration. International Journal of Food Science & Technology*, 2008. 43(12): pp. 2278–88.

29 Ferreira, R.E.C., Y.K.; Steel, C.J., *Influence of wheat bran addition and of thermoplastic extrusión process parameters on physical properties of corn-based expanded extruded snacks*. Alimentos e nutricao, 2001. 22(4): pp. 507–20.

30 Heiniö, R.L., et al., *Sensory characteristics of wholegrain and bran-rich cereal foods – A review. Trends in Food Science & Technology*, 2016. 47: pp. 25–38.

31 Heiniö, R.L., *Influence of processing on the flavour formation of oat and rye*, In *VTT Biotechnology*. 2003. *Universtiy Helsinki.*

32 Heiniö, R.L.L., K.-H.; Myllymäki, O.; Pihlava, J.-M.; Poutanen, K., *Quantities of phenolic compounds and their impacts on the perceived flavour attributes of rye grain*. Journal of Cereal Science, 2008. 47(3): pp. 566–75.

33 Jiang, D. and D.G. Peterson, Identification of bitter compounds in whole wheat bread. Food Chem, 2013. 141(2): p. 1345–53.

34 Vadivambal, R.J., D.S. , *Food Safety Considerations for Cereal Grains*, in *Food Supplies and Food Safety: Production, Conservation and Population Impact*, M.B. Walsch, Editor. 2010. Nova Science Publisher. pp. 249–266 .35. Jones, J.M., *REVIEW: Regulatory aspects of whole grain and whole grain foods: Definitions and labeling. Cereal Chemistry*, 2010. 87(2): pp. 150–54.

36 Englyst, K.N., et al., *Glycaemic index of cereal products explained by their content of rapidly and slowly available glucose. Br J Nutr*, 2003. 89(3): pp. 329–40.

37 Feng, Y.L., Y., *Effect of specific mechanical energy on in-vitro digestion and physical properties of extruded rice-based snacks*. Food andNutrition *Sciences*, 2014. 5(19).

38 Pekkinen, J., et al., *Disintegration of wheat aleurone structure has an impact on the bioavailability of phenolic compounds and other phytochemicals as evidenced by altered urinary metabolite profile of diet-induced obese mice. Nutr Metab (Lond)*, 2014. 11(1): p. 1.

39 Slavin, J.L., D. Jacobs, and L. Marquart, *Grain processing and nutrition. Crit Rev Food Sci Nutr*, 2000. 40(4): pp. 309–26.

40 Manzocco, L., et al., *Review of non-enzymatic browning and antioxidant capacity in processed foods. Trends in Food Science & Technology*, 2000. 11(9): pp. 340–46.

41 Michalska, A., et al., *Effect of bread making on formation of Maillard reaction products contributing to the overall antioxidant activity of rye bread. Journal of Cereal Science*, 2008. 48(1): pp. 123–32.

22 Global Regulation and Labeling, Claims and Communication with Consumers

Heddie Mejborn[1] and Caroline Sluyter[2]

[1]National Food Institute, Technical University of Denmark, Kgs. Lyngby, Denmark
[2]Oldways Whole Grains Council, Boston, Massachusetts, USA

22.1 Introduction

In many countries worldwide, whole grain food traditions have been forgotten and refined grains have taken their place in the general diet. Consumers are not even always aware that whole grain options exist, and they may not fully understand the nutritional benefits of switching to whole grains. Even if consumers know about whole grains, there may be barriers to the consumption of whole grain foods. Because these barriers are different for various consumer subgroups, it can be complicated changing consumer attitudes towards whole grains. To those unfamiliar with the flavor of whole grains, these foods may be perceived as less tasty than foods made from refined grains. Availability of whole grain food options is a problem in some places, and it can be difficult for consumers to identify whole grain foods, even when the option exists. However, globally there is an increasing interest in whole grains. This is largely due to the fact that the health benefits associated with high whole grain intake are becoming increasingly well understood. Over the past decade or so, many health authorities have moved to include recommendations for increased whole grain intake in their official dietary guidelines.

Despite the growing momentum for whole grains, few countries have defined whole grains and whole grain foods in their legislation. This lack of officially recognized definitions means that industry groups and health organizations are often left to create their own definitions and standards. Whole grains are frequently included as ingredients in compound foods (e.g., breads, crackers, breakfast cereals, etc.), but without clear and consistent labelling it is difficult for consumers to identify which ingredients are whole or determine how much whole grain there is in a serving. Consumers may lose confidence in foods labelled "whole grain" when they cannot be sure whether, and how much, whole grain is actually contained in the food. Without standardized definitions, it's difficult for food producers to communicate with consumers and differentiate their products from those made primarily from refined grain.

These same issues impact the field of nutrition science as well. Since there are many products on the market claiming to be whole grain foods, even if they contain only a small quantity of whole grains, it can be challenging for researchers to accurately measure intake. Establishing an internationally recognized definition of *whole grain foods* and making

Whole Grains and Health, Second Edition. Edited by Rikard Landberg and Nathalie Scheers.

Additional materials available for download online at https://www.wiley.com/en-gb/Whole+Grains+and+Health-p-9781118939437

information about the actual whole grain content of foods available would benefit researchers, food producers and consumers alike (Ferruzzi *et al.* 2014).

22.2 Global regulation on whole grain labelling

In 1999, the American Association of Cereal Chemists International (AACCI) officially defined *whole grains* as follows: "Whole grains shall consist of the intact, ground, cracked or flaked caryopsis, whose principal anatomical components – the starchy endosperm, germ, and bran – are present in the same relative proportions as they exist in the intact caryopsis" (AACCI 1999). This definition applies to all cereal grains and pseudocereals (e.g., quinoa, amaranth, buckwheat). The HealthGrain Forum, a European-based health and science organization, proposed an update to this definition in 2014, in an effort to bring it in line with advances in industrial production practices (van der Kamp *et al.* 2014). This version clarifies that bran, germ and endosperm separated during the milling process may be recombined into whole grain flour as long as the three parts of the grain are recombined in the same relative proportions, as they exist in the intact kernel. It also allows for small losses of grain components (less than 2% of the grain or 10% of the bran) that occur through processing.

These definitions have played a huge role in creating widespread international agreement about what counts as a whole grain, but reaching a consensus about what should count as a whole grain food has been more difficult. An international scientific working group recommended in 2014 that an international standard definition for whole grain foods be adopted with the goal of increasing global whole grain consumption (Ferruzzi *et al.* 2014). The group suggested that any food containing at least 8g of whole grain per 30g of product should count as a whole grain food.

Since this characterization of whole grain foods was released, there has been further international collaboration and debate on this topic. In July 2017, the HealthGrain Forum proposed that whole grain food products should contain at least 30% whole grain ingredients (by dry weight) and that the product should contain more whole grain than refined-grain ingredients (again, by dry weight) in order to be labelled "whole grain" (Ross *et al.* 2017). At the November 2017 Whole Grain Summit in Vienna, it was decided that an International Working Group for Whole Grain Definitions would be convened in an effort to further refine this definition and reach more widespread international consensus. Despite the fact that no governmental regulatory body has legally defined what constitutes a whole grain food, some authorities have an accepted "code of practice" for use of the term *whole grain*, and in some countries, private organizations (e.g., bakers' organizations) have defined whole grain foods. These definitions and codes of practice are established primarily to make it easier for consumers to identify whole grain foods when making purchasing decisions.

22.2.1 Canada

The Canadian Food Inspection Agency (CFIA) has ruled that foods can be labelled "100% whole grain" only when *all* of their ingredients are whole grain. This means that a bag of brown rice could be labelled 100% whole grain, but bread made from whole grain whole-wheat flour, water and salt could not be so labelled because of the presence of water and salt in the ingredients list (Canadian Food Inspection Agency 2018).

In this context, it is also helpful to note a peculiarity of Canadian law under which "whole wheat" flour is allowed to be missing up to 5% of the original kernel. To be sure that they are getting whole grain flour, consumers in Canada must therefore look for the words "whole grain whole-wheat," which would be redundant in most countries (Health Canada 2013).

22.2.2 Europe

22.2.2.1 Germany

In Germany, whole grain guidance exists specifically around the labelling of bread products. "Vollkornbrot" (whole grain bread) must contain at least 90% whole grain flour (Bundesministerium für Ernährung und Landwirtschaft 1994). The criterion applies to both rye bread and wheat bread, including toast bread, and for bread where rye and wheat flour have been mixed.

22.2.2.2 Italy

In Italy, there is whole grain guidance that targets pasta in particular. Pasta made entirely from whole grain ("integrale") flour can be labelled "pasta de semola integrale di grano duro" (Ministero delle politiche agricole alimentari e forestali 1994). However, according to Italian regulations, "integrale" flour does not have to contain the germ portion of the grain, so in Italy "integrale" pasta may not be truly whole grain.

22.2.2.3 The Netherlands

According to Dutch law (De Staatssecretaris van Volksgezondheid, Welzijn en Sport 1998) bread can only be labelled "100% whole grain" if all the flour in the recipe is whole grain. There is no similar law for other cereal products, but the law requires that food labelling not be misleading to consumers. Thus, it is understood that if a product is labelled "whole grain," at least 50% of the cereal part of the product must be whole grain.

22.2.2.4 The Nordic countries

In 2008, the National Food Institute, Technical University of Denmark, published a report in which whole grains and whole grain foods were defined, and a recommendation for whole grain intake was made (Mejborn *et al.* 2008). The National Food Institute suggested that, by definition, whole grains and whole grain flour should be 100% whole grain, and that foods should contain at least 51% whole grain on a dry-weight basis in order to be labelled a "whole grain" product. Calculating the whole grain percentage of a product on a dry-weight basis allows a level playing field for foods with different levels of moisture content – otherwise, food groups with higher water content, such as bread, would have to meet a higher standard than drier foods, like crisp bread or pasta. Most of the Nordic countries (Denmark, Iceland, Norway and Sweden) use the Keyhole label on foods (see Figure 22.1). The Keyhole label is considered a nutrition claim and is meant to help consumers identify healthier food alternatives within more than 20 food groups. Use of the label is voluntary for food manufacturers, and foods carrying the Keyhole label must meet

Figure 22.1 The Nordic Keyhole Label. (Source: The Nordic Council 2018).

certain nutrition standards (see Table 22.1). Food groups that include a grain component, such as cereal foods (e.g., bread and breakfast cereals) and ready-prepared dishes (e.g., sandwiches and pizzas), must meet a certain minimum whole grain content that varies depending on food group. The criteria were notified with the European Commission in 2014 and went into effect in March 2015. These criteria set a minimum fibre content for all cereal food groups as well as a maximum content of total fat, saturated fat, sugars and salt for relevant groups. It is important to note that meeting the whole grain content criteria for the Keyhole label does not necessarily mean the food qualifies as a whole grain food under the Danish National Food Institute's definition.

22.2.2.5 United Kingdom

The Institute of Grocery Distribution (IGD), a private industry organization, recommends that foods wishing to communicate the presence of whole grain, for example, by stating "contains whole grain" or "with whole grain" on packages should contain a minimum of 8g of whole grain per serving (IGD 2007).

22.2.3 The United States of America

While there is no official definition of a whole grain food in the United States, if a food producer wants to make an authorized health claim referring to whole grains, the food must contain at least 51% whole grain (as a % of total weight) and meet other requirements for fat and cholesterol content (FDA 1999, 2003). The American Association of Cereal Chemists International (AACCI), based on work performed by its Whole Grains Working Group, proposed a characterization of a whole grain product, recommending that a whole grain food should contain 8g or more of whole grain per 30g of product. The characterization (which the organization does not consider a definition) was adopted by AACCI's Board of Directors in May 2013. The board states that this level of 8g of whole grains per 30g "strikes a balance, promoting sufficient whole grain to be nutritionally significant and minimally penalizing foods containing whole grains" and reports that the Whole Grains Working Group "thought that expanding the characterization further could dilute its effectiveness" (letter from AACCI to the Whole Grains Council 13 February 2014).

Table 22.1 Nutrient criteria required of whole grain products using the Nordic Keyhole label. (Source: The Nordic Council 2018).

Product	Criteria
Cereal flour, flakes, grains and crushed cereal containing at least 100% whole grain calculated on the basis of the product's dry matter content, also cereal brands and sprouts.	-Minimum fibre 6g/100g
Rice containing at least 100% whole grain calculated on the basis of the product's dry matter content.	-Minimum fibre 3g/100g
Breakfast flakes and muesli containing at least 55% whole grain calculated on the basis of the product's dry matter content. Gluten-free breakfast flakes and muesli shall contain at least 20% whole grain calculated on the basis of the product's dry matter content.	-Maximum fat content 8g/100g -Maximum sugars 13g/100g, of which a maximum of 9g/100g added sugars -Minimum fibre 6g/100g -Maximum salt 1.0g/100g
Porridge and porridge powder prepared in accordance with the manufacturer's instructions, containing at least 55% whole grain calculated on the basis of the product's dry matter content.	-Maximum fat content 4g/100g -Maximum sugars 5g/100g -Minimum fibre 1g/100g -Maximum salt 0.3g/100g (These criteria refer to the products as ready-to-consume products.)
Soft bread and bread mixes where only liquid and yeast are to be added and bread containing a minimum of 30% whole grain calculated on the basis of the product's dry matter content. Gluten-free bread and bread mixes shall contain at least 10% whole grain calculated on the basis of the product's dry matter content.	-Maximum fat content 7g/100g -Maximum sugars 5g/100g -Minimum fibre 5g/100g -Maximum salt 1.0g/100g (These criteria refer to the products as ready-to-consume products.)
Rye bread, bread mixes and other products based on rye, where only liquid and yeast are to be added. The product shall contain at least 35% whole grain, calculated on the basis of the product's dry matter content. The grain element shall contain at least 30% rye.	-Maximum fat content 7g/100g -Maximum sugars 5g/100g -Minimum fibre 6g/100g -Maximum salt 1.2g/100g (These criteria refer to the products as ready-to-consume products.)
Crisp bread and crusts containing at least 50% whole grain calculated on the basis of the product's dry matter content. Gluten-free hard bread and crusts shall contain at least 15% whole grain calculated on the basis of the product's dry matter content.	-Maximum fat content 7g/100g -Maximum sugars 5g/100g -Minimum fibre 6g/100g -Maximum salt 1.3g/100g
Pasta (without filling) containing at least 50% whole grain calculated on the basis of the product's dry matter content. Gluten-free pasta (without filling) has no whole grain requirements.	-Minimum fibre 6g/100g -Maximum salt 0.1g/100g (These criteria refer to the product's dry matter content.)

If the Food and Drug Administration (FDA) were to adopt the AACCI characterization as a definition of a whole grain food, it would mean that foods containing more refined grains than whole grains could qualify as whole grain foods. This has been criticized by the US-based Oldways Whole Grains Council (WGC), which suggests that only foods containing more whole grain than refined grain should be called whole grain foods (letter from WGC to FDA 17 January 2014). As of July 2018, the FDA had not officially defined whole grain foods.

In 2012, the Food and Nutrition Service (FNS) division of the US Department of Agriculture (USDA) released a definition of "whole grain rich" foods as part of its grain requirements for the National School Lunch and School Breakfast Programs (USDA 2012). It defines a whole grain rich food as one where at least 50% of its grain is whole grain.

Although this definition was established for use in national school meals programs, it could also become a standard in other government nutrition programs. Whole grain rich foods must meet one of three requirements: 1) Contain at least 8g of whole grain per serving; or 2) Qualify for the FDA whole grain health claim; or 3) For non-mixed dishes (e.g. breads, cereals), whole grain must be the primary ingredient by weight; for mixed dishes (e.g., pizza, corn dogs), whole grain must be the primary *grain* ingredient by weight (United States Department of Agriculture 2014). In 2016, the FNS adopted this whole grain rich standard for use in its Child and Adult Care Food Program as well (USDA 2016).

The FDA regulates the content of certain foods by establishing a "standard of identity" for them. For example, there is a standard of identity for whole-wheat bread that states exactly which ingredients are allowed in order for a product to be labelled "whole-wheat bread." Note, however, that the standard of identity for whole-wheat bread applies only to breads made with whole-*wheat* flour and not to breads made with other whole grains.

The FDA has established standards of identity for whole-wheat bread, rolls and buns (21 CFR 136.180, CFR 1993a); for whole-wheat macaroni products (21 CFR 139.138, CFR 1993b); for whole-wheat flour/graham flour (21 CFR 137.200, CFR 1993d); and for whole-durum flour (21 CFR 137.225, CFR 1993c). Other standards of identity define terms that describe refined grains. For instance, according to the standard of identity for "wheat flour," this term always refers to refined wheat flour (21 CFR 137.105, CFR 1993e).

22.3 Nutrition and health claims

In an effort to support international trade as well as food safety, the Codex Alimentarius Commission, created by the Food and Agriculture Organization (FAO) and World Health Organization (WHO), has established standard guidelines for nutrition and health claims (2004) that can be used in countries where national standards do not exist. Some countries and governing bodies (e.g., the European Union) have their own definitions and guidance in national legislation that differ from the Codex standards (European Commission 2006).

22.3.1 Nutrition claims

The term *nutrition claim* is defined by Codex as "any representation which states, suggests or implies that a food has particular nutritional properties, including but not limited to the energy value and to the content of protein, fat and carbohydrates, as well as the content of vitamins and minerals." A nutrient content claim "is a nutrition claim that describes the level of a nutrient contained in a food."

Since whole grains are food ingredients and not nutrients, claims on foods referring to their whole grain content are considered by some countries to be ingredient claims, rather than nutrition claims. Some countries allow ingredient claims referring to the level of whole grain in the food ("contains," "high in," "very high in"), while others do not.

22.3.1.1 Australia

The Australian Grains & Legumes Nutrition Council (GLNC) has developed a "Code of Practice for Whole Grain Ingredient Claims" (GLNC 2017). The primary aim of the code is to guide the food industry in providing consumers with clear, consistent messaging on

Table 22.2 Whole grain ingredient claims that can be used in Australia. (Source: Grains & Legumes Nutrition Council 2017).

Claim	Criteria
"Contains whole grain"	Minimum 8g of whole grain per manufacturer-defined serving
"High in whole grain"	Minimum 16g of whole grain per manufacturer-defined serving
"Very high in whole grain"	Minimum 24g of whole grain per manufacturer-defined serving

the whole grain content of foods and to complement existing food standards and consumer protection regulation as Food Standards Australia/New Zealand (FSANZ) do not regulate claims describing the amount of whole grain in foods. The code covers the use of the whole grain Daily Target Intake statement, whole grain ingredient content claims, the GLNC logo, the GLNC certification mark and GLNC certification statements on food packages, and in advertising in Australia and New Zealand. The code includes requirements for whole grain ingredient content claims. Three levels of claims are permissible (see Table 22.2).

To use the claims, a company must become a Registered User of the Code, and each food carrying the claim must be registered with GLNC. The company must provide verification of the food's whole grain content by demonstrating adherence to the recommended calculation of the whole grain content that aligns with the Australia New Zealand Food Standards Code. The code permits use of synonyms for the whole grain ingredient content claims. Instead of "Contains whole grain," companies may state "With whole grain," "Made with whole grain" or "Source of whole grain." As an alternative to "High in whole grain, companies may use "Rich in whole grain" or "Good source of whole grain," and finally, "Very high in whole grain" can be replaced with "Very good source of whole grain," "Excellent source of whole grain" or "Great source of whole grain." Alternatively, factual statements about whole grain content in grams or as a percentage of the finished food are permitted, for example, "Made with 67% whole grain." To carry these statements of whole grain content, a food must contain at least 8g of whole grain per serving. Products that are registered with GLNC can be searched in its online database.

A special GLNC certification can be obtained for food products that are core foods according to Australian Dietary Guidelines and are either "high in" or "very high in" whole grain and that are considered healthier choices within the relevant categories. To promote this message, a food may only carry the GLNC logo or certification statement if it meets specific nutrient criteria via the Nutrient Profile Scoring Calculator (NPSC) developed by FSANZ to identify healthier food choices. Verification of whole grain content and proof of the NPSC must be provided. Cereal foods that may carry the GLNC logo or certification statement are: whole grains, milled grains, breads, breakfast cereals, crisp breads, English muffins, crumpets, scones, noodles, pasta, semolina and couscous. Cereal foods for which the GLNC logo or certification statement is not permitted, but which may carry a whole grain ingredient content claim or the DTI statement are: muesli bars, rice cakes, rice crackers, grain-based chips, cakes/muffins/sweet buns, sweet biscuits, spring rolls/dim sums/chiko rolls, pies/pastries/pizzas/burgers, burritos/enchiladas/nachos, pancakes/pikelets/crepes/waffles and doughnuts.

22.3.1.2 Europe

Within the European Union, the expression "Contains whole grain" is considered an ingredient claim, at least in some European countries. The approved nutrition claims "Contains [Name of the nutrient or other substance]" cannot be used for whole grain since it can only be used for "nutrients and other substances," not for food ingredients (European Commission 2006). The nutrition claims "source of" and "high in" can only be used for compounds listed as nutrients in the Nutrition and Health Claim Regulation (EC) 1924/2006 such as dietary fibre, vitamins and minerals. Instead, factual statements such as "Made with whole grain", "X% whole grain" and "Xg whole grain per serving" can be used as long as they are true and not misleading to the consumer. The latter means that foods carrying the claim should contain a certain minimum amount of whole grain, but it is left up to each individual European country to decide what that minimum amount of whole grain should be.

22.3.1.3 The United States of America

In the United States, it is legal to use factual statements about whole grain content on the label of foods. For example, a manufacturer can claim a product is "100% whole grain" when all the grain in the product is whole grain. Similarly, a package can state the amount of whole grain in the product by claiming "10g of whole grain" (FDA 2006). Manufacturers are not allowed to imply a particular level of the ingredient, however, (e.g., "high" or "excellent source").

22.3.2 Health claims

A health claim is any statement included on the packaging or in the representation of a food or beverage product that says consumption of that food, or an ingredient in that food, provides (or may provide) a particular health benefit. In many countries, these statements are carefully regulated by government and health organizations and must be supported by substantial, credible scientific evidence. In order to qualify for health claims, foods are often required to meet nutrient content level requirements. The claims permitted and the criteria required vary widely from country to country.

22.3.2.1 Canada

Health Canada has accepted a health claim for oat and barley products containing beta-glucan and their cholesterol-lowering effect. Foods that contain at least 1g of beta-glucan from barley, or at least 0.75g of beta-glucan from oats per serving, and which meet several other nutrient requirements for cholesterol, sodium, fat, and so on may use the following health claim. "[Serving size from Nutrition Facts table in metric and common household measures] of (Brand name) [name of food] [with name of eligible fibre source] supplies/provides X% of the daily amount of the fibre shown to help reduce/lower cholesterol" (Government of Canada 2010, 2012).

Based on a systematic review, Health Canada (2012) concluded that the evidence to date from clinical trials and prospective cohort studies was not sufficient to support a whole grains and coronary heart disease risk reduction claim in Canada. The review found an overall effect of whole grains on total and LDL cholesterol when the results from controlled clinical trials were pooled, but sensitivity analysis showed that the effect was largely attributable to trials that tested single grains high in beta-glucan fibre and trials judged to be of poor quality. It was concluded that cholesterol-lowering effects caused by grains high in beta-glucan fibre cannot be generalized to other grains, including wheat, the predominant grain consumed in Canada. Therefore, a whole grain and coronary heart disease health claim would be misleading if applied to grains that are not high in beta-glucan fibre.

22.3.2.2 Europe

In the European Union, health claims for dietary fibres from specific grains – namely, oat grain fibre, barley grain fibre, rye fibre and wheat bran fibre – have been approved by the European Commission (2012) but no health claim on whole grains as such has been approved. This is partly because the commission has not defined whole grain, and partly because different varieties of whole grains have shown differential health effects. Thus, scientific substantiations have only been accepted for specific grain fibres. According to the European Food Safety Authority (EFSA) (2010), the food constituent "whole grain," which was the subject of several health claim applications, is not sufficiently characterized in relation to the claimed effects, and therefore it was not possible to perform a scientific evaluation of the documentation related to the health effects stated in the claims.

22.3.2.3 Singapore

In Singapore, the Agri-Food and Veterinary Authority regulates health claims on food products. There are a few health claims relating to the whole grain content of foods.

Whole grain foods that meet requirements for fat and fibre may use the following health claim (Agri-Food and Veterinary Authority 2017): "A healthy diet rich in whole grains, fruits, and vegetables that contain dietary fibre, may reduce the risk of heart disease. [Name of food] is low/free of fat and high in dietary fibre." Similarly, whole grain foods meeting specific standards for fat, fibre and sodium content may state (Agri-Food and Veterinary Authority 2017): "A healthy diet rich in fibre containing foods such as whole grains, fruits and vegetables may reduce the risk of some types of cancers. [Name of food] is free/low in fat and high in dietary fibre." Convenience meals (i.e., sandwiches, ready-to-eat rice-based meals, instant noodles, frozen pizzas, etc.) that meet certain criteria for calorie, fat, sodium and whole grain content can qualify as "Higher in whole grains," which, in turn, makes them eligible to include the following health claim on their packaging (Health Promotion Board 2018): "Whole grains are [an] essential part of a nutritious diet. As whole grains contain all parts of the grain (germ, bran and endosperm), [they are] healthier than refined grains."

In order to use this health claim or label a product as "Higher in whole grains," manufacturers must additionally include a declaration of the whole grain content in the product's ingredients list. For example, a compliant ingredients list might say, "Rice (20% brown rice), fish, cheese, salt, flavoring." The package must also include a statement expressing the amount of whole grain per serving as a percent of the 50g/day whole grain requirement established by the Health Promotion Board (e.g., "1 serving of [name of product] provides [x]g of whole grain, which meets [x%] of your daily whole grain requirement").

22.3.2.4 The United States of America

In the United States, the FDA regulates health claims in the labelling of food products under the Nutrition Labeling and Education Act of 1990. Health claims must be "complete, truthful, and not misleading" and must "enable the public to comprehend the information provided and to understand the relative significance of such information in the context of a total daily diet" (FDA 2017). There are a few health claims referring to grains and whole grains that are allowed under FDA.

Health claims regulated by the FDA fall into three categories:

1. Claims that meet significant scientific agreement (SSA) among experts that the diet-disease relationship purported by the health claim is supported by the totality of publicly available evidence;
2. Claims under the 1997 Food and Drug Administration Modernization Act (FDAMA), which further defined acceptable processes for making health claims by referring to an authoritative statement or document from an established and reputable scientific body; and
3. Qualified Health Claims, designed for claims based on emerging science that do not yet meet the SSA standard; these are given qualifying language to reflect the limitations in existing evidence.

There are two SSA claims that relate to fibre-containing foods, including grains (see Table 22.3). In order to use either of these claims, a food must qualify as a good source of fibre (without fortification) and must be low in fat. Additionally, SSA health claims for dietary fibres from specific whole grains (namely, oats and barley) have been approved. Under FDAMA, two whole grain health claims have been established (see Table 22.3). The first, in 1999, allowed a health claim to be used on foods in which 51% or more of the total weight is made up of whole grain ingredients, as long as the food also meets other requirements for fibre content, fat content, and so on. (See Table 22.3). This original whole grain health claim required that products be low in both total fat and saturated fat. In 2003, a modified whole grain health claim was allowed under the FDAMA process, so that foods moderate in total fat – but still low in saturated fat – could use the whole grain health claim. The approved claims do not specify which whole grains are subject of the claims. Some grains that are naturally lower in fibre were originally thought not to qualify for these two FDA whole grain health claims. Brown rice, for example, does not meet the levels of fibre shown in Table 22.3. In May 2008, the FDA clarified that its requirement for a fibre "marker" was necessary only in products where the whole grain nature of the food would otherwise be uncertain; single-ingredient foods like brown rice that meet FDA's definition of *whole grain* can indeed use the whole grain health claim. To date, only one qualified claim has been approved by the FDA in reference to whole grains. In September 2013, the FDA ruled that it would allow a qualified claim for whole grains and diabetes. However, based on FDA's consideration of the scientific evidence submitted with the petition and other pertinent evidence, the FDA concluded that there is very limited scientific evidence for the claim. Thus, in order not to mislead consumers, the FDA considered this wording for the claim acceptable: "Whole grains may reduce the risk of type 2 diabetes, although the FDA has concluded that there is very limited scientific evidence for this claim," or "Whole grains may reduce the risk of type 2 diabetes. FDA has concluded that there is very limited scientific evidence for this claim."

Table 22.3 Approved health claims meeting significant scientific agreement among experts and related to grain foods in the United States.

Approved claim	Requirements for the food	Claim requirements	Model claim, Statements
Fibre-Containing Grain Products, Fruits, and Vegetables and Cancer *(21 CFR 101.76)*	A grain product, fruit, or vegetable that contains dietary fibre; Low fat, and Good source of dietary fibre (without fortification)	*Required terms*: "Fibre," "Dietary fibre or "Total dietary fibre" "Some types of cancer" or "Some cancers" Does not specify types of dietary fibre that may be related to risk of cancer.	Low-fat diets rich in fibre-containing grain products, fruits and vegetables may reduce the risk of some types of cancer, a disease associated with many factors.
Fruits, Vegetables and Grain Products that contain Fibre, particularly Soluble Fibre, and Risk of Coronary Heart Disease *(21 CFR 101.77)*	A fruit, vegetable, or grain product that contains fibre; Low saturated fat, Low cholesterol, Low fat, At least 0.6 grams of soluble fibre per RACC (without fortification), and Soluble fibre content provided on label	*Required terms*: "Fibre," "Dietary fibre," "Some types of dietary fibre," "Some dietary fibres" or "Some fibres" "Saturated fat" and "Cholesterol" "Heart disease" or "Coronary heart disease" Includes physician statement ("Individuals with elevated blood total – or LDL – cholesterol should consult their physicians") if claim defines high or normal blood total – and LDL – cholesterol.	Diets low in saturated fat and cholesterol and rich in fruits, vegetables and grain products that contain some types of dietary fibre, particularly soluble fibre, may reduce the risk of heart disease, a disease associated with many factors.
Whole grain Foods and Risk of Heart Disease and Certain Cancers *(Docket No. 1999P-2209)** (1999)	Contains 51% or more whole grain ingredients by weight per RACC, and Dietary fibre content at least: • 3.0g per RACC# of 55g • 2.8g per RACC of 50g • 2.5g per RACC of 45g • 1.7g per RACC of 35g Low-saturated fat, low cholesterol, low fat	*Required wording of the claim:* "Diets rich in whole grain foods and other plant foods and low in total fat, saturated fat and cholesterol may reduce the risk of heart disease and certain cancers."	

(continued)

Table 22.3 Approved health claims meeting significant scientific agreement among experts and related to grain foods in the United States. (*continued*)

Approved claim	Requirements for the food	Claim requirements	Model claim, Statements
Whole grain Foods with Moderate Fat Content and Risk of Heart Disease *(Docket No. 03Q-0547)** (2003)	Contains 51% or more whole grain ingredients by weight per RACC, and Dietary fibre content at least: • 3.0g per RACC of 55g • 2.8g per RACC of 50g • 2.5g per RACC of 45g • 1.7g per RACC of 35g • Low-saturated fat, low cholesterol	*Required wording of the claim*: "Diets rich in whole grain foods and other plant foods, and low in saturated fat and cholesterol may help reduce the risk of heart disease."	-

*FDAMA (FDA Modernization Act) Health Claims (Health Claims Authorized Based on an Authoritative Statement by Federal Scientific Bodies).
#RACC = Reference Amount Customarily Consumed.
(Source: FDA 2006, 2013).

22.4 Communication with consumers

Many consumers associate dark-colored baked goods with being whole grain and assume that products that are high in fibre must be full of whole grain ingredients. Unfortunately, it is not always that simple. The fact that a food is brown or claims a high fibre content does not necessarily mean it's a whole grain food. This is why informative, trustworthy labelling is so important. Providing information about the whole grain content of foods is significantly more effective if the consumers interpreting this information have some basic knowledge about what makes a grain whole and why whole grains are good for them. Many of the organizations creating whole grain food labels and packaging symbols to help consumers identify whole grains also work to educate consumers by explaining recommended intake levels and informing them of the demonstrated health benefits. Lately, increasing scientific consensus about the health benefits associated with regular consumption of whole grains (see previous chapters) has led to increased public awareness and a renewed focus by governments on promoting increased whole grain intake.

In some countries, recommendations for whole grain intake are now included in the official dietary guidelines. Recommendations are often supported by non-governmental organizations like Heart Associations, Cancer Associations and Dietetic Associations, and in some places, private campaigns supported or initiated by the food industry inform consumers about whole grains. Increasingly, Public Private Partnerships, which bring together health organizations or non-profits, and industry (often alongside government representatives and academics), are creating collaborative efforts to promote whole grains. Many players take part in this communication, from newspapers and magazines to governments, health professionals and health organizations. But providing information and advice to consumers is not always enough to change dietary habits; these consumers must also be persuaded to act on the information. When it comes to changing consumer attitudes and habits around whole grain consumption, the availability of whole grain options is key. If it's difficult for consumers to find or identify whole grain foods, they will not buy them. That's where the importance of whole grain labelling comes in. Most people already eat cereals in one form or another, so encouraging consumers to simply exchange refined cereal products for their whole grain counterparts would go a long way towards changing overall dietary habits. Many creative initiatives directed toward making this change are taking place around the world.

22.4.1 Australia

The 2013 Australian Dietary Guidelines recommend Australians eat grain (cereal) foods, mostly whole grain and/or high cereal-fibre varieties, such as breads, cereals, rice, pasta, noodles, polenta, couscous, oats, quinoa and barley (National Health and Medical Research Council 2013). Recommendations range from four to seven servings per day for children, from three to six servings per day for women and from 4.5 to six servings per day for men. A serving equates to 1 slice of bread; 1/2 cup of cooked rice, pasta or noodles; 1/2 cup of porridge; 2/3 cup of cereal flakes; or 1/4 cup of muesli. In 2006, the Grains & Legumes Nutrition Council (GLNC) developed an industry standard in grams for whole grain Daily Target Intake (DTI), which outlines a DTI of 48g per day for adults and children 9 years and older. DTI for children 2–3 years is 24g, and DTI for children 4–8 years is 32–40g. To use the whole grain DTI statement on a food, the food producer must be a Registered User of the Code of Practice for Whole Grain Ingredient Content Claims, also developed by GLNC (GLNC 2017), and provide verification of the whole grain content in its food. Registered Users need to notify GLNC of any product carrying the whole grain DTI statement, and they have to use specific GLNC-approved statements about the whole grain content in their foods in relation to the whole grain DTI. Foods with DTI statements must contain at least 8g of whole grain per serving. This minimum amount of whole grain is required for adults to achieve the whole grain DTI, if they follow the Australian Dietary Guideline Recommendation of six servings of grain foods per day.

The code allows the following statements:

"One [product serve descriptor] serve/s of [insert registered product name] contributes XX% of the 48g whole grain Daily Target Intake"; or

"One [product serve descriptor] serve/s of [insert registered product name] contributes XX% towards the Grain & Legumes Nutrition Council™ 48g whole grain Daily Target Intake."

On products for children, the text must state:

"One [product serve descriptor] serve/s of [insert registered product name] contributes XX% of the 32–40g whole grain Daily Target Intake for children 4–8 years"; or

"One [product serve descriptor] serve/s of [insert registered product name] contributes XX% towards the Grain & Legumes Nutrition Council™ 32–40g whole grain Daily Target Intake for children 4–8 years."

The GLNC Code includes different types of certification badges that can be presented with the DTI statement or with a whole grain content claim. The badge can be in black and white, or in colors specified in the code. Badge examples are available for viewing in the Code of Practice for Whole Grain Ingredient Content Claims (GLNC 2017).

22.4.2 Canada

Canada's Food Guide (Health Canada 2011) recommends that Canadians make at least half of their grain products whole grain each day. The Food Guide suggests consumers eat a variety of whole grains such as barley, brown rice, oats, quinoa and wild rice, and whole grain foods such as whole grain breads, oatmeal or whole-wheat pasta. At least three servings of whole grains per day are recommended for all Canadians age 9 and up. For children 2–3 years old, the recommendation for whole grain intake is 1.5 servings per day and for children 4–8 years old, 2 servings per day. The Whole Grain Stamp (see Figure 22.2) from the US-based Oldways Whole Grains Council, has been used in Canada since 2008. All three Stamps (100%, 50%+ and Basic) are used in a bilingual English/French format (WGC "Canadian Stamp"). Apart from that, the Canadian Stamps look like the American Stamps (Fig. 22.6). In Canada, the 100% Stamp can only appear on products where 100% of the *ingredients* are whole grain. (In contrast, in the United States and most other countries, products where 100% of the *grain ingredients* are whole can use the 100% Stamp). This means that in Canada, only foods like a bag of whole grain flour or brown rice, or a box of oatmeal can use the 100% Stamp, as long as these products have no added non-whole grain ingredients, while a bread cannot use the 100% Stamp. Similarly, in Canada, the

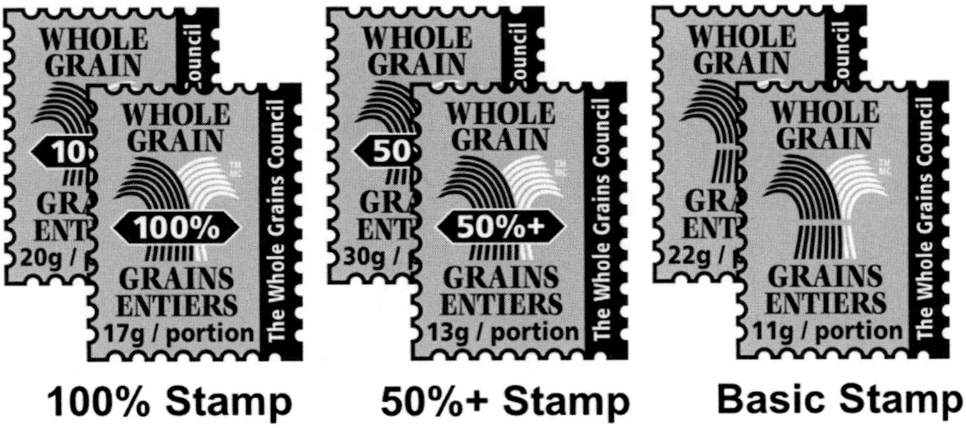

Figure 22.2 The Canadian Whole Grain Stamp. The stamp comes in three versions, the 100% Stamp, the 50%+ Stamp and the Basic Stamp, each with different criteria for whole grain content. (Source: Whole Grains Council 2018).

50%+ Stamp can only appear on products where at least half of the product (by weight) is whole grain (whereas in the United States, products where at least half of the grain is whole grain can use the 50%+ Stamp). As in the United States, Canadian products carrying the Basic Stamp must contain at least 8g of whole grain per serving – all requirements for using the Basic Stamp are the same in Canada as in the United States.

22.4.3 Europe

22.4.3.1 Denmark

Since 2008, the Danish Veterinary and Food Administration (DVFA), which is responsible for the official Danish dietary guidelines, has recommended consumers "choose whole grains first" and reach a daily whole grain intake of 75g/10 MJ (Danish Veterinary and Food Administration 2013). This recommendation is based on the National Food Institute, Technical University of Denmark's suggested level of whole grain intake (Mejborn *et al.* 2008), which it put forth based on a scientific review of the health benefits of consuming whole grains (Ovesen 2008). In 2009, a public-private partnership, the Danish Whole Grain Partnership ("Fuldkornspartnerskabet"), was founded to disseminate knowledge about whole grains and the Danish dietary guidelines' whole grain recommendation to the Danes. The partnership includes collaboration between the DVFA, major health organizations (the Cancer Society, the Heart Association, the Diabetes Association, the Dietetics Association) and food producers, including mills and food retailers. Due to the participation of the DVFA and these well-known health organizations, the Danish Whole Grain Partnership is highly respected among Danes. The vision of the partnership is to improve public health through increased whole grain intake. The partners work for product development and increased availability of whole grain foods and by a coordinated communication of the whole grain recommendation by the use of a "Whole Grain Logo" (See Figure 22.3) (Fuldkornspartnerskabet 2015). The Whole Grain Logo is not considered a health or nutrition claim since it simply uses wording from the official dietary guidelines: "Choose whole grains first."

Figure 22.3 The Danish Whole Grain Logo ("Fuldkornsmærket"). The text says "Choose whole grain first." (Source: The Danish Whole Grain Partnership 2013).

Table 22.4 Whole grain content criteria required of products using the Danish Whole Grain Logo. Foods carrying the logo must also meet standards for total fat, fibres, sugars and salt.

Product	Criteria
Flour, grains and rice	100% whole grain (dry matter basis)
Flour mixes for home baking	≥60% whole grain (dry matter basis)
Bread, except rye	≥50% whole grain (dry matter basis) AND ≥30% whole grain according to Quantitative Ingredient Declaration (QUID)
Bread, rye	≥50% whole grain (dry matter basis) AND ≥ 30% whole grain according to Quantitative Ingredient Declaration (QUID). At least 30% of cereals must be whole grain rye
Crisp bread	≥60% whole grain (dry matter basis)
Breadcrumbs	≥60% whole grain (dry matter basis)
Breakfast cereals	≥65% whole grain (dry matter basis)
Pasta and noodles	≥60% whole grain (dry matter basis)
Porridge	≥70% whole grain (dry matter basis)

(Source: The Danish Whole Grain Partnership 2015).

Only members of the partnership can use the Whole Grain Logo. It can be used on flour, grains and rice; bread; crisp bread; breakfast cereals; pasta and noodles; and porridge as long as these products meet the specified minimum whole grain content for their food group (see Table 22.4). The Whole Grain Logo can also be used on pre-packed ready meals if the grain portion of the meal meets the criteria for the food category it belongs to, for example, if the whole grain pasta in a ready-to-eat lasagna has at least 60% whole grain.

The Whole Grain Logo can only be used on foods that are considered a healthy choice, meeting a number of nutrient profile requirements. Each product must meet the Nordic Keyhole qualification criteria for total fat, sugar, fibre and salt as outlined for its food group.

The Danish Whole Grain Partnership has been very successful in its educational pursuits, increasing Danes' knowledge about the health benefits of whole grains through creative campaigns and events. The food producers involved in the partnership have made a committed, innovative effort to develop delicious new whole grain products that consumers like, and by June 2018, there were 800 food products carrying the Whole Grain Logo. As a result, the availability of whole grain foods is very good in Denmark – whole grain products can be found in most bakeries, retail markets, convenience stores, in-work canteens and in many restaurants. The Danish Whole Grain Partnership has proven to be a very efficient tool for increasing Danes whole grain consumption. Before there was an official recommendation for whole grain intake and before the partnership was formed, Danes (4–75 years old) had an average whole grain intake of 32g per day, and only 6% met the 75g per day level (Biltoft-Jensen *et al.* 2008). However, results from the 2011–2013 National Danish Survey on Diet and Physical Activity indicate that Danes (4–75 years old) have increased their intake to an average of 58g per day with 30% meeting the daily recommendation of 75g per 10 MJ (Mejborn *et al.* 2014). More children (43%) than adults (27%) meet the Danish whole grain recommendation. These figures have been further improved since 2011–2013, and in 2019, a study found that Danes eat, on average, 82 g of whole grain per day and 50% of the survey population now eat the recommended amount of 75 g whole grain per day. Danes with the lowest whole grain intake have now doubled their intake compared to their previous average (www.fuldkorn.dk). Furthermore, in 2019, 1097 products existed that carried the orange whole grain logo compared to 150 when the partnership started in 2009. In 2019, the whole grain partnership was awarded EUs Best Case-certificate for having achieved extraordinary results during the last 10 years.

22.4.3.2 Hungary

The Dietary Guidelines to the Adult Population in Hungary (Rodler 2001) say: “The basis for healthy nutrition is regular consumption of cereals. One should eat cereal products – 6–11 units – several times a day and choose from the assortment of such products the so-called whole grain ones that are made from flour that contains bran and also have seeds in them”. The dietary guidelines define *whole grain cereals* as “food products and nutriments prepared from wholemeal flour that preserve the nutritional value of seeds and contain bran also, complemented with other grains; and this term also includes brown rice.”

One unit of cereal is equivalent to 1 slice of bread (40g); 1 crescent roll (40g); 50g (half portion) of pearl-shaped pasta or dumplings; 100g (half portion) of ready-cooked rice or pearled barley; corn flakes or cooked pasta; 50g of maize; 1 pancake; 1 small scone (30g); 1 slice of pizza (40g); 3 tablespoons of muesli; 1 thin slice of milk bread.

22.4.3.3 The Netherlands

The Netherlands has no official dietary recommendation for whole grain intake. However, there is a recommendation to eat 5–7 slices of whole grain bread per day, depending on age and sex. In addition, the official guidelines for a healthy diet states: “Eat 30 to 40g a day of dietary fibre, especially from sources such as fruit, vegetables and whole grain cereal products” (Health Council of the Netherlands 2006).

In 2011, the Dutch Bakery Centre, supported by the two bakery associations in the Netherlands (the Association for Industrial Production, and the Association for Artisanal Bakers), has developed a Whole Grain Logo to help consumers recognize whole grain bread (See Figure 22.4). To use the logo, the bread must be made from 100% whole grain flour. Use of the logo is free to Dutch bakers, but bakers outside the Netherlands must pay

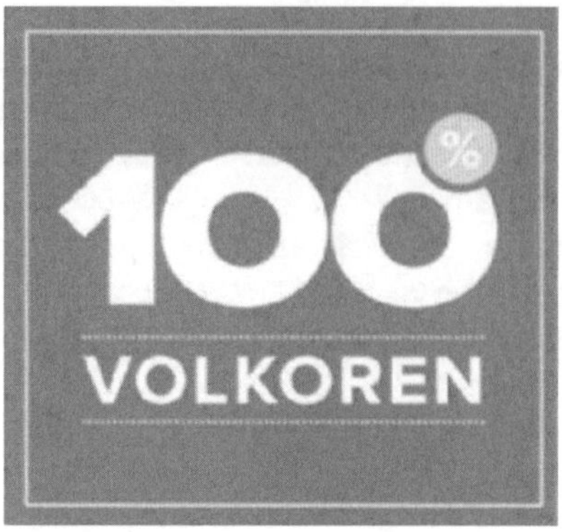

Figure 22.4 The Dutch Whole Grain Logo "100% whole grain." (Source: Dutch Bakery Centre 2018).

a fee if they want to use it. The fee is determined on an individual case-by-case basis according to the intended use.

In modern grain mills (roller mills), fractions of the kernels are separated during milling and then recombined at the end to produce whole grain flour. In an effort to ensure that flour labelled "whole grain" contains the appropriate levels of bran and germ that correspond with the content of the full kernel, the Dutch Bakery Centre, in close collaboration with Dutch millers, has created a voluntary testing protocol. This protocol includes criteria for ash levels (>1.45%; ICC 104 method) and fat content (>1.85%; Soxhlet) and mills that opt in for certification are enrolled in a yearly audit, where flour samples are taken at the mill for analysis. Additionally, control samples are taken from the bakers using their flour. If the analyses show that the flour meets the ash and fat standards established by the Dutch Bakery Centre, the mill gets a certificate and is granted a license to deliver whole grain flour to the members of the bakers' organization.

22.4.4 Singapore

The Health Promotion Board (HPB) in Singapore recommends that Singaporeans consume 50g of whole grain daily (Health Promotion Board 2018). In an effort to help consumers make healthier food choices, the HPB created the Healthier Choice Symbol, a labelling tool for packaged foods (see Figure 22.5). In order to use this symbol, foods must meet a whole range of criteria specific to their food category, which include targets for whole grain content, calories, fat, sodium, sugar, and so on. As of July 2018, the Healthier Choice Symbol was used on more than 2600 different products across a wide variety of food categories.

All intact grains, including brown rice and rice mixes that include at least 20% unpolished whole grain rice, are eligible to use the symbol. In addition, 100% whole grain flour may use the symbol as long as there is no added sodium and it contains least 5g of fibre per 100g weight. Instant oats and oatmeal qualify as long as they have no added sodium or sugar. Mixed foods like breakfast cereals, noodles, muffins, buns and crackers must meet certain whole grain thresholds (different for each food category) and must adhere to additional requirements for fat, sodium, fibre, sugar and overall calorie content. In addition to creating this packaging tool to help consumers make healthier choices when buying

Higher in Wholegrains

Figure 22.5 The Singaporean Healthier Choice Symbol. (Source: Health Promotion Board 2018).

packaged foods, the HPB runs campaigns and promotional events to increase whole grain consumption. HPB regularly partners with noodle suppliers and food vendors at local hawker centers, which are open-air food courts with multiple stalls offering inexpensive meals. By offering partial whole grain noodles and mixed brown-and-white-rice dishes (often at a reduced price, thanks to HPB funding), these hawker center meals increase awareness about whole grains and offer consumers about half their daily whole grain requirement in one portion. The HPB has also worked with supermarkets to offer discounts and promotions on brown rice in a country where less than 20% of the population eats brown rice regularly. They have seen impressive results with these campaigns, with white rice sales steadily decreasing while brown rice sales rise. In fact, in 2018, one supermarket chain reported a record-breaking 40% increase in brown rice sales over a six-month period (Channel NewsAsia 2018).

22.4.5 The United States of America

The 2015–2020, Dietary Guidelines for Americans recommends that Americans consume at least half of all grains as whole grains, and that they increase their whole grain intake by replacing refined grains with whole grains. The recommended whole grain intake is 3 ounce-equivalents per day. One ounce-equivalent of grain is equal to: 1 one-ounce slice of bread; 1 ounce uncooked pasta or rice; 1/2 cup cooked rice, pasta or hot cereal; 1 tortilla (6" diameter); 1 pancake (5" diameter) or 1 ounce ready-to-eat cereal (about 1 cup cereal flakes). Three ounce-equivalents (servings) of whole grain correspond to a minimum of 48g of whole grain ingredients. The recommendations of the US Dietary Guidelines are based on eating three servings (ounce-equivalents) of 100% whole grain foods per day. However, most consumers are unsure which foods are 100% whole grain foods, and many prefer to get their recommended whole grains from foods made with a mix of whole and refined grains. In both cases, it's difficult for consumers to be sure that they are getting enough whole grains.

The United States has no official definition of a *whole grain food*, except that a food carrying an authorized health claim must contain at least 51% whole grain (as a % of total weight). Although this health claim began appearing on foods in 1999, whole grain intake did not increase during the period 1999–2005, indicating that this type of labelling was unlikely to steer consumers towards eating more whole grains. To respond to this need for clearer labelling that could potentially influence consumer behavior, the US-based educational non-profit Oldways created an initiative called the Whole Grains Council (WGC) in 2003. The WGC's two initial goals were to create a definition of *whole grains* that was understandable to consumers and to develop a packaging symbol to help consumers more readily identify foods contributing significant amounts of whole grain to the diet.

In January 2005, the WGC introduced the Whole Grain Stamp. Originally, the stamp had three versions: the "Good Source" Stamp (minimum whole grain content 8g per serving), the "Excellent Source" Stamp (minimum 16g whole grain per serving) and the "100%/ Excellent Source" (minimum 16g whole grain and all grains must be whole grain). Based on consumer and regulatory input, the WGC introduced an enhanced version of the Whole Grain Stamp in June 2006 in two versions: the Basic Stamp and the 100% Stamp. In January 2017 a third version, the 50%+ Stamp, was added to the lineup (WGC "Whole Grain Stamp") (see Figure 22.6). The 100% Stamp is used on products where all the grain is whole grain, and there is a minimum of 16g of whole grain content per serving. The 50%+ Stamp is used on foods that make at least half their grain whole grain, and which contain a minimum of 8g of whole grain per serving. And the Basic Stamp is used on products that contain at least 8g of whole grain, but which are made with primarily refined grain.

All three stamps clearly state the number of grams of whole grain content per serving, so the gram amount shown on the Stamp is often much higher than the minimum amount required to qualify for stamp use. Although the information on the Whole Grain Stamps is comprehensive, the WGC recognizes that most consumers will not tally up the grams of whole grain in each food they eat. Instead, the message to consumers is simple: "Eat three products labeled '100% whole grain' or six products bearing any Whole Grain Stamp each

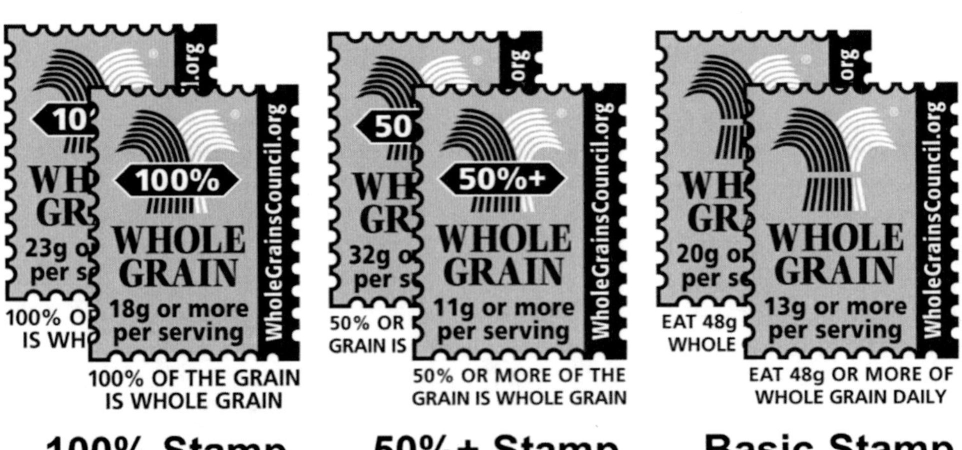

Figure 22.6 The American Whole Grain Stamp. The stamp comes in three versions, the 100% Stamp, the 50%+ Stamp and the Basic Stamp, each with different criteria for whole grain content. (Source: Whole Grains Council 2018).

day" to get the recommended three servings (48g) or more of whole grain. The Whole Grain Stamp is successful and sought by consumers, who are trying to improve their health by eating more whole grains. Evidence for the success of the Whole Grain Stamp as a consumer awareness tool is growing. While whole grain consumption was unchanged from 1999–2005, before the Whole Grain Stamp was created, in the first three years after the introduction of the Whole Grain Stamp (2005–2008) whole grain consumption rose 20% and that trend has continued. According to US National Survey Data (NHANES), whole grain intake increased 50% between 2003 and2004 and between 2013 and 2014 (USDA ARS 2017). As of July 2018, the Whole Grain Stamp was on more than 12 000 products in seven languages and in 58 countries: Argentina, Australia, Barbados, Bahrain, Belgium, Belize, Brazil, Canada, Chile, China, Colombia, Costa Rica, Denmark, Dominican Republic, Ecuador, El Salvador, Egypt, France, Germany, Ghana, Greece, Guatemala, Honduras, India, Ireland, Israel, Italy, Jamaica, Japan, Kuwait, Lebanon, Maldives, Mauritius, Mexico, The Netherlands, New Zealand, Nicaragua, Oman, Panama, Paraguay, Peru, Poland, Portugal, Qatar, Romania, Saudi Arabia, Singapore, South Korea, Spain, Sri Lanka, Taiwan, Tanzania, Trinidad and Tobago, U.A.E., United Kingdom, United States, Uruguay and Venezuela (WGC "It's working").

In addition to administering the Whole Grain Stamp program and reviewing product applications to use the stamp, the WGC carries out extensive education programs to support its three-part mission: to help consumers find whole grains and understand their benefits; to help manufacturers and restaurants create delicious whole grain foods; and to help the media write accurate, compelling stories about whole grains. The WGC funds its free consumer educational programs and administration of the Whole Grain Stamp program through annual fees paid by food industry members; food producers must be members of the WGC to use the stamp, but can use the WGC's educational materials without paying a fee.

22.5 Conclusion

More than three decades of nutrition research have demonstrated that increased whole grain consumption contributes to many positive health outcomes. However, globally, intake still falls well below recommended levels. Many countries have made progress in establishing recommended intake levels, and in many places, requiring that products labelled "whole grain" contain a minimum level of whole grain, so as not to be misleading to consumers. For the same reason, many governments strictly regulate the use of nutrition and health claims on food packages. Expanding on these efforts made by government regulators, many health organizations and other non-governmental organizations (NGOs) have pursued large consumer education campaigns that have been very successful in raising awareness about the health benefits of whole grains. The impact has been even greater in countries where there has been wide adoption of third-party-approved packaging labels calling out products that provide consumers with significant amounts of whole grain and making it easy for consumers to find and compare these products when shopping. As these efforts continue, the establishment of clear, consistent product labelling remains a priority and has benefits to stakeholders at every level – for consumers seeking whole grain products, for food producers who wish to communicate the whole grain content of their foods and for researchers working to quantify actual whole grain intake and the measure the associated health benefits.

22.6 Acknowledgments

The authors are grateful to Cynthia Harriman, Oldways Whole Grains Council, USA; Sara Grafenauer and Michelle Broom, Grains & Legumes Nutrition Council™, Australia; Flip van Straaten, Nederlands Bakkerij Centrum, The Netherlands; Carola Buller and Michael Gusko, GoodMills Innovation GmbH, Germany; and Jan-Willem van der Kamp, TNO, The Netherlands for information regarding their organizations' effort to inform consumers about whole grain foods and for proof reading part of the manuscript.

22.7 References

AACCI (1999) Standard Definitions & Resources: Whole Grains. [Online], Available: http://www.aaccnet.org/initiatives/definitions/pages/wholegrain.aspx [27 July 2018].

Agri-Food & Veterinary Authority, Singapore (2017) *A Guide to Food Labelling and Advertisements*, Updated April 2017. [Online], Available: http://www.ava.gov.sg/docs/default-source/tools-and-resources/resources-for-businesses/aguidetofoodlabellingandadvertisementsversionjuly2 [25 July 2018].

Australia New Zealand Food Standards Code – Standard 1.2.7 – Nutrition, Health and Related Claims – F2013L00054, 2013.

Biltoft-Jensen A., Ygil K.H., Kørup K., Christensen T. (2008) Danskernes indtag af fuldkorn. In: *Whole grain. Definition and scientific evidence for recommendation of whole grain intake in Denmark* (Fuldkorn. Definition og vidensgrundlag for anbefaling af fuldkornsindtag i Danmark) (eds Mejborn H., Biltoft-Jensen A., Trolle E., Tetens I.) National Food Institute, Technical University of Denmark, Søborg.

Bundesministerium für Ernährung und Landwirtschaft (1994) Leitsätze für Brot und Kleingebäck, [Online], Available: http://www.bmel.de/SharedDocs/Downloads/Ernaehrung/Lebensmittelbuch/LeitsaetzeBrot.pdf;jsessionid=0B4F4829081A5FE84AFC8841E5E3BF29.2_cid288?__blob=publicationFile [20 July 2018].

Canadian Food Inspection Agency (2018), *Composition and quality claims*, Last updated 23 May 2018. [Online], Available: http://inspection.gc.ca/food/labelling/food-labelling-for-industry/composition-and-quality-claims/eng/1391025998183/1391026062752?chap=2#s1c2 [19 July 2018].

Channel NewsAsia (2018), *More Singaporeans choosing brown rice as grain of choice*, Published 24 March 2018. [Online], Available: https://www.channelnewsasia.com/news/singapore/more-singaporeans-choosing-brown-rice-as-grain-of-choice-10074026 [24July 2018].

Code of Federal Regulations (1993a) *21 CFR 136.180*, [Online], Available: https://www.gpo.gov/fdsys/pkg/CFR-2011-title21-vol2/pdf/CFR-2011-title21-vol2-sec136-180.pdf [13 July 2018].

Code of Federal Regulation (1993b) *21 CFR 139.138*, [Online], Available: https://www.gpo.gov/fdsys/pkg/CFR-2011-title21-vol2/pdf/CFR-2011-title21-vol2-sec139-138.pdf [13 July 2018].

Code of Federal Regulation (1993c) *21 CFR 137.225*, [Online], Available: https://www.gpo.gov/fdsys/pkg/CFR-2011-title21-vol2/pdf/CFR-2011-title21-vol2-sec137-225.pdf [13 July 2018].

Code of Federal Regulations (1993d) *21 CFR 137.200*, [Online], Available: https://www.gpo.gov/fdsys/pkg/CFR-2012-title21-vol2/pdf/CFR-2012-title21-vol2-sec137-200.pdf [13 July 2018].

Code of Federal Regulation (1993e) *21 CFR 137.105*, [Online], Available: https://www.gpo.gov/fdsys/pkg/CFR-2011-title21-vol2/pdf/CFR-2011-title21-vol2-sec137-105.pdf [13 July 2018].

Codex Alimentarius Commission (2004) Guidelines for use of nutrition and health claims. Guideline 23-1997. Revised 2004, Last Amended 2013.

Danish Veterinary and Food Administration (2013) Danish Dietary Guidelines.

Food and Drug Administration (1999) *Health Claim Notification for Whole Grain Foods*, Last updated 3 January 2018, [Online], Available: https://www.fda.gov/food/labelingnutrition/ucm073639.htm [13 July 2018].

De Staatssecretaris van Volksgezondheid, Welzijn en Sport (1998) *Warenwetbesluit Meel en brood*, Updated 1 October 2017 [Online], Available: http://wetten.overheid.nl/BWBR0009669/2017-10-01 [23 July 2018].

European Food Safety Authority (2010) EFSA Panel on Dietetic Products, Nutrition and Allergies (NDA); Scientific Opinion on the substantiation of a health claim related to whole grain (ID 831, 832, 833, 1126, 1268, 1269, 1270, 1271, 1431) pursuant to Article 13(1) of Regulation (EC) No 1924/2006. EFSA Journal **8**, 1766.

European Commission (2006) REGULATION (EC) No 1924/2006 OF THE EUROPEAN PARLIAMENT AND OF THE COUNCIL of 20 December 2006 on nutrition and health claims made on foods.

European Commission (2012) COMMISSION REGULATION (EU) No 432/2012 of 16 May 2012 establishing a list of permitted health claims made on foods, other than those referring to the reduction of disease risk and to children's development and health.

Food and Drug Administration (2003) *Health Claim Notification for Whole Grain Foods with Moderate Fat Content,* Last updated 3 January 2018, [Online], Available: https://www.fda.gov/Food/LabelingNutrition/ucm073634.htm [13 July 2018].

Food and Drug Administration (2006) *Draft guidance: whole grain label statement. Guidance document for industry and FDA staff.* Last updated 04 November 2017, [Online], Available: http://www.fda.gov/Food/GuidanceRegulation/GuidanceDocumentsRegulatoryInformation/ucm059088.htm [13 July 2018].

Food and Drug Administration (2017) Code of Federal Regulations Title 21. 21 CFR 101.14(c)-(d), 101.70. Updated 1 April 2017, [Online], Available: https://www.accessdata.fda.gov/scripts/cdrh/cfdocs/cfcfr/CFRSearch.cfm?fr=101.14 [16 July 2018].

Ferruzzi M.G., Jonnalagadda S.S., Liu S., Marquart L., McKeown N., Reicks M., Riccardi G., Seal C., Slavin J., Thielecke F., Kamp J.-W. van der, Webb D. (2014) Developing a standard definition of whole-grain foods for dietary recommendations: summary report of a multidisciplinary expert roundtable discussion. *Am Soc Nutr* 5, 164–76.

Fuldkornspartnerskabet (The Danish Whole Grain Partnership) (2015) *Manual for the use of the Whole Grain Logo, March* 2015, [Online], Available: www.fuldkorn.dk [16 July 2018].

Government of Canada (2010) *Summary of Assessment of a Health Claim about Oat Products and Blood Cholesterol Lowering.* [Online], Available: https://www.canada.ca/en/health-canada/services/food-nutrition/food-labelling/health-claims/assessments/products-blood-cholesterol-lowering-summary-assessment-health-claim-about-products-blood-cholesterol-lowering.html [19 July 2018].

Government of Canada (2012) *Summary of Health Canada's Assessment of a Health Claim about Barley Products and Blood Cholesterol Lowering.* [Online], Available: https://www.canada.ca/en/health-canada/services/food-nutrition/food-labelling/health-claims/assessments/assessment-health-claim-about-barley-products-blood-cholesterol-lowering.html [19 July 2018].

Grains & Legumes Nutrition Council (2017) *Code of Practice for Whole Grain Ingredient Content Claims,* [Online], Available: http://www.glnc.org.au/wp-content/uploads/2013/12/GLNC-Code-of-Practice-for-Whole-Grain-Ingredient-Content-Claims-2017.pdf [19 July 2018].

Health Canada (2011) *Eating well with Canada's Food Guide,* [Online], Available: https://www.canada.ca/content/dam/hc-sc/migration/hc-sc/fn-an/alt_formats/hpfb-dgpsa/pdf/food-guide-aliment/print_eatwell_bienmang-eng.pdf [19 July 2018].

Health Canada (2012) *Summary of Health Canada's Assessment of a Health Claim about Whole Grains and Coronary Heart Disease,* [Online], Available: http://www.hc-sc.gc.ca/fn-an/alt_formats/pdf/label-etiquet/claims-reclam/assess-evalu/grains-heart-coeur-eng.pdf [19 July 2018].

Health Canada (2013) *Whole grains – Get the facts,* [Online], Available: http://www.hc-sc.gc.ca/fn-an/nutrition/whole-grain-entiers-eng.php [19 July 2018].

Health Council of the Netherlands (2006) *The Guidelines for a healthy diet* 2006, [Online], Available: https://www.gezondheidsraad.nl/sites/default/files/200621E_0.pdf [23 July 2018].

Health Promotion Board (2018) *Healthier Choice Symbol Nutrient Guidelines,* Updated January 2018. [Online], Available: https://www.hpb.gov.sg/docs/default-source/default-document-library/hcs-guidelines-(january-2018) 9ab599f6468366dea7adff00000d8c5a.pdf?sfvrsn=2d36ff72_0 [24 July 2018].

Institute of Grocery Distribution (2007) *UK Whole Grain Guidance Note,* [Online], Available: https://www.igd.com/Portals/0/Downloads/Charitable%20Impact/UK%20Whole%20Grain%20Guidance%203433.pdf [17 July 2018].

Mejborn H., Biltoft-Jensen A., Ygil K., Trolle E., Tetens I. (2008) Anbefalet indtag af fuldkorn. In: Whole grain. Definition and scientific evidence for recommendation of whole grain intake in Denmark (Fuldkorn. Definition og vidensgrundlag for anbefaling af fuldkornsindtag i Danmark) (eds Mejborn H., Biltoft-Jensen A., Trolle E., Tetens I. National Food Institute, Technical University of Denmark, Søborg.

Mejborn H., Ygil K.H., Fagt S., Trolle E., Kørup K., Christensen T. (2014) Danskernes fuldkornsindtag 2011-2013 (Wholegrain intake of Danes 2011-2013). E-article no. 4, 2014 from National Institute of Food, Technical University of Denmark, Søborg.

Ministero delle politiche agricole alimentary e forestali (2001) Decreto del Presidente delle Repubblica 9 febbraio 2001, n. 187. Regolamento per la revisione della normative sulla produzione e commercializzione de sfarinati e paste alimentary, a norma dell'articolo 50 della legge 22 febbraio 1994, n. 146.

National Health and Medical Research Council (2013) *Australian Dietary Guidelines 2013. Eat for health.* [Online], Available: https://www.nhmrc.gov.au/_files_nhmrc/file/publications/n55_australian_dietary_guidelines1.pdf [19 July 2018].

Oldways Whole Grains Council, [Online], Available: http://wholegrainscouncil.org [17 July 2018].

Oldways Whole Grains Council *Whole Grain Stamp*, [Online], Available: http://wholegrainscouncil.org/whole-grain-stamp [17 July 2018].

Oldways Whole Grains Council *It's working*, [Online], Available: http://wholegrainscouncil.org/whole-grain-stamp/its-working [17 July 2018].

Oldways Whole Grains Council *Canadian Stamp*, [Online], Available: http://wholegrainscouncil.org/whole-grain-stamp/canadian-stamp [17 July 2018].

Ovesen L (2008) Indtag af fuldkorn og sygdomsrisiko – en systematisk gennemgang. In: *Whole grain. Definition and scientific evidence for recommendation of whole grain intake in Denmark* (Fuldkorn. Definition og vidensgrundlag for anbefaling af fuldkornsindtag i Danmark) (eds Mejborn H., Biltoft-Jensen A., Trolle E., Tetens I.) National Food Institute, Technical University of Denmark, Søborg.

Rodler I (2001) Dietary Guidelines to the Adult Population in Hungary. Public Health Programme for a Healthy Nation.

Ross, A.B., van der Kamp, J.W., King, R., Lê, K.A., Mejborn, H., Seal, C.J., Thielecke, F. (2017) Perspective: A Definition for Whole-Grain Food Products—Recommendations from the Healthgrain Forum. *Adv Nutr* 2017;8:525–31.

United States Department of Agriculture, Food and Nutrition Service (2012) *Grain Requirements for the National School Lunch Program and School Breakfast Program.* [Online], Available: https://wholegrainscouncil.org/sites/default/files/atoms/files/SP30-2012os_FNSApril30.pdf [13 July 2018].

United States Department of Agriculture, Agricultural Research Service (2017) *Food Patterns Equivalents Intakes by Americans: What We Eat in America, NHANES 2003-2004 and 2013-2014.* [Online], Available: https://www.ars.usda.gov/ARSUserFiles/80400530/pdf/DBrief/17_Food_Patterns_Equivalents_0304_1314.pdf [19 July 2018].

United States Department of Agriculture (2014) *Whole grain resource for the National school lunch and school breakfast programs. A guide to meeting the whole grain-rich criteria.* [Online], Available: http://www.fns.usda.gov/sites/default/files/WholeGrainResource.pdf [13 July 2018].

United States Department of Agriculture, Food and Nutrition Service (2016) *Child and Adult Care Food Program Final Rule: Meal Pattern Revisions Related to the Healthy, Hunger-Free Kids Act of 2010.* [Online], Available: https://www.gpo.gov/fdsys/pkg/FR-2016-04-25/pdf/2016-09412.pdf [13 July 2018].

United States Department of Health & Human Services and United States Department of Agriculture (2015) *2015-2020 Dietary Guidelines for Americans.* 8th Edition, [Online], Available: http://health.gov/dietaryguidelines/2015/guidelines/ [17 July 2018].

van der Kamp, J.W., Poutanen, K., Seal, C.J., Richardson, D.P. (2014) The HEALTHGRAIN definition of 'whole grain.' Food Nutr Res 2014;58:22100.

Summary

Rikard Landberg and Nathalie Scheers

The future of whole grains and health

The literature on the health effects of whole grains has become massive, not the least during the past 13 years since the first edition of this book was published in 2007. Not only the body of evidence on the link between whole grains and specific disease outcomes such as type 2 diabetes, cardiovascular disease, some cancers and total mortality have become stronger, but also several large and well-controlled studies to evaluate the effects on established risk factors have emerged and shed more light on the role of whole grains for specific intermediate risk factors. However, these studies have also taught us that there is large heterogeneity in the effects obtained across studies and that results in different studies may not always converge. This points to a larger complexity that needs to be considered for the evaluation of the health effects of whole grains and for an improved understanding of underlying mechanisms in future studies.

The lack of global definitions of whole grains and whole-grain foods have to some degree hampered not only the possibility to convey clear consumer messages, but probably also the research on the health effects of whole grains. Different definitions have resulted in a diversity of cereals and pseudocereals included in the different studies and different cut-off values of the whole-grain content in whole-grain products have been used across studies. Although there is still no uniform and global definition of *whole grains* or *whole grain products*, useful definitions have been suggested recently (see Chapter 3). With such definitions, along with information about whole-grain content in foods incorporated in national food databases, whole-grain intakes could probably be more uniformly estimated across studies in the future.

One aspect that has been acknowledged and incorporated in scientific investigations lately, is that cereal grains differ substantially in terms of chemical composition and physiochemical properties, not the least regarding the composition and characteristics of the dietary fibre complex and the pool of bioactive compounds. For example, the dietary fibre content in rye can reach >25%, whereas it is seldom higher than 6% in rice. Moreover, beta-glucans in oats are viscous forming, which arabinoxylans in wheat are not, which results in widely different properties of relevance for physiological responses with implications for health. Based on this, it is likely that the different grains have differential effects on, for example, gut fermentation and cholesterol lowering. Furthermore, grain processing and differential food processing will have further impact on the composition and properties

Whole Grains and Health, Second Edition. Edited by Rikard Landberg and Nathalie Scheers.

Additional materials available for download online at https://www.wiley.com/en-gb/Whole+Grains+and+Health-p-9781118939437

of whole grains and needs to be studied in more detail in the years to come. For example, processing methods that reduce starch digestibility have the potency to influence health-related processes not only by modulating glycaemia directly, but also by modulating the insulin and incretin response. Processing allows a great possibility to tailor the food traits needed for specific outcomes.

In order to get more detailed insights on how the grain-food properties affect physiological responses, and thereby provide the blueprint for development of foods for specific purposes, grains need to be studied separately in relation to health outcomes and not just as "total whole-grain intake." Both observational studies and intervention trials conducted lately support the need to study their effects separately, and this is something that should be emphasised for future studies.

The need for accurate assessment of whole-grain intake is becoming even greater, when the health effects of different grains are to be investigated. The self-reported intakes through questionnaires, typically used in epidemiological studies, have limitations in this aspect and there is a need for specific biomarkers of whole-grain intake. There has been considerable advancement in this area. Alkylresorcinols and their metabolites have been evaluated and found useful as biomarkers of whole-grain wheat, rye and quinoa intake, in dietary intervention trials for assessment of compliance as well as for observational studies as objective measures of intakes in relation to disease endpoints. The challenge now remains to find specific biomarkers of other whole grains such as oats, barley and rice. Promising candidate biomarkers of oat intake, avenocosides and avenanthramides, have been suggested recently and needs to be followed up in future studies.

The rapid development of OMICs techniques has opened greater possibilities to provide detailed mechanistic understanding that could both help explain the observed health effects as well as the potential differences across studies and individuals. This is well illustrated by the number of metabolomics and gene expression studies that have emerged since the first edition of the book.

Metabolomics has emerged as a powerful technique not only to evaluate the global effects of whole-grain interventions on intermediates of the host metabolism, but also to characterize the large pool of metabolites derived from the whole grain intake and its interaction with gut microbiota. Metabolomics techniques have also been important to characterize bioactive compounds in whole grains and their foods. In the HealthGrain-diversity screen, a large number of wheat varieties, and to a limited extent also rye, oats and barley varieties from Europe, were characterized with regards to several bioactive compounds. This provided important information about the compounds that may be of relevance to health, how they were affected by genetics, the environment and their interaction.

Metabolomics has also been useful to discover novel compounds in cereal grains. For example, a new group of potent bioactive compounds have been identified in wheat and rye, the benzoxazinoids. These compounds are allopathic compounds that are also similar to compounds used for different drug targets. Studies have been undertaken to study their presence in foods, effects of processing and their absorption, distribution, metabolism and excretion in animal and human trials. Moreover, their potential beneficial effects for prostate cancer has been a major focus lately. More studies are needed to elucidate their pharmacodynamics in humans.

The role of gut microbiota in modulating gut and systemic health is another field that has emerged since the last edition, which has already provided new insights to some mechanisms that may link the gut fermentation of the dietary fibre complex with physiological effects that may underline some of the health benefits observed in epidemiological studies.

More detailed knowledge on the role of specific fibres on the gut microbiota composition and activity is warranted and will be an important future area of research.

Utilization of comprehensive OMCIs data, not the least gut microbiota data, along with study designs that allows frequent repeated sampling, will open for new possibilities to develop new personalized nutrition concepts, that is, tailor the right whole-grain foods to the right individual at the right time. Studies have already emerged recently, showing a major impact of gut microbiota on metabolic effect responses to whole grains and dietary fibre-rich dietary interventions. It has, for example, been demonstrated that postprandial glucose responses differ substantially among individuals under standardized food intakes, but that such differences can be predicted by taking information about the individual's gut microbiota into account. Along the same lines, it has been shown that baseline gut microbiota is associated with differential response to weight loss of high-fibre diets and on blood lipid profiles in different studies. This suggests large potential for personalized nutrition and for development of tailored foods targeted to modify specific aspects of gut microbiota to maximize beneficial physiological responses. Development of personalized concepts using OMICs data along with tailored foods to be matched against such concepts will likely emerge during the coming years. Testing such approaches against general advice will be crucial to determine whether potential improvements are large enough to motivate such costly personalization concepts for the general public.

Although most consumers would benefit from increasing their consumption of whole grain cereals and bran-rich fractions, it is important to keep in mind that such consumption may also have adverse effects, including allergenic proteins and proteins that provoke food sensitivity, toxic effects of the heavy metal cadmium, phytate and phenolic compounds for their inhibition of iron absorption, and acrylamide, which is a heat-generated class II carcinogen. The scientific community and the food sector need to continue developing and implementing methods that can reduce the production of acrylamide during processing, without at the same time comprising other food safety and nutritional or health promoting aspects such as those beneficial effects associated with whole grain cereals. As for the other compounds, research is needed to better identify the levels that may contribute to negative effects on long-term consumption.

Despite the huge progress in improving our understanding of the health effects of whole grain foods during the last decade, as evidenced by the chapters in this edition, there are a number of remaining challenges to be addressed in the years to come. This includes but are not restricted to:

- Dissecting the role of whole grains from different cereals as part of a healthy and sustainable diet. A diet does not only need to be healthy; it shall also be sustainable, that is, its production should be kept within the planetary boundaries. There is a need for improved knowledge how cereal grains shall be consumed (type and amount) as part of a healthy and sustainable diet at different regions of the globe.
- More knowledge on how to enhance the nutritional value as well as improving the eating quality of whole-grain foods. This includes challenges not only for the food industry in finding new ways of processing cereals, but it also includes effective raw material selection and utilization.
- Further characterization and studies to evaluate health effects of minor cereals such as ancient grains and pseudo cereals. Many of them have interesting nutrient and bioactive compound profiles that may be of relevance to health.

- Worldwide definitions of *whole grains* and *whole-grain products* would be desirable to facilitate research on the health effects of grains and communication towards consumers.
- Improved understanding of the specific role of *different* whole grains, that is, different grain types, on health outcomes. Studies should be made on well characterized grains and different grains separately.
- Further utilization of comprehensive OMICs techniques to allow in-depth studies of changes in metabolism and physiological events of importance to health in response to whole-grain interventions
- Utilization of frequent repeated sampling in both epidemiological studies and in dietary interventions. This would allow studies of trajectories that may lead to adverse or beneficial health effects in response to whole-grain interventions or followups.

We are proud to have provided a comprehensive summary of the development of our current understanding of the role of whole grains for human health through the current edition and we hope that the reading has been useful.

We are excited to continue our own efforts to contribute to the research in the field of whole grains and health the years to come and hope that many will do the same!

Index

Note: Figures are indicated by f; Tables are indicated by t. Including the index header is not a part of our standard guidelines.

Whole Grains and Health, Second Edition. Edited by Rikard Landberg and Nathalie Scheers.

Additional materials available for download online at https://www.wiley.com/en-gb/Whole+Grains+and+Health-p-9781118939437

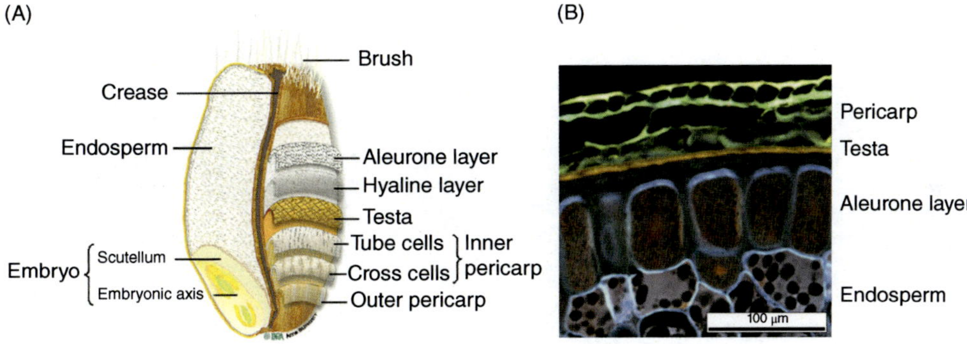

Figure 1.1 A: General structure of a cereal grain); B: Epifluorescence micrograph of parts of rye grain. The sections were stained with Acid Fuchsin and Calcofluor: protein appears red, cell walls rich in β-glucan appear light blue and lignified cell walls of the pericarp appear yellowish-orange. Structure of cereal foods (Source: Hemery et al. 2007).

Whole Grains and Health, Second Edition. Edited by Rikard Landberg and Nathalie Scheers.

Additional materials available for download online at https://www.wiley.com/en-gb/Whole+Grains+and+Health-p-9781118939437

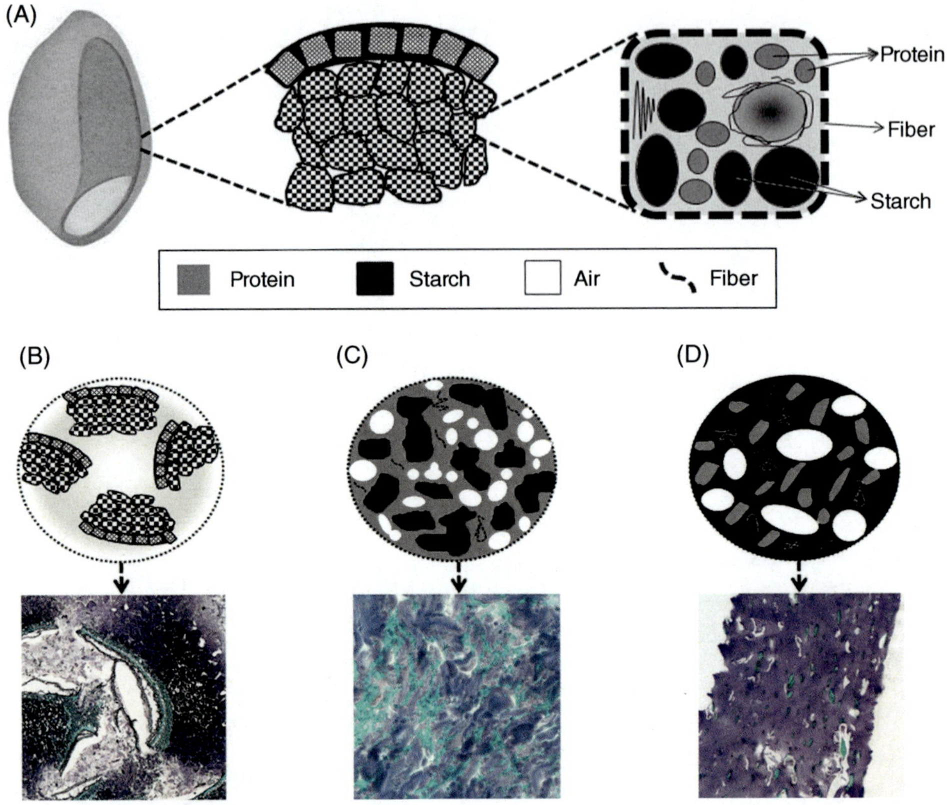

Figure 1.2 Schematic representation of a typical endosperm cell (A) and microstructure of different cereal products such as rye porridge (B), wheat bread (C) and extruded rye breakfast cereal (D). Starch and protein can be observed in blue/purple and green, respectively.

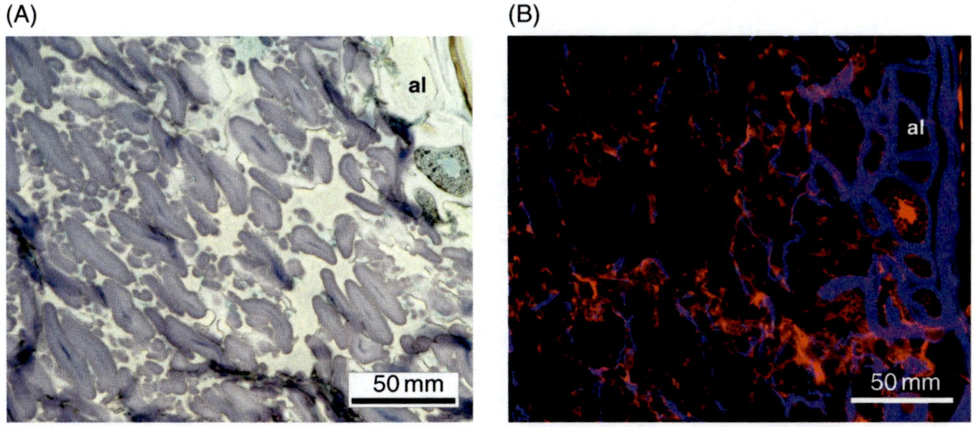

Figure 1.3 Microstructure of rolled rye grain. A: bright field micrograph with iodine and light green staining for observation of starch (purple) and protein (green), respectively; B: epifluorescence micrograph with Calcofluor and Acid Fuchsin staining for observation of cell walls (blue) and protein (red), respectively.

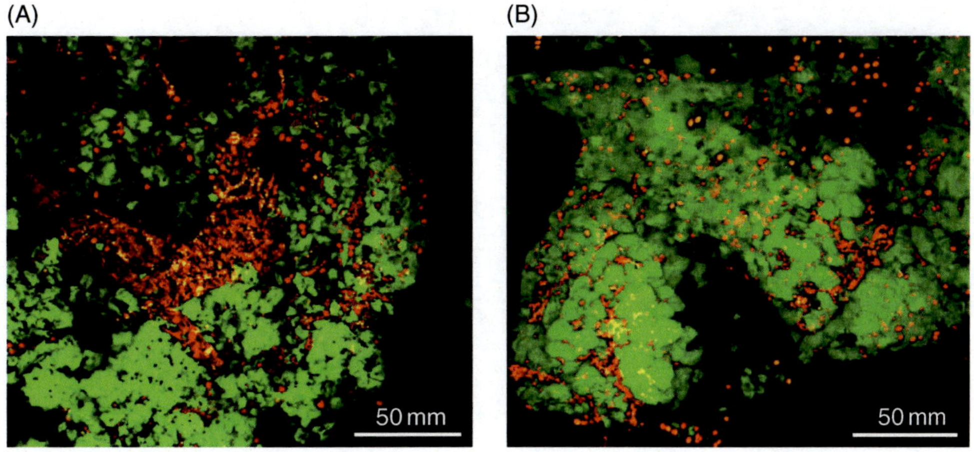

Figure 1.4 CLSM images of untreated (A) and 0.01% protease-treated (B) brown rice bread crumbs (40x magnification) showing starch (green) and proteins (red-yellow). Adapted from Renzetti and Arendt 2009.

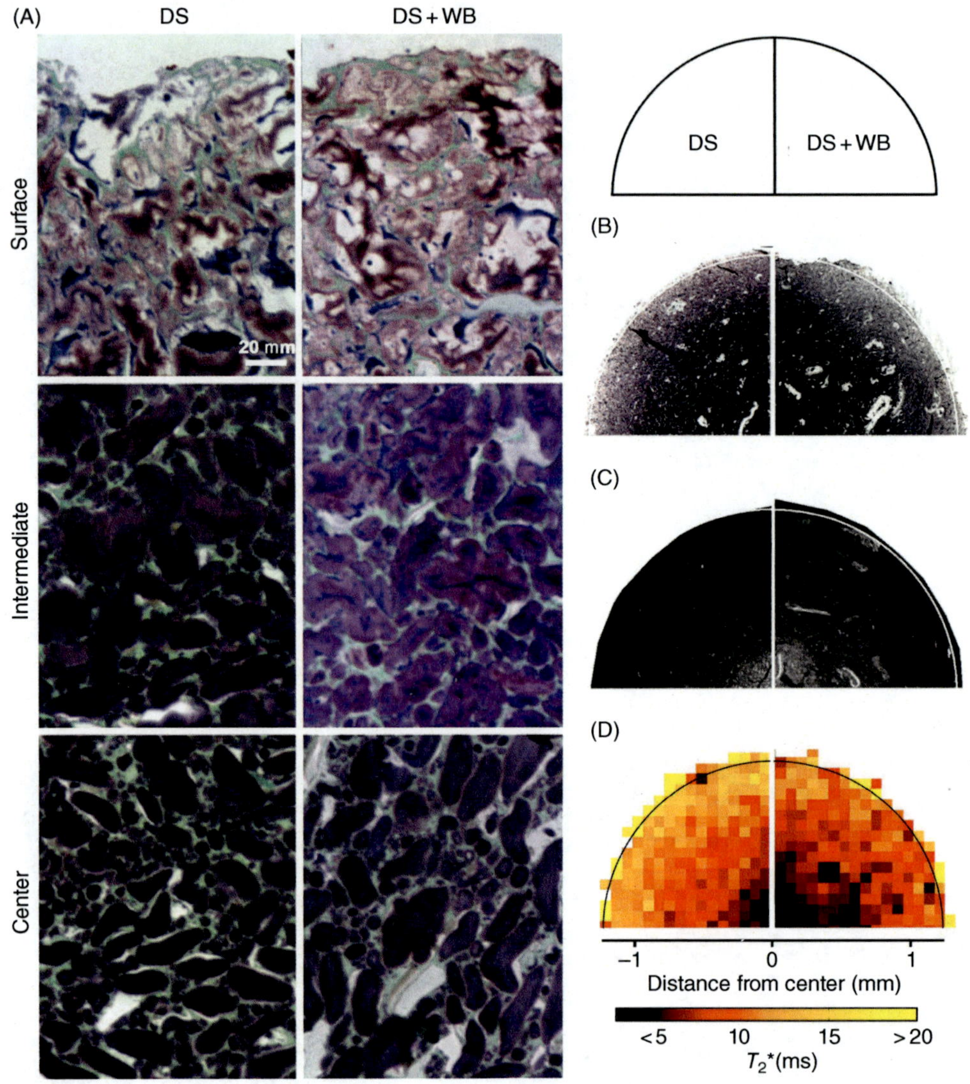

Figure 1.5 Representative cross-sections of 10-min cooked spaghetti made of 100% fine durum wheat semolina (DS) and durum whole grain flour (DS+WG). A: Bright field light micrographs at high magnification from three regions; B–D: Bright field light micrographs (B), polarized light micrographs (C), and T_2^* maps (D) of cross-sections at lower magnification. Sections in A and B were stained with Light Green and Lugol's iodine solution for observation of protein (green) and starch (blue/violet), respectively, while fibre particles were not stained (Source: (B) and (D): Modified from Steglich et al. 2014).

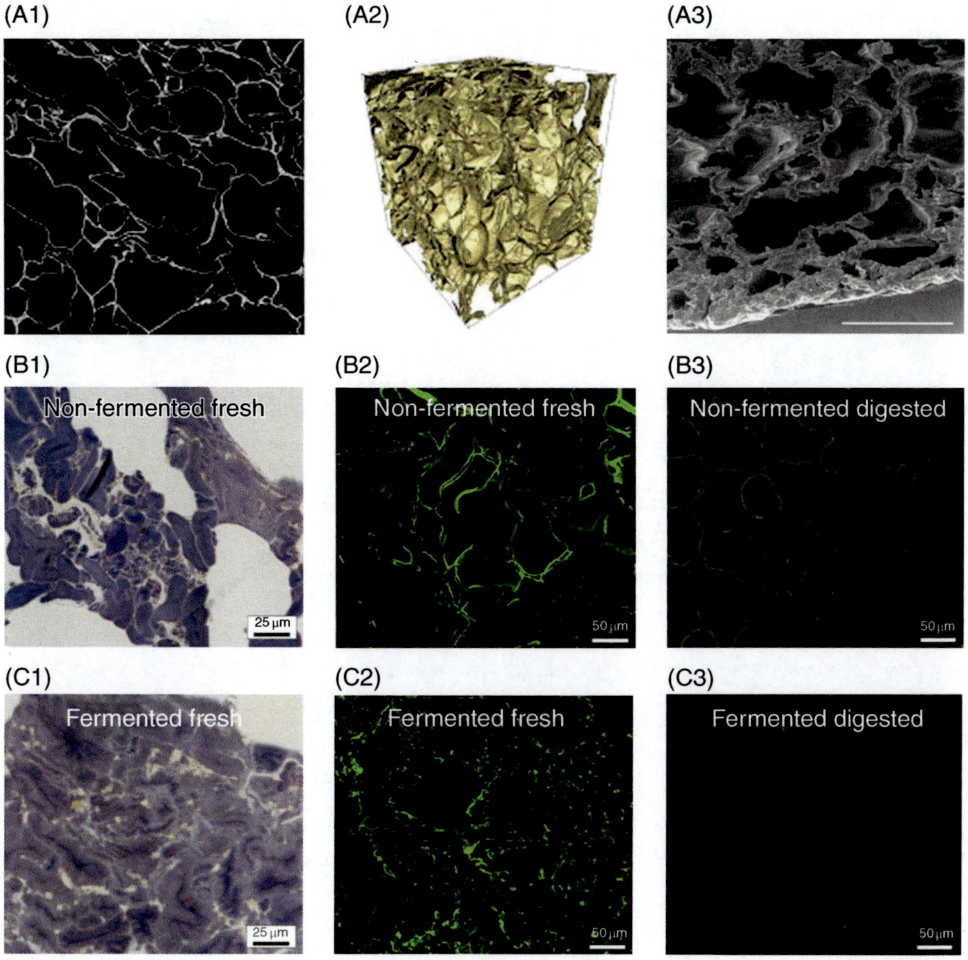

Figure 1.7 Microstructure of rye crisp bread. A1 and A2: Reconstructed X-ray micro-CT cross-sections and 3-D structure of extruded rye crispbread (Gondek et al. 2013). A3: Scanning electron micrograph of extruded rye crispbread (Marzec et al. 2007). B1–C3: bright field (B1 and C1) and confocal (B3, B3, C2, C3) micrographs of non-fermented and fermented (yeast leavened) rye crisp bread before and after in vitro digestion. Amylose in blue, amylopectin in purple, protein in yellow, β-glucan in green fluorescence. Images from B1 to C3 kindly provided by Daniel Johansson (Source: Department of Molecular Sciences, SLU, Uppsala).

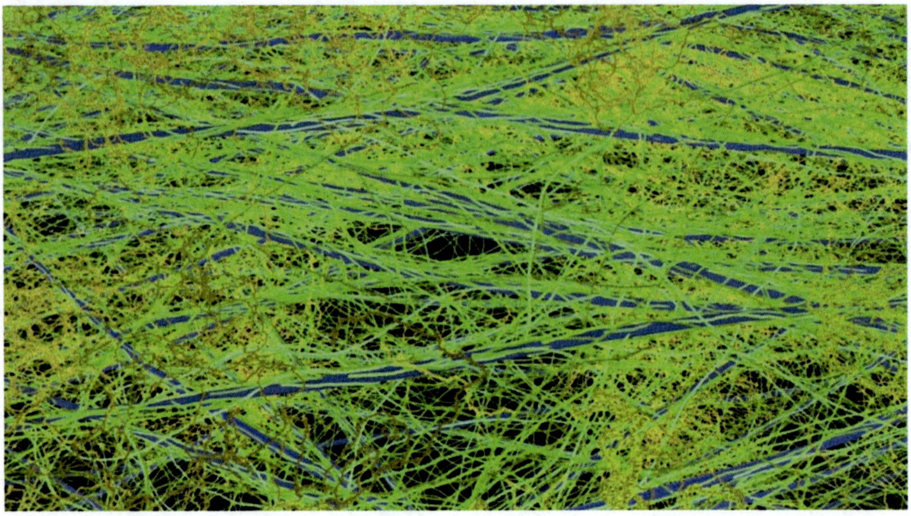

Key
- *Blue: Cellulose microfibrils (MFs)*
- *Greens: Non-cellulosic polysaccharides (Hemicelluloses)*
- *Yellow/Brown: Pectins*

Illustration by Drew Berry
The Walter and Eliza Hall Institute of Medical Research
Melbourne VIC Australia

Figure 4.1 Depiction of plant cell wall structure consisting of cellulose microfibrils (blue), non-cellulosic polysaccharides, termed hemicelluloses (green), and pectins (yellow/brown). Source: Johnson et al. 2018.

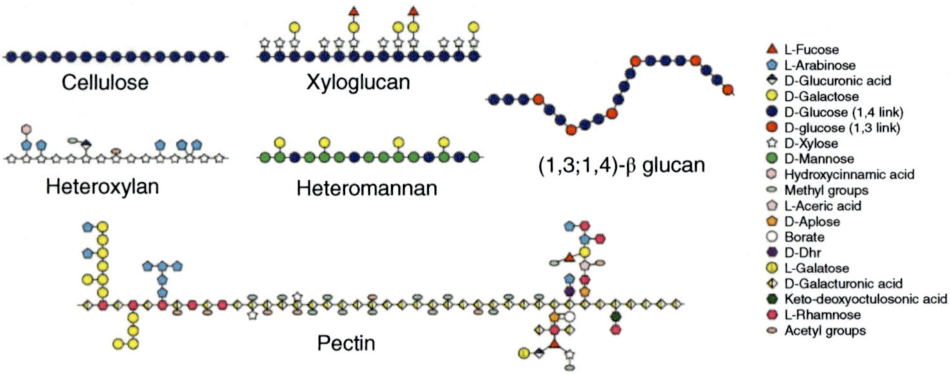

Figure 4.3 The molecular structure of the major non-starch polysaccharides found in plant cell walls. Heteroxylan (arabinoxylan), (1,3/1,4)-β-glucan and cellulose are the major non-starch polysaccharides in whole grain cereals; and pectin, xyloglucan, and cellulose are the major non-starch polysaccharides in whole grain pseudocereals (amaranth, quinoa). Source: Burton et al. 2010. © 2010 Springer Nature.

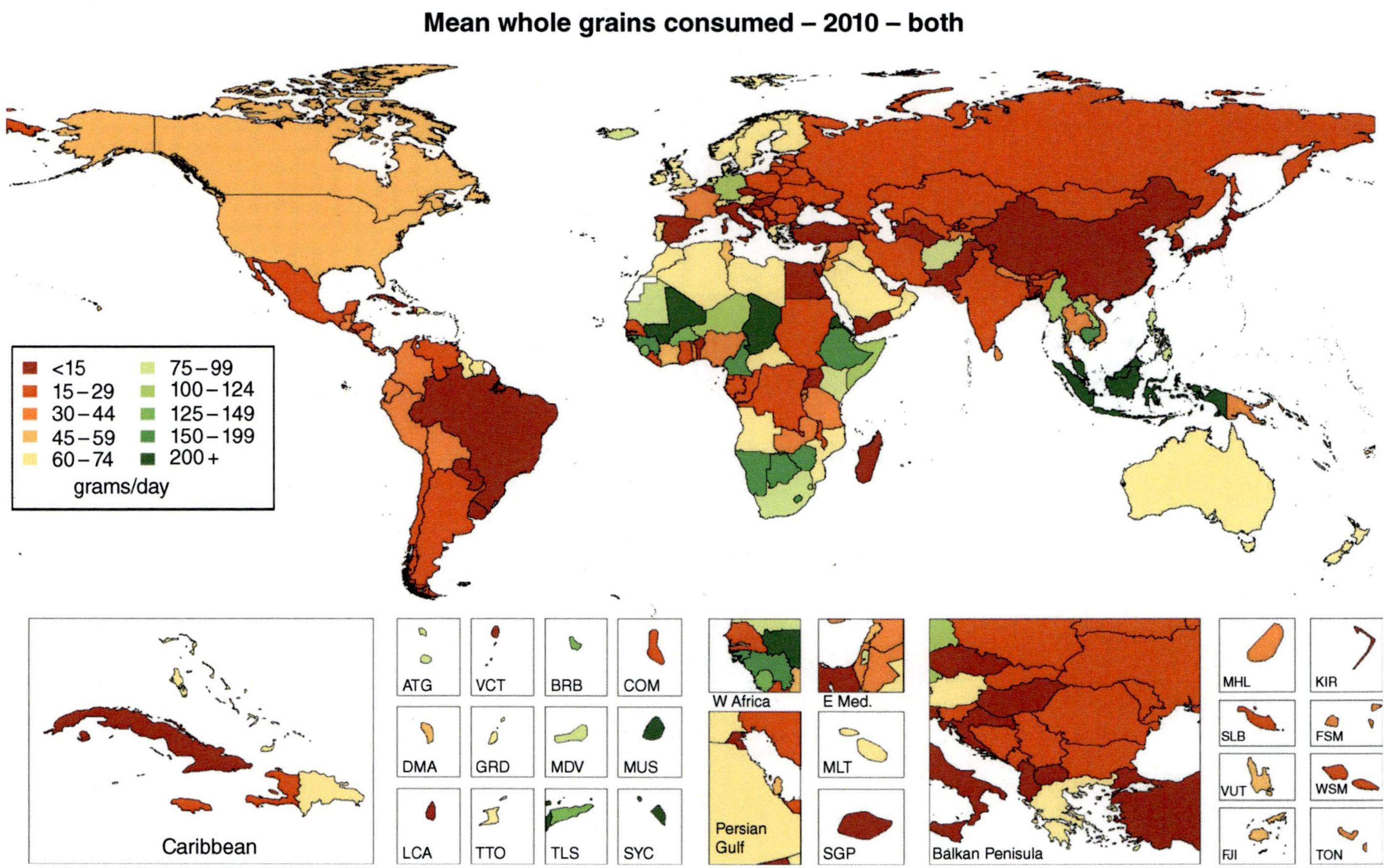

Figure 6.1 Global and regional mean whole grains consumed (g products/day) in 2010 for adults ≥20 years of age. (Source: Micha et al. [2015]).

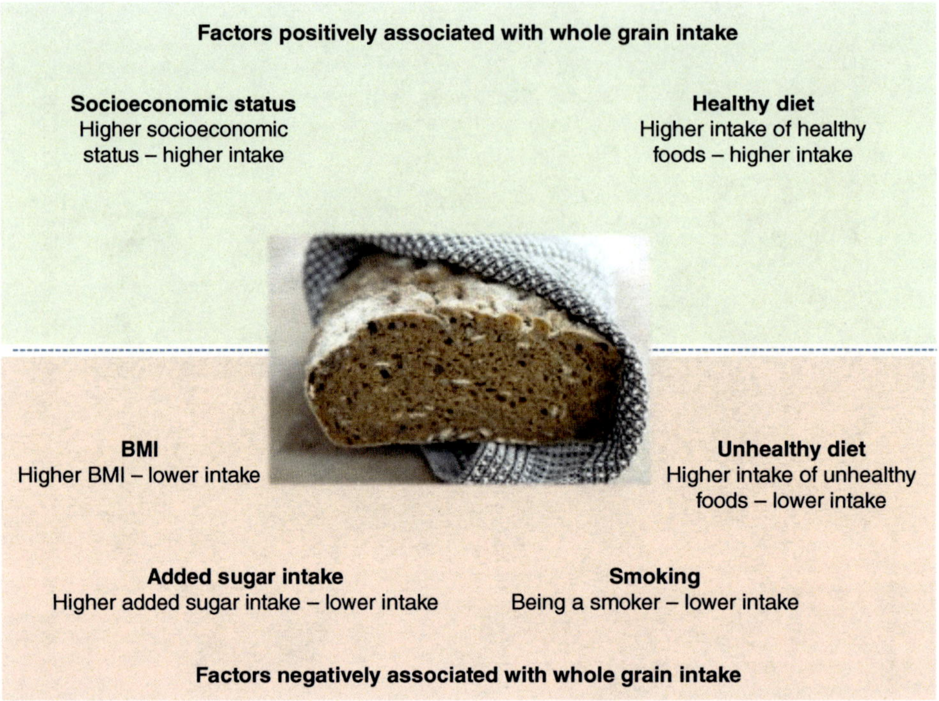

Figure 6.4 Dietary and lifestyle factors suggested to be associated with whole grain intake. BMI; body mass index.

Made in the USA
Las Vegas, NV
15 September 2026

76afe74a-2c9c-489b-92d6-ca38bc5a8b2cR03